The Birth of Bioethics

D0090741

The Birth of Bioethics

Albert R. Jonsen
School of Medicine
University of Washington

New York   Oxford
OXFORD UNIVERSITY PRESS
1998

Oxford University Press

Oxford   New York   Toronto
Delhi   Bombay   Calcutta   Madras   Karachi
Petaling   Jaya   Singapore   Hong Kong   Tokyo
Nairobi   Dar es Salaam   Cape Town
Melbourne   Auckland

and associated companies in
Berlin   Ibadan

Library of Congress Cataloging-in-Publication Data
Jonsen, Albert R.
The birth of bioethics / Albert R. Jonsen.
p.   cm.
Includes bibliographical references and index.
ISBN 0-19-510325-4
1. Medical Ethics—United States—History. 2. Bioethics—United States—History.
I. Title.
R724.J657   1998
174'.2'0973—dc21   97-41154

9 8 7 6 5 4 3 2 1

Printed in the United States of America
on acid-free paper

Contents

Preface

Bioethics is "the systematic study of the moral dimensions—including moral vision, decisions, conduct and policies—of the life sciences and health care, employing a variety of ethical methodologies in an interdisciplinary setting."[1] A systematic study, necessarily, is carried out by scholars dedicated to thinking, writing, and teaching about a subject. These scholars, now called "bioethicists," appeared on the scene in the late 1960s, usually as migrants from other academic disciplines, and developed bioethics as a new way of viewing the traditional ethics associated with medicine. In the intervening years, bioethics has attracted attention from the health professions and interest from the public. The three professional associations for bioethics now count about 1,000 members; almost 200 centers, departments, and programs exist, most of them in academic institutions; and the 1996 *Bibliography of Bioethics* lists 3,620 books, essays, and articles on bioethics.[2]

During the week this preface was being composed, the esteemed scientific journal *Nature* reported that the bioethics "industry" was booming: governments and industries were soliciting advice; and bioethicists were offering it—in commissions, at conferences, and through scholarly literature and media comments. The author argued, however, that "despite their growing prominence, it is far from clear whether US bioethicists have substantially shaped either the culture of science or the political decisions of recent years."[3] As the article elaborated this skeptical view, citing fragments of history and quoting several self-depreciating bioethicists, it teetered on the edge of factual and interpretative inaccuracies. It is not quite correct that "the new prominence of bioethicists can be traced to the 1988 launch of the human Genome Programme." It is inaccurate to state that bioethics was "cloistered 30 years ago in university departments of theology and philosophy." It is not entirely true that the National Commission for the Protection of Human Subjects of Biomedical and Behavior Research was "set up in response to the 1972 revelation that the US had for 40 years funded the notorious Tuskegee Syphilis Study." It is an exaggeration to claim that "everybody before would have identified . . . as theological literature" the earlier bioethical writings. And it is questionable that "apart from a couple of early, significant, victories, 'it is hard to show any concrete influence on policy by US bioethicists.'" Certainly, it is not easy to assess the influence of bioethics, now some thirty years old, on thought, culture, policy, and practice. Such assessments are haunted by the Missionaries' Fallacy: much preaching is done and many converts counted but how many hearts and minds are won? Still, an assessment demands an accurate historical recounting of why and how the field came into being. It is time to write that history.

In 1992, I invited sixty pioneer bioethicists to the University of Washington in Seattle to recall the beginnings of bioethics.[4] Everyone responded enthusiastically and forty-six attended the conference, which I called "The Birth of Bioethics." Before an audience of some three-hundred persons from various scholarly disciplines and from the public, each speaker addressed a bioethical topic on which he or she had done original work—death and dying, human experimentation, genetic engineering, reproductive technology, and organ transplantation—and explained how they and that topic came together. The participants at this conference were pioneers in the most proper sense: they blazed trails into a field of study that was unexplored and built conceptual roads through unprecedented problems. They were the first settlers of a new medical ethics that was named bioethics. Many of the ideas in this book were borrowed, with permission, from these colleagues.[5]

Despite the conference title, my colleagues and I knew that disciplines are not born; they grow slowly, gradually taking a shape distinct enough to merit a name. In truth, bioethics emerged in the years after World War II, beginning as an amorphous expression of concern about the untoward effects of advances in biomedical science and gradually forming into a coherent discourse and discipline. Although it addressed ethical issues in medicine and science, bioethics diverged in striking ways from the discourse about morality and medicine, commonly called "medical ethics," that had run through twenty-five centuries of Western history. The purpose of this book is to trace the origins and evolution of the ideas and institutions that have acquired the name "bioethics."

Bio of a Bioethicist

The biographies of the pioneer bioethicists and the birth of bioethics are entwined. Turns in personal careers move with events in the surrounding world of medicine and science and morality; the events are analyzed through the eyes of persons whose academic careers educated them to see those events in certain ways. Each of the early bioethicists has his or her own story to tell. Uniquely personal as each would be, the stories have some common features. Almost all of us are academics educated in the classical disciplines that the medieval university bequeathed to modern higher education: philosophy, theology, law, and medicine. Most of us were not interested in the ethical issues in medicine and the biological sciences until we encountered an intriguing problem that drew us closer to them. Most of us had to find our way in the foreign world of medical science and health care, and win acceptability there. Many of us opened new academic units that were often, but not exclusively, inside medical schools. We began to meet at conferences and symposia and on panels. We wrote and lectured and taught, leaving a record of our reflections that grew into a literature and a field of discourse that now has a name and a place in the academic and public policy world. I judge, then, that it is not inappropriate to begin this book with my own story. My autobiography, like those of my colleagues, reveals in a personal way how bioethics came to be.[6]

I was born in San Francisco, California, in 1931 and, like many a well brought-up Catholic boy of that era, I was convinced that I had a vocation to the Catholic priesthood. I entered a seminary of the Society of Jesus (Jesuits) as an eighteen-year-old novice and over the next thirteen years I enjoyed a splendid classical education. I read Latin, Greek, and English literature, studied ancient, medieval, and modern philosophy, did a little science and a lot of biblical and scholastic theology. After taking my Master's degree in philosophy, with a heavy concentration on Aristotle, Aquinas, and Maritain, I was assigned for three years to teach philosophy at a Jesuit college, Loyola University of Los Angeles. I then entered theological studies, and after my ordination to the priesthood, my superiors acceded to my request to study religious ethics in an ecumenical context. In 1964, I began doctoral studies at Yale University's Department of Religious Studies.

My professor at Yale, James M. Gustafson, was an ecumenical theologian, learned not only in his own Protestant tradition but also in Roman Catholic moral theology. Professor Gustafson had noticed the ferment of ideas that was beginning to boil around advances in the biomedical sciences, particularly in genetics and the neurosciences. In a 1970 essay he wrote: "The 'new biology' and developments in medical science and technology have aroused a great deal of public interest. Nothing less than the future of human development seems at stake."[7] Although Professor Gustafson called his students' attention to these questions, we did not concentrate on them. We were absorbed in the theoretical realms of theological ethics, reading the masters—St. Paul, St. Augustine, St. Thomas, Luther, and Calvin and the moderns, Barth, Brunner, Tillich, and the Niebuhrs. Still, from Professor Gustafson's students came many of the pioneers of bioethics.

Two chance encounters drew me toward the nascent bioethics. The first took place on a May day in 1967, when I delivered my doctoral dissertation to Yale's Hall of Graduate Studies.[8] Stepping onto the street with a fine feeling of relief, I met a friend, Dr. F. Patrick McKegney, who directed the psychiatric liaison service at Yale-New Haven Hospital. Dr. McKegney invited me to lunch at Morey's to celebrate the completion of the great labor. During lunch he said, "You've been reading and writing all this theoretical stuff about ethics. Why not come down to the hospital and I'll show you what an ethical problem really looks like."

I accepted his invitation and accompanied Dr. McKegney, as a sort of ethical intern, over the next two months. He had recently encountered a problem that he considered truly ethical and truly unique: some patients whose lives were maintained by the new process of chronic hemodialysis wished to "turn off the machine" and be left to die. He and others who had encountered the problem wondered whether this decision was equivalent to suicide and whether a physician who acceded to it became an accomplice. As a psychiatrist he asked whether "dialysis suicide" was, as many suicidal wishes are, a psychopathology or whether, given the unprecedented situation of chronic life support, it should be analyzed differently. McKegney explained the problem to me and asked me to reflect on it. I discovered that a small literature had only recently accumulated about the ethical problems of chronic hemodialysis. I learned the story of the Seattle Artificial Kidney Center around which many of those problems revolved. I never imagined that twenty-five years later, I would be a faculty member of the medical school where chronic hemodialysis had originated and be a friend of its originator, Dr. Belding H. Scribner.

After the ecumenical experience at Yale, my Jesuit superiors re-immersed me in Catholic theology with a year at the Institut Catholique in Paris and the Gregorian University in Rome. They then assigned me to teach moral theology and philosophical ethics at the University of San Francisco (USF). Again, a chance meeting revived my interest in medical ethics. I met Dr. J. Engleburt Dunphy, Chairman of the Department of Surgery at the University of California, San Francisco (UCSF) at a dinner party in 1969. Dr. Dunphy asked me what I did. When I responded that I taught ethics at USF, he exclaimed, "Terrific! We have a serious ethical problem in medicine—how is death defined?" When I commented that doctors, if anyone, should know the answer to that question, he told me that the growing practice of organ transplantation was forcing reconsideration of the criteria for declaring death. A committee at Harvard Medical School had suggested a "brain death definition" during the previous year and the UCSF Medical School had formed a committee to evaluate the Harvard definition. If the committee judged the definition suitable, it would adopt it for use in the new UCSF renal transplant program. Would I join the committee as a consultant? I did so eagerly (and ignorantly) and, during a year of evening meetings with a small group of physicians, learned about neurology, organ transplantation, and the conceptual confusion that surrounded life's ending.

During my graduate studies and my tenure at USF, very real ethical problems were agitating the national conscience. Persons who chose to study academic ethics, philosophical or religious, could not immure themselves within classical treatises. The Civil Rights movement stirred passions. In March 1965, several of my fellow Jesuits at Yale and I were preparing to travel to Selma but were deterred by news of the savagery at the Pettus Bridge. Sentiment against the war in Southeast Asia grew during the late sixties and had reached fever pitch by the time I was a professor at USF. Many of my students sought my advice about conscientious objection to military service. This was a peculiarly difficult problem for Catholics. Roman Catholic theology taught a doctrine of "just war": warfare was ethically justified under certain conditions. American courts had recognized conscientious objection only for the traditional "peace churches," such as the Quakers and the Mennonites, which repudiated all warfare. I served as confessor and advisor to many of these perplexed young Catholics. I knew how complex the moral issue was because my graduate student colleague, Jim Childress, had written a brilliant dissertation on conscientious objection. My uncle, Federal Judge William T. Sweigert, was among the first to declare the war unconstitutional.[9] So, during my first year as a student and teacher of ethics, I became deeply and personally engaged in very real ethical issues. As we shall see, many of the early bioethicists had similar experiences.

My internship with Dr. McKegney in the wards of Yale-New Haven Hospital, supplemented by my service with the UCSF brain death committee, had started a transmutation from ethicist to bioethicist. I actually became a bioethicist—with a title and a salary—in the spring of 1972. Dr. Philip R. Lee, Chancellor of the University of California, San Francisco, the senior medical school of the University of California, invited me as visiting professor to a newly established UCSF Institute of Health Policy. I eagerly accepted, and with my Jesuit superior's permission, moved across Golden Gate Park from the USF to UCSF. I spent my year as visiting professor doing more learning than professing. Suspecting that I might want to specialize in this field, I attended lectures with the medical students, dissected a cadaver in the anatomy course, and joined discussions about health policy and about the evolving forms of medical care. I conversed with two eminent figures in medical ethics, Dr. Otto Guttentag and Dr. Chauncey Leake, "senior statesman of medical ethics."[10]

At the end of the year, the Dean of the School of Medicine, Dr. Julius R. Krevans, offered me the position of Adjunct Associate Professor of Bioethics at the Medical School. A professor of bioethics was an odd creature. Only one other ethicist was appointed to a medical faculty, K. Danner Clouser at Penn State Hershey Medical School. Bioethics was not a recognized academic field. There was no curriculum and the literature was sparse. Even the world "bioethics" caused confusion; not only was it a neologism but it also invited association in the San Francisco Bay Area where I lived with the biorhythms and biofeedback and macrobiotics that had become the cant of the New Age philosophies burgeoning there. My task at UCSF was not to impart the facts and methods of an established discipline but to create something that would deserve academic respect and public recognition. I was now set on an academic track that led within a few years to tenured faculty status within a leading medical school. I became a bioethicist, just at the time bioethics was being born.

In 1975, I requested and was granted release from the vows of the Society of Jesus and the Roman Catholic priesthood. I became a happily married layperson. I was hardly alone; in those years, many Catholic priests no longer felt called to that vocation. Several of the early bioethicists have a similar entry in their biography. Men trained in ethics and experienced in helping persons deal with perplexing moral issues were seeking a place in secular life. The opening world of bioethics provided that place. I remained at UCSF until 1987, when I migrated to the Pacific Northwest to become Professor of Ethics in Medicine at the University of Washington School of Medicine.

The Scope of this History

The history of bioethics weaves together personal stories like my own with remarkable advances in medical science and technology and with the social climate of the second half of the twentieth century in the United States. The advances raised questions in the minds of reflective persons and sometimes occasioned events that prompted wonder and worry. That response was shaped by the attitudes about personal and social ethics that prevailed in post-World War II America and by the deeper values of the American ethos. Persons like myself, formed not only by those attitudes and values but also educated to reflect on them, hoped to shape the concerns into articulate questions that could be carefully analyzed and sometimes even resolved. Bioethics is the systematic study that works at this task. It is also a discourse—that is, the discussion and debate—that surrounds the advances and events to which many parties contribute, from professionals to private citizens.

This book designates the forty years between 1947 and 1987 as the era during which bioethics emerged as a distinct discipline and discourse. In 1947, the Nuremberg Tribunal convicted twenty-three physicians of war crimes committed under the guise of medical experiments, and it promulgated the Nuremberg Code. That event, dramatizing the most egregious violation of medicine's traditional ethic, opens my history because it initiated an examination by professional persons in science, medicine, and law of one of modern medicine's central features: scientific research. The next two decades were prologue to bioethics, during which questions accumulated and scientists, physicians, and sometimes the public expressed genuine but diffuse concern about the ethical problems raised by medical and scientific advances.

The opening chapter of this book recalls the long tradition of medical ethics that precedes bioethics and the public expression of concern by many scientists during the 1960s. By the second half of that decade, these diffuse concerns fell under concentrated analysis by scholars trained not in the biomedical sciences but in the two classic disciplines that deal with ethics, theology and philosophy, and in several other fields that dwell close to ethics, such as law and the social sciences. The second and third chapters examine why these scholars were ready and willing to join the discourse and what they brought to it. The next chapter records how the United States government became engaged in bioethics, drawing the reflections of scholars into the realm of public policy. Five chapters are devoted to topics that became the focus of bioethical analysis: research with human subjects, genetics, care of terminally ill persons, organ transplantation, and artificial reproduction. Each of these chapters starts long before 1947, in the conviction that the bioethical shape of these modern problems must be seen within the evolution of thought about their analogues in the past. Two chapters reflect on the nature of bioethics as a discipline and as discourse. Finally, after a brief review of international bioethics, Chapter 12 places the four decades of bioethics within the larger sweep of the American ethos, in the hope that this larger picture might explain why bioethics appeared in the United States during the latter decades of the twentieth century.

Writers of history, I am told, should not get too close to the present, lest perspective be lost. So I conclude this history at the end of 1987. This closure is arbitrary but reasonable. I propose that the seeds of bioethics were sown and the seminal work of bioethics accomplished during the forty years between 1947 and 1987 (one of those nicely rounded-out eras that professors love). Those years show the medical and biological sciences advancing with astonishing rapidity and record many questions about such wondrous advances. Bioethics is now firmly established in the world of academic medicine, medical practice, and public policy. Since 1987, bioethics has taken on new questions, new forms, and new methods. Its younger scholars are critically reviewing the work of their teachers and undertaking new ventures in ethical methodology and policy. All that will be told in the next history of bioethics.

Seattle, Washington   A. R. J.
November 1997

Notes

1. Warren T. Reich, "Introduction," in Reich (ed.), *The Encyclopedia of Bioethics,* revised ed. (New York: Simon Schuster Macmillan, 1995), p. xxi.

2. The American Association of Bioethics has 613 members (1997), the Society for Health and Human Values has 842 (1995), and the Society for Bioethics Consulation, 149 (1995). These organizations have many overlapping members yet when all three combined into the American Society for Bioethics and Humanities in 1998 some 1500 persons enrolled. Centers are listed in Anita Nolen and Mary Carrington Coutts (eds.), *International Directory of Bioethics Organizations* (Washington, D.C.: Kennedy Institute of Ethics, Georgetown University, 1993) and literature is referenced in LeRoy Walters and Tamar Joy Kahn. *Bibliography of Bioethics,* vol. 22 (Washington, D.C.: Kennedy Institute of Ethics, 1996).

3. Meredith Wadman, "Business booms for guides to biology's moral maze," *Nature* (1997), 389: 658–659; Editorial, "Trust and the bioethics industry," p. 647.

4. The pioneers were selected from those persons still living and working in bioethics whose publications were listed in the first edition of LeRoy Walters (ed.), *The Bibliography of Bioethics,* vol. 1 (Detroit: Gale Research Co., 1975).

5. "The Birth of Bioethics: A Conference to Celebrate the Past 30 Years of Bioethics in the United States." University of Washington, September 23–24, 1992. A summary of the conference appeared in Albert R. Jonsen (ed.), "The Birth of Bioethics," *Hastings Center Report,* suppl. 23, no. 6 (1993).

6. The biographies of many of the leading figures in American and European bioethics are related in Sandro Spinsanti, *La bioetica. Biographie per una disciplina* (Milan: Franco Angeli, 1995).

7. James M. Gustafson, "Basic ethical issues in the bio-medical fields," *Soundings* 53, no. 2 (1970): 151–180, p. 151.

8. Albert R. Jonsen, *Responsibility in Modern Religious Ethics* (Washington, D.C.: Corpus Books, 1968).

9. James F. Childress, *Civil Disobedience and Political Obligation: A Study in Christian Social Ethics* (New Haven: Yale University Press, 1971); *Mattola v Nixon* 318 F. Supp 538 (ND Cal 1970).

10. This accolade was awarded to Dr. Leake by Paul Ramsey in *Patient as Person* (New Haven, Yale University Press, 1970), p. xv. Leake's story is told in Chapter 1; Dr. Guttentag appears in Chapter 5.

Acknowledgments

This book was conceived after a conference "The Birth of Bioethics," held at the University of Washington, September 23–24, 1992. Many of the pioneers of bioethics were present to tell their stories about the origins of the field and they all gave me permission to use their remarks as building blocks for this book. Many other pioneers welcomed interviews. I thank them all and apologize if I have distorted their words. I thank the readers who reviewed all or part of the draft: Darrel Amundsen, Robert Baker, Dan Callahan, James Childress, Maurice de Wachter, James Gustafson, Diego Gracia, John Ladd, Richard McCormick, Jonathan Moreno, Sandro Spinsanti, Robert Veatch, James Whorton, and one *anonyme*. All added to clarity, correctness, and conciseness. The staff of the National Reference Center for Bioethics Literature at Georgetown University responded generously to requests for documents difficult to find. My graduate assistant, Kelly Edwards, hunted indefatigably for sources and references; Lauri Shannon and Barron Learner helped with research. Toni Reinicke gave invaluable assistance in formatting the text. Jeffrey House of Oxford University Press, was encouraging and judiciously critical. My wife, Mary Elizabeth, is my best editor. The time and resources to write this long book were a gift from the John Simon Guggenheim Foundation, which granted me a prized Fellowship for 1995–96, and from the Charles E. Culpeper Foundation, whose support of medical history is unique. I appreciate the sabbatical provided by the University of Washington and the people of Washington State, which still understands that good teaching flows from the leisure for study. To all, my gratitude!

I

BIOETHICAL BEGINNINGS: THE PEOPLE AND PLACES

1

Great Issues of Conscience: Medical Ethics Before Bioethics

Bioethics did not begin with a Big Bang. Even though medical ethics, bioethics' predecessor, was shaken by notable and notorious events, it was a slow accumulation of concerns about the ambiguity of scientific progress that turned the old medical ethics into the new paths of bioethics. Contributors to scientific progress began to express their concerns during the 1960s, in occasional writings and at professional meetings and public conferences. They worried that the old tradition of medical ethics was too frail to meet the ethical challenges posed by the new science and medicine.

The Long Tradition of Medical Ethics

Picture a country doctor trudging through a field under a stormy sky. Black bag in hand, his body droops in weariness and his face is marked with worry about the little girl whose serious injury he has been summoned to treat. This cover shot for a 1948 *Life* photoessay, "Country Doctor," "created an earnest, empathetic portrait of an American folk hero."[1] Dr. Ernest Ceriani, the story's Colorado country doctor, probably never considered himself a folk hero, but in 1948, he was part of a profession held in high esteem. Dr. Ceriani was a competent physician: he could diagnose and offer good advice about many illnesses. He could even treat a few of them. He could set a fracture and suture a wound. But beyond these skills, his earnestness and empathy won him respect. He was on call twenty-four hours a day. When called, he responded; when he undertook care, he stayed to the end. He was gentle but firm, honest but discreet, a thoroughly trustworthy confidante. He expended energy and time, often compensated only with gratitude. He practiced alone, his medical judgment unfettered by any supervisor. The doctor's ethics, even more than his power to cure, made him, if not an American folk hero, at least a paradigm of moral probity.

This was one portrait of the American doctor at the end of the first half of this century. The aura of moral probity surrounded not only the country doctor but also the Park Avenue specialist and the medical school professor. All physicians basked in the light of the fictional physicians of the time. Sinclair Lewis's 1925 novel *Arrowsmith*, while critical of the profession's ignorance and venality, eulogized an idealistic young physician torn between a scientific career and care of the poor. Two hit plays during the 1933–1934 Broadway season, *Men in White* and *Yellow Jack*, showed American doctors as "embodying the virtues of independence, integrity and dedication, even patriotism, in the service of the American public."[2] Dr. Kildare, appearing first in a 1936 short story and then in popular films, was a competent and altruistic physician, beloved by millions of would-be patients.[3] Unquestionably, actual doctors were sometimes selfish and occasionally scoundrels, but the image of the profession in the public mind, and in its own, was one of moral probity.

Dr. Ceriani probably did not think much about "medical ethics." He may have recited the Hippocratic Oath at his graduation from Loyola University Medical School. Although its actual words may have faded from memory, he probably believed that the Oath imposed upon him certain firm duties: he was to heal, not harm; if asked to extinguish life, either at its beginning or at its end, he must refuse; he must keep the strictest confidence. If he attended his county medical society meeting, he heard the AMA's indictment of prepaid group practices cropping up here and there as unethical, because their arrangements compromised the physician's judgment about what was best for the patient. He would have also learned that the proposals for compulsory health insurance surfacing in a few state legislatures were equally unethical, because government would dictate the conditions for care.[4] But oaths, codes, and the fulminations of the AMA were probably not the primary sources of Dr. Ceriani ethics. His moral beliefs and character most likely came from exemplars he knew as colleagues or professors—medical men who exhibited the virtues described by the almost universal model, Sir William Osler, "to do the day's work well . . . to act the Golden Rule toward my professional brethren and toward the patients committed to my care . . . to cultivate such a measure of equanimity as would enable me to bear success with humility."[5]

This moral image, and the public esteem that it inspired, had not always adorned the American physician. One hundred years before Dr. Ceriani was making his rounds, physicians were often perceived as "jealous, quarrelsome men, whose chief delight is in the annoyance and ridicule of each other." Even more seriously, they were widely seen as dangerous, doing little more for the sick than "poisoning" and "butchering" them. Some regarded the whole profession as "a stupendous humbug."[6] During the intervening century, medical education had improved, the profession had organized itself and adopted a code of ethics, licensure had been regularized, organized medicine supported public health measures, quackery had been stigmatized, and nostrums exposed. By the turn of the century, most doctors were familiar enough with the Code of Ethics of the American Medical Association to know that their primary duty to their patients implied that they should repudiate unorthodox, uneducated, and unethical practitioners, avoid institutional entanglements, whether with the government or with commerce, that would compromise their independent judgment, and refrain from unsavory financial deals and from advertising. By the time Dr. Ceriani entered practice, he joined a profession held in high esteem by the public.

For doctors like Ernest Ceriani, medical ethics was incarnate in their behavior and character and in the social arrangements that sustained the solidarity, respectability, and educated competence of the profession. There were ethical battles to be fought, such as those against quackery, but there were few ethical dilemmas about the doctor's duties. As late as 1966, a series of editorials commenting on the AMA Principles of Medical Ethics contains no hint of moral perplexity: each phrase of the Principles is lucid and "represents a facet of the complete physician . . . a portion of the character and personality of a Doctor of Medicine!" Only one caution appears: "With the advent of Medicare (enacted one year before the articles were written) let doctors be bold. . . . Ethics and decent behavior have not, as yet, been abrogated by the new Federalism."[7] Medical ethics had a clear conscience. Yet, by the end of the 1960s, this optimism about the lucidity and sufficiency of the old ethics had begun to waver. A 1970 medical journal editorial entitled "A new ethic for medicine and society" proclaimed: "The traditional Western ethic . . . is being eroded at its core and may eventually even be abandoned. This will produce profound changes in Western medicine and in Western society."[8] The traditional Western ethic, the author claimed, had enjoined an absolute respect for the sanctity of life and this imperative supported the ethics of medicine; modern developments, particularly the population explosion and the appearance of new medical technologies, would force society and its doctors to relativize that absolute value. The clear conscience of medical ethics began to be troubled. What had happened during the years between the eulogy for the sturdy ethics of the American doctor and the misgivings of the author of that editorial?

Those misgivings anticipated bioethics and the bioethics that soon appeared was a "new ethic," a break from the old medical ethics. A review of traditional medical ethics will prepare the way for the new bioethics. It is possible, within the compass of this book, to sketch the history of medical ethics only in the most schematic fashion.[9] Even the phrase "medical ethics" is difficult to define: it is a relatively modern designation that may not accommodate much of the discourse about the relationship between medicine and morality that has taken place in the past and, indeed, the words "medical" and "ethics" bear different meaning at different times. It seems, however, that the work of healing and convictions about right and wrong behavior have always been tightly linked.

In all cultures, individuals apply remedies and bring solace to their sick relatives and friends. In many cultures special practices of healing are reserved for certain individuals who have learned therapeutic skills and rituals. These individuals are distinguished from the people as a whole and are respected, venerated, and sometimes feared for their powers and knowledge. Illness is seen as the consequence of a knowing or an unknowing infraction of the order and law of nature or society; the healer must apply remedies that restore order and reintegrate the sick person into conformity with that order. The work of healing, then, often carries strong religious and moral tones and the healer must observe the metaphysical rules and the rituals that reflect the beliefs of the culture.[10] The work of the healer must not only be correct, that is, the proper remedy for the illness is used, but it must also be right and good, done in conformity with rules, customs, and beliefs that constitute the meaning of life for the society. Thus on the basis of anthropological evidence, it is possible to say that the work of human healing is commonly associated with ethics.

Ethics refers not only to the rules, customs, and beliefs of a society; it also names the scholarly effort to articulate and analyze those rules, customs, and beliefs. Three persistent themes can be discerned in the vast literature about morality produced in the Western cultural tradition. First, moral philosophers have described the character or qualities of persons that might win them praise or blame. Second, moral philosophers and theologians meditate on the duties and obligations that bind humans to perform, and to refrain from performing, certain actions. Finally, philosophers who have reflected on character and duties have also linked individuals to social communities, inquiring how the existence of communities is related to the purposes of individuals. These three topics—character, duty, and social responsibility—are constant topics of ethical reflection and discourse.

These same three topics appear in the literature on medicine and morality that has accumulated during twenty-five centuries of Western medicine. That literature begins with the collection of writings attributed to the School of Hippocrates in the third and fourth centuries before the Christian era and continues to modern times. Much of that literature describes the qualities of "the good physician," the decorum and the deportment that the doctor should exhibit toward patients. A doctor should be gentle, pleasant, comforting, discreet, firm. These qualities attract and keep patients, give them confidence, make them grateful, and even contribute to their healing. While these qualities can be feigned, they should reflect true virtues. These "bedside manners" remain remarkably steady throughout the entire history of Western medicine, and they have their counterparts in the medical ethics of other cultures.[11]

Alongside the ethics of medical decorum stands a more grave morality: certain injunctions that define the duty of the good physician. Sometimes incorporated in solemn affirmations such as oaths, or in stringent rules dictated by church, state, or profession, these duties enjoin the physician "to benefit the sick and do them no harm," to keep confidences, to refrain from monetary and sexual exploitation of patients, and to show concern for those in need of medical help, even at cost to one's own health and wealth. These duties, which are stressed with varying emphasis, are more profoundly linked to deep moral beliefs than are the admonitions of decorum. The paradigm of these duties is the so-called Hippocratic Oath, which, according to some scholars, emerged not from the general milieu of Greek medicine but from a philosophical-religious cult,

Pythagoreanism, that inculcated clear moral imperatives on all its believers and thus on its believers who practiced medicine.[12] The Judeo-Christian religious tradition, with its strong emphasis on divine commands that enforce respect for the sanctity of life, enhanced the prohibitions of abortion and euthanasia that are obscurely expressed in the Oath and prescribed caring compassion for the poor and even for enemies. The literature of medical duty is profoundly marked by these moral traditions.[13]

A third type of advice appears in the literature of medical ethics: physicians must define their place in society. They must show themselves as worthy of social trust and deserving of social authority and reward. This "social ethics," hardly noted in the ancient medical world, began to assume importance during the Middle Ages, as medicine was being taught in universities, guilds and colleges were being established, and civic authorities were taking notice of the dangers of untrained practitioners. The marks of the profession began to appear: the privilege to educate, examine, license, and discipline their members, and the tacit pledge of public service. This social ethics of medicine served both as a regulator of professional relationships and as a demonstration of professional reliability; it also encouraged professional monopoly over healing. The first book to bear the title *Medical Ethics*, was written by the English physician Thomas Percival in 1803. It combined the traditional virtues of medical decorum with novel injunctions about the behavior of physicians among themselves. Percival, who wrote to regulate the relationships between physicians and surgeons in England's charity hospitals, insisted that the duties of "office" had been granted to doctors by society as "public trusts." By encouraging "urbanity and rectitude" among physicians, Percival hoped to render the profession worthy of that public trust.[14]

This social ethics finds its most extensive expression in the ethical codes produced by the American Medical Association from its inception in 1847 through the mid-twentieth century. The founders of the AMA hoped to reform medical education and to improve the ethics of physicians. It initiated the latter effort by issuing a Code of Medical Ethics at the Second National Medical Convention held in Philadelphia, May 5–7, 1847. The Code was largely based on Percival's *Medical Ethics*, as adapted to American needs and tastes. One chapter, reflecting the American scene, repudiated quackery, forbade advertising, and prohibited consultation with doctors "whose practice is based on an exclusive dogma, to the rejection of the accumulated experience of the profession, and of the aids actually furnished by anatomy, physiology, pathology and organic chemistry." Those words not only endorsed the scientific medicine that was emerging; they banished from "the regular profession" all doctors who practiced forms of "sectarian" medicine, such as homeopathy, naturopathy, and hydropathy. According to a medical historian, that one chapter "became the heart of the code and the source of the profession's subsequent troubles during the 19th century."[15] Trouble they did cause but, more importantly, they encouraged professional cohesion around the goal of an effective medicine.

The expansive Code of 1847 was revised under the new name, *Principles of Medical Ethics*, in 1903 and again in 1912, each time becoming briefer and less rhetorical. In

1957, a major revision cut the *Principles* down to ten terse statements that in form were reminiscent of the biblical decalogue (these were reduced again in 1966 to seven principles). Stated in very general terms, the Principles urge physicians to respect the rights of their patients, to keep up their skills, to accept the discipline of the profession, to consult when necessary, to keep confidences, and to be good citizens. They also forbid physicians to practice in circumstances where their independent medical judgment might be restricted or to obtain professional income other than remuneration for services. Ethics becomes almost synonymous with rules for professional cohesion and respectability.[16]

In the United States, two unconventional figures introduced novelty into these traditional patterns of medical ethics. Dr. Richard Cabot (1869–1939), professor of clinical medicine at Harvard Medical School and of social ethics in Harvard College, was acutely sensitive to the changes American medicine was undergoing at the turn of the century: the shift of care into the hospital, the use of "ancillary professions," such as social work, in the care of the patient, and the increasing contribution of biological science to the understanding of disease.[17] Dr. Cabot formed a particularly modern view of medical ethics in the evolving world of medicine. Medical historian Chester Burns describes Cabot's place in that world:

> As much as any other physician of his day Richard Cabot demonstrated the validity of the new bases for professional goodness. . . . Whether or not the practitioner went to church on Sunday, knew the 'Star Spangled Banner,' swore the Hippocratic Oath, or adhered to precepts about consultation in the AMA Code of Ethics were not the important criteria for judging professional propriety. What counted (for Cabot) was whether a practitioner understood the specific diseases, their causes, signs, symptoms, courses, prognoses, treatments—and whether each practitioner applied this understanding in the assessment and management of each individual patient.[18]

In a short article, "Medical ethics in the hospital,"[19] Cabot enumerated the duties of the modern physician working in the hospital setting. Extensive cooperation between physicians and all other professionals involved in the care of patients was required. Accurate records of patient care had to be kept and analyzed. The number of patients assigned to doctors was not to compromise attention to all patients. Patients should be informed of their diagnosis and their treatments explained to them by their attending physicians. Patients should not be exploited for teaching purposes. Senior physicians should not exploit their junior colleagues, either by assigning them work they themselves should do or by taking credit for their scientific contribution. Disputes over appropriate care should be settled in committees. This list of ethical duties initiates what might be called "an ethic of competence."[20]

Since ancient times, physicians had been warned that they had a moral obligation to attain knowledge and skill, but through most of medical history, few ways to measure knowledge and skill were available. As the medicine of the nineteenth century absorbed the advances in physiology, pathology, and bacteriology and learned to use the "numerical method" to evaluate results of treatment, knowledge and skill became more measurable. Cabot analyzed 1,000 consecutive autopsies at the Massachusetts General Hospital and demonstrated a high rate of error in diagnosis. His publication of this analysis and a later similar study dismayed and angered many of his colleagues, who accused him of the ethical breach of "publicly advertising the faults of the general practitioner."[21] But for Cabot, this *was* ethics: moral practice was competent; incompetent practice was unethical. Clinical competence had moved to the center of medical education and even of medical ethics. Clinical competence, in Dr. Cabot's view, was not a cold, calculating skill. It had to include not only mastery of science but also appreciation of the personal and social needs of the patient. He recognized what we now call the humanistic qualities of the physician, not as mere decorations on clinical competence but as intrinsic to it. In dealing with the distressed and the sick, "Someone must win the affection of each sufferer, penetrate the past and guide the future better."[22] Richard Cabot stands at an important turning point in American medicine, when scientific medicine had taken a firm hold and when it was reasonable to insist that the practitioner's highest moral duty was mastery of that scientific medicine for the benefit of the patient.[23]

Dr. Chauncey Leake (1896–1978) also challenged the traditional medical ethics. A pharmacologist by training, he became interested in medical ethics as a graduate student when he came upon the writings of Thomas Percival. He prepared and published a modern edition of that classic. Although Leake admired much in the Manchester physician's writings, he judged that Percival had misconceived medical ethics from the beginning. He accused Percival of ignoring the philosophical literature on ethics and thus of elaborating an "etiquette" rather than an "ethic," a sort of "Emily Post guide to proper professional conduct." Leake begins the prefatory essay to his edition of Percival with the remark, "The term 'medical ethics,' introduced by Percival is really a misnomer. Based on Greek traditions of good taste and on Thomas Percival's 'Code,' it refers chiefly to the rules of etiquette developed in the profession to regulate the professional contacts of its members with each other. . . . Medical ethics should be concerned with the ultimate consequences of the conduct of physicians toward their individual patients and toward society as a whole."[24] In his view, this error had infected the American view of professional ethics.

Dr. Leake insisted that professional ethics be rebuilt on a foundation of moral philosophy. In an article that appeared the year after his Percival volume, he wrote: "Changing conditions in medical practice are making the matter (of teaching medical ethics) acute. It is becoming apparent that group practice, health insurance and periodic health examinations, as well as various aspects of public health measures, are profoundly altering the view of the physician." With a prescience that anticipated the bioethics of four decades later, he outlined the ideal ethics course for medical students. The course should open with three lectures on the chief questions of moral philosophy, given by a member of the philosophy faculty, followed by an historical survey of ethics in medicine. Then the students should meet with experienced physicians for an informed discussion and debate of actual cases that raise ethical questions.[25]

Leake's advocacy of a philosophically based ethics education went unheeded until bioethics came into its own. However, Cabot's insistence on clinical competence as an ethical duty entered into the medical ethos, reinforced by the growing confidence that science could convert medicine into an effective healing art. Although rarely listed among ethical duties, competence, which was based on continually updated scientific knowledge, achieved primacy in the moral repertoire. American physicians assumed a professional persona that was shaped by an appreciation of scientifically dictated duties. The primary duty of competence was supplemented by a concept of fiduciary responsibility, inherited from common law, that required all professionals to serve their client's interests rather than their own. Although applicable to lawyers, accountants, and architects, the concept seemed particularly suited to physicians because it echoed the Hippocratic injunction to help and do no harm.

Another ancient duty, fostered in medieval medicine, lingered in ghostly form: the duty of gratuitous care for the sick poor. The first and second editions of the AMA Code took this duty for granted, saying, "There is no profession, by the members of which eleemosynary services are more liberally dispensed than the medical."[26] The 1912 revision makes the duty explicit: "The poverty of a patient and the mutual professional obligation of physicians should command the gratuitous services of a physician."[27] The 1957 revision passes over this duty in silence. Many good doctors had incorporated that duty into their work. In its most prestigious form, the duty was fulfilled by a doctor guiding medical students in their clinical education without taking a salary. In a less prestigious way, doctors often dispensed with fees from patients whom they knew to be hard pressed. Some physicians served gratuitously for one day each week in public hospitals. Little notice was given, however, to the multitudes of potential patients whose poverty prevented them from approaching a physician. When health insurance became common after World War II, and when Medicaid and Medicare were initiated in the 1960s, "charity medicine" disappeared and the old duty of gratuitous care for the poor faded from the physician's ethic.

By the 1950s, medical ethics had become tranquil. The wars over consultation and competition had been won. The medical marketplace was being allotted to the new specialties, state licensure laws were back in force and specialty certification was emerging, hospitals were largely under the control of their medical staffs, contract and group practice were rare anomalies. Above all, twentieth-century physicians had attained the respectability and the social authority that their nineteenth-century predecessors yearned for. Along with that respectability came enhanced income. By mid-century, words that Dr. Cabot had written in 1918 were no longer true: "Among the rewards which the doctor must not expect is wealth. . . . I have known few physicians fail to get a living in medicine, but the number who make comfortable incomes is equally few."[28] The aims of the founders of the American Medical Association—to organize medicine into a profession that merits public respect and holds authority in society—

seem to have been achieved. The professional decorum, now surrounded with the aura of science, satisfied the public that doctors were decent, responsible, and competent. The ethical and legal duty of fiduciary responsibility inspired trust.

The extensive literature that expounds on the decorum, duties, and social ethics of the physician had been written almost exclusively by physicians. Although civil authorities had decreed some rules and religious authorities imposed some obligations, physicians drew on their experiences and from their cultural and religious values to articulate the standards of conduct appropriate to the good physician. Much of the literature is in the voice of exhortation (and occasionally sanction) rather than explanation. Detailed analyses of problems are rare and the elaborate reasoning of moral philosophy almost nonexistent. While these writers appreciated the Hippocratic maxim, "Life is short, the art long, opportunity fleeting, experiment treacherous, judgment difficult,"[29] they seldom expressed perplexity before moral dilemmas. In all of this, the medical ethics of the past differs from the bioethics described in this book.

The New Medicine

In the decades after World War II, medical ethics took a turn as medical science advanced and medical interventions became increasingly technical. The decorum was challenged by impersonal machines that intervened between doctor and patient. Traditional duties were challenged because it was no longer clear what is benefit and what is harm: is life sustained a benefit when that life is bereft of consciousness or wracked with pain? Is it harm to experiment on a dying person to generate better ways of curing disease? The social ethics was challenged by the growing intricacy of medicine with government, commerce, and the producers of new technologies. A medicine grown so technical became expensive; who assumes the duty of caring for those who cannot pay? Cultural and religious changes led to doubts about the authority that had been the privilege of the professional. The untroubled medical conscience began to feel some qualms.

New intellectual resources were summoned to struggle with the new questions: What is benefit? What is harm? Who should live? Who should die? How should the expensive resources of health care be distributed? Who should decide? Life, death, and justice are issues long pondered by theologians and philosophers, and long contemplated by the law. Theologians and philosophers, who in the past were hardly cognizant of medicine and its ethics, were invited in—or came unbidden—into these discussions. The law, an old enemy of medicine badly practiced, now struggled with the same dilemmas of life and death faced by the physicians. Bioethics was born, inheriting some of the ideas and values of the old medical ethics but encountering unprecedented problems, evolving through unique styles of analysis, and embracing many more participants than the old medical ethics ever had. In large part, the appearance of a new medicine that offered promise of great benefit initiated the examination of medicine's conscience.

After World War II, the long, slow progress of the biological sciences was spurred by the effort to improve military medicine and spilled over into the medicine and the health care of subsequent decades.[30] In *Two Centuries of American Medicine,* McGehee Harvey and James Bordley describe the three decades, 1946–1976, as the "Period of Explosive Growth."[31] Reading down their chronological summary of major events for only the first few years of that period reveals how explosive it was. In 1946, streptomycin began to be given on a wide scale to patients with tuberculosis, closing hundreds of sanitoria during the next decade. Penicillin, discovered in 1928 and first applied clinically during the war, was produced synthetically, making this rare drug the treatment of choice for pneumonia and other serious infections. In 1947, the drug methotrexate was first used to treat acute leukemia, initiating the era of cancer chemotherapy. In 1949, polio virus was cultivated in human tissue, making possible the development of the polio vaccines that were introduced in the mid-fifties; and lithium was administered to patients with manic disease. Effective anti-hypertensive drugs were discovered—the malignant hypertension that killed President Roosevelt in 1945 could have been treated only five years later. In 1952, chlorpromazine became available for agitated schizophrenia. The external cardiac pacemaker was applied for cardiac arrhythmias and its implantable transistorized form appeared eight years later. Also in 1952, the first open-heart surgery was performed, a human heart valve was replaced for the first time, and external cardiac stimulation reversed acute myocardial infarction; the electrical defibrillator was to come four years later and full cardiopulmonary resuscitation in 1958. Cardiac catheterization allowed visualization of heart defects. Chronic hemodialysis was initiated in 1962. These dramatic clinical changes were at the surface of a boiling sea of research in which the secrets of metabolism, the endocrine system, the mechanisms of immunity and wound healing, the biology of reproduction and, most exciting of all, the secrets of the genetic code were revealed.

The 1950s reveled in the progress of medicine and these medical advances were seen as undiluted goods. As the 1960s dawned, this unalloyed optimism began to falter and qualms began to tweak the conscience of those who were responsible for the advances in medicine and science. Some public opinion expressed qualms about the way in which the introduction of medical technologies damages the relationship between physicians and patients by encouraging the growth of new specialties to the detriment of general practice and by making the relationship more impersonal. A few books and articles appeared that pushed "the M.D.'s off their pedestal."[32] The scientific training of which modern medicine was so proud seemed to transform the healer into the technician who was remote, difficult to see, and even more difficult to understand. The profession's long opposition to reforms in the financing of medical care, stigmatized as "socialized medicine," also made physicians seem uncaring, greedy, and self-interested.[33] *Harper's* carried a special supplement in 1960 with the shocking title, "The Crisis in American Medicine." Although American medicine was unquestionably the best in the world, it was troubled: doctors were in critically short supply, the family doctor was becoming extinct, the costs of care were soaring, the government was ready to enter the private world of medicine. "Among themselves, worried doctors frequently talk about such questions—but they seldom mention them to their patients and other laymen," wrote the editor.[34] Privately, medical scientists debated over the growing use of patients as human subjects of research and the rationing of scarce remedies, such as penicillin.[35]

The Decade of Conferences

During the 1960s, a few leading medical scientists broke their silence. They aired their qualms of conscience at unprecedented conferences, ruminating before their colleagues and even lay audiences about the social and ethical problems involved in medical and scientific progress. Although their consciences were not as tortured as those of many atomic scientists who had seen their theories used to incinerate 100,000 people, the biomedical scientists nonetheless initiated serious dialogue about their work.[36] Here we shall visit a few of those conferences to catch the tenor of the discussions.

A conference that opened the decade was aptly called, "Great Issues of Conscience in Modern Medicine," held at Dartmouth College, Hanover, New Hampshire, September, 8–10, 1960.[37] An impressive array of medical scientists gathered to discuss what their consciences told them were the great issues. René Dubos, Professor of Microbiology at Rockefeller Institute, served as chair. He was an appropriate choice, for he had written a thoughtful book, *Mirage of Health: Utopias, Progress and Biological Change*, that had appeared in the previous year. Dubos presided over lectures by scientific leaders of the day: Sir George Pickering, Regius Professor of Medicine at Oxford University, Brock Chisholm, recently Director-General of the World Health Organization (WHO), Wilder Penfield, the father of neurosurgery, Walsh McDermott, one of America's leading physicians, Hermann J. Muller, a Nobelist in physiology and medicine for his work in genetic effects of radiation, and George Kistiakowsky, Assistant to President Eisenhower for Science and Technology. C. P. Snow and Aldous Huxley represented the humanities. Dr. S. Marsh Tenney, Dean of Dartmouth Medical School, opened the conference: "Although [medicine's] foundations have become more rational, its practice—the welding of science and humanism—is said to have become more remote and indifferent to human values, and once again medicine has been forced to remind itself that it is often the human factors that are determinant." The purpose of the convocation, said Dr. Tenney, was "to examine the issues of conscience in medical and scientific progress . . . not simply the question of the survival or the extinction of man, but *what kind* of survival? a future of what *nature?*"[38]

The speakers addressed large questions: the effects of ionizing radiation, the pollution of water and air, and chemical adulteration of food. The medical advance most in view was the "conquest of infectious disease."[39] This thrilling victory had its adverse side; it lowered the death rate without decreasing the birth rate. The Honorable Mohamedali Chagla, Indian Ambassador to the United States, asserted that "one of the most important issues of conscience in modern medicine" is that, while medicine must advance to improve hygiene and public health, it increases population among the most impoverished.[40] Although Professor Dubos and Dr. McDermott challenged the contention that overpopulation was the result of medical advance, most participants seemed to agree with the ambassador and returned repeatedly to that thesis. The claim that medical advances had contributed to the population explosion and to the pollution of the gene pool became a common theme of the conferences during the 1960s.

René Dubos called "prolongation of the life of aged and ailing persons" and the saving of lives of children with genetic defects "the most difficult problem of medical ethics we are likely to encounter within the next decade. . . . To what extent can we afford to prolong biological life in individuals who cannot derive either profit or pleasure from existence, and whose survival creates painful burdens for the community? . . . this is not a decision for the physician whose duty is to save and prolong life. . . . It will be for society to redefine these ethics, if the problem becomes one that society is no longer willing or able to carry."[41] Geneticists worried that the gene pool was becoming polluted because the early death of persons with certain genetic conditions was now preventable: in addition to antibiotics, insulin for diabetes and diet for phenelkytonuria were frequently mentioned. A unique solution was offered by Nobelist Hermann J. Muller, who promoted his concept of a bank of healthy sperm, together with the "new techniques of reproduction," to prevent the otherwise inevitable degeneration of the race. The novel proposal was sharply repudiated by Aldous Huxley, whose imagination had once created a similar bank for *Brave New World*; he argued that such efforts to control "human breeding lends itself to totalitarian manipulation."

Sir Charles Snow summed up the conference: there were "two kinds of problems of conscience with which modern medicine is concerned." The first is the old set of problems "that beset any practicing physician in the course of his relations with his patients." About this "private morality" the conference said little, "because we were all pretty satisfied with what is generally established in this relationship." The second problem, "a much more difficult kind of morality," is what one speaker, Mr. Warren Weaver of the Sloan Foundation, had called "statistical morality . . . one can perform acts which are in themselves innocent . . . [but which] bring the risks or indeed the certainty of disease and death to people who are anonymous." The way to deal with such problems is by foresight and intelligence and, above all, by scientists telling the truth, but "it is not enough for scientists to make statements of the greatest possible truth," concluded Sir Charles; "they must have the courage to carry those statements through because they alone know enough to be able to impress their authority upon a world which is anxious to hear."

Many questions had been raised; many wise observations had been made; few answers had been given. This seemed right to Chairman Dubos: "We are not assembled here to solve problems. Our purpose is to air problems . . . to state our problems as clearly and thoughtfully as we can, so that they can be better analyzed by the scientific community and so that the community at large—lay people—can struggle under our guidance to form its own opinions, often to be based on judgments of values."[42] "Great Issues of Conscience in Modern Medicine" was an impressive occasion: men of science, joined by a few humanists, reflected in public about the troubling issues they saw hidden within the wonderful inventions of modern science. They "aired problems" rather than analyzing them. They spoke with confidence in the power of their own intelligence and honesty to deal with the problems. The "ethics" was common sense and commonplace with not a hint of the "moral sciences," philosophy and theology. Moral problems were stated in generic terms, with little effort to refine the exact nature of the ethical issue. The public was only rarely invited to partake in resolving these great problems. Dubos does say that the problem of prolonging life is a matter for society to determine but, for the most part, the public is seen as an audience, waiting for scientists to bring solutions to the problems they have created. The more mature bioethics, still a decade in the future, will invite more participants from the humanities, who will employ the methods of the moral sciences to analyze problems and who will be less confident in the ability of scientists to solve the problems of their own making. Still, the Dartmouth Convocation was a signal event in the move toward bioethics.

"Man and His Future," sponsored by the Ciba Foundation in London, November 27–30, 1962, replicated the style and themes of the Dartmouth conference. The Ciba proceedings begin: "The world was unprepared socially, politically and ethically for the advent of nuclear power. Now, biological research is in a ferment, creating and promising methods of interference with 'natural processes' which could destroy or could transform nearly every aspect of human life which we value. It is necessary for . . . every intelligent individual of our one world to consider the present and imminent possibilities."[43] As at Dartmouth, the gathering was glittering. Drs. Brock Chisholm and Hermann Muller were again invited. Aldous Huxley's scientific brother, Julian, lectured, as did Joshua Lederberg, J. B. S. Haldane, and Albert Szent-Gyorgyi. Francis Crick, Jacob Bronowski, and Peter Medawar participated in the discussions. Five of the twenty-seven participants were Nobel prize winners. As at Dartmouth, generic and global issues were discussed: agricultural productivity, world resources, and environmental degradation.

Sir Julian Huxley opened the conference with a wide-ranging lecture entitled "The Future of Man—Evolutionary Aspects." He painted a picture of evolution that for the first time had become conscious of itself in humankind and thus was responsible for its own direction. This evolution, he proclaimed, had significant implications for ecology, population, economics, education, and above all, for the exploration of "inner space— the realm of our own minds and the psychometabolic processes at work in it." The problems of overpopulation and the dysgenic effects of progress had to be overcome to assure the realization of human fulfillment: "Eventually, the prospect of radical eugenic improvement could become one of the mainsprings of man's evolutionary advance." Man was, he triumphantly proclaimed, "the trustee . . . of advance in the cosmic process of evolution."[44]

Few among the distinguished audience disagreed with Huxley's words. One after another, the savants chronicled medical progress. Nobelist Szent-Györgyi concluded: "You may wish for anything: a cure-all for cancer, a mastery of mutation, an understanding of hormone action, or a cure of any disease you have in mind. None of your wishes need remain unfulfilled, once we have penetrated deep enough into the foundations of life. This is the real promise of medicine."[45] Yet, repeatedly, the participants admitted that advances brought in their beneficial wake unintended problems. It was not difficult to educe examples, ranging from the agricultural revolution's effect on overpopulation to the worry expressed by the microbiologist, Koprowski, that eradication of the polio virus might "lead to the replacement of its commonly innocuous gastrointestinal form by other, unrelated viral agents which might treat the human host much less mercifully (Good old polio days!)."[46] While they admitted the problems attendant on progress, they expressed confidence in the ability of their kind to overcome them. Along with the recognition of adverse effects of progress, humanity had to recognize our responsibility for the direction of the future.

Sessions devoted to genetics and brain sciences incited a turmoil: scientists took sides for and against programs of eugenics and thought control; loud protests against totalitarianism were heard. J. B. S. Haldane was not daunted by these protests. He gave the final lecture of the conference, in which he described a vision of "his own utopia," imagining the biological possibilities in the next ten thousand years. He admitted that some might consider his utopia "his own private hell." It included broad control of physiological and psychological processes, achieved largely by pharmacological and genetic techniques, including cloning and deliberate provocation of mutations, to suit the human product for special purposes in the world of the future. "Men who had lost their legs by accident or mutation would be specially qualified as astronauts . . . preparing the crew of the first spaceship to Alpha Centauri by reducing not only their weight but their food and oxygen requirements."[47] It is difficult to discern whether Professor Haldane was playing the serious prophet or the ironic critic.

The panel discussion devoted to "ethical considerations" was a rambling conversation between a group of highly intelligent men, most of whom shared the profession of science and a broad common culture, but little else. Bronowski delivered a long speech, extolling the ways in which science, which is a search for truth, could improve the morals of humankind. Most speakers espoused ethical relativity. The sole representative of religion, a pediatrician turned priest, Rev. Dr. Hugh Trowell, suggested that those who accepted Christian beliefs had a broad agreement with those who did not when it came to "basic ethical considerations that concern all humanity." Francis Crick retorted that while there might be some agreement on values, "they do not necessarily coincide . . . for practical purposes . . . there is bound to be a conflict of values. . . . I think that in time the facts of science are going to make us become less Christian."[48] Medawar had the last word, saying, "Groups of this kind usually end up by agreeing on one thing, namely, that more education is what is wanted. I am unable to see how that view can be reconciled with the incredible diversity of opinion which has been expressed here. . . . We scientists proceed in society as we do in science . . . by a process of exploration from which we sometimes learn to do better."[49]

Several conferences sponsored by small American liberal arts colleges "did better." Gustavus Adolphus College in Minnesota inaugurated a series of conferences at which Nobel Prize winners joined other scholars from many fields to discuss the implications of science in the modern world. The first Nobel Conference, held January 5–8, 1965, was devoted to "Genetics and the Future of Man." Dr. William Shockley, who had won the Nobel prize for physics, presented his views on eugenics, suggesting that, since intelligence was largely genetically determined, serious efforts to improve human intelligence should be pursued by various means, including sterilization, cloning, and artificial insemination. Shockley praised Hermann Muller's advocacy of sperm banks.

Muller's proposal had been attacked at Dartmouth and at the Ciba conference, but never before had it met an analytic refutation from a scholar trained in ethics. The next speaker was such a scholar, Paul Ramsey, Professor of Religion at Princeton University, making his first appearance on the stage (or, some might say, in the pulpit) of bioethics that he was to dominate for many years. That confrontation will be chronicled in Chapter 9. Ramsey's Nobel Conference lecture may be counted as one, and perhaps the first, genuine example of bioethics. It goes beyond "airing the issue" to analyzing it in light of distinctly expressed principles and values.

Later Gustavus Adolphus Nobel Conferences contributed important pieces to the emerging bioethics. At the 1967 conference, "The Human Mind," theologian James Gustafson spoke on "Christian Humanism and the Human Mind." Professor Gustafson was deeply impressed by the reports of neurobiologists about the biochemical bases of memory and learning. Gustafson felt that theological ethicists should reflect upon "the brain we are coming to know and understand in biological terms." The scientific community had to be vigilant about the potential misuses of its knowledge and the religious community had to participate in the processes through which the uses of new knowledge would be determined. Together, these communities had to work toward a "a much more detailed and clearer formulation of those values to be preserved and developed in human existence . . . so that these may indicate the direction that uses of research ought to take, and the limitations of those uses that ought to be firmly formed.[50] These principles anticipate the agenda for the nascent bioethics: broader participation in deliberation about scientific advances and a clearer formulation of values to be served by those advances.

In 1966 Reed College of Portland, Oregon held a conference entitled "The Sanctity of Life." This conference took one more step toward the "doing better" that Sir Peter Medawar had hoped for at the 1962 Ciba conference. Fortunately, Sir Peter was in the auditorium of Reed College on March 12, 1966, lecturing on "Genetic Options: An Examination of Current Fallacies." On the same platform, the prominent sociologist Edward Shils, Norman St. John-Stevas, a distinguished British barrister and member of Parliament, and Abraham Kaplan from the Philosophy Department at the University of California, Los Angeles, joined two others who would become stars in the bioethical firmament: theologian Paul Ramsey and Harvard professor of anesthesia, Henry Beecher. Although the topics covered a broad range, from Shils' eloquent disquisition, "The Secular Meaning of Sanctity of Life," to St. John-Stevas's learned lecture, "Law and Moral Consensus," three issues that would eventually emerge as canonical questions of bioethics were broached: Ramsey spoke on the morality of abortion, Medawar on eugenics, and Beecher on medical research involving human subjects.

Chairman Daniel Labby opened the conference with the remark that sanctity of life seemed an appropriate topic because "an unpopular war was threatening to escalate insanely, and the use of nuclear power in war was a world-wide anxiety. The problems of racism and rioting were again aflame, the wounds of the thalidomide tragedy were still unhealed, and contraception and abortion were troublesome moral dilemmas." However, after this reference to the cataclysms of the time, Labby cited a comment by Medawar: "The mischief . . . grows just as often out of trying to do good . . . as out of actions intended to be destructive." These remarks mingle two aspects of the emerging bioethics: the broad statement of "troublesome moral dilemmas" and the more precise recognition that these dilemmas appear in bioethics as the result of attempting and even achieving great goods.[51]

The Reed conference "did better" because the issues were more closely defined and because a proper theologian and a proper philosopher were invited to do some scholarly ethics. Ramsey had initiated the bioethical debate at Gustavus Adolphus; now Professor Kaplan (whose philosophical forte was logic rather than ethics) appeared as the first philosopher to join the discourse. His task was to summarize the conference presentations and he did so in a properly philosophical fashion, opening with the comment, "Bertrand Russell once characterized the real task of philosophy as being twofold: first, to make complicated things simple and, second, to make simple things complicated. . . . [I will] supplement what has already been said, not only by simplifying what was complicated, but also by complicating what appear to me to have been oversimplifications."[52] Prophetically, Kaplan described the function that many philosophical bioethicists would later perform, namely, the exposé of ethical oversimplifications. Kaplan concluded his summary with a remark that presaged a dominant principle of future bioethics: "The moral judgment must accord with the principle of moral autonomy, as it has been known in philosophy since Immanuel Kant. The moral will must be a lawgiver unto itself; . . . in that case, we are committed to respecting the moral autonomy of other moral agents as well."[53]

On December 3, 1967, Dr. Christiaan Barnard performed the world's first heart transplantation in Capetown, South Africa. Dr. Michael E. DeBakey, America's most prominent cardiac surgeon and then Chancellor of the University of Texas, Houston Medical Center, encouraged Kenneth Vaux, a young theologian on the staff of the Institute of Religion, Texas Medical Center, to organize "a platform for discussion of the vital issues" raised by transplantation and other "unprecedented medical events that give rise to reconsideration of medical ethical codes."[54] Dr. Vaux brought together a splendid scholarly panel: his own teacher, German Protestant theologian Helmut Thielicke,

Paul Ramsey, Joseph Fletcher, Jesuit lawyer Robert Drinan, Emmanuel Mesthene, Director of the Harvard Program on Science and Technology, and, as keynote speaker, the irrepressible anthropologist, Margaret Mead.

In his concluding address, "The Doctor as Judge of Who Shall Live and Who Shall Die," Professor Thielicke gave a prophetic account of the future bioethics, illustrating the "ambiguity of progress" with a number of examples, such as the ability to save the lives of children with genetic defects who go on to propagate those genes in their progeny (using phenylketonuria as his example). He found the "origins of this fateful ambiguity" in the human condition as interpreted in the Biblical religions, which "see in this ambiguity a manifestation of the halflight between creation and fall, between man as he was meant to be and as he presently is, standing in sinful contradiction to his intended destiny; . . . there is an ambiguity about man's creativity."[55] Even stripped of its theological idiom, the concept of moral ambiguity would remain a theme in the bioethics to come: bioethics would recognize that the evils to be avoided are inextricably bound with the goods to be enjoyed. At the same time, bioethical ambiguity was not an excuse to abandon inquiry but an invitation to explore, refine, and resolve to the extent possible the difficult questions raised. Only ten days after this excellent conference closed, Dr. DeBakey's protégé, Dr. Denton Cooley, exemplified this moral ambiguity by implanting the first artificial heart in Mr. Haskell Karp on April 4, 1968.

The conferences of the 1960s prepared the materials for the emerging bioethics. Scientific and medical advances which, at first sight, promised undiluted benefits, were seen to have certain disadvantages, inconveniences, and harms associated with them. These unwanted effects were recognized not simply as technical problems that could easily be fixed (although some scientists found it difficult to admit this) but as ethical questions that required serious reflection and discussion. That serious reflection and discussion was accomplished in a series of conferences, symposia, and colloquia, at which the scientists and medical professionals "aired" the issues. At first, there was little effort to define with care what constituted an ethical problem or to analyze in detail the nature of the problem. It seemed sufficient, if not entirely satisfying, to discuss the problems frankly and honestly. Gradually, persons with some academic credentials in the moral sciences were invited to these events. They began to press for clearer definitions and to offer arguments for or against various positions. The "doing better" at the articulation of issues was apparent. An unprecedented discourse was inaugurated: scientists and ethicists, along with many others, were talking with each other and beginning to understand each other's language.

From Conferences to Centers

By the end of the decade, a small library of conference proceedings and collections of essays existed.[56] James Gustafson, in reviewing the volume from the Reed College Symposium, noted that medical ethics was being discussed at many meetings. "Such conferences," he wrote, "and the papers that are published from them are important at this stage of the discussion. . . . But one hopes we can move beyond the conference procedure to a more disciplined, careful, long range way of working in which areas of disagreement can not only be defined, but in part at least overcome. What is needed, it seems to me, is interdisciplinary work within universities or centers that have personnel and resources for the arduous tasks of intensive and long-term work."[57]

As the 1960s ceded to the 1970s, Gustafson's hope began to be realized. Conferences continued, but from this time on their results were less ephemeral. The free-floating bioethical concern that the conferences had inspired began to coalesce into pieces of scholarly analysis. The discourse of the conferences was now fitted into a general framework of research fostered by several new permanent centers: the Institute of Society, Ethics and the Life Sciences (The Hastings Center) and the Kennedy Institute of Ethics at Georgetown University. A third organization, The Society for Health and Human Values, also encouraged interdisciplinary activity. These organizations were the culmination of the decade of conferences: they gave permanent homes to the discourse of bioethical concern.

The Hastings Center

In the mid-1960s, Dan Callahan, a recent graduate in philosophy from Harvard and employed as editor at the Catholic journal of opinion, *Commonweal*, began a book on the burning question of abortion. He realized that he needed more than philosophical background and acumen to write about abortion. He knew that he had to view the problem from many perspectives with which he was not familiar, such as demography, law, medicine, and public policy. He later wrote, "I was trying to be an interdisciplinary one-man band, working my way, more or less unassisted, through a wide range of literature, most of it unfamiliar." He realized that, with the lengthening list of controversial moral questions appearing in the biomedical world, and with the many conferences and wide media coverage, there was no provision for concentrated interdisciplinary study "to explore these problems in a serious and systematic way."[58] He determined to create a center dedicated to this task.

At a Christmas party, he mentioned the idea to a Hastings-on-Hudson neighbor, Dr. Willard Gaylin, a psychiatrist on the faculty of Columbia University's College of Physicians and Surgeons. Over the next several months, they discussed the idea intensely, contacted acquaintances in philosophy, theology, medicine, and science who might be supportive and, in March 1969, helped by a loan from Callahan's mother, they gathered a group at the Princeton Club in New York City. The group formed itself into "A Center for the Study of Value and the Sciences of Man." The Center incorporated and in September, changed its name to The Institute of Society, Ethics and the Life Sciences. By the end of the year, the Institute had garnered financial support from two individuals, John D. Rockefeller III and Elizabeth Dollard, and from two foundations, the National Endowment for the Humanities and the Rockefeller Foundation.

Callahan and Gaylin enticed an extraordinary group of scientists and scholars to serve as the first Board of the Institute. Among them were Henry Beecher, Robert Coles, Theodore Dobzhansky, André Cournand, René Dubos, and Renée Fox. Robert Morison, Distinguished Professor of Biological Sciences at Cornell, served as first chair. Theologians Ramsey and Gustafson represented ethics. Senator Walter F. Mondale served on the Advisory Council. Robert M. Veatch, who was completing his doctorate at Harvard, was hired as the first staff member and literally unlocked the doors of the new Institute in space rented from a Hastings-on-Hudson dentist in September, 1970. Almost from the beginning, the cumbersome title was abbreviated to The Hastings Center. Generous grants enabled quick expansion. A staff of young scholars was assembled: Veatch was named Associate for Medical Ethics, Marc Lappé, a graduate student in physiology at the University of California, was hired as Associate for Biological Sciences, Robert Neville, a philosopher, was Associate for Behavioral Sciences, and Peter Steinfels, with a doctorate in Intellectual History, was Associate for Humanities. Bruce Hilton, coming from a theological background, supervised publications.[59] Willard Gaylin directed the Program on Teaching Medical Ethics and New York University philosopher Martin Golding was Senior Associate. This was a fortuitous assembly of very bright minds. I benefited from their intense and enthusiastic engagement in the problems of new medicine and biology, for during the winter of 1973, when I was a Fellow at the National Library of Medicine in Washington, D.C., Dan Callahan invited me to journey to Hastings-on-Hudson twice a month to discuss the conjunction of ethics and public policy.

The activities of the Center were assigned to four research groups: death and dying, behavior control, genetic engineering and counseling, and population control. Each group consisted of scholars from diverse fields and was led by one of the staff associates. They met regularly to work through their topics in a systematic way. The research groups presented the results of their studies in articles published in many influential journals. The Center realized the importance of having its own publication for the dissemination of research group products and to stimulate scholarly and popular interchange on topics of interest. The first issue of the *Hastings Center Report* appeared in June 1971, containing such articles as "Values, facts and decision making" by Dan Callahan, "Experimental pregnancy" by Bob Veatch, and "On not facing death alone," by William May. A larger journal, *Hastings Center Studies*, appeared in 1973, but it was soon folded into an expanded *Hastings Center Report*. The index of the *Hastings Center Report* over the next years defines the range of topics that were becoming bioethics and constitutes a roll call of the authors who would become its proponents.[60]

Callahan and his colleagues avoided affiliation with academic institutions. They feared the stultifying effect of academic practices such as tenure and they desired to do what universities rarely do well: traverse between theoretical issues and practical policy, between experts and professionals and the broader public. Callahan says, "we felt it would be much easier to run an interdisciplinary center outside the university, and I think it is fair to say that in twenty years we have never doubted the wisdom of the decision to remain independent."[61]

Callahan understood that the discourse that the early conferences had encouraged among scholars was an important stimulus to serious analysis. He therefore organized symposia, including "Problems on the Meaning of Death" at the December 1970, American Association for the Advancement of Science (AAAS) meeting, and a 1971 conference co-sponsored by the Center and the Fogarty Center, National Institutes of Health (NIH), entitled "Ethical Issues in Genetic Counseling and the Use of Genetic Knowledge." The Center's first annual meeting in June 1971 was called "Heart Transplants and Public Policy" and featured Dr. Theodore Cooper, Director of the National Heart and Lung Institute. The following June, the Center sponsored a National Conference on the Teaching of Medical Ethics.[62] These conferences drew scientists and non-scientists together for serious discussion of ethical questions that were now more focused and interdisciplinary than at the earlier conferences, and they began to put "bioethics" on the intellectual map.

The Kennedy Institute

André E. Hellegers, M.D., was a man of ingenuity and creativity. Born in the Netherlands, educated at the venerable Jesuit College of Stonyhurst in England, and trained in medicine at the University of Edinburgh, he joined the faculty of obstetrics and gynecology at The Johns Hopkins School of Medicine as a research scientist in fetal physiology. His work, which explored the prenatal etiology of mental retardation, won him a Fellowship from the Joseph P. Kennedy, Jr. Foundation, and he formed a friendship with Eunice Kennedy Shriver, sister of President John F. Kennedy. In 1967, he was lured to Georgetown University School of Medicine. An avid reader of philosophy and theology, Hellegers found the atmosphere of the Jesuit university congenial.

Hellegers was a prime mover in organizing a conference on abortion in 1967, jointly sponsored by the Harvard Divinity School and the Kennedy Foundation. He felt that occasional conferences were not sufficient to deal with the momentous issues associated with the reproductive sciences. During 1970, he discussed the idea of a center for the scholarly study of these issues with Rev. Robert J. Henle, S.J., the President of Georgetown University. Father Henle, whose academic discipline was philosophy, encouraged Hellegers to pursue this idea. I was a member of Georgetown's Board of Directors at that time, and I recall Henle's enthusiastic recommendation of the concept to the Board. A proposal to fund an institute was submitted to the Kennedy Foundation on December 30, 1970. It was to be called The Kennedy Center for the Study of Human Reproduction and Development. Hellegers was already Director of Georgetown's Center for Population Research, which was supported by a Ford Foundation Grant, and it was envisioned that the new institute would become part of that unit, with emphasis on prenatal and genetic studies. During the spring of 1971, ongoing discussions within the University and with the Foundation shifted attention to ethical studies and by the opening date, July 1, 1971, the official title was The Joseph and Rose Kennedy Center for the Study of Human Reproduction and Bioethics. Within a few years, the title was changed to The Kennedy Institute of Ethics. Father Henle gave credit to Hellegers for making that transition and for convincing the Kennedys and the Shrivers of its importance.[63]

The Kennedy Institute opened on July 1, 1971, with two Research Scholars: LeRoy Walters, a Mennonite theologian fresh from graduate studies in ethics under James Gustafson, who was soon given the title Director of the Center for Bioethics within the Kennedy Institute, and Warren Reich, who had left the moral theology faculty at Catholic University and later became Professor of Bioethics at the Georgetown University School of Medicine. Funding was available for visiting scholars who were left to do their own research in the general area of ethical issues in medicine and science. The first scholars were all theologians: Charles E. Curran, Richard A. McCormick, Gene A. Outka, and John Connery, each of whom produced a book or article during their time at the Institute.[64] Many more visiting scholars from a variety of disciplines and from different countries spent time at the Institute. An intensive summer course in bioethics for physicians was initiated in 1974 which has educated hundreds of physicians and other health professionals. A graduate degree program, in collaboration with the university's philosophy department, was inaugurated in the late 1970s, producing a steady stream of Ph.D.s with special concentration in bioethics.

LeRoy Walters' first task was to build a research library, which was no easy task in a field that had barely come into being. By October 1971, he was able to issue a bibliography of the Core Ethics Library that contained 641 titles, a valuable index of the available literature for scholarly research. The library continued to be built into the premier research library in bioethics. When Walters suggested to Hellegers that they publish an annual list of acquisitions, Hellegers countered with the suggestion that an annual bibliography of all publications in bioethics would be valuable. Walters picked up that suggestion and applied for funding from the National Library of Medicine, NIH. In March 1974, a $280,000 grant enabled the Kennedy Institute to establish a comprehensive information retrieval system. In 1975, the first product of that system, *Bibliography of Bioethics*, was published and in the following years, the system expanded into a National Reference Center for Bioethics Literature.[65]

Warren Reich brought Hellegers a similar modest proposal that Hellegers magnified. It had occurred to Reich that a dictionary of bioethics might be useful; Hellegers proposed that an encyclopedia should be prepared. Although the field was young, many issues were not new; furthermore, an encyclopedia would establish some benchmarks for further exploration of issues. Reich accepted this challenge, successfully sought funding from the National Endowment for the Humanities, and in 1978, produced *The Encyclopedia of Bioethics* in four volumes.[66]

In 1973, Dr. Hellegers and Fr. Henle convinced the Kennedy Foundation to support several faculty Chairs in bioethics. Father McCormick became the first Rose F. Kennedy Professor of Christian Ethics. The Kennedy Professorships provided prominent positions for excellent scholars who were given freedom to expand the intellectual dimensions of bioethics. After McCormick, theologian James F. Childress was lured from the University of Virginia in 1975, and H. Tristram Engelhardt, Jr., the Institute's first trained philosopher and a physician, came from Texas Medical Branch in Galveston in 1977. In December of 1979, Robert Veatch moved from The Hastings Center to The Kennedy Institute; William May came from the University of Indiana in 1980. Each of these scholars was highly productive. The most influential of their products was the collaborative work of Childress and Georgetown philosopher Tom Beauchamp, *Principles of Biomedical Ethics*, which was conceived in 1976 and published in 1979. It was the first "systematic analysis of the principles that should govern a wide range of decisions affecting biomedicine."[67]

André Hellegers died in 1979. After interim leadership, one of bioethics' prominent physicians, Dr. Edmund D. Pellegrino, became Director of the Institute, a position he held until he was succeeded by Veatch in July 1989. The Kennedy Institute and The Hastings Center were indispensable organizations for the new field of bioethics. Both organizations assembled scholars from science and the moral disciplines; both gave focus to questions. The Kennedy Institute took the more academic path, enabling research by providing professorships, fellowships, and courses and by creating the tools for research in *The Bibliography of Bioethics*, *The Encyclopedia of Bioethics*, and the National Reference Center for Bioethics Literature. The Hastings Center fostered interdisciplinary discourse by arranging working groups and task forces. Its *Hastings Center Report* brought that discourse to the wider educated public. Both organizations contributed scholars and ideas to the federal activities in bioethics that we shall review in Chapter 4.

The Society for Health and Human Values

The third organization that fostered development of the field of bioethics, the Society for Health and Human Values, was of a different sort. The staff of the United Ministries in Education, a collaboration of the Methodist and Presbyterian Churches, initiated discussions on the nature of religious ministry in medical schools. In 1965, a Committee on Medical Education and Theology emerged from those discussions. The Committee included four ministers, three physicians, and one psychologist. They were concerned about "the depersonalization of medical students" and "the teaching of mechanistic medicine," and for several years they discussed the means through which these perceived problems could be remedied. In February 1968, the Committee sponsored a Conference on Human Values in Ministry and Medical Education at the University of Florida, Gainesville, where one of its founders, Sam Banks, was on the faculty.

One month after the conference, the committee changed its name to the Committee on Health and Human Values, added several new members, and determined to seek funding for demonstration projects in the medical humanities. Prominent medical administrators, such as Dr. George Harrell, founding Dean of Hershey Medical School, and Dr. Paul J. Sanazaro, Director of The National Center for Health Services Research, were members. In February 1969, the Committee decided to transform itself into a society and to apply for a grant from the National Endowment for the Humanities "to identify explicitly the human values that are lacking or inadequately represented in the study and practice of medicine and to begin to remedy the deficit."[68] The application was successful and, with a second grant from the Russell Sage Foundation, the new Society for Health and Human Values (SHHV) held its first annual meeting in October 1970, with 67 invited members—a mixed lot of ministers, medical academic administrators, and scholars. Membership was opened to subscription in 1972.

The Society announced its purpose as follows: "Advances in medical science . . . are introducing a great array of new human problems. This Society sees its task as identifying these problems, in forming groups that will develop methods to clarify and assist in solving them, and in developing change in both professional attitudes and public awareness in relation to them."[69] The NEH grant enabled the Society to establish the Institute on Human Values in Medicine. Seminarian Thomas K. McElhinney was hired as administrator and a board was selected with Dr. Edmund Pellegrino as chair. The Institute began to define the medical humanities and to find ways to incorporate them in medical education. "Medical humanities" meant art, philosophy, history, and literature, as they were relevant to understanding health, disease, and healing. The Institute arranged conferences of humanists and medical educators, holding the first one in April 1971. It initiated a program of visits to medical campuses by persons with competence in the humanities and in medicine to advise faculty on ways of introducing humanities into the curriculum. Some 85 visits were made over ten years. It sponsored a summer fellowship program in which humanities scholars and physicians spent several months in a medical setting, learning from each other. Many major figures in the emerging bioethics, such as Ron Carson, Larry Churchill, Loretta Kopelman, Mark Siegler, and David Thomasma, found their way into the field through these fellowships.

The Society for Health and Human Values was focused not only on ethical issues in health care but rather on the medical humanities, or the broader questions of human values that can be addressed from literature and art as well as from philosophy and theology. Yet, by bringing together many of the persons who were devoting themselves to teaching ethics in medical schools, SHHV created a community in which common interests were recognized and fostered. During the next decade, the Society was the meeting place for those otherwise lonely figures, the bioethics professors. With Warren Reich, Peter Williams, Larry McCullough, and a few others, I helped organized an SHHV Section for Faculty in which those who taught ethics and humanities in medical schools could discuss their work.

The story of the three organizations makes it obvious that there was financial support for the emerging study of ethical issues in the new biology and medicine. Callahan has noted, "the main obstacle (to obtaining funding) initially was the use of the word 'ethics.' . . . problems of morality were thought to be 'soft,' elusive, and not subject to rational analysis or resolution. Potential donors had to be persuaded that the founders (of the Hastings Center) believed just the opposite to be the case and that in any event, however difficult, the emerging moral problems of medicine and biology had to be confronted."[70] It did not hurt, of course, that the "founders" of The Hastings Center, the group of scientists and scholars that Callahan and Gaylin had assembled, were drawn from America's best scientists and scholars. Consequently, donors were persuaded. The Hastings Center found support from the Rockefeller, Ford, and other foundations; The Kennedy Institute received funding from the Kennedy Foundation and the National Library of Medicine.

The National Endowment for the Humanities (NEH) was the munificent benefactor of bioethics. The NEH, established by Congress in 1965 to provide federal funding for studies in the humanistic disciplines, was asked by President Nixon in 1970 to add comparative religion and ethics to its definition of humanities. Grant applications from the emerging bioethics groups allowed the NEH to fulfill the Presidential request. In 1973, the Program on Science, Technology and Human Values, established in collaboration with the National Science Foundation, provided a focus for applications in bioethics. In addition to grants to the Hastings and Kennedy Institutes and to the Society for Health and Human Values, NEH funds supported new academic units, such as those at the University of Florida, Penn State at Hershey, and Texas Medical Branch, Galveston. It funded summer workshops in bioethics, conducted by many of the early scholars in bioethics and attended by many of the later ones. Stephen Toulmin and I received a generous grant for the research that led to the publication of our book, *The Abuse of Casuistry*. Without the NEH, bioethics would have been penurious and possibly died at birth. NEH Chairman Joseph D. Duffey was the presiding benefactor whose largess watered the field of bioethics.

A Conversation

The "poet's pen . . . gives to airy nothing a local habitation and a name," wrote Shakespeare.[71] The centers gave to the airy speculation of the conferences "a local habitation," but no one had yet come up with a name. A name may have been conjured up in a conversation one night during 1970. Mr. R. Sargent Shriver, the first director of the Peace Corps, his wife, Mrs. Eunice Kennedy Shriver, Dr. André Hellegers, and several others sat in the living room of the Shrivers' Bethesda, Maryland home. They were discussing the possibility that the Joseph P. Kennedy Jr. Foundation might sponsor Dr. Helleger's hope for an institute devoted to the study of the religious and ethical aspects of advances in the biological and medical sciences. Years later, Mr. Shriver recalled a moment of that meeting:

Because of the need to bring biology and ethics together, I thought of "bioethics." And the people in the room latched onto it as the name of the Institute. Our idea was that we were starting an ethics institute regarding this new science, with primary emphasis on biology with ethics. . . . I know full well I proposed the word. But I don't think it was a stroke of genius. It was as easy to come up with the word "bioethics" as falling off a log.[72]

It wasn't quite this easy, according to Warren Reich, who believes that the word had a "bilocated birth" in the years 1970–1971. Van Rensselaer Potter, a research oncologist at the University of Wisconsin, published an article in 1970 entitled "Bioethics, the science of survival"[73] and in 1971, followed it with his book, *Bioethics: Bridge to the Future*.[74] He defined his neologism as "a new discipline that combines biological knowledge with a knowledge of human value systems."[75] This new science was to identify and promote an optimum changing environment and an optimum human adaptation within that environment, so as to sustain and improve the civilized world. To achieve that objective, Potter proposed a "new science of survival," which Reich describes as an "open-ended biocybernetic study of self-assessment toward evolutionary, physiological and cultural adaptation."[76] The word appeared in the popular media when the April 19, 1971 issue of *Time* published a long article, titled "Man into superman: the promise and peril of the new genetics," in which Potter's book was cited.

Dr. André Hellegers had also occasionally used the word in conversation and on October 1, 1971, when the University announced that the Kennedy Foundation would fund the Institute, the press release noted that the Institute would "pioneer in the development of a new field of joint research which the institute's founders have named 'bioethics.'"[77] It is unclear whether Hellegers knew Potter's scholarly work. Yet, by late 1971, bioethics had been translated from a neologism in a scholarly article into the title of an institution and was on its way toward becoming the name of a new discipline.

Drs. Potter and Hellegers probably both understood the implications of the prefix "bio" in the same way: both were physicians and researchers in the biological sciences. They probably understood the suffix, "ethics" somewhat differently: Potter used it as a general term for human values; Hellegers, as a Jesuit-educated Catholic, knew ethics as a rigorous examination of the grounds for moral norms. This ambiguity about ethics lingers, but "bioethics" caught on and its meaning narrowed from Potter's ample embrace of the global future to Helleger's concentration on the problems of biomedicine. In 1972, Warren Reich decided to entitle the encyclopedia he was about to edit, *The Encyclopedia of Bioethics*, defining bioethics in the introduction as "the study of the ethical dimensions of medicine and the biological sciences."[78] The word was given canonical status in 1974 when the Library of Congress entered it as a subject head, citing as authority "Bioethics as a discipline," by Daniel Callahan.[79]

By 1971, a word had been invented and used to christen a wide discourse about the problematic side of the new medicine and new science. The next two chapters will examine how the two moral sciences, theology and philosophy, helped to transform the conversations of the era of conferences into a disciplined study.

Notes to Chapter 1

1. Richard Flaste, *Medicine's Great Journey. One Hundred Years of Healing* (Boston: Little, Brown, 1992), p. 104; W. E. Smith, "Country doctor. A photographic essay," *Life*, September 20, 1948, pp. 115–125.

2. Estelle Raben, *"Men in White* and *Yellow Jack* as mirrors of the medical profession," *Literature and Medicine* 12 (1993): 19–41, p. 20.

3. Chester R. Burns, "Fictional doctors and the evolution of medical ethics in the United States, 1875–1900," *Literature and Medicine* 7 (1988): 39–55; Richard Malmsheimer, *"Doctors Only." The Evolving Image of the American Physician* (New York: Greenwood Press, 1988).

4. See Paul Starr, *The Social Transformation of American Medicine* (New York: Basic Books, 1983), especially Book II, chapters 1–3.

5. Robert B. Bean and William B. Bean (eds.), *Sir William Osler. Aphorisms* (Springfield, Ill.: Charles C. Thomas, 1951), #155.

6. Richard Harrison Shryock, "The American physician in 1846 and 1946," *Journal of the American Medical Association* 134 (1947): 417–424; reprinted in Shryock, *Medicine in America* (Baltimore: The Johns Hopkins Press, 1966), pp. 151, 176. Shryock quotes from the *Cincinnati Medical Observer* 2 (1857), p. 129; *The Philadelphia Item*, Nov. 6, 1858; and *Medical and Surgical Reporter* 1 (1859), 356. See also William Rothstein, *American Physicians in the Nineteenth Century: From Sects to Science* (Baltimore: Johns Hopkins University Press, 1973). Shryock's 1947 address should be compared with the addresses presented at the 150th anniversary of the Code, Philadelphia, (March 14–15, 1997) published in Robert Baker, Linda Emanuel, and Steven Latham, *The American Medical Ethics Revolution* (Baltimore: Johns Hopkins University Press, 1998). Here the shift from medical ethics to bioethics is obvious.

7. Roland F. Schoen, John W. Kennedy, William McGrath, "Principles of medical ethics," *Arizona Medicine* 23 (1966): 601, 677, 761, 873, 941.

8. C. Malcolm Watts, "A new ethic for medicine and society," *California Medicine* 113 (1970): 67–68.

9. Medical ethics has been neglected by medical historians. Although some historians have recently shown an interest in medical ethics, few studies of particular topics, eras, or authors have been published and no comprehensive scholarly work exists. The easiest way to survey the history of medical ethics is to consult the articles under "Medical ethics history of," in Warren Reich (ed.), *The Encyclopedia of Bioethics*. (New York: Simon & Schuster, 1995).

10. Arthur Kleinman, *Patients and Healers in the Context of Culture: An Exploration of the Borderland Between Anthropology, Medicine, and Psychiatry* (Berkeley: University of California Press, 1980); Arthur J. Rubel and Michael Haas, "Ethnomedicine," in Thomas M. Johnson and Carolyn F. Sargent (eds), *Medical Anthropology: Contemporary Theory and Method* (New York: Praeger, 1990), pp. 115–131.

11. Brief descriptions of the medical ethics of other cultures can be found under the heading, "Medical ethics, history of," in Reich, *The Encyclopedia of Bioethics*.

12. Ludwig Edelstein, "The Hippocratic Oath: text, translation and interpretation," *Bulletin of the History of Medicine*, suppl. 5 (1943): 1–64, reprinted in Oswei Temkin and C. Lilian Temkin (eds.), *Ancient Medicine: Selected Papers of Ludwig Edelstein* (Baltimore: The Johns Hopkins Press, 1967), pp. 3–65. For a different perspective, see Vivian Nutton, "Beyond the Hippocratic Oath," in Roger K. French, Andrew Wear, and Johanna Geyer-Kordesch (eds.), *Doctors and Ethics: the Earlier Historical Setting of Professional Ethics* (Amsterdam: Rodopi, 1993), pp. 10–37.

15. Darrel W. Amundsen, "The early Christian Tradition" and "The medieval Catholic tradi-

tion," in Ronald L. Numbers and Darrel W. Amundsen (eds.), *Caring and Curing: Health and Medicine in the Western Religious Tradition* (New York: Macmillan, 1986), pp. 40–64, 84–91. See Robert M. Veatch and Carol G. Mason, "Hippocratic vs. Judeo-Christian medical ethics: principles in conflict," *Journal of Religious Ethics* 15 (1986): 86–105.

14. Thomas Percival, *Medical Ethics: or, a Code of Institutes and Precepts, Adapted to the Professional Conduct of Physicians and Surgeons* (London: S. Russell, 1803). References here are to Chauncey Leake (ed.), *Percival's Medical Ethics* (Baltimore: Williams and Wilkins, 1927), preface, p. 67 and chapter 2, p. 111. See Robert Baker, "Deciphering Percival's code," in Robert Baker, Dorothy Porter, and Roy Porter (eds.), *The Codification of Medical Morality: Historical and Philosophical Studies of the Formalization of Western Medical Morality in the Eighteenth and Nineteenth Centuries*, vol. 1 (Dordrecht/Boston: Kluwer Academic Publishers, 1993), pp. 179–212.

15. 1847 *Code of Medical Ethics*, chapter 2, article iv, in Leake, *Percival's Medical Ethics*, pp. 228–229; John S. Haller, Jr., *American Medicine in Transition: 1840–1910* (Urbana: University of Illinois Press, 1981), p. 237.

16. See Baker et al., *The Codification of Medical Morality*, vol. 1 and Robert Baker (ed.), *The Codification of Medical Morality*, vol. 2 (Dordrecht/Boston: Kluwer Academic Publishers, 1995).

17. Richard C. Cabot, *Social Work: Essays on the Meeting Ground of Doctor and Social Worker* (Boston/New York: Houghton-Mifflin Company, 1919). Dr. Cabot educated himself in moral philosophy and produced a number of books on that subject: *The Meaning of Right and Wrong* (New York: Macmillan Company, 1933), *What Men Live By* (Boston and New York: Houghton-Mifflin Company, 1914); *Honesty* (New York: Macmillan Company, 1938).

18. Chester Burns, "Richard Cabot and reformation in American medical ethics," *Bulletin of the History of Medicine* 51 (1977): 353–368, quote on p. 368.

19. Richard Cabot, "Medical ethics in the hospital," *Nosokomeion* 2 (1931): 151–161.

20. Albert R. Jonsen, *The New Medicine and the Old Ethics* (Cambridge, Mass.: Harvard University Press, 1990), p. 27.

21. Burns, "Richard Cabot," pp. 358–359; Richard Cabot, "A study of mistaken diagnosis," *Journal of the American Medical Association* 55 (1910): 1343–1350; "Diagnostic pitfalls identified during a study of three thousand autopsies," *Journal of the American Medical Association* 59 (1912): 2295–2298.

22. Cabot, *What Men Live By*, pp. xi, xii.

23. On Cabot's influence, see Ida Maud Cannon, *On the Social Frontier of Medicine: Pioneering in Medical Social Service* (Cambridge: Harvard University Press, 1952); T. F. Williams, "Cabot, Peabody and the care of the patient," *Bulletin of the History of Medicine* 24 (1950): 462–481; Burns, "Richard Cabot," pp. 353–368.

24. Leake, *Percival's Medical Ethics*, p. 18. The distinction between "ethics" and "etiquette" was made by W. H. S. Jones, *The Doctor's Oath: An Essay in the History of Medicine* (Cambridge: The University Press, 1924).

25. Chauncey D. Leake, "How is medical ethics to be taught?" *Bulletin of the Association of American Medical Colleges* 3 (1928): 341–343, quote from p. 343.

26. AMA Code, 1847, III, article 1, 3; 1903, II, article iv, 1. In Leake, *Percival's Medical Ethics*, pp. 235, 254.

27. AMA Code, 1912, II, article 6, 1. In Leake, *Percival's Medical Ethics*, p. 270.

28. Richard C. Cabot, *Training and Rewards of the Physician* (Philadelphia: J. B. Lippincott Company, 1918), pp. 133, 136.

29. Hippocrates, in W. H. S. Jones (trans.), *Hippocrates with an English Translation*, Aphorisms I, (Cambridge, Mass: Harvard University Press, 1959), vol. 4, p. 99. There are notable

exceptions to the generality that the physician authors of medical ethics books were not philosophical, for example, Rodrigo a Castro (1557?–1637) and John Gregory (1724–1773). On the former, see Winfred Schleiner, *Medical Ethics in the Renaissance* (Washington, D.C.: Georgetown University Press, 1995); on the latter, see Laurence McCullough, *John Gregory and the Invention of Professional Medical Ethics and the Profession of Medicine* (Dordrecht: Kluwer Academic Publishers, 1998).

30. David J. Rothman, *Strangers at the Bedside* (New York: Basic Books, 1991), chapter 2; E. C. Andrus, D. W. Brock, G. A. Carden, Jr., et al. (eds.), *Advances in Military Medicine; Made by American Investigators Working Under the Sponsorship of the Committee on Medical Research*, 2 vols. (Boston: Little, Brown, and Company, 1948).

31. McGehee Harvey and James Bordley, *Two Centuries of American Medicine* (Philadelphia: Saunders, 1976), part III, pp. 385–771.

32. H. Maurer, "The M.D.'s are off their pedestal," *Fortune*, February 1954, p. 138; Richard Carter, *The Doctor Business* (New York: Doubleday, 1958).

33. John Burnham, "American medicine's Golden Age: what happened to it?" *Science* 215 (1982): 1474–1479; see Paul Starr, *The Social Transformation of American Medicine* (New York: Basic Books, 1982).

34. Foreword, "The crisis in American medicine," *Harper's*, 221, special suppl., October, 1960, p. 123.

35. Ruth R. Faden (ed.), *The Human Radiation Experiments: Final Report of the President's Advisory Commission* (New York: Oxford University Press, 1996). Gladys L. Hobby, *Penicillin. Meeting the Challenge* (New Haven: Yale University Press, 1985) only hints at the debates about rationing penicillin. I have been unable to verify the story told by Paul Ramsey, who based his remarks on an unsupported comment by Paul Freund, that an official decision to ration penicillin to soldiers with venereal disease in preference to those with war wounds was made in the North African war theater during World War II. See Paul Ramsey, *The Patient as Person. Explorations in Medical Ethics* (New Haven: Yale University Press, 1970), p. 257; Paul A. Freund, Introduction to the issue "Ethical Aspects of Experimentation with Human Subjects," *Daedalus* 98 (1969), p. xiii.

36. Morgon Grodzins and Eugene Rabinowitch (eds.), *The Atomic Age. Scientists in National and World Affairs: Articles from the Bulletin of Atomic Scientists, 1945–1962* (New York: Simon and Schuster, 1965); John C. Bennett, *Nuclear Weapons and the Conflict of Conscience* (New York: Scribner, 1962).

37. Other conferences were held prior to the Dartmouth Convocation, such as the 1951 symposium on research with human subjects at the University of California, San Francisco and the 1959 conference on human experimentation at Boston University Law Medicine Research Institute. These are discussed in Chapter 5.

38. S. Marsh Tenney, "Opening Assembly," from the *Dartmouth Convocation on Great Issues of Conscience in Modern Medicine* (September 8–10, 1960), published in *Dartmouth Alumni Magazine* 53(2) (1960):7–8; René Dubos, *Mirage of Health: Utopias, Progress and Biological Change* (New York: Harper and Row, 1959).

39. C. E. A. Winslow, *The Conquest of Epidemic Disease: A Chapter in the History of Ideas* (Princeton: Princeton University Press, 1943). In 1967, only a few years later, the Surgeon General of the United States, Dr. William Stewart, would declare that it was time to close the book on infectious diseases. Cited in Laurie Garrett, *The Coming Plague. Newly Emerging Diseases in a World Out of Balance* (New York: Penguin, 1994), p. 33.

40. Mahomedali Currim Chagla, "Address to the Evening Assembly," in *Dartmouth Convocation on Great Issues of Conscience in Modern Medicine* (September 8–10, 1960), p. 20.

41. *Dartmouth Convocation on Great Issues,* pp. 8, 9.

42. *Dartmouth Convocation on Great Issues,* p. 24, 37.

43. Ciba Foundation was established by an endowment from the Swiss chemical company CIBA (now CIBA-GEIGY) in 1949 to foster international cooperation among scientists. The Foundation, which had sponsored 72 conferences on highly technological topics across all the biomedical sciences, considered "Man and His Future" "unusual" and "extraordinary." G. E. W. Wolstenholme (ed.), *Man and His Future* (Boston: Little, Brown, and Co., 1963).

44. Sir Julian S. Huxley, "The future of man-evolutionary aspects," in Wolstenholme, *Man and His Future*, pp. 20–22. Huxley acknowledges his debt to the Jesuit anthropologist and theologian, Pierre Teilhard de Chardin, whose similar views about evolution to the "noösphere" were then fashionable. See de Chardin's *The Phenomenon of Man* (New York: Harper and Row, 1959).

45. Albert Szent-Györgi, "The promise of medical science," in Wolstenholme, *Man and His Future*, p. 195.

46. Albert Szent-Györgi in Wolstenholme, *Man and His Future*, p. 201.

47. J. B. S. Haldane, "Biological possibilities for the human species in the next ten thousand years," in Wolstenholme, *Man and His Future*, p. 354.

48. Francis Crick, "Discussion: Ethical considerations," in Wolstenholme, *Man and His Future*, p. 380.

49. Peter Medawar, "Discussion: Ethical considerations," *Man and His Future*, p. 382.

50. James M. Gustafson, "Christian humanism and the human mind," in John D. Roslansky (ed.), *The Human Mind. A Discussion at the Nobel Conference* (Amsterdam: North Holland Publishing, 1967), p. 108.

51. Daniel H. Labby (ed.), *Life or Death: Ethics and Options* (Seattle: University of Washington Press, 1968), pp. vii, xix, 96.

52. Abraham Kaplan, "Social ethics and the sanctity of life: a summary," in Labby, *Life or Death*, p. 153.

53. Abraham Kaplan, "Social ethics," in Labby, *Life or Death*, p. 164. The theme of autonomy also surfaced at the first conference sponsored by a major medical organization, the American College of Physicians. Dr. J. Russell Elkington was intensely interested in ethics and organized "A Colloquium on Ethical Dilemmas from Medical Advances" at the annual meeting of the College in San Francisco, April 12, 1967, at which Lederberg, Medawar, Dubos, McDermott, Starzl, and Leake lectured on experimentation, contraception, abortion, artificial prolongation of life by resuscitation, dialysis and transplantation, and genetics and overpopulation. In conclusion, Dr. Elkington said that despite different opinions on all these matters, "throughout the discussion there appeared the common agreement on the importance of the dignity and quality of human life and of the basic principle that human beings should be treated as ends and not just as means to an end." J. Russell Elkington, "Preface," "The changing mores of biomedical research," *Annals of Internal Medicine* 67, suppl. 7 (1967), p. 4.

54. Michael E. DeBakey, "Forword," in Kenneth Vaux (ed.), *Who Shall Live? Medicine, Technology, and Ethics* (Philadelphia: Fortress Press, 1970), p. vii.

55. Helmut Thielicke, "Ethics in modern medicine," in Vaux, *Who Shall Live?*, p. 155.

56. Dr. J. Russell Elkington prepared three articles entitled "The literature of ethical problems in medicine" which appeared in the *Annals of Internal Medicine* 73 (1970): 495–497; 662–666; 863–869. The literature review covered population, contraception, abortion, eugenics, genetic counseling, genetic engineering, experimentation, use of artificial and transplanted organs, care and prolongation of life in the dying, definition of death, and euthanasia. In 1970 another extensive bibliography was compiled by James Carmody: *Ethical Issues in Health Services: A Report*

and Annotated Bibliography (Washington, D.C.: Department of Health, Education, and Welfare [DHEW], 1970). The articles cited in both bibliographies were largely lectures and reports from the conferences of the decade. Ten years later, Christine Cassel, Bernard Lo, and Henry Perkins, physicians studying ethics under my tutelage, prepared "The ethics of medicine: An annotated bibliography," *Annals of Internal Medicine* 92 (1980): 136–141. This later bibliography shows many more independently written, analytic articles.

57. James M. Gustafson, "Review of *Life or Death: Ethics and Options*," *Commonweal* 89 (Oct 4, 1968): 27–30, quote on p. 27.

58. Daniel Callahan, "The Hastings Center. Origin and History," unpublished manuscript, 1981.

59. A series of Associates followed these first Associates: scholars such as Ruth Macklin (philosophy of science), Thomas Murray (social psychology), Jon Moreno (philosophy of social science), and Peter William (philosophy of law) would become important contributors to bioethics.

60. "How the Report Made a Difference," special supplement, *Hastings Center Report* 16, no. 5 (1986).

61. Daniel Callahan, personal communication, December 11, 1996.

62. Robert Veatch, Willard Gaylin, Councilman Morgan (eds.), *The Teaching of Medical Ethics* (Hastings-on-Hudson: The Hastings Center, 1973).

63. Interview with Warren Reich, October 2, 1992. Warren T. Reich, "Revisiting the launching of the Kennedy Institute: re-visioning the origins of bioethics," *Kennedy Institute of Ethics Journal* 6 (1996): 323–328.

64. Charles E. Curran, *Politics, Medicine and Christian Ethics: A Dialogue with Paul Ramsey* (Philadelphia: Fortress Press, 1973); Richard McCormick, "Notes on moral theology: the abortion dossier," *Theological Studies* 35, no. 2 (1974): 312–359; McCormick, "To save or let die: the dilemma of modern medicine," *Journal of the American Medical Association* 228 (1974): 172–176; Gene A. Outka, "Social justice and equal access to health care," *Journal of Religious Ethics* 2 (1974): 11–32; John Connery, *Abortion: The Development of the Roman Catholic Perspective* (Chicago: Loyola University Press, 1977).

65. Information on the origins of the National Reference Center was supplied by its librarian, Doris Goldstein, in an interview on May 13, 1996.

66. Warren T. Reich (ed.), *The Encyclopedia of Bioethics*, 4 vols. (New York: The Free Press, 1978).

67. Tom L. Beauchamp and James F. Childress, *Principles of Biomedical Ethics* (New York: Oxford University Press, 1979), p. xi.

68. Daniel M. Fox, "Who are we: the political origins of the medical humanities," *Theoretical Medicine* 6 (1985): 327–341, quote from p. 334.

69. Fox, "Who are we," p. 338.

70. Callahan, "The Hastings Center."

71. William Shakespeare, *A Midsummer Night's Dream*, V, i, 15–17.

72. Warren T. Reich, "The word 'bioethics': its birth and the legacies of those who shaped its meaning," *Kennedy Institute of Ethics Journal* 4 (1994): 319–336, quote from p. 325; Reich, "The word 'bioethics': the struggle over its earliest meanings," *Kennedy Institute of Ethics Journal* 5 (1995): 19–34.

73. Van Rensselaer Potter, "Bioethics, the science of survival," *Perspectives in Biology and Medicine* 14 (1970): 127–153; Potter, "Bioethics," *Bioscience* 21 (1971): 1088.

74. Van Rensselaer Potter, *Bioethics: Bridge to the Future* (Englewood Cliffs, N.J.: Prentice-Hall, 1971).

75. Potter, *Bioethics: Bridge to the Future*, p. 2. Biophysicist Leroy Augenstein of Michigan State University published *Come, Let Us Play God* (New York: Harper and Row, 1969), in which

he described in more popular fashion, the ethical issues posed by the new genetics, population control, behavior manipulation, and organ transplants; he called for society to decide who should make decisions about these issues. Ironically, Augenstein was in Seattle as Science Coordinator for the 1961 World's Fair at the time the Seattle renal dialysis program was initiated.

76. Potter, *Bioethics*, p. 4; Warren Reich, "How bioethics got its name" (paper presented at the Birth of Bioethics Conference, Seattle, Wa., September 23–24, 1992), transcript p. 157. For a revised version of Reich's talk, see the *Hastings Center Report* 23, no. 6 (1993): 56–57.

77. News from Georgetown University, press release, October 1, 1971, cited in Reich, "The word 'bioethics'" 1994, p. 325; "Institute for bioethics established at Georgetown University," *BioScience* 21 (1971): 1090.

78. Warren T. Reich, "Introduction," in *The Encyclopedia of Bioethics*, vol. 1, pp. xix–xx.

79. Daniel Callahan, "Bioethics as a discipline," *Hastings Center Studies* 1, no. 1 (1973): 66–73. Despite being one of its progenitors, Callahan has always professed to dislike the word "bioethics" and seldom uses it in his writings.

2

The Theologians: Rediscovering the Tradition

The scientists who gathered at the conferences of the early 1960s confessed their concerns about the problems raised by the new medicine and biology, and they often called those problems "ethical." Like their fellow scientist Van Renssellaer Potter, they probably understood that word in its broadest sense, describing the values that should frame human life. When scholars from the classical disciplines of theology and philosophy joined those early conversations, they brought a sharper concept of ethics, one more like that of André Hellegers: the critical, analytic study of the norms for human behavior. These professional students of ethics molded these conversations into a shape designed by their disciplines, their traditions, and their personalities. The bioethics that began to appear during the 1970s, while generated by the new medicine and science encountering human values and customs, was their creation. Theologians were the first to appear on the scene. This chapter will provide a brief summary of theological ethics and will identify the theological pioneers.[1]

To theologically astute observers, it was obvious that behind the questions raised by the new biology there loomed even larger questions of the sort that have always preoccupied theologians. In a 1965 lecture, leading Catholic theologian Karl Rahner noted that we live in a scientific age in which the "experiment was man himself." Humans are consciously, deliberately changing themselves, discovering that the human itself is "operable, open to self-manipulation in every dimension of physical, psychological and social life. Man is question for all disciplines, even for theology, because it cannot be assumed that man's salvation is independent of this self-manipulation . . . and thus he can never say in advance what concrete possibilities man himself, in the course of his history, will include in his formal theological outline of himself." Father Rahner advised "Christian coolheadedness in the face of man's future, as individuals and society controls and manipulates itself to a degree that was previously undreamed of. . . . he can do no other if he wishes to exist. . . . he must wish to be 'manipulable' . . . for, whatever the form of this world, it will still be the world of creation, sin, promise, judgment and blessing. . . . there is nothing possible for man that he ought not to do."[2] An eminent Protestant theologian, Helmut Thielicke, gave what might be deemed the theological inaugural address for bioethics. In his lecture to the 1968 Houston conference "Who Shall Live," he said, "We run into the question as to the nature and destiny of man in connection with almost all the problems we confront in the field of medicine, particularly as regards the direction of medical and biological progress."[3] Yale theologian James Gustafson also noted the interest in the new medicine: "Precise specification of the meaning of the human cannot be avoided when we confront issues such as abortion, genetic manipulation and behavior control."[4]

These theologians speak of "the nature and destiny of man." Theology is literally the study of God, but within the Western religious traditions, theologians study God by pondering the history of God's dealings with humans and seeking "precise specification of the meaning of the human" in light of that history. Thus, theologians saw the new biology and the new medicine as appropriate subject matter for their thinking about God. The fit between theology and the questions raised by the new biology depended on the form of theology being used. Although Christian theology has a long and complex history, some common strands are visible.[5] The study of theology falls into two general categories. One category, designated by such terms as doctrinal, dogmatic, systematic, or speculative theology, seeks to understand the fundamental notions that define the relation between God and humans: creation, redemption, grace, justification, divine providence, and human freedom. The second kind of theology, called practical, pastoral, or moral theology, studies the manner of life and behavior expected of believers. A few doctrinal theologians (Catholic Karl Rahner and Protestant Karl Barth were among them[6]) were moved to comment on the broad theological implications of the new medicine. For the most part, however, theologians who focused on practical theology—often called Christian ethics in Protestant circles and moral theology among Roman and Anglo-Catholics—became the theological voices in the emerging field of bioethics, speaking with the accents of different traditions within Christianity (the Judaic tradition, as we shall see, was less frequently heard in the early days). These theologians delved into their religious traditions, rediscovering within them directions for bioethics.[7]

Roman Catholic Moral Theology

Roman Catholic theologians were well prepared for venturing into the emerging bioethics. Although medicine had attracted the church's attention since earliest Christian times, moral theology, which appeared as a distinct discipline in the fifteenth century, treated medical matters quite explicitly. Intended as guidance for priests hearing confession and for the faithful in fulfilling the duties of their station in life, its volumes were divided into chapters on each of the Ten Commandments and under the Fifth Commandment, "Thou shalt not kill," were listed the duties of doctors and obligations of the sick.[8] Moral problems arising in the work of healing were closely analyzed in a casuistry that examined the aim and intent of the agents, the nature of the actions, and their circumstances to render a judgment on the moral probity of a course of action.[9] For example, the distinction between "ordinary" and "extraordinary" medical interventions first appeared in the writings of sixteenth-century theologians as they analyzed the question whether a person has a moral obligation to preserve his own life?[10] A genre of moral theology, sometimes called "pastoral medicine," appeared in the nineteenth century to guide pastors as they assisted their sick parishioners and to advise doctors on the moral dimensions of their duties as they cared for the sick. In the twentieth century, as Catholic hospitals became widespread in North America, moral theologians began to devote special treatises to medical and nursing ethics.[11] The first of these, *Moral Principles and Medical Practice: The Basis of Medical Jurisprudence*, contained the lectures delivered to medical students at Creighton Medical College, Omaha, Nebraska, by Jesuit professor Charles Coppens at the end of the last century. He lectured on the duties and rights of physicians, on abortion, sexuality, eugenics, euthanasia, insanity, and hypnosis.[12]

The volumes on medical ethics authored by Catholic moral theologians during the first half of this century followed a general pattern: they gave an exposition of fundamental moral principles derived from natural law and divine revelation, followed by a casuistic analysis of specific topics, invariably including abortion, contraception, sterilization, euthanasia, and various types of surgery, such as amputation, lobotomy, and corneal transplants. A recent study of these authors has described their method as "physicalism" and "ecclesiastical positivism."[13] Physicalism refers to the interpretation of natural law doctrine in terms of the apparent physical structure and purpose of human functions. For example, the ethics of sexuality is derived from the "natural orientation" of the sexual act to effect reproduction. Ecclesiastical positivism means that moral theologians sought the final justification of all moral teaching in the *magisterium,* the teaching authority of the Church, constituted by the bishops under the supreme authority of the Pope. When the *magisterium* pronounced on an issue, such as abortion or contraception, the final word had been said and the theologians respectfully concluded their debates.

Magisterial teaching on medico-moral matters had been relatively rare until Pope Pius XII took an intense interest in such questions. Over his long reign (1939–1958), he frequently addressed medical audiences on a wide range of topics. With the advice of a German Jesuit moral theologian, Father Franz Huth, the Pope spoke learnedly on an incredible range of medical topics (the index to the 724 pages of his collected speeches to physicians and scientists begins with "abbreviation of life, abortion, antibiotics" and ends with "ultrasound, virus, willing acceptance of suffering").[14] The Holy Father did not simply air issues, he spoke with an authoritative voice about the moral rightness or wrongness of many medical innovations. The Catholic moral theologians, faced with this plethora of Papal statements, could do little more than respectfully comment. Thus, in the 1950s, the moral theology of medicine was colored by ecclesiastical positivism as well as by the more traditional physicalism. Even the best of the Catholic moralists of that era followed this pattern.[15]

Catholic moral theology considered not only the personal morality of individuals but also the social morality of institutions. The American Catholic Church was a church of immigrants; its faithful were among the exploited and despised. Their pastors became social activists on their behalf, fostering the labor movement and creating social supports, such as schools and hospitals. After Pope Leo XIII issued the Encyclical *Rerum Novarum* (1891) on the condition of the laboring class, moral theologians wrote treatises on social justice that formed the beliefs of clergy and faithful about the duties of employers and politicians and the rights of workers and citizens.[16] Medicine, too, could be placed within this social context.

As the era of bioethics opened, Catholic theologians began to reflect on the new biology and the new medicine in ways that challenged the tradition. Richard McCormick, Charles E. Curran, and Bernard Häring (a German theologian who taught frequently in the United States) criticized the physicalism of their predecessors and interpreted in a more nuanced way the pronouncements of the *magisterium*.[17] These authors were inspired to challenge the tradition not only by the novelty of the questions regarding bioethics but also by events within their church. Controversies over contraception and abortion agitated the church. The *aggiornamento* occasioned by the papacy of Pope John XXIII and by Vatican Council II (1962–1965) that he convened brought fresh ideas into moral theology, drawing it away from the physicalism of natural law toward a more biblical and pastoral perspective on moral life. According to Father McCormick, this led to "a new willingness to reexamine some traditional formulations that were authoritatively proposed to the Catholic community."[18]

Several issues troubled Catholic theologians. The question of abortion needed to be reexamined—not in itself, for Catholic theologians almost unanimously agreed that it was intrinsically wrong—but in relation to civil law. Contraception was even more problematic, for Catholic theologians were not unanimous on its moral status. After the invention of hormonal contraception in the late 1950s, debate over the prohibition of "artificial" birth control stirred the church. In 1968, Pope Paul VI attempted to close that debate by issuing an encyclical prohibiting artificial birth control but this only instigated a worldwide theological and pastoral crisis.[19]

As bioethics was coming into being, Roman Catholic moral theology was in turmoil. It was undergoing an inner debate about its methods and suffering from dissension about some of its central doctrines. The debate about method was not only over the general redirection of moral theology away from physicalism and ecclesiastical positivism toward ethics based more on biblical, historical, and personalistic tenets but also over certain methods and concepts that had long served the moralists well. Among these concepts was the venerable doctrine of "double effect." As we shall see later in this chapter, the debate over the meaning and application of that doctrine forced moral theologians to think deeply about the justification of ethical claims made in situations of moral perplexity. The turmoil within the tradition may have stimulated its contribution to the emerging bioethics. Theologians were now rethinking familiar moral questions that were under pressure from the advances in medicine and science, and they were compelled by the renewal of their doctrinal tradition and by the questions of a perplexed and informed laity to address such questions.

Protestant Theological Ethics

Protestant theological ethics is more difficult to characterize than that of the Roman Catholic tradition. Although both flow from a common scriptural source and from fifteen centuries of common theological reflection and ecclesiastical life, they diverged five centuries ago. Since then, the Catholic tradition has run largely within the same banks, while Protestant thought has branched off into many channels, carved by the distinct thought of the Reformers, Luther, Calvin, and Zwingli, and then furrowed again by many communities of the faithful. Each community held rather different views of the nature of the Christian church, of the central doctrines of sin, redemption, and justification, and of the form and goal of the moral life. All Protestants, however, repudiated the Catholic doctrine of a *magisterium* charged with teaching and preserving faith and morals; most Protestant theologians either repudiated or greatly diminished the role of natural law in moral analysis. Thus, neither the ecclesiastical positivism nor the physicalism that marked Catholic thought are found in Protestant thought. Furthermore, Protestant churches, with the exception of Anglicanism, abandoned the practice of sacramental confession, which had pushed Catholic moral theology toward its practical, casuistic form. Although Protestant authors did not neglect the religious dimensions of medicine and health (John Wesley was interested in medicine and skeptical of doctors!), their writings never attained the detailed moral analysis found in Roman Catholic moral theology.[20]

The tenor of Protestant theology, unlike Catholic moral theology, dwelt on the significance of large Biblical themes for the moral life. Justification and Covenant, Law and Grace, Providence and Freedom were notions with scriptural roots that inspired reflection on the attitudes and actions appropriate to Christians. Protestant theologians, however, hardly ignored the practical aspects of life; indeed, they wrote detailed prescriptions of how Christians should behave. In America, the initial prominence of the Calvinist tradition assured a careful attention—in theological literature, preaching, and community life—to behavior that often influenced civic and legal arrangements. Other evangelical traditions inspired attempts to found perfect Christian communities in which the entire life of believers was ruled by the Gospel.

The strong evangelical strain in American Protestantism, which had its sources in the revivals of the eighteenth and nineteenth centuries and in the missionary preaching of itinerant ministers, stressed conversion of heart, an acceptance of Jesus as personal savior, and a strict observance of a simple morality based on the Ten Commandments and on Jesus' teaching, which often extended to abstinence from frivolous entertainment, particularly dancing and gaming, and sometimes from alcohol. Toward the end of the nineteenth century, Protestant moral teaching and preaching dwelt on personal morality, and obedience to God's law as announced in the Bible and as demonstrated in the exemplary lives of white, middle-class Americans. Church historian Martin E. Marty writes that popular preachers "tried to please everybody, in their accent on minor vices, even as they christened the business world as it was and pronounced benedictions on the doings of the great industrialists."[21] John D. Rockefeller, who had amassed millions from the most rapacious exploitation, was a devout Presbyterian whose conscience was apparently never assailed by a preacher's accusations. *The Protestant Ethic and the Spirit of Capitalism*, the title of German sociologist Max Weber's famous treatise, described a relationship that seemed compatible and mutually reinforcing.[22]

Although some social work was fostered, such as the establishment of Settlement Houses in the teeming immigrant sectors of the cities, evangelical Protestantism was not oriented toward social reform. Inner belief and conviction, it was affirmed, would create an improved society. As the social injustices of industrial America became more manifest, figures within the major denominations, which had been too allied with the commercial classes to harbor much zeal for reform, began to urge their churches and congregations toward more direct social concern. Dismayed by the conventionality of Christian churches and shocked by prevailing social and economic injustices, a few theologians searched the Bible for guidance. Rather than seeing an easy conformity between faith and the social world, they discovered in the Scriptures an internal conflict between institutional structures and ethical imperatives. In the early decades of the 1900s, a "Social Gospel," articulated by Walter Rauschenbusch, laid out a peaceful rather than revolutionary plan for ". . . bringing into harmony [the social order] with the ethical convictions which we identify with Christ."[23] The family, the church, the economy, and the state must be reformed to reflect in their very structures the laws of love, liberty, and service. The Social Gospel, contemporary with the Progressive movement in politics, drew the attention of Protestant theologians to social ethics but was often criticized for its naive optimism.

One critic came from within its own ranks: Reinhold Niebuhr, who labored as a pastor in industrial Detroit before turning to academic theology, deepened and strengthened the theological basis of the Social Gospel, while instilling a trenchant realism about political and economic power. He criticized the pacifism that frequently was associated with Christian social thinking and insisted that, in all human relations, justice with its coercion must accompany love in its conciliatory role. Reinhold Niebuhr convinced many clergy and congregations that Christian belief had social and political implications; he convinced even great statesmen that theology was strong enough to criticize policy.[24]

Reinhold Niebuhr was a powerful public theologian. His brother, H. Richard, was a quieter theologian and appeared much less frequently in the pulpit or in public and political places. Spending most of his career as Professor of Christian Ethics at Yale Divinity School, his profundity and originality as a theologian of ethics touched many students and many readers of his extensive writings. H. Richard's final statement of his theological ethics appeared in a posthumously published book, *The Responsible Self*, which is based on lectures given at the University of Glasgow in 1960. This short book proposes a basic thesis about the ethical life: the ethical life is the responsible life and "the idea . . . of responsibility may summarily and abstractly be defined as the idea of an agent's action as response to an action upon him in accordance with his interpretation of the latter action and with his expectation of response to his response; and all of this is in a continuing community of agents."[25] The Christian "interpretation of the latter action" should reflect fundamental Christian beliefs about God as Creator, Governor, and Redeemer, and responses should be crafted that are creative, ordering, and redemptive. In this view, the moral life is not a static one of obedience to principle but a continuing dialogue within a community. Responses that curtail or stifle response are irresponsible; responses that open the opportunity to respond are responsible and ethical. The simplicity and fluidity of the concept of responsibility as the center of the moral life provides an approach to an ethics that both liberates the ethicist from rigid patterns of principled analysis and bestows a sense of direction and order. Although I came to Yale in the year following Niebuhr's death, Professor Niebuhr's influence was still palpable. James Gustafson, his successor in the Chair of Christian Ethics, conveyed Niebuhr's spirit and method to his students, who acknowledge the Niebuhrian influence on their work in bioethics.[26]

Just as Catholic moral theologians re-examined a central doctrine, "the double effect," Protestants debated the application of general moral rules to particular situations, under the rubric "norm vs. context." Some Protestant theologians, dismayed by the ease with which Christians could claim fidelity to generalities, demanded much deeper engagement in the "context" of real life: rules were not enough; love must engage in acts.[27] Joseph Fletcher's situationism, discussed later in this chapter, was built on the preeminence of the situation and of the loving act over rules and principles. Paul Ramsey issued a strong rebuttal to situationism in a series of essays entitled *Deeds and Rules in Christian Ethics*.[28] A debate followed, in which Protestant theologians were drawn more fully into philosophical analysis than ever before (just as their Catholic brethren had been drawn into Biblical moral teachings by the new theology of Vatican II).[29] The Catholic debate about double effect and the Protestant debate about situationism prepared both groups to enter the array of practical questions that the new bioethics would raise.

The Catholic and the Protestant traditions, divergent for so long, began to meet in tentative fashion during the 1960s. The ecumenical movement that for several decades had cautiously beckoned theologians from both sides to talk with each other became bold under the genial inspiration of Pope John XXIII, who invited all faiths to share their common riches, while preserving their unique traditions. The password for those who would cross the historic divide was "dialogue." This word designated not merely the willingness to converse but a conviction that truth could be uncovered by that conversation. The era of dialogue between Catholic and Protestant ethicists prepared the way for dialogue during the era of bioethics: scholars and professionals who had rarely talked to each other began to converse. Even more, it fostered the belief that common moral ground could be discovered beneath the moral pluralism of modern America.

The Catholic and the Protestant traditions entered the era of bioethics with a rich heritage of theoretical reflection and practical admonition about the moral life. Both traditions brought an indelible conviction that all humans are uniquely valued by their Creator and Redeemer, that each person is responsible for his or her life and choices, and that human choices can be designated as right and wrong, according to certain norms. Both traditions called for serious engagement in political, social, and economic life, bringing Christian inspiration into daily life. Theologians, in contrast to philosophers, speak about morality not in the abstract, but within particular communities seeking the right way to live. The traditions differed in their view of the authority of the church over individuals, in the detail with which moral problems were analyzed, and in their resolution of many moral issues. Yet both traditions brought to bioethics a wisdom about the moral life and a dexterity in discourse about moral behavior.

The theologians mentioned in this chapter come from Christian denominations. Judaism also has a rich tradition of teaching about medical morality. Because the tradition was written in Hebrew, little of it was known to scholars of other faiths until Rabbi Immanuel Jakobovits published *Jewish Medical Ethics. A Comparative and Historical Study of the Jewish Religious Attitude to Medicine and Its Practice*.[30] As bioethics began to evolve, Jewish scholars and physicians brought the riches of their tradition to the discussion.[31] Rooted in scriptural texts and rabbinic commentary, this tradition is profound but complex and difficult to penetrate in language and style of argument. Through the complexity, however, shines an almost unconditional devotion to the sanctity of human life. Although Jewish scholars have actively participated in bioethical debates, Jewish bioethics remains largely within the Jewish community as expressions of obligation on the observant. Nevertheless, as philosopher Baruch Brody has said, those teachings can be "a source for ideas about medical ethics which can be defined independently of their origins."[32]

A Trinity of Theologians

Three theologians presided over the creation of bioethics: Joseph Fletcher, an Episcopal minister; Paul Ramsey, a Methodist professor; and Richard McCormick, a Jesuit moral theologian. This trinity, unlike the divine Trinity of Christian theology, was not "one and undivided," but rather, formed a spectrum of opinion that ranged from the liberal Fletcher to the conservative Ramsey, with McCormick standing in the moderate middle. Each man represented his theological tradition in a unique way; each made major intellectual contributions to the formulation of bioethical questions, sometimes in shaping substantive positions that have endured, often by setting contrasting perspectives within which subsequent debate has continued.

Joseph Fletcher [1905–1991]

Joseph Fletcher, Professor of Pastoral Theology and Christian Ethics at Episcopal Theological School in Cambridge, Massachusetts, was invited to present the 1949 Lowell Lectures at Harvard University and subsequently published his lectures as a book, *Morals and Medicine*. He chose as topic for those lectures "certain problems of conscience, certain ethical issues, which arise in the course of medical care." He hoped to "show a way to a field of ethical inquiry clamoring for attention, although too long neglected" (except, as Fletcher acknowledges, by Roman Catholic moralists).[33] Fletcher shed little light on why he chose medical ethics as the topic of the Lowell Lectures.[34] Medical ethics was not a burning issue: no dramatic incidents had drawn public attention, no scandals had tainted medicine's good reputation. Fletcher himself had not previously shown any interest in the field; he had dedicated his energy and ethical reflection to social problems such as economic equity, and he had engaged, somewhat to the embarrassment of his ecclesiastical superiors, in vigorous labor activism and peace advocacy. Yet, "it is high time," Fletcher thought, "that we brought our ethical and spiritual experience, and its new dimensions of understanding, to bear upon the care of the sick."[35]

Joseph Fletcher was an unusual moral theologian. His autobiography reveals a young man from the mining country of West Virginia, deeply concerned about social and economic inequities. Raised with no formal religion, he joined the Episcopal Church because he saw the church as a launching ground for social reform. Although ordained with the purpose of serving the working classes, which he did for several years, Fletcher turned to scholarship with the hope of informing the church, in a theologically compelling way, of its social responsibilities. His mature writings, however, are somewhat slim on theology. His occasional references to scriptural texts are used more as illustration than as justification of his arguments. He makes little use of the classical themes of sin and salvation; indeed, even in his more explicit theological moods, he refers to these doctrines as "Christian mythology." He does invoke a doctrine central to Christian ethics, the Scriptural concept of *agape*, or God's loving concern for humankind which implies that humans must have loving concern one for another. However, Fletcher believed that this Biblical doctrine can and should be translated into its secular counterpart, utilitarian beneficence.[36] Fletcher's theological scholarship rode lightly on his deeper moral commitments: from the quiet ambiance of the seminary he sallied out, often among the first, to stand in picket lines, march in protests, and put himself in jeopardy in civil rights confrontations, where he was more than once the victim of brutal beatings. He sometimes said that he turned to "the comfort of bioethics because everything else was so vicious."[37]

Morals and Medicine has a peculiar look to the present-day reader who opens a book on medical ethics expecting to find an ethical dissection of some extraordinary medical or scientific advance. A decade after the Lowell Lectures were given, Fletcher stated in his preface to the paperback edition of *Morals and Medicine*, "medicine is making tremendous and exciting advances; and these advances constantly provide new depth and new circumstances for the moral discussion."[38] But when the Lowell Lectures were given, those advances were not yet on the scene. Although Fletcher listed among the reasons for problems of conscience in medicine "changes in technology and scientific advances," his only examples of these advances were the rather primitive technology of artificial insemination and the "conflicts of value and sentiment such as those between the personal ministrations of the general practitioner and the efficient but relatively impersonal specialization of practice." He illustrated "advances in science" by "doubts as to whether medical researchers who are also physicians, under the Hippocratic Oath to fight illness and pain, should turn over their knowledge of botulisms to militarists for bacteriological warfare." He also mentioned the problem of compromised loyalty arising in group practice.[39] The topics Fletcher treated differ little from those treated by Father Coppens in his pioneer medical ethics of fifty years before. The medicine of 1949, with a few notable exceptions, such as use of insulin and penicillin, and refinements of technique, was not notably different from the medicine of 1900.

Fletcher's challenges were launched against received ethical doctrines within the medical profession, such as the old belief that physicians should withhold unpleasant truths from their patients or, more often, against the received doctrines of the Roman Catholic moralists. Despite his admiration for the Catholics' "painstaking analyses," he consistently refuted their arguments against sterilization, contraception, artificial insemination, and euthanasia. Their teachings constrained the human freedom and responsibility that Fletcher set at the heart of ethics. The rights that Fletcher claimed for patients are less against their doctors than against the "otiose dogmas of religious moralists."[40]

Physicians were rarely the target of his critique. Apart from his criticism of the practice of withholding diagnostic truth from patients, Fletcher had little to say about what later was characterized as "medical paternalism." He had almost unstinting praise for modern medicine: "medical science, we can be certain, has as its motive only the protection and fulfillment of human values. It gives us more control over health and life and death, and therefore raises man to a loftier moral level."[41] Thus *Morals and Medicine* does not show signs of the two principal contentions of later bioethics, namely, physician paternalism as an offense to patient autonomy and the imperialism of medical technology. Although *Morals and Medicine*, as Fletcher himself remarks, "is generally said nowadays to be the pioneering work of a new discipline, biomedical ethics,"[42] it is, curiously, more a book that ends the past than one that opens the future.

In one crucial respect, however, *Morals and Medicine* was the harbinger of the future bioethics because of its central theme: "the demands the patient has a right and duty to make upon his physicians. It is from this . . . perspective, from the patient's point of view, that we shall try in this book to examine the morals, principles and values at stake in medical care." Fletcher believed that the moral rights and interests of patients should weigh as heavily in the medical scales as do physical needs and conditions:

> we shall attempt, as reasonably as may be, to plead the ethical case for our human rights (certain conditions being satisfied) to use contraceptives, to seek insemination anonymously from a donor, to be sterilized, and to receive a merciful death from a medically competent euthanasiast. We believe we can show, at the very least, that any absolute prohibition of these boons of medicine is morally unjustified, subversive of human dignity, and most serious of all, spiritually oppressive.[43]

Joseph Fletcher consistently based his ethical analysis on his conception of human freedom: "Choice and responsibility are the very heart of ethics and the sine qua non of a man's moral status. . . . The dimensions of our moral responsibility expand, of necessity, with the advances made in medical science and medical technology." Those advances mean "control over health, life and death" and "control is the basis of freedom and responsibility, of moral action, of truly human behavior. . . . In any discussion of morals and medicine, it becomes necessary to trace our moral freedom, our human action, in a number of decisions over life and death."[44] This strong endorsement of human rights in medical care, and the call for personal responsibility in medical and scientific choices, is the new voice in medical ethics.

It is not easy to discern any consistent ethical theory that underlies Fletcher's thesis. He does explicitly identify "the basis of my ethical standpoint, apart from its frame of reference in Christian faith . . . as personalist . . . the doctrine that personality is a unique quality in every human being, and that it is both the highest good and chief medium of our knowledge of the good."[45] Fletcher does not explain the doctrine of personalism in any detail. Although the final chapter of *Morals and Medicine* is entitled "The Ethics of Personality," it hardly illuminates the philosophical or theological background of "personalism." Rather, Fletcher affirms what the attentive reader already suspects: "Deliberately we have relied upon a cumulative support for our central thesis, choosing to bring out what it means in a clinical style by examining concrete problems rather than by presenting a contrived and systematic construction of ethical doctrine. It is better, after all, to let doctrine weave itself in and out of real life and practical questions in medical care. In the end, all ethical issues are concrete." Fletcher strongly affirms that neither nature nor custom must determine the ethical view: "Our principle of personal integrity . . . asserts that there is a place for the doctrine of human agency in the scheme of creation, which is a process as well as an event."[46]

This statement points toward Fletcher's later and very popular book, *Situation Ethics,* in which he did explicate his moral theory.[47] After that book was published in 1966, Joseph Fletcher was identified with the ethical theory called "situationism." Indeed, it almost seemed that Fletcher had invented the theory and given it its name, although Pope Pius XII had condemned the situation ethics of European existentialism in 1956.[48] In Fletcher's version of the doctrine, situationism asserts that, apart from the agent's intention, which must be directed by concerned love, only the features of an actual situation could determine the rightness or wrongness of any action. Framed against what Fletcher characterized as the *apriorism* of an ethic of absolute rules and principles, situationism placed concern for human need, as discerned in the particular situation, at the center of ethics. Again and again in his writing one finds expressions such as, "Whether and when genetic control could be right would depend on the situation. Let's look at a few cases. . . ."[49] Considerable controversy attended the publication of *Situation Ethics*. It was highly praised and roundly condemned. Fletcher later reflected on the controversy:

> My main principle, that concern for human beings should come before moral rules, and that particular cases and situations are more determinant of what we ought to do than "universal" norms are, was applauded in the helping professions (medicine, social work, public administration, clinical psychology, and so on) but generally condemned by Christians, Jews, and Muslims—most of all by the orthodox ones.[50]

Fletcher's ethics is theoretically thin, working with a few key notions such as responsibility, freedom, and choice, which are not explicated in depth. If one were to seek congenial theoretical grounds for Fletcher's situationism, John Dewey's philosophy, which we will examine in the following chapter, might be a candidate. Fletcher's biographer states, "He borrows Dewey's naturalist conception of ethics, modifies his process of moral deliberation . . . and adopts his reconstructive social philosophy, which embraces the belief that the human condition can be changed, via the efficacious use of intelligence and choice and that persons have a responsibility continually to reconstruct their experiences." Yet the influence of Dewey, as well as other philosophers favored by Fletcher, such as William James and John Stuart Mill, is diffuse: Fletcher is, his biographer remarks, "a synthesizer, not a philosopher . . . he was adept at appropriating particular components of various philosophical and theological doctrines and fashioning them into a unique conception. He was a creator of positions and perspectives, not theories."[51] The popularity of *Situation Ethics* is due less to its theoretical strength than to the appeal of its message in the libertarian and anti-authoritarian era in which it appeared.

Twenty years after *Medicine and Morals*, Fletcher produced his second book on ethics in medicine, *The Ethics of Genetic Control: Ending Reproductive Roulette*.[52] In those intervening 20 years, everything, it seemed, had changed. In his foreword to the book, Joshua Lederberg remarks, "Dr. Fletcher comments how quickly things change. Indeed, this book may already be overtaken by changes in the process of science. . . ."[53] Fletcher himself had changed. He had left Episcopal Theological School to take the post of Visiting Professor of Medical Ethics in the School of Medicine, University of Virginia. He had not only left the setting of a church institution; he had intellectually and emotionally departed from church life and belief. He had "de-Christianized himself,"[54] and was now free to expound his humanistic ethic without scandalizing his believing brethren.

Immersed in a medical setting, Fletcher saw firsthand the remarkable changes in science, technology, technique, and delivery of service that had taken place since his first entry into medical ethics. He could spend his time doing what he had recommended in *Morals and Medicine*: "Moralists who spend little or no time in the terminal wards of a modern hospital cannot contribute much in the way of realistic opinion or relevance on the subject of euthanasia."[55] Fletcher was now comfortable identifying himself as an "act-utilitarian" whose sole criterion of the rightness or wrongness of an act was the informed calculation of whether the consequences of this act in this situation would improve the aggregate well-being of humankind: "What is right will be what is most humane, what is most conducive to human welfare and happiness. It is based on loving concern."[56] He agreed with philosopher William Frankena's characterization of his ethics as "modified act-agapism . . . a form of utilitarianism and consequentialist ethical decision making,"[57] and was untroubled by the criticisms launched against such a position by philosophers and theologians.

From this standpoint, it was not difficult for Dr. Fletcher to champion the moral goodness of every technological advance, finding grounds for criticism only when, in particular circumstances, the human harm that might result from them outweighed the human benefits for society as a whole. He decried the nay-saying of many ethicists as a priori commitment to unexamined rules, often supported by "theological spookery."[58] In *The Ethics of Genetic Control* and in the subsequent collection of essays entitled *Humanhood: Essays in Biomedical Ethics*,[59] he defended not only abortion, sterilization, and contraception, as he had in the past, but also genetic screening that was both voluntary and mandatory, negative and positive eugenics and euphenics, and human cloning and the creation of human-animal hybrids; and, going beyond his advocacy of euthanasia, he argued for infanticide. All of these practices, of course, were defensible only insofar as they reduced human suffering and enhanced the human good.

Dr. Fletcher hesitated to describe in any great detail the content of the "human good," as he was concerned that specificity might encourage rigid prescriptivism. He was persuaded to become more explicit by the constant criticism that his highest moral goal was too vague. His essay "Humanhood," written for a conference of The Hastings Center, became famous (or notorious). Humanhood, Fletcher proposed, consists of a profile of characteristics: minimum intelligence, self-awareness, self-control, a sense of time—of futurity and of the past, the capability to relate to others, concern for others, communication, control of existence, curiosity, changeability, balance of rationality and feeling, idiosyncrasy, and neocortical function. Excluded from the profile were several other characteristics: man is not anti-artificial, not essentially parental, not essentially sexual, not a bundle of rights, not a worshipper. This profile obviously ruled out embryos and fetuses, as well as the retarded, the moribund, and the senile, from humanhood or, as Fletcher qualified, from personal status. This profile seemed plausible to many readers, but its implications were troubling to many others.

Joseph Fletcher was criticized by many ethicists. It was impossible to dislike him personally—he was genial, gentlemanly, and witty—but the growing group of bioethicists generally repudiated his enthusiastic endorsement of almost everything they considered ambiguous and dangerous. They criticized what they considered his naive espousal of act-utilitarianism. Still, Fletcher was a figure of influence. He wrote in a swift, breezy style that laypersons could read with pleasure. His manner of argument was not the sustained, logical analysis favored by philosophers. Rather, he argued his case as an experienced homilist: stating a common sense thesis, marshaling objections to the thesis, then lancing them as fallacies or as obscurantism, asking rhetorical questions and summoning prominent witnesses from science and letters, past and present (in ten lines, for example, he calls up Aldous Huxley, C. S. Lewis, Henry David Thoreau, and George Beadle).[60] His style irritated the analytically inclined but appealed to the intelligent, interested reader.

Many physicians and scientists found his philosophy congenial. It generally endorsed both their altruism and their conviction that science was uniformly beneficial (although he did occasionally gently chide them for "their blind faith that facts will be used for good purposes, not for evil"[61]). Physicians often failed to notice how antithetical his utilitarianism was to the traditional ethic of allegiance to their patient (although he was not shy about noting the antithesis).[62] Fletcher was a welcome figure among renown leaders of science and medicine. His friend, Dr. Thomas Hunter of the University of Virginia, wrote in the introduction to *Humanhood*, "Not a scientist, he has brainstormed with many of the best of them . . . Garrett Hardin, Joshua Lederberg, Robert Sinsheimer, Bernard Davis, Robert Wagner, and many, many others."[63] Fletcher estimated that by 1980, he had spoken in 415 universities and medical schools and had been a lecturer or visiting professor in 45 schools in Europe, Asia, and Australia.[64] Hundreds of his articles appeared in the medical and ethical literature. Over some 40 years, his voice was heard in bioethics, often as an *agent provocateur* against established moralities but, perhaps most memorably, as the first vigorous advocate of human rights, the rights of the patient, in medical care. Theological ethicist Kenneth Vaux has said of Joseph Fletcher, "Throughout his career, Fletcher struggled against the absolutist inclinations of ethics, especially when these were expressed in inhumane ideologies. . . . Transcending virtue, acts of love and hope, sacrifice and faith, the incredible dignity of the human spirit, as these are manifested in our daily life . . . this has been the genius of Joe Fletcher's contribution."[65]

Paul Ramsey [1913–1988]

Paul Ramsey, Harrington Spear Paine Professor of Religion at Princeton University, was the second theologian to enter the nascent world of bioethics. A more scholarly and committed theologian than Joseph Fletcher, Ramsey brought to the questions of the new biology and medicine a powerful analytic mind and a relentless, often rough, polemic spirit. Coming from the Methodist tradition, educated at Yale under H. Richard Niebuhr, and influenced by the neo-orthodox Calvinism of Karl Barth, he maintained throughout his career that he did "not hesitate to write as a Christian ethicist . . . to invoke ultimate appeal to scripture or theology and to warrants such as righteousness, faithfulness, canons of loyalty, the awesome sanctity of a human life, humankind in the image of God, holy ground, *hesed* (steadfast covenant love), *agape* (or charity), as these standards are understood in the religions of our culture, Judaism and Christianity."[66] Although this confession of his ethical faith is certainly genuine, theological themes and warrants are not always visible in his ethical analysis. They frame, limit, and ultimately ground all his analysis, but they are rarely visible in the texts which, for the most part, vigorously wrestle with the definitions of terms, the logic of arguments, and the factual referents of moral claims. Ramsey wrestles an ethical argument to the ground (he once said "the Protestant Christian should wrestle with his Catholic brother"[67]). Although theological style occasionally dominates, the religious skeptic or the theological illiterate can usually appreciate the force of his ethical argumentation.[68]

Professor Ramsey expressed his fundamental theological ethics in *Basic Christian Ethics*,[69] in which he places the concept of "God's steadfast love" at the center of Christian ethics. That love is manifested in God's faithful covenant with humankind to which all humans must consent in obedient love toward God and in faithful neighborly love toward all fellow humans. Ramsey's starting place, then, is quite like that of Joseph Fletcher—the *agape* of God toward humankind. Indeed, *Basic Christian Ethics* has a tone not unlike Fletcher's rejection of legalism, the belief that the moral life is bound by rules. In the Augustinian spirit of "love and do whatever you will," Ramsey strongly affirms that "everything is lawful, absolutely everything is permitted which love permits . . . and absolutely everything is commanded which love commands." However, Ramsey interprets God's *agape* in a way radically distinct from Fletcher's interpretation: it does not will humankind's good, but commands humankind's obedience. Fletcher's theology leads to a utilitarian ethic; Ramsey's theology implies a deontological ethic. "Christian ethics is a deontological one," he states, "[it is] radically non-teleological."[70] This different interpretation has major implications for Ramsey's later work in bioethics: a rigorous backbone of principles upholds his every analysis of a moral problem in medicine.

His conception of those principles was sharpened by his studies of *Nine Modern Moralists*, in which he explored the thinking of figures as different from each other as Dostoevski and Jean-Paul Sartre.[71] Working through the thought of these moralists, Ramsey enriched his conception of covenant love with a notion of "inprincipled love," in which the tradition of natural law, with its claim of an innate sense of justice, becomes a framework in which the work of love can be guided. In two significant essays, "Deeds and rules in Christian ethics"[72] and "The case of the curious exception,"[73] Ramsey elaborated a defense of the central place of "almost exceptionless rules" within the ethic of *agape* that had appeared almost unfettered in his earlier *Basic Christian Ethics*. He found classical Roman Catholic moral theology a useful starting place for his analysis of practical ethics. His earliest concerns about the problem of war were il-luminated by Catholic doctrines of "just war," and particularly by the use of "the prin-ciple of double effect," In *War and the Christian Conscience,* he carefully applies this principle to the ethics of war and, in so doing, discusses its application in quite another problem, abortion.[74]

Ramsey's short exursus into the problem of abortion was expanded into a major lec-ture at the Reed College Symposium, "The Sanctity of Life." This lecture initiated a se-ries of reflections on abortion that Ramsey expanded and deepened over the rest of his career. Ramsey was also the first ethicist to enter the debate over genetic engineering. He challenged the proposals of Nobelist Hermann Muller about positive eugenics and sperm banking at the 1965 Gustavus Adolphus Nobel Conference. Several years later, Ramsey engaged in combat with another Nobel prizewinner in genetics, Joshua Leder-berg, over the issue of human cloning.[75] When human cloning again leapt into the headlines in the 1990s, the debate echoed Ramsey's thoughts of almost 30 years be-fore.[76] Until Ramsey turned his attention to the genetic debate, no theologian or philosopher had carefully examined its moral premises. After he did so, many theolo-gians began to attend to questions on genetics, realizing that these questions, as scien-tifically daunting as they were, touched the essence of the human condition. We shall revisit Ramsey's thoughts on these matters in the chapters on genetics and on repro-duction.

Ramsey moved deeply into the nascent field of bioethics as he prepared to present the 1969 Lyman Beecher lectures at Yale University. Yale professor Gustafson had noticed Ramsey's writing on medical ethics and had suggested to the Beecher Lec-ture committee that he be invited and that a university-wide symposium, including the Divinity School, the Law School, and the Medical School, be organized around his lectures. During the week of April 14–17, 1969, a distinguished group from Yale and other institutions gathered to discuss "The Patient as Person," as expounded by Paul Ramsey. Ramsey had prepared for this auspicious occasion by spending the spring se-mesters of 1968 and 1969 as the Joseph P. Kennedy Jr. Foundation Visiting Professor of Genetic Ethics at Georgetown University Medical School. This opportunity, he said, "enabled me, a Protestant Christian ethicist, to be located in the middle of a medi-cal school faculty—not on its periphery—and to begin some serious study of the moral issues in medical research and practice." In biweekly conferences, medical faculty would present topics and Ramsey "could put questions to experts in many fields of medicine, overhear discussions among them and begin to learn how teach-ers of medicine, researchers and practitioners themselves understand the moral as-pects of their practice."[77] In light of this experience, he wrote, "Medical ethics today must, indeed, be 'casuistry'; it must deal as competently and exhaustively as possible with the concrete features of actual moral decisions of life and death and medical care."[78]

By the time Ramsey delivered the Beecher Lectures, he had prepared himself thor-oughly in five "cases": research with human subjects, care of the dying, the definition of death, transplantation, and the allocation of scarce resources. For each topic, Ramsey endeavored to articulate the problems clearly and to analyze the arguments that he had encountered about how these practices should be conducted ethically. Ramsey offered his own arguments in favor of certain positions and worked them out thoroughly. The lectures were published the next year as *The Patient as Person: Explorations in Medical Ethics,* a book that deserves to be ranked as the first truly modern study of the new ethics of science and medicine.

Ramsey forthrightly states his theological premises in the preface of *Patient as Person* but then moves them into the background, where they are always influential but barely visible, as he wades into the particular problems. He justifies this move with the words, "This is a book about ethics, written by a Christian ethicist. I hold that medical ethics is consonant with the ethics of a wider human community . . . the moral requirements governing the relationship of a physician to patients and researcher to subjects are only a special case of the moral requirements between man and man." Ramsey contends that human life in general, and the medical relationship in particular, is governed by covenants of loyalty and fidelity between humans and that these covenants can be envisioned and discussed "in an actual community of moral discourse concerning the claims of persons . . . [in which] an ethicist finds he has been joined— whether in agreement or some disagreement—by men of different persuasions, often quite different ones."[79]

Under the covenant of faithful love God offers to humankind, human individuals are "a sacredness in bodily life. . . . The sanctity of human life prevents ultimate trespass upon him even for the sake of treating his bodily life, or for the sake of others who are also only a sacredness in their bodily lives."[80] Ramsey makes clear that, for him as a Christian ethicist, the good of the individual ought never be dominated by the good of society. He believes that even those who do not share his religious beliefs can appreciate this view and repudiate the relativism and utilitarianism so commonly found in modern thought. As he investigates the ethics of research, of death and dying, and of transplantation, this emphasis on individual inviolability and on faithfulness between persons is consistently heard. He intended *Patient as Person* "to explore the meaning of care, to find the actions and abstentions that come from adherence to covenant, to ask the meaning of the sanctity of life, to articulate the requirements of steadfast faithfulness in which some decision must be made about how to show respect for, protect, preserve and honor the life of fellow man." Ramsey was convinced that all this is compatible with the tradition of medical ethics, for "there is no profession that comes close to medicine in its concern to inculcate, transmit and keep in constant repair its standards governing the conduct of its members."[81] Traditionally, the ethics of medicine has been strongly deontological, for loyalty to one's patients dominates any concern for overall social benefits that might be produced by its interventions.

Research with human subjects was a burning topic during the days that Ramsey was preparing himself to be a bioethicist. Dr. Henry Beecher's exposition of the problem had been published in 1966, and several important conferences on the topic had been held. In addition, a few notorious examples of questionable research had become public. Subsequently, the National Institutes of Health published new policies to guide researchers. Ramsey was familiar with all this. He devoted the first chapter of *Patient as Person* to human research and titled it "Consent as a canon of loyalty with special reference to children in medical investigation." The chapter opens with a definitive thesis: "Medical ethics has not its sole basis in the overall benefits to be produced. It is not a consequence-ethics alone." On the contrary, "a crucial element in the answer to the question, what constitutes right action in medical practice? is the requirement of a reasonably free and adequately informed consent. In current medical ethics, this is the chief canon of loyalty (as I shall call it) between the man who is patient/subject and the man who performs medical investigations."[82]

Here, Ramsey states the theme for much of what follows not only in subsequent pages but in subsequent bioethics. Medical ethics is not, in its essence, utilitarian. Rather, it has as a "crucial element," a deontological requirement expressed as a "canon of loyalty" between physician and anyone whom they engage as patients or as experimental subjects. His brief exposition of the canon of loyalty suggests both the covenant theology that long reigned in American Protestantism and the democratic ethos of American political life; Reinhold Niebuhr and Abraham Lincoln are both cited in this passage. Consent, he says, expresses "fidelity between man and man in these procedures. . . . fidelity is the bond between consenting man and consenting man. . . . In this requirement, faithfulness among men—the faithfulness that is normative for all the covenants or moral bonds of life with life—gains specification for the primary relations peculiar to medical practice."[83] Then Ramsey explores the covenant in the context of medical research, taking as his "prismatic" case what is perhaps the most difficult problem in the ethics of human research: experimentation with children. We will follow his arguments on this point in Chapter 5.

Perhaps Paul Ramsey's most influential contribution to bioethics is his thought on the care of the dying patient. He entitled the third chapter of *Patient as Person* "On (Only) Caring for the Dying Patient." The opening paragraphs list a series of interventions that had become routine in the twenty years since Joseph Fletcher had discussed the dying patient: extensive use of the respirator, heart-lung circulatory bypass and cardiac surgery, organ transplantation, and renal dialysis (he might have added cancer chemotherapy). Ramsey asks rhetorically, "Is there no end to the doctor's vocation to maintain life until the matter is taken out of his hands? Alternatively expressed, ought there to be any relief for the dying from a physician's search for exquisite triumphs over death in a sort of salvation by works?"[84] His answer to the latter question was yes and his effort was to state precisely the point at which the doctor's vocation to cure ends, without relaxing in any way the doctor's (and our) duty to care for the dying patient in our ultimate fidelity. We shall follow his arguments on these points in Chapter 8.

Richard A. McCormick, S.J.

Father Richard A. McCormick, a Roman Catholic theologian and member of the Society of Jesus (Jesuits), was teaching moral theology at the Jesuit seminary in West Baden, Indiana, when he was invited to be a discussant of Paul Ramsey's Beecher lectures at Yale in 1969. Father McCormick was well known in the world of Catholic theology as the editor of "Notes on Moral Theology," a regular review of current literature that appeared in the leading American Catholic theological journal, *Theological Studies*. He had shown himself to be both a faithful expositor of the Catholic tradition and a respectful but convincing reformer of that tradition. He said of himself, "I was trained in and for some years taught a moral theology with deep roots in what is now called a 'classicist mentality' . . . [but I am] conscious of both its strengths and weaknesses—and the need to correct or modify the latter."[85]

As we have noted, the Catholic tradition maintained both a strong theoretical basis for moral judgment and an interest in medico-moral questions. Because of his fidelity to that tradition and his openness to revision where he deemed necessary, Father McCormick became an articulate spokesman of his tradition as it approached bioethics. Since that tradition had always endorsed the natural law thesis that moral judgments based on reason were comprehensible to all reasonable persons, regardless of their religious faith, McCormick could enter the bioethical dialogue with ease. In terms of his stance within his own church, McCormick has been described as "'moderately progressive'—loyal to Catholic tradition's essential values, but slightly left of center in relation to current official teaching. . . . He maintains that religious premises need not be brought explicitly into the discussion if this would hinder public discourse. Reason can be used to discover and debate the moral aspects of the human reality that the Christian story more fully discloses."[86]

As a student of moral theology in the early 1960s, I had become familiar with McCormick's moderate reforming stance, which appealed to many of us who appreciated the fresh air that Pope John XXIII had allowed to blow through the ancient corridors of Catholic theology. I first met him at an extraordinary meeting of Catholic theologians summoned by the Kennedy family to Hyannisport to discuss how a Catholic candidate for political office should confront the issue of abortion policy. No more difficult issue can be posed to a Catholic theologian, given the Church's resolute opposition to abortion. As we shall see in Chapter 9, McCormick's moderate and mediating instincts prompted him to frame this adamant doctrine, to which he personally adhered, within the context of moral pluralism consistent with a democratic society.[87]

McCormick took a similar mediating position in another bioethical controversy that raged within the Catholic church, namely, contraception. Although American society in general had come to accept contraception and American law restricting access to contraception had been struck down by the Supreme Court's 1964 Griswold decision, Catholics remained deeply divided. Many Catholic laity considered the Church's condemnation of all reproductive planning, except total or periodic sexual abstinence, irrelevant to their lives. Many Catholic theologians had anticipated some relaxation of the strict doctrine. When Pope Paul VI reaffirmed traditional teaching in the encyclical *Humanae Vitae*, many Catholics suffered a *crise de conscience* and moral theologians aligned themselves as orthodox conservatives or liberal "heretics." McCormick typically moved to neither side: he attempted to formulate an orthodox position that was liberal.[88]

Father McCormick moved away from the intraecclesial discussion of abortion and contraception and into the larger realm of bioethics by engaging two principal issues of that emerging field: human experimentation and care of the dying patient. He did so not by composing essays in quiet reflection but by entering the clash of debate with the most polemical of ethicists, Paul Ramsey. Ramsey and McCormick had become close friends; each respected the other's integrity and scholarship. Thus, they made excellent debaters. Two controversial questions, the use of children in research and the legitimacy of quality-of-life judgments in allowing a patient to die, provided topics for debate. At the heart of both questions lay moral principles of foundational importance to bioethics. Their debate over pediatric research appears in Chapter 5.

The two theologians challenged each other over the ethical legitimacy of quality-of-life judgments. Ramsey, having borrowed the Roman Catholic doctrine of ordinary/extraordinary means as the basis for his own analysis of the ethics of allowing a patient to die, later retracted one feature of that doctrine, namely, the use of quality-of-life measures to assess medical means as extraordinary. Father McCormick, who interpreted the traditional Catholic doctrine as allowing such considerations, entered the lists with his friend. McCormick's stated his view in a 1974 essay, "To save or let die: the dilemma of modern medicine," which appeared in the *Journal of the American Medical Association* and in the Catholic journal of opinion, *America*. In McCormick's usual style, that essay steered "a middle course between sheer concretism and dogmatism"—that is, between the claim that the terrible decisions that allow a patient to die could be made only in the specific circumstances of each unique case and the insistence that such decisions confirm to certain absolute rules. The "middle course" was discovered through an exegesis of Pope Pius XII's teaching that preservation of life is not morally obligatory "if it would render the attainment of the higher, more important good too difficult." McCormick interprets "higher, more important good" as the "love of God and neighbor . . . [which is] the meaning, substance, and consummation of life from a Judeo-Christian perspective." He then suggests that when a life can be saved only under conditions that render "human relationships—which are the very possibility of growth in the love of God and neighbor . . . so threatened, strained, or submerged that they would no longer function as the heart and meaning of the individual's life, it is no longer obligatory to save that life."[89] Quality of life is defined by the capacity for living within these fundamental human relationships, and its absence can justify a decision to forego life support. This position offended the reformed Ramsey, who severely criticized McCormick in *Ethics at the Edges of Life*. McCormick's analysis, he wrote, "erodes the distinction between voluntary and involuntary euthanasia, and between letting die and actively accelerating death," and ultimately deprives living human beings of their intrinsic value.[90]

Richard McCormick also made a major contribution at the theoretical level of bioethics. In an intraecclesial debate over a revered principle of moral theology called "the principle of double effect or indirect voluntary," he refined and expanded the principle as a general method of analyzing moral dilemmas. This doctrine, first formulated in Thomas Aquinas' analysis of justifiable homicide, proposes that any action that necessarily causes two inextricably linked effects, one good and the other evil, is morally justifiable only if (among several other conditions) the good effected is intended, while the evil effect is permitted or tolerated.[91] Moral theologians had applied the doctrine to many problems, most notably to warfare and to certain medical questions, such as sterilization. In the 1960s, several Catholic theologians questioned what they believed to be an excessively physicalist interpretation that stressed physical causation and psychological motivation.[92] The debate that ensued helped to free Catholic moral theology from its rigid and narrow application of natural law concepts and shaped a much more subtle instrument of moral analysis.

In 1973, Father McCormick delivered a major lecture at Marquette University "Ambiguity in Moral Choice."[93] The lecture judiciously analyzed the recent Roman Catholic literature on the double effect doctrine and concluded that the revered formula came down to the ability to provide a "proportionate reason" for choosing the action with unavoidably bad effects. "Proportionate reason," said McCormick, "means three things: (*a*) a value at stake at least equal to that sacrificed; (*b*) no other way of salvaging it here and now; (*c*) its protection here and now will not undermine it in the long run."[94] Six years later, McCormick and Paul Ramsey collaborated on a study of the question. They invited the Catholic theologian who had initiated the intraecclesial discussion, German Jesuit Bruno Schüller, and two moral philosophers, Baruch Brody and William Frankena, to comment on the propositions of the original Marquette lecture. In a provocative volume, *Doing Evil to Achieve Good*, both philosophers found it difficult to avoid seeing "proportionate reason" as anything other than a reduction to utilitarian reasoning. All three theologians, including Ramsey, who was strongly committed to deontological reasoning, defended "proportionate reasons."[95] The original bioethical issues, genetic engineering and experimentation, as well as the later ones concerning prolongation of life, all involved the paradox of effecting goods inextricably bound with risks and burdens. The cogency of the double effect doctrine as an instrument of analysis of such paradoxes continues to be debated.

In 1974, Father McCormick left his position as seminary professor to accept the Rose F. Kennedy Professorship in Christian Ethics at the Kennedy Institute of Ethics, Georgetown University, a commanding position in the world of bioethics. During the twelve years that he held that position, his voice was heard in almost every bioethical debate, and it was always a voice for reason. He was appointed to the Ethics Advisory Board of the Department of Health, Education and Welfare which, during its short life

(1978–1980), produced a report on *HEW Support of Research Involving Human In Vitro Fertilization and Embryo Transfer*, a topic on which McCormick's Catholic commitments might have inhibited his contributions. On the contrary, while forced to dissent on some points, he helped to construct a reasonable public policy on that controversial issue, as we shall see in Chapter 9.

Joseph Fletcher and Paul Ramsey stood at opposite ends of a spectrum of doctrine and opinion. Both were Protestant theologians, but Fletcher was a theologian "lite" who took as Gospel little more than one theological truth, "God is love," and rushed quickly into a personalist and situationist view of ethics that was profoundly humanistic and utilitarian. Ramsey was a "heavy" theologian who plunged into scripture and doctrine for a range of truths applicable to ethics and resisted any reduction of Christian ethics to humanistic and consequentialist views (even though he admitted the compatibility of Christian and secular ethics at many points). Both theologians became thoroughly familiar with the language, practices, and theories of medicine and science. Joe Fletcher found in medicine and science almost nothing but praiseworthy contributions to human welfare. Paul Ramsey, even though he admired the humanity of physicians and scientists, worried always that "what can be done will be done," often leading to transgressions of the sanctity of the individual created and redeemed by God.[96]

Richard McCormick stood solidly between Joseph Fletcher and Paul Ramsey in the first decades of bioethics. A committed Catholic theologian, he had a talent for translating the doctrines of his faith into reasonable arguments that reasonable persons could consider and often accept. Although he was sometimes accused of being a covert utilitarian, he consistently adhered to principles that protect the values of human life, human individuality, human freedom and human sociability. Although a skillful debater, he did not become a polemicist. McCormick came from a highly articulate and often dogmatic tradition of moral theology, but he brought to bioethics proficiency in analysis of ethical problems and an ecumenical openness to the well-argued opinions of others.[97]

Other scholarly theologians made forays into the emerging field of bioethics, sometimes with a single book and sometimes with occasional essays. Many theologians participated in the increasingly frequent conferences and became familiar figures at The Hastings Center or faculty at The Kennedy Institute. Some were as conservative as Ramsey, attempting to keep the analysis of the new problems close to the themes of the revered tradition; others were as liberal as Fletcher, rejoicing in divine creativity and human freedom. All these theologians, regardless of denomination or inclination, shared an appreciation that new moral problems were, despite their novelty, embedded in moral traditions, and they shared the conviction that moral problems could be subject to careful analysis. At the deepest level, these theologians honored the Judeo-Christian belief that human individuals are endowed with an inalienable value and dignity that is manifested in their freedom and responsibility. Many of these theologian-bioethicists will appear in later pages of this story.[98]

The Education of the Ethicists

During the 1960s, religious studies had migrated out of the divinity schools dedicated to the training of ministers into graduate programs committed to the education of scholars. Harvard, Yale, Princeton, the University of Chicago, and Union Theological Seminary of New York formed fine faculties and attracted promising students who studied not only denominational doctrines but also the critical analysis and comparative history of those doctrines, as well as their relation to systematic theology, philosophical ethics, and the social sciences. The faculty of these programs began to notice the ethical questions raised by the new biology and medicine and called their students' attention to them. At Yale, James Gustafson began to contribute to the bioethical debates: from 1970 to 1975, Gustafson authored notable essays on bioethical issues.[99] Although bioethical questions were seldom the topic of courses or lectures, his students were sensitized to them. Several of his students from Yale and from the University of Chicago, to which Gustafson moved in the early 1970s, became major figures in the early bioethics. At Harvard, Professors James Luther Adams, Arthur Dyck, and Ralph Potter encouraged interest in population ethics and the moral questions of medicine, and they sent forth another cadre of bioethicists.[100]

One of bioethics' most prominent figures, Robert M. Veatch, emerged from this educational milieu. Other early bioethicists studied one of the traditional moral disciplines and then, either by intention or by accident, moved into the maelstrom of bioethical questions. Veatch trained himself as a medical ethicist. In his college years at Purdue University, he developed an interest in the relation between medicine and religion. He considered preparing himself as a medical missionary for the Methodist church but decided that he did not want to practice medicine. Instead, he chose a career in research pharmacology, matriculating at the University of California Medical School in San Francisco and winning his master of science degree in 1962. His research interest was in neuropharmacology, particularly the neurological basis for the affective and "valuing" effects of morphine. He joined the Peace Corps and spent two years teaching biology and chemistry in Nigeria.

Instead of continuing to a doctorate in science, he decided to pursue studies in ethics, selecting Harvard Divinity School as the venue most compatible with his interests. He studied with Arthur Dyck, Ralph Potter, and, while Professor James Luther Adams was on sabbatical, with visiting professor Joseph Fletcher. In 1964, he shifted to the graduate school, where he was allowed to fashion his own program toward a unique doctoral degree in medical ethics. Roderick Firth ("Ideal Observer Theory") and John Rawls (*Theory of Justice*) were his philosophical mentors; Renée Fox and Talcott Parsons guided him in medical sociology. As he studied, he was engaged in a civil rights project in a largely African-American community in Boston's South End. He found himself "transferring his interest in civil rights to patients' rights."[101]

Professor James Luther Adams had acquainted him with the history and doctrines of the Anabaptists and the Zwinglians, who constituted a "left wing" of the Reformation.

This study gave Veatch a theological framework within which he could reflect on the moral problems of civil disobedience and resistance to political authority. During his graduate studies, an ad hoc Harvard committee was fashioning the criteria for brain death. On many occasions, Veatch and Professor Potter, who was a committee member, discussed what they saw as the intrinsic problem posed to the committee: not the definition of death as such, which was a technical matter, but the values that the committee brought to that technical task. There were metaethical assumptions underlying the claims of expertise by scientists making value judgments. These reflections inspired Veatch's choice of a topic for his dissertation, "Value Freedom in Science and Technology," in which he analyzed the moral status of physicians' advice to patients about the use of contraceptives.

Professor Potter introduced Veatch to Dan Callahan, who hired him as the first employee of The Hastings Center in September 1970. He had, by good fortune, found the perfect locus for the skills certified by his idiosyncratic Ph.D. in medical ethics. At the first meeting of the Hastings Fellows in spring 1971, a decision was made to establish several "task forces" for concentrated study of particular issues. Associate for Medical Ethics Veatch was assigned supervision of the task forces (later renamed research groups) on death and dying and on behavior control. During his years at The Hastings Center, Robert Veatch made an indelible mark on bioethics. His championing of the rights of patients moved the principle of respect for autonomy to the pinnacle of bioethics' principles. In 1979, Veatch left Hastings to assume the Professorship in Medical Ethics at the Kennedy Institute and, in 1989, he became its director. Neither theologian nor philosopher, Veatch might be called the original bioethicist.

A strange thing happened to Christian ethicists on their way to bioethics. Educated in theological traditions, and sometimes ordained as clergy in their denominations, their theological and denominational identities often faded as they migrated into the bioethical world. Professor Gustafson, who mentored many of these ethicists, noted this transmutation. In a 1975 lecture, *The Contributions of Theology to Medical Ethics*, he proposed that theology and theologians had much to offer bioethics but that "for most persons involved in medical care and practice, the contributions of theology is likely to be of minimal importance, for the moral principles and values needed can be justified without reference to God, and the attitudes that religious beliefs ground can be grounded in other ways."[102]

Several years later, Gustafson co-edited, along with his former student, Stanley Hauerwas, an issue of the *Journal of Medicine and Philosophy* devoted to theology and medical ethics. They noted that while the initial literature in the field was largely written by theologically trained and religiously affiliated persons, "as medical ethics became a growth industry in the academic world, and as the traditional religious and theological bases for the work apparently lost significance, many of the theologically trained speakers and writers repressed, denied, or became indifferent to theology as a field. The historic religious communities of our culture, which are the bearers of symbols and traditions and of patterns of thought about practical moral questions, were seen even by persons who belonged to them to be divisive."[103] There were good reasons for this fall from faith. Some early bioethicists resigned their ordinations in the church. Many of them found employment at medical schools where a secular and scientific culture dominated. Most bioethicists quickly discovered that, while rumination about human nature and destiny invites the transcendent references of theology, discussion of the practical problems of bioethics, such as regulation of research or allocation of resources, can be carried out quite satisfactorily in more mundane terms. Although in recent years, some theologians have summoned theologically trained bioethicists back to their roots, they remain, in their bioethical analyses, outside the faith.[104] With few exceptions, the theologians and the philosophers, who were partners in the early medical ethics, merged into one—the bioethicist.

Notes to Chapter 2

1. Allan Verhay and Stephen E. Lammers (eds.), *Theological Voices in Medical Ethics* (Grand Rapids, Mich.: Eerdmans, 1993); Paul E. Camenisch (ed.), *Religious Methods and Resources in Bioethics* (Dordrecht: Kluwer Academic Publishers, 1994). Two special issues of *The Journal of Medicine and Philosophy* have been devoted to the relationship between theology and bioethics: vol. 4, no. 4 (December 1979) and vol. 17, no. 3 (June 1992).

2. Karl Rahner, "Experiment with man: theological observations on man's self-manipulation," in *Theological Investigations IX*, trans. Graham Harrison (New York: Herder and Herder, 1972), pp. 206, 211. Many theologians noted Rahner's lecture: James Gustafson praised it, Paul Ramsey criticized it as a "priestly blessing on everything," and Richard McCormick mediated between the two positions by noting that Rahner's effusiveness is modulated in a more sober essay on genetic manipulation, "The problem of genetic manipulation" (*Theological Investigations IX*). See James M. Gustafson, "Basic ethical issues," in *Theology and Christian Ethics* (Cleveland: Pilgrim Press, 1974), p. 246; Paul Ramsey, "Parenthood and the future of man," in *Fabricated Man: The Ethics of Genetic Control* (New Haven: Yale University Press, 1970), pp. 139–143; and Richard A. McCormick, "Notes on genetic medicine," in *How Brave a New World: Dilemmas in Bioethics* (Garden City: Doubleday, 1981), p. 294.

3. Helmut Thielicke, "The doctor as judge of who shall live and who shall die," in Kenneth Vaux (ed.), *Who Shall Live* (Philadelphia: Fortress Press, 1970), p. 184.

4. James M. Gustafson, "What is the normatively human," in *Theology and Christian Ethics*, p. 230.

5. See Jaroslav Pelikan, *The Christian Tradition: A History of the Development of Doctrine* (Chicago: University of Chicago Press, 1971–1989). For an accessible treatment of "God's dealings with humans," see Jack Miles, *God: A Biography* (New York: Vantage Books, 1995).

6. Karl Barth, *Church Dogmatics*, trans. G. W. Bromiley and R. J. Ehrlich (Edinburgh: T. & T. Clark, 1961), III. 4 (*The Doctrine of Creation*), pp. 324–470.

7. In their introduction to *Theological Voices in Medical Ethics*, Verhay and Lammers state, "Theologians—and the religious traditions they rediscovered—played an important role in the emergence of the field of modern medical ethics" (p. 3).

8. John Mahoney, *The Making of Moral Theology* (Oxford: Oxford University Press, 1987).

9. Albert R. Jonsen and Stephen Toulmin, *The Abuse of Casuistry: A History of Moral Reasoning* (Berkeley and Los Angeles: University of California Press, 1988).

10. Dominico Soto and Dominico Banez appear to have invented the distinction. See J. J. Mc-

Cartney, "The development of the doctrine of ordinary and extraordinary means of preserving life in Catholic moral theology," *Linacre Quarterly* 47 (1980): 215.

11. David F. Kelly, *The Emergence of Roman Catholic Medical Ethics in North America: A Historical-Methodological-Bibliographical Study* (New York and Toronto: The Edwin Mellen Press, 1979).

12. Charles Coppens, *Moral Principles and Medical Practice: The Basis of Medical Jurisprudence* (New York: Benziger Brothers, 1897).

13. Kelly, *Emergence of Roman Catholic Medical Ethics*, chapter 3.

14. F. Angelini (ed.), *Discorsi ai Medici* (Rome: Orrizante, 1959). Many of these allocutions are collected in *Papal Teachings: The Human Body,* eds. The Monks of Solesmes (Boston: St. Paul Editions, 1960).

15. The principal authors were Gerald Kelly, *Medico-Moral Problems,* 5 parts (St. Louis: The Catholic Hospital Association of the United States, 1949–1954); Thomas J. O'Donnell, *Morals in Medicine* (Westminster, Md.: Newman Press, 1956); Charles J. McFadden, *Medical Ethics* (Philadelphia: F. A. Davis, 1949); John P. Kenny, *Principles of Medical Ethics* (Westminster, Md.: Newman, 1952); Edwin P. Healy, *Medical Ethics* (Chicago: Loyola University Press, 1956).

16. Aaron I. Abell, *American Catholicism and Social Action. A Search for Social Justice.* (Notre Dame: Notre Dame University Press, 1963); Jean-Yves Calvez and Jacques Perrin, *The Church and Social Justice: The Social Teaching of the Popes from Leo XIII to Pius XII, 1878–1958* (Chicago: Regnery, 1961); Charles E. Curran, *Directions in Catholic Social Ethics* (Notre Dame: University of Notre Dame Press, 1985).

17. Richard A. McCormick, "The new medicine and morality," *Theology Digest* 21 (1973): 308–321; *How Brave a New World*; Charles Curran, *Medicine and Morals* (Washington, D.C.: Corpus, 1970); *Politics, Medicine and Christian Ethics: A Dialogue with Paul Ramsey* (Philadelphia: Fortress, 1973); Curran (ed.), *Contraception, Authority and Dissent* (New York: Herder, 1969); Bernard Häring, *Medical Ethics,* trans. Gabrielle L. Jean (Slough: St. Paul Publications, 1972); *Ethics of Manipulation: Issues in Medicine, Behavior Control and Genetics* (New York: Seabury Press, 1975).

18. McCormick, *How Brave a New World,* p. x.

19. Pope Paul VI, *Humanae Vitae* (1968). I tell the story of this crisis and its relation to bioethics in Chapter 9.

20. See Martin E. Marty and Kenneth Vaux (eds.), *Health/Medicine and Faith Traditions: An Inquiry into Religion and Medicine* (Philadelphia: Fortress Press, 1982; 15 volumes to 1992).

21. Martin E. Marty, *Righteous Empire: The Protestant Experience in America* (New York: Dial Press, 1970), p. 199. It should not be ignored that early evangelical preachers denounced slavery and subjugation of women; see Christine Leigh Heyrman, *Southern Cross. The Beginnings of the Bible Belt* (New York: Knopf, 1996).

22. Max Weber, *The Protestant Ethic and the Spirit of Capitalism,* trans. Talcott Parsons (London: Allen and Unwin, 1930).

23. Walter Rauschenbusch, *Christianizing the Social Order* (New York: The Macmillan Company, 1912), p. 125; *A Theology for the Social Gospel* (New York: Abingdon Press, 1917); Ronald C. White, *The Social Gospel: Religion and Reform in Changing America* (Philadelphia: Temple University Press, 1976).

24. Reinhold Niebuhr, *Moral Man and Immoral Society: A Study in Ethics and Politics* (New York: C. Scribner's Sons, 1932); *Christian Realism and Political Problems* (New York: C. Scribner's Sons, 1953); *The Nature and Destiny of Man: A Christian Interpretation* (New York: C. Scribner's Sons, 1941). For a discussion of Niebuhr's theological and political positions, see

Charles W. Kegley, *Reinhold Niebuhr: His Religious, Social and Political Thought* (New York: Macmillan, 1956).

25. H. Richard Niebuhr, *The Responsible Self* (New York: HarperCollins Publishers, 1963), p. 65. See also Albert R. Jonsen, *Responsibility in Modern Religious Ethics* (Washington, D.C.: Corpus Books, 1968).

26. See Paul Ramsey (ed.), *Faith and Ethics: The Theology of H. Richard Niebuhr* (New York: HarperCollins Publishers, 1957). Interviews with LeRoy Walters (October 25, 1995) and James Childress (August 4, 1996).

27. Paul L. Lehmann, *Ethics in a Christian Context* (New York: Harper and Row, 1963).

28. Paul Ramsey, "Deeds and rules in Christian ethics," *Scottish Journal of Theology Occasional Papers* 11 (Edinburgh: Oliver and Boyd, 1965).

29. Gene H. Outka and Paul Ramsey, *Norm and Context in Christian Ethics* (New York: Scribner's, 1968). James Gustafson wrote a objective analysis of the debate in "Context versus principles: a misplaced debate in Christian ethics," *Harvard Theological Review* 58 (1965): 171–202.

30. Immanuel Jakobovits, *Jewish Medical Ethics. A Comparative and Historical Study of the Jewish Religious Attitude to Medicine and Its Practice* (New York: Bloch, 1959). This book had its origins in a doctoral dissertation presented to the University of London in 1955.

31. J. David Bleich and Fred Rosner, *Jewish Bioethics* (New York: Hebrew Publishing, 1979); Fred Rosner, *Modern Medicine and Jewish Law* (New York: Yeshiva University Press, 1972); *Modern Medicine and Jewish Ethics* (New York: Yeshiva University Press, 1986); David M. Feldman and Fred Rosner (eds.), *A Compendium on Medical Ethics: Jewish Moral, Ethical and Religious Principles in Medical Practice* (New York: Federation of Jewish Philanthropies, 1984).

32. Baruch Brody, "Halakhic material in medical ethics discussions," *Journal of Medicine and Philosophy* 8:(1983) 317–328 (special issue, "Medical Ethics from the Jewish Perspective," ed. Isaac Franck).

33. Joseph Fletcher, *Morals and Medicine. The Moral Problems of: the Patient's Right to Know the Truth, Contraception, Artificial Insemination, Sterilization, and Euthanasia* (Princeton, N.J.: Princeton University Press, 1954), pp. xix, xxii.

34. In his autobiography, "Memoir of an ex-radical," Fletcher remarks, a propos of his choice, that he had seen a shift in the field of ethics from an interest in the social and psychological sciences in the 1920s and 1930s to the physical sciences in the 1940s and 1950s, "due chiefly perhaps to two things, nuclear power and various ecological imbalances. . . . we could see their impact on human beings and values, and out of that phase emerged a new sensitivity about nuclear energy, weaponry and protection of the environment" (p. 83). Joseph F. Fletcher, "Memoir of an ex-radical," in Kenneth Vaux (ed.), *Joseph Fletcher: Memoir of an Ex-Radical* (Louisville: John Knox Press, 1993), p. 83.

35. Fletcher, *Morals and Medicine*, p. 224.

36. Joseph F. Fletcher, *Situation Ethics: The New Morality* (Philadelphia: Westminster Press, 1966), pp. 49–50.

37. Kenneth Vaux, "Tribute to Joseph Fletcher," (paper presented at the Birth of Bioethics Conference, Seattle, Wa., Sept. 23–24, 1992), transcript, p. 487.

38. Fletcher, *Morals and Medicine*, p. xv.

39. Fletcher, *Morals and Medicine*, p. 27.

40. Fletcher, *Morals and Medicine*, p. 225.

41. Fletcher, *Morals and Medicine*, p. 116.

42. Fletcher, "Memoir of an ex-radical," p. 82.

43. Fletcher, *Morals and Medicine*, pp. 6, 8, 25.

44. Fletcher, *Morals and Medicine*, pp. 10, 11, 12.

45. Fletcher, *Morals and Medicine*, p. xx. As an Episcopal theologian, Dr. Fletcher was familiar with the tradition of Angelican moral theology. That tradition, similar in many ways to Roman Catholic moral theology but more open to personal freedom, offered solid grounds for analysis of practical moral problems. Yet Fletcher pays little attention to his own tradition. He refers to its leading modern practitioner, Bishop Kenneth Kirk, only once in *Morals and Medicine* and then only to criticize him. See Fletcher, *Morals and Medicine*, p. 61, citing Kenneth Kirk, *Conscience and Its Problems: An Introduction to Casuistry* (London: Longmans, Green and Co., 1927).

46. Fletcher, *Morals and Medicine* pp. 214, 215.

47. *Situation Ethics* (Phila: Westminster Press, 1966).

48. "Allocution," (March 23, 1952) *Acta Apostolicae Sedis* 44 (1952): 270; see also Instruction of the Holy Office, February 2, 1956 in Henry Denzinger and Adolf Schönmetzer, *Enchiridion Symbolorum Definitionum et Declarationum de Rebus Fidei et Morum* (Rome: Herder, 1965), 33rd ed., #3918.

49. Fletcher, *Humanhood: Essays in Biomedical Ethics* (Buffalo: Prometheus Books, 1979), p. 84.

50. Fletcher, "Memoir of an ex-radical," p. 82; Mary Faith Marshall, "Fletcher the matchmaker," in Vaux, *Joseph Fletcher*, pp. 25–54. See also Albert R. Jonsen, "Casuistry, situationism and laxism," in Vaux, *Joseph Fletcher*, pp. 10–24; Harvey Gallagher Cox (ed.), *The Situation Ethics Debate* (Philadelphia: Westminster Press, 1968).

51. Marshall, "Fletcher the matchmaker," p. 36.

52. Fletcher, *The Ethics of Genetic Control: Ending Reproductive Roulette* (Garden City: Doubleday, 1974; 2nd ed., 1988).

53. Fletcher, *Ethics of Genetic Control*, p. vii.

54. Fletcher, "Memoir of an ex-radical," pp. 85–86.

55. Fletcher, *Morals and Medicine*, p. 26.

56. Fletcher, *Ethics of Genetic Control*, p. 120.

57. Fletcher, *Humanhood*, p. 147; William K. Frankena, *Ethics*, 2nd ed. (Englewood Cliffs, N.J.: Prentice-Hall, 1973), pp. 36, 55–56. The term "agapism" was coined by Frankena to indicate that the goal and end of Fletcher's utilitarianism was the creation of a loving (*agape*) relationship.

58. Fletcher, *Ethics of Genetic Control*, p. 99.

59. "Humanhood" first appeared under the title "Medicine and the nature of man," in Robert M. Veatch, William Gaylin, and Councilman Morgan (eds.), *The Teaching of Medical Ethics* (Hastings-on-Hudson, N.Y.: Institute of Society, Ethics, and the Life Sciences, 1973), pp. 47–58. It was reproduced in reduced form in "Four indicators of humanhood: the enquiry matures," *Hastings Center Report* 4, no. 6 (1974): 4–7, and in full form in Fletcher's *Humanhood: Essays in Biomedical Ethics* (Buffalo: Prometheus Books, 1979).

60. Fletcher, *Humanhood*, p. 80.

61. Fletcher, *Humanhood*, p. 86.

62. Fletcher, *Humanhood*, pp. 46–53.

63. Thomas Hunter, Introduction, Fletcher, *Humanhood*, p. xi.

64. Fletcher, "Memoir of an ex-radical," p. 83.

65. Kenneth Vaux, "Tribute to Joseph Fletcher," transcript pp. 482–490.

66. Paul Ramsey, *Ethics at the Edges of Life. Medical and Legal Intersections* (New Haven: Yale University Press, 1978), p. xiii; see also, *The Patient as Person: Explorations in Medical Ethics* (New Haven: Yale University Press, 1970), pp. xi, xii.

67. Paul Ramsey, "The morality of abortion," in Daniel H. Labby (ed.), *Life or Death: Ethics and Options* (Seattle: University of Washington Press, 1968), p. 81.

68. For one essay in which theological style dominates, see Ramsey, "Indignity of 'death with dignity'," *Hastings Center Studies* 2, no. 2 (1974): 47–62.

69. Paul Ramsey, *Basic Christian Ethics* (New York: Scribner's 1950).

70. Ramsey, *Basic Christian Ethics*, p. 89.

71. Paul Ramsey, *Nine Modern Moralists* (Englewood Cliffs, N.J.: Prentice Hall, 1962).

72. Paul Ramsey, "Deeds and rules in Christian ethics," *Scottish Journal of Theology Occasional Papers*, No. 11 (Edinburgh: Oliver and Boyd, 1965).

73. Paul Ramsey, "The case of the curious exception," in Gene H. Outka and Paul Ramsey (eds.), *Norm and Context in Christian Ethics* (New York: C. Scribner's Sons, 1968), pp. 67–139.

74. Paul Ramsey, *War and the Christian Conscience: How Shall Modern War Be Conducted Justly?* (Durham, N.C.: Duke University Press, 1961), pp. 171–186.

75. Ramsey, "The morality of abortion"; "Moral and religious implications of genetic control," in John Roslansky (ed.), *Genetics and the Future of Man* (Amsterdam: North-Holland Publishing Company, 1966); Ramsey, "Shall we clone a man?" in *Fabricated Man: The Ethics of Genetic Control* (New Haven: Yale University Press, 1970), pp. 66–103.

76. Allan Verhey, "Cloning: revisiting an old debate," *Kennedy Institute of Ethics Journal* 4 (1994): 227–234.

77. Ramsey, *The Patient as Person*, p. xx.

78. Ramsey, *The Patient as Person*, p. xvii; see also Ramsey, *Ethics at the Edge of Life. Medical and Legal Intersections* (New Haven: Yale University Press, 1978), p. xiv, and with Richard A. McCormick (eds.), *Doing Evil to Achieve Good: Moral Choice in Conflict Situations* (Chicago: Loyola University Press, 1978), p. 4.

79. Ramsey, *The Patient as Person*, pp. xi–xii.

80. Ramsey, *The Patient as Person*, pp. xiii.

81. Ramsey, *The Patient as Person*, p. xiii, p. 2.

82. Ramsey, *The Patient as Person*, p. 2.

83. Ramsey, *The Patient as Person*, p. 5.

84. Ramsey, *The Patient as Person*, p. 115.

85. McCormick, *How Brave a New World?* p. x.

86. Lisa Cahill, On Richard McCormick: "reason and faith in post-Vatican II Catholic ethics," in Verhey and Lammers, *Theological Voices*, pp. 80, 98.

87. Richard A. McCormick, "Public policy on abortion," *Hospital Progress* 60 (1979): 26–30; *How Brave a New World?* p. 200.

88. Richard A. McCormick, "The encyclical Humanae Vitae," *Theological Studies* 29 (1968): 718–741; *How Brave a New World*, pp. 209–237; "The tenth anniversary of Humane Vitae," *Theological Studies* 40 (1979): 80–97; also included in *How Brave a New World*, pp. 238–259.

89. Richard A. McCormick, "To save or let die," *Journal of the American Medical Association* 229 (1974): 172–177, also in *America* 130 (1974): 6–10 and *How Brave a New World*, pp. 346–347; see also McCormick, "The quality of life, the sanctity of life," *Hastings Center Report* 8, no. 1 (1978): 30–36.

90. Paul Ramsey, "'Euthanasia' and dying well enough," in *Ethics at the Edges of Life*, pp. 171–181.

91. Thomas Aquinas, *Summa Theologiae* II–II, Q. 64, a. 7; J. T. Mangan, "An historical analysis of the principle of double effect," *Theological Studies* 10 (1949): 40–61.

92. P. Knauer, "The hermeneutic function of the principle of double effect," *Natural Law Forum* 12 (1967): 132–162; B. Schüller, "Direkte Totung—Indirekte Totung," *Theologie und Philosophie*, 47 (1972), 341–357; C. Van der Poel, "The principle of double effect," in Charles Curran (ed.), *Absolutes in Moral Theology* (Washington: Corpus Books, 1967) pp. 186–210;

Richard A. McCormick, *Ambiguity in Moral Choice* (Milwaukee: Marquette University Press, 1973).

93. McCormick, *Ambiguity in Moral Choice*.

94. McCormick, *Ambiguity in Moral Choice*, p. 69; Ramsey and McCormick, *Doing Evil to Achieve Good*, p. 35.

95. Baruch Brody "The Problem of exceptions in medical ethics," pp. 54–68, and William Frankena, "McCormick and the traditional distinction," pp. 145–164. in McCormick and Ramsey, *Doing Evil to Achieve Good*, pp. 145–164. The double effect debate was resuscitated in the wake of a renewed interest in assisted suicide, in which the widely accepted distinction between direct and indirect killing was challenged. However, even apart from that context, double effect poses fascinating intellectual challenges. See Lee W. Quinn, "Actions, intentions and consequences: the doctrine of double effect," *Philosophy and Public Affairs* 18 (1989): 334–351; Joseph Boyle, "Who is entitled to double effect," *Journal of Medicine and Philosophy* 16 (1991): 475–494; Alan Donagan, "Moral absolutism and the double-effect exception," *Journal of Medicine and Philosophy* 16 (1991): 495–509; Frances M. Kamm, "The doctrine of double effect: reflections on theoretical and practical issues," *Journal of Medicine and Philosophy* 16 (1991): 571–585.

96. Lisa S. Cahill, "Paul Ramsey: covenant fidelity in medical ethics," *Journal of Religion* 55 (Oct. 1975): 470–476; David H. Smith, "On Paul Ramsey: a covenant centered ethic for medicine," in Verhey and Lammers, *Theological Voices*, pp. 7–29; Curran, *Politics, Medicine and Christian Ethics;* James T. Johnson and David. H. Smith (eds.), *Love and Society: Essays in the Ethics of Paul Ramsey* (Missoula, Mont.: Scholars Press, 1974).

97. McCormick, *How Brave a New World*; Lisa Cahill, "On Richard McCormick: reason and faith in post-Vatican II Catholic ethics," in Verhey and Lammers, *Theological Voices*, pp. 78–105.

98. Episcopal theologian Harmon L. Smith of Duke University Divinity School published *Ethics and the New Medicine* (Nashville: Abington Press, 1970) in the same year that Ramsey's *Patient as Person* appeared. Smith's book, which reviewed abortion, reproductive technology, organ transplantation, experimentation, and care of the dying, is theologically tinged but not dogmatic, and presents a competent statement of the issues. However, Ramsey's more aggressive style and analysis overshadowed what would have been an excellent survey of the state of the issues at the turn of the decade. William May, who was Joseph P. Kennedy Sr. Professor of Christian Ethics at the Kennedy Institute from 1980 to 1985 produced several classic articles: "Attitudes toward the newly dead," *Hastings Center Studies* 1, no. 1 (1973): 3–13, and "Code, covenant, contract, or philanthropy," *Hastings Center Report* 5, no. 6 (1975): 29–38. Two major theologians of the renewed Catholic moral theology wrote books on medical ethics: Charles Curran produced a study of the thought of Paul Ramsey, *Politics, Medicine, and Christian Ethics. A Dialogue with Paul Ramsey* (Philadelphia: Fortress Press, 1973), and Bernard Häring, a German theologian who often taught in the United States, authored *Medical Ethics* (Notre Dame: Fides, 1973) and *Ethics of Manipulation: Issues in Medicine, Behavior Control and Genetics* (New York: Seabury Press, 1975). Father Häring's views are often hardly distinguishable from those of Joseph Fletcher in their openness to human freedom and embrace of human creativity.

99. James Gustafson, "Basic ethical issues in the biomedical fields," *Soundings* 53 (1970): 151–180; "What is the normatively human," *American Ecclesiastical Review* 165 (1971): 192–207; "Genetic engineering and the normative view of the human," in Preston Williams (ed.), *Ethical Issues in Biology and Medicine* (Cambridge: Shenkman, 1972), pp. 46–58; "Mongolism, parental desires and the right to life," *Perspectives in Biology and Medicine* 16 (1973): 529–557; *The Contributions of Theology to Medical Ethics: The 1975 Pere Marquette Lecture* (Milwaukee: Marquette University Press, 1975); James Gustafson, Marc Lappé, and Richard Roblin, "Ethical

and social issues in screening for genetic disease," *New England Journal of Medicine* 286 (1972): 1129–1132.

100. Among Gustafson's students at Yale in the 1960s were James Childress, Stanley Hauerwas, and LeRoy Walters, and me, and at Chicago, Lisa Cahill, Allan Verhey, and Stephen Post. From Harvard came Robert Veatch, Charles Reynolds, Karen Lebacqz, Ruth Purtillo, Preston Williams, and Roy Branson. John Fletcher was educated at Union Theological Seminary under Roger Shinn; David Smith studied at Princeton with Paul Ramsey.

101. Interview with Robert Veatch, October, 1995.

102. Gustafson, *The Contributions of Theology to Medical Ethics*, p. 93.

103. James Gustafson and Stanley Hauerwas (eds.), "Editorial: theology and medical ethics," *Journal of Medicine and Philosophy*, 4 (1979): 345; see Gustafson, "Theology confronts technology and the life sciences," *Commonweal* 105 (June 16, 1978): 386–392.

104. See Verhay and Lammers, *Theological Voices*. The journal *Christian Bioethics* appeared in March, 1995, dedicated to the examination of "the traditional content-full commitments of the Christian faiths with regard to the meaning of life, sexuality, suffering, illness, and death within the context of medicine and health care." See H. Tristram Engelhardt, Jr., "Toward a Christian bioethics," *Christian Bioethics* 1 (1995): 1. The Park Ridge Center, founded in 1985 under sponsorship of the Lutheran General Health System, fosters multifaith theological analysis "of the religious elements in every aspect of human well-being, especially as they relate to prevention of disease, care and treatment, interpretation of illness and health, and the ethical issues connected with these and other matters," (Park Ridge Center for the Study of Health, Faith and Ethics, Fact Sheet). Even before the Center was opened, Martin Marty and Kenneth Vaux began to edit a splendid series, *Health/Medicine and Faith Traditions: An Inquiry into Religion and Medicine* (Philadelphia: Fortress Press, 1982; 15 volumes to 1992).

3

The Philosophers: Clarifying the Concepts

"In the early days," recalls Dan Callahan, "the theologians were a powerful force. They were articulate and had thought much about the problems . . . but philosophers, who had started to realize that philosophy should have something to say about real life, brought a different set of concepts and strategies, a different vocabulary than theological ethics."[1] The theologians had discovered that the concepts and vocabulary imported from their traditions required translation for bioethical debates. The philosophers had an even more difficult task: they were compelled to move beyond their training to speak cogently in the bioethical debates. The philosophers who came into bioethics had been trained in the philosophical idiom of the 1950s. That idiom was not congenial to the kind of analysis that the new questions seemed to require—an analysis that could facilitate practical decisions and contribute to policy. Those who made the transition from academic philosophy to bioethics had to venture from their disciplinary home without losing touch with its intellectual heritage. This chapter traces that heritage from its beginnings in Western philosophy through a characteristic American version during the nineteenth and early twentieth centuries and ends in the academic departments of the 1950s and 1960s. We shall then introduce some of the persons who applied their philosophical training and acumen to the questions of the new medicine and biology.

Moral Philosophy

The word "ethics" is used in many ways. It may designate the moral beliefs and behavior of individuals, the rules devised to prevent political conflict of interest, the mores of society, and, as the *Oxford English Dictionary* quaintly states, "the department of study concerned with the principles of human duty." That department was founded by Greek and Roman thinkers—Socrates, Plato, Aristotle, Cicero, Seneca, and others—who attempted to describe the best form of human life and the best recipes for living it. As the classical era ceded to the Christian era, the study of ethics was done less by philosophers than by Christian theologians who interpreted the commandments and counsel of the Ancient and the New Covenant to Christian believers. They pondered the question, how should persons destined for salvation behave in a sinful world? These theologians, such as Ambrose, Jerome, Augustine, Aquinas, Luther, Calvin, and Melancthon, often relied on the pre-Christian philosophical moralists—sometimes as allies whose noble ideas could be christened, sometimes as adversaries whose terrestrial vision needed celestial correction. When theology and philosophy both worked within the department of study concerned with the principles of human duty, moral philosophy was hardly distinct from moral theology.

The late Scholastic theologians began to address questions about the nature of voluntary activity that presaged a more independent moral philosophy. During the Renaissance and Enlightenment, the desire to accord human reason an independent domain in all human enterprises favored an autonomous moral philosophy. The pre-Christian philosophers, particularly Cicero and the Stoics, were studied for themselves rather than for their affinity to Christian theology. Christian scholars speculated on questions that revelation did not directly address: by what faculty of soul are moral truths known? under what circumstances are praise and blame attributed? what is the nature of human virtues and human passions? Most of these scholars studied such questions in the belief that their speculation was compatible with Christian faith. Other authors, such as Thomas Hobbes and Baruch Spinoza, departed explicitly from the perspective of religious faith and attempted to erect ethics on a thoroughly rational base. By the seventeenth century, moral philosophy was mature enough to leave its theological home and take up residence as a standard subject, beside natural philosophy and metaphysics, in the philosophy curriculum. Moral theology and moral philosophy were henceforth distinct departments of moral science.[2]

Moral Philosophy in America

Moral philosophy has long held an honored place in American intellectual life and education. The Puritan theologians who dominated colonial culture were reluctant to admit an autonomous moral philosophy into moral teaching. Cotton Mather called "Ethicks" a "vile Peece of Paganism."[3] However, the premier intellectual of the colonial era, Jonathan Edwards, resolute Puritan theologian though he was, generously invited "natural conscience and virtues" into his moral theology. He and many of his theological colleagues appreciated (not uncritically) the description of this "natural moral order" as given by the British moral philosophers Henry More, Samuel Price, Francis Hutcheson, Antony Ashley, and Bishop Joseph Butler.[4] These moralists, all committed Protestants, described moral character, conscience, freedom, and duty in ways conformable to Christian piety. They generally opposed Thomas Hobbes, who was considered by Anglican and Puritan divines to be an enemy of faith and moral rectitude.

These authors, despite their differences, agreed that humans possessed a moral sense, coupled with powers of reasoning, that could discover in human nature standards of goodness and justice that intimated God's will. Although Puritan theology was fiercely committed to a doctrine of divine predestination, its theologians were able to espouse a notion of human moral freedom that was defined, in the words of Richard Price, as "the power of following, in all circumstances, our sense of right and wrong, or of acting in conformity to our reflecting and moral principles, without being controlled by any contrary principles."[5] The doctrines of the moral sense and of human freedom featured prominently in subsequent American moral philosophy.

As the colonial era came to a close, the leading American intellectuals added to their libraries of English moralists European writers who were distant from the Puritan tradition: John Locke, Hugo Grotius, Samuel Pufendorf, Cesar Beccaria, Jean-Jacques Rousseau, and Charles-Louis Montesquieu, finding in their books ideas about liberty, natural law, and natural rights that suited the revolutionary temper. As one author says, "It is impossible to recount accurately the intellectual history of colonial America in the eighteenth century without prominently featuring the teaching of moral philosophy, since it engaged the best minds of the time. . . ."[6]

In the first decades of the new Republic, moral philosophy assumed preeminence in the college curriculum. At Harvard, Yale, and Princeton, and in the many small colleges that founded as the country spread westward, a course in moral philosophy was taught in the senior year, often by the college president, as the capstone of education. The presidents were seen as "the custodians of certain truths necessary to the successful function of civilized society . . . [whose] job was to convey these truths to the youth who would one day assume positions of leadership."[7] As scholars, public figures, and preachers (most were ordained ministers), the presidents addressed the serious questions of the day: military adventures and territorial expansion, temperance, prison reform, suffrage, free trade, and, most serious of all, slavery and abolition.[8] Although the courses were called "moral philosophy" and the topics were elaborated with the arguments of classical moral philosophers, the academic moral philosophers of the early Republic made no effort to hide their Christian beliefs. Their work was Christian ethics in thin disguise. They urged Sabbath observance and the duty of daily prayer in their texts of moral philosophy and, without embarrassment, justified virtues by reference to Scripture. Still, the presidential philosophers encouraged rational discourse about moral matters and attempted to instill a high sense of moral probity that would affect the public life of the nation.[9]

Despite the prominence of the presidential moralists, the most influential "public philosophers" of antebellum America lived outside academe. William Ellery Channing, Ralph Waldo Emerson, and Henry David Thoreau expounded from the pulpit, podium, and by pen a view of human life that urged vigorous self-reliance and independence of thought and action. The new Republic was to be built by men who lived imaginatively in nature and encountered it creatively. These "public philosophers" were outspoken commentators on the political and cultural life of the nation. Although their thought was rarely framed in the classical categories of moral philosophy, it infiltrated American views of the good life. Thoreau's teaching on civil disobedience, "Resistance to Civil Government," unpopular as it was in his day, echoed down to the era of Martin Luther King and the Vietnam War protests.[10] A biographer of Thoreau calls the essay "Thoreau's most read—and taught—essay and one of the great Western statements on the importance of conscience."[11]

The golden era of American philosophy spanned the last quarter of the nineteenth century and the first quarter of the twentieth. William James and Josiah Royce at Harvard, and John Dewey and George Herbert Mead at the University of Chicago, cultivated a style of philosophizing that combined an erudite appreciation of the classic philosophers with an appealing public voice about contemporary issues. Each of them believed that philosophy should make a difference in the life of the people. Vividly conscious of the appeal of Darwinian thought, each scholar adapted the dynamism of the evolutionary concept to the moral life and, at the same time, repudiated its deterministic and materialistic implications. Each of them celebrated the dignity and value of the individual who creatively met life's challenges. The American pragmatism that flowed from their thoughts reflected American vigor and practicality and elevated these qualities to philosophic doctrines. The tradition of the public philosopher culminated with these men, who incessantly addressed the public about the life of the nation and its affairs. Yet, even as these public philosophers were thriving, philosophy was becoming more technical, more academic, and more reticent about public affairs.[12]

William James was the dominant figure in American philosophy from the 1870s until his death in 1910. Scion of a distinguished family, James trained in medicine at Harvard and then became a member of its faculty, first in psychology and then in philosophy (subjects often joined in those times). A man of prodigious learning and intense intellectual curiosity, he shaped original positions across the spectrum of philosophical thought, from empirical psychology to religious and mystical knowledge. Although his thought touched ethics at many points, James spoke most expansively about morality in an 1891 address to the Yale Philosophical Club entitled "The Moral Philosopher and the Moral Life."[13] James begins the address by repudiating "any ethical philosophy dogmatically made up in advance. . . . there can be no final truth in ethics any more than in physics, until the last man has had his experience and said his say." He then describes three questions in ethics: the psychological question about the origin of moral ideas, the metaphysical question about the meaning of such words as "good," "evil," and "obligation," and the casuistic question about the "measure" of the goods and evils that people recognize. He affirms an experiential and intuitional origin of moral ideas and gives to moral words a meaning rooted in the experience of the demands that persons make upon each other. The casuistic question arises when we realize that the demands we make upon each other are multiple, various, and often incompatible, and we are forced to ask how they can all be fulfilled. After reviewing the various answers given by philosophers, he proposes that "the essence of good is simply to satisfy demand . . . (and) since all demands cannot be satisfied in this poor world, the guiding principle for ethical philosophy must be simply to satisfy at all times as many demands as we can." James then issues an imperative: "Invent some manner of realizing your own ideals which will also satisfy the alien demands—that and that only is the path of peace!"[14]

The imperative is characteristically Jamesian: he located the deepest roots of philosophy in human striving and action. Persons must live, encounter problems, devise solutions, and design ways of living. Despite this encomium for human moral creativity, James warns that the "laws and usages . . . in our civilized society" demonstrate the most satisfying solutions to problems, so that "the presumption in cases of conflict must be in favor of the conventionally recognized good." Experience will show again and again that new solutions to new problems must be invented, so as to assure the continued mutual satisfaction of as many demands as possible So, he concludes, "ethical science is just like physical science, and instead of being deductible all at once from abstract principles, must simply bide its time, and be ready to revise its conclusions from day to day." While the moral life may remain in "the easy going mode," of avoiding present ills, it is called from time to time to "the strenuous mode . . . [to] attain the highest ideal . . . endurance, courage and capacity for handling life's evils." Belief in a "divine thinker with all-enveloping demands" must be postulated to sustain the rigor of the strenuous ethical life.[15]

William James's ethics is preeminently American. It is conservative and religious, though not credal or denominational. At the same time, it is inventive, creative and strenuous. It accepts the worlds of nature and society, yet is eager to renew them. It recognizes problems in the facts of situations and resolves them by understanding the facts and by exerting the energy of human intelligence and will. James was an outstanding public philosopher. In innumerable lectures and letters, he expressed his opinions on "the position of blacks, women, immigrants, the care of the insane, vivisection, medical legislation and the temperance movement."[16] On all of these topics, he held what would today be considered liberal views. Toward the end of his life, he became deeply concerned about American imperialism and militarism. Although James, together with almost all the classical American philosophers, ceased to be read in formal academic philosophy for many decades, his genius somehow diffused itself and became an anonymous tone in the American ethos.

John Dewey was America's public philosopher for the first fifty years of the 20th century. His philosophical work is enormous and protean and, like that of William James, touches ethics at many points. He commented on, and engaged in, public affairs through a constant stream of articles on public education, woman's suffrage, industry and labor, politics and economics, and international affairs. These contributions appeared in scholarly books and journals, but much of his work was aimed at the general reader, especially in the pages of *The New Republic*, of which he was a contributing editor for over 20 years. He agonized over America's participation in both World Wars and, in 1937, he chaired an international commission of inquiry into the charges levied by the Soviet Union against Leon Trotsky. One student of American political culture has commented, "So faithfully did Dewey live up to his own philosophical creed that he became the guide, the mentor and the conscience of the American people: it is scarcely an exaggeration to say that for a generation no issue was clarified until Dewey had spoken."[17]

Although his *Ethics* of 1909, co-authored with James Tufts, is a rather conventional exposition of the classical problems of moral philosophy, those classical problems are illuminated by a fundamental Deweyan insight:

> The moral act is one which sustains a whole complex system of social values; one which keeps vital and progressive the industrial order, science, art, and the State. . . . It is not the business of moral theory to demonstrate the existence of mathematical equations, in this life or another one, between goodness and virtue. It is the business of men to develop such capacities and desires, such selves as to render them capable of finding their own satisfaction, their invaluable value, in fulfilling the demands which grow out of their associated life. . . . Such a person has found himself and has solved the problem in the only place and in the only way in which it can be solved: in action.[18]

Another Deweyan thesis states, "A moral principle is not a command to act or forbear acting in a given way: it is a tool for analyzing a special situation, the right or wrong being determined by the situation in its entirety and not by the rule as such."[19] Writing a decade later, he expanded that notion: "Morals must be a growing science if it is to be a science at all, not merely because all truth has not yet been appropriated by the mind of man, but because life is a moving affair in which old moral truth ceases to apply. Principles are methods of inquiry and forecasts which require verification by the event. . . . Principles exist as hypotheses with which to experiment."[20] He saw "moral science, not as a separate province, [but as] physical, biological and historical knowledge placed in a human context where it will illuminate and guide the activities of men."[21] Like James, Dewey repudiated a finished system of ethics. The ethical response was always a reflective and creative solution to a problem that presented itself in a unique way.

Dewey, however, emphasized more than James the utility of scientific information and reasoning in the resolution of moral problems. He considered scientific thinking the paradigm of rational thought and believed that its investigative methods could clarify values and valuing. In addition, the results of scientific investigations illuminated moral problems. Professor John Smith explains Dewey's instrumentalist view of moral reasoning: morality arises with desire and is fulfilled in critical assessment of desire. That critical assessment is the work of intelligence. "Between a problem and its solution," writes Smith, "we must always interject a rational method. In the moral situation this means that between casual desire and values approved on reflection there must come a process of knowledge and critical inquiry. Science—in this case, knowledge of the potentialities and powers of things together with basic insight into the na-

ture of man and his needs—instead of being alien to ethics, turns out to be indispensable."[22]

Neither William James nor John Dewey created a system of moral philosophy;
rather, they created a style. Moral philosophy was an incessant inquiry into the way humans, conceived as bundles of habits vitalized by a curious intelligence and creative
freedom, could live in the world of physical nature and cultural creation and could
change and challenge that world to meet human purposes. The critical edge of moral
philosophy was set against barriers and boundaries in thought, culture, and religion that
obstruct human openness and the expansion of mind and mores.

James and Dewey were unquestionably the dominant intellectuals in America for
decades. Their thought was not merely speculative but highly practical and, as recent
commentators have convincingly shown, their contributions to public philosophy
flowed logically from their philosophical convictions.[23] Strangely, their philosophical
dominance left little in the way of a formal legacy in academic philosophy. Perhaps the
vigorous optimism that inspired their thought could not survive the gloom of the Depression and the devastation of two World Wars. The cultural ideal of progress that had
flourished in the nineteenth century lost favor with intellectuals. American pragmatism,
homegrown though it was, survived more as a spirit and a style than as either a system
of philosophical thought (this would, of course, have suited its authors) or as a program
for the moral life (which would not have pleased them).

The spirit of American philosophy, says Professor Smith, is encapsulated in three
dominant beliefs. First, thinking is primarily an activity in response to a concrete situation and this activity is aimed at solving problems. Second, ideas and theories must
make a difference in the conduct of people who hold them. Third, the earth can be civilized and obstacles to progress overcome by the application of knowledge. "From this
perspective, all things derive their value from the contribution they make to the founding and securing of the good life."[24] To these characteristics might be added: American
moral philosophy was respectful of religious feeling, enthusiastic about democracy,
and convinced of the power of individual freedom. It was also, in its epistemological
foundations, naturalistic and intuitionist—that is, moral notions arise from sentiments
innate in human nature, grasped first by intuition and then cultivated by reason and experience. I have made this lengthy tour through American moral philosophy because I
believe that bioethics inherited from its distant and almost forgotten forebearers, the
American philosophers, some of its most distinctive traits, as I shall argue in Chapters
10 and 12. But between the philosophical forebearers and the bioethicists intervened an
interloper called metaethics.

Metaethics

At the beginning of the twentieth century, foreign currents began to flow into American
moral philosophy that over time would have critical, even destructive, effects on its

prevailing style. The critique had begun abroad in a friendly fashion. In 1903, British philosopher G. E. Moore published *Principia Ethica*, in which he advocated the possibility of sound moral philosophy but challenged the idea that the notion "good" could be defined by reference to any natural property. To claim that "good" means pleasure, or the satisfaction of desires or interests, or the attainment of a more evolved state, was to commit "the naturalistic fallacy." Good, like the color yellow, is undefinable; unlike yellow, it is a "non-natural property," perceived by intuition. American philosophers— naturalists almost to a man—either ignored or refuted Moore's position, which seemed to them incompatible with moral experience and ethical argument.[25]

Moore's friendly critique of naturalistic ethics was superseded by a critique antagonistic to all ethical discourse. In 1934, Oxford philosopher A. J. Ayer brought to the English-speaking world the doctrines of the Vienna Circle, a coterie of philosophers and scientists who affirmed that meaningful statements must be either tautologies or verifiable by empirical methods. Applied to ethics, this thesis concluded that any ethical statement is nothing more than a speaker expressing a feeling of approval or disapproval at some event, object, or person. As such, ethical terms are "pseudo-concepts and ethical statements cannot be true or false or argued for or against."[26]

Charles L. Stevenson imported Ayer's thinking to the United States. While a Harvard graduate student in the 1930s, Stevenson had visited Cambridge University where Continental logical positivism, with its radical critique of ethical concepts and language, was popular. Stevenson incorporated these ideas in his doctoral dissertation, "The Emotive Meaning of Ethical Terms," which, in 1944, he published as *Ethics and Language*.[27] This epochal book asserted, in logical positivist fashion, that ethical statements are not factual statements that can be called true or false; they are persuasive ejaculations, expressing emotions of approval or disapproval and attempting to convince others to approve or disapprove what the speaker approves or disapproves. *Ethics and Language* pushed the dominant approach to ethics—namely, that ethical claims rested on a rationally discernible set of natural facts—off its base. John Dewey himself attempted to refute Stevenson's thesis as "a theoretical error and, when widely adopted in practice, a source of moral weakness."[28] Nevertheless, Stevenson's argument either persuaded many philosophers that the traditional search for the ground of morality in objective, empirical fact was erroneous or stimulated others to advance counterarguments that would give to ethical terms some empirical reference. Thus the era of "metaethics" began.

Metaethics, a term coined by A. J. Ayer in 1949, named a new approach to moral philosophy. It became common to distinguish first-order moral discourse from second-order discourse—the former comprising discussions and arguments about what kinds of actions or policies were morally right or wrong, or what characteristics of persons were good or evil; the latter consisting of reflections about what people mean when they use words like "right" or "wrong," "good" or "evil," or when they attribute blame or praise. First-order discourse was the business of normative ethics; second-order discourse was the subject of metaethics. Metaethical questions had to be distinguished and separated from normative ethics. Indeed, some philosophers maintained that metaethics alone was the proper business of philosophers; normative ethics was the business of "journalists, politicians and preachers."[29] It became common to distinguish "fact" from "value," and to claim that it was impossible to clamber over "Hume's hurdle," the barrier between "is" and "ought." Normative ethics had, of course, been the central concern of moral philosophy; questions of metaethics, when they arose, had been left almost unnoticed. Now attention shifted, moving metaethical questions to the center of attention. Normative ethics was not only neglected but spurned, since much of the metaethical discussion cut at its very foundations.

Surveying the scene in moral philosophy at mid-century, William Frankena lamented, "the tendency of recent moral philosophers to avoid the normative task of guiding human action [leads] to a certain sterility which has often been remarked." He speculated that "a venture into normative ethics would help us in our theorizing, for example, in our attempt to see what sort of evidence is relevant to the support and confutation of ethical judgments."[30] A decade later, in her survey of moral philosophy from 1900, British philosopher Mary Warnock agreed:

> One of the consequences of treating ethics as the analysis of ethical language is . . . that it leads to the increasing triviality of the subject. . . . One aspect of the trivializing of the subject is the refusal of moral philosophers in England to commit themselves to any moral opinions. . . . The concentration upon the most general kind of evaluative language, combined with the fear of committing the naturalistic fallacy, has led too often to discussions of grading fruit, or choosing fictitious games equipment, and ethics as a serious subject has been left further and further behind. But I believe that the most boring days are over. . . .[31]

Even though metaethics dominated the scene for more than a quarter century, some moral philosophers struggled to keep normative ethics alive. Men trained under the "old philosophers," such as Ralph Barton Perry and C. I. Lewis, were critical of the dominance of metaethics or were concerned to locate precisely where metaethics and normative ethics met. William Frankena, Richard Brandt, Marcus Singer, John Ladd, Henry Aiken, John Rawls, and others continued to think about normative ethics, although even they were absorbed by the task of refuting or accommodating the metaethical critique.[32]

These philosophers were interested in refurbishing the objective grounds for ethical judgments. In 1951, John Rawls opened an article entitled "Outline of decision procedure for ethics" with the premise, "to establish the objectivity of moral rules, and the decisions based upon them, we must exhibit the decision procedure, which can be shown to be both reasonable and reliable. . . ."[33] Rawls went on to outline a set of conditions for designating a class of competent moral judges and for defining the class of considered moral judgments that foreshadowed his famous "Original Position," in *A Theory of Justice*, published twenty years later.[34] In the following year, another Harvard philosopher, Roderick Firth, published a provocative article in which he attempted to defend the objectivity of moral judgments. Borrowing from eighteenth-century philosophers David Hume and Francis Hutcheson, Firth sketched out the epistemic conditions for an "ideal observer" thesis. This thesis proposed that the assertion "x is right" means "if anyone were, in respect to x and y [two moral options], fully informed and vividly imaginative, impartial, in a calm frame of mind and otherwise normal, he would approve x."[35] Although Firth's formulation itself was much debated, the ideal observer thesis worked its way into the new normative moral philosophy.

Some philosophers pursued that new moral philosophy by concentrating more on the reasons offered for moral judgment than on the words used in the judgment itself.[36] In 1950, Stephen Toulmin, in *An Examination of the Place of Reason in Ethics*, urged a closer examination of the relation between ethical assertions and the reasons and justifications people offer to support them.[37] There are, he suggests, two kinds of moral reasoning. In one type, an accepted moral code provides premises that can be applied to actions; the conclusion of this syllogistic reasoning provides the good reason for action. In the second type, the good reason for action comes from the evaluation of the social consequences of an action; social harmony is the ideal that ultimately justifies all action. Toulmin later repudiated the simplicity of this explanation as well as its utilitarian tone, but he continued to explore the role of reasons in justifying action. Another British philosopher, Richard M. Hare, also investigated the logical and ethical function of "good reasons." In two books, *The Language of Morals*, and *Freedom and Reason*, Hare elaborated a theory of the universality of moral imperatives as an alternative to the irrationality of emotivist approaches to ethical language.[38] Both Toulmin and Hare became frequent contributors to bioethics, bringing a fresh philosophical analysis to practical moral judgments.

In 1951, William Frankena confessed that he yearned for "moral philosophy on a book-size scale again."[39] Twenty years later, that book-length moral philosophy appeared as John Rawls's *A Theory of Justice*. Although not a complete moral philosophy, the tome was a complete theory of one of the central elements of a moral philosophy: justice. This impressive work elaborated the classical contractarian theory of ethics as the basis for an articulation of the principles of justice that rational persons, blinded to their future condition in life, would choose as the moral conditions to enter a society. Rawls's thesis excited many moral philosophers, restored faith in a rational approach to ethics, provided a carefully articulated version of contractarianism, and bequeathed to some future bioethicists the basis for a theory of the allocation of medical resources.[40]

A graduate student studying philosophy during the 1960s would have been unlikely to choose moral philosophy as an exciting specialty. Epistemology was the center of interest, in particular, the epistemological questions raised by science and mathematics. Indeed, it had become popular to suggest that "philosophy" as such was nothing more than a set of analytic tools with which various realms of discourse could be dissected; philosophy of science, law, art, or language became modish. Graduate students who did take a course in moral philosophy might glance at Thomas Hobbes, John Locke, and Immanuel Kant, then plunge into the "analytic" debates of the first fifty years of the century, beginning with Moore's *Principia Ethica*, which was considered the starting point for a correct way of thinking about ethics, namely, the metaethical way. A quick swing through metaethics would touch on the naturalistic fallacy, non-naturalism, and emotivism, a tour sufficient to suggest to the bright student that moral terms could be evacuated of meaning and that moral reasoning could be (to use contemporary language) deconstructed. Despite this devastation, the principal theories of normative ethics would be reviewed, often grouped as two major theories of obligation—teleological and deontological.[41] Approaches to ethics other than theories of obligation would be ignored. The main example of a teleological theory, utilitarianism, would be presented as ostensibly compelling but, on closer examination, as suffering from conceptual weaknesses. The deontological approaches would be revealed as standing on the shifting sands of intuition.[42]

The perceived impotence of normative theories discouraged forays into real problems. A philosophy student of that era could pass an ethics course without wrestling any dark angel of moral perplexity. Stephen Toulmin recalls a graduate seminar in ethics at Oxford in the 1950s in which discussion focused largely on the question, "whether and under what conditions could we describe wearing the wrong colored tie as 'morally offensive.'"[43] G. E. Moore had pronounced "casuistry . . . a much less respectable" branch of ethics, which aims at a more particular and detailed investigation of ethical behavior. He admitted that casuistry is "the goal of ethical investigations," but he contended that casuistry, which concerns itself with the practical problems of the moral life, from major public questions about justice to quite personal ones such as adultery, could not be attempted until "true answers" to the fundamental questions about the meaning of the words "good" and "right" had been secured.[44] While moral philosophy struggled with the metaethical questions, the Holocaust, the Nuremberg trials, Hiroshima, nuclear armament, the McCarthy purges and the Kinsey Report occurred, with barely a whisper from most of the practitioners of metaethics. A few political philosophers, such as Hanna Arendt and Sidney Hook, spoke vehemently about some of these events, but the moral philosophers held their peace.[45]

When Mary Warnock said in 1960 that "the most boring days" of moral philosophy were over,[46] she was correct—a new vitality was stirring in moral philosophy—but not for the speculative reasons that an Oxford philosopher might suspect. Rather, the strongest impetus for the new life was a public disaster: the American military involvement in Southeast Asia. The public agony over the war reached its apogee in 1968–1969, and that agony swarmed into the ordinarily sedate annual meeting of the Western Division of the American Philosophical Association. A non-philosopher, linguist Noam Chomsky, had been invited to open a symposium entitled "Philosophers and Public Policy." After delivering a stinging attack on the American government for its pursuit of the war and for its imperialism, and on the general dominance of a power elite wielding technological mastery that it proclaimed to be "value-free," Chomsky challenged the audience of philosophers: "These are the typical questions of philosophy . . . philosophers must take the lead in this effort."

Only a non-philosopher could believe that such issues had been "typical questions of philosophy," at least during its recent history. The philosophers on the panel strongly disagreed with Chomsky's challenge. University of Texas professor John Silber responded, "As philosophers we can assist in the formation of sound public policy by distinguishing appropriately different kinds of ethical theories and kinds of moral and political obligation."[47] Yet the genie was out of the bottle; some moral philosophers were determined to show the relevance of their discipline. A new journal, sponsored by many of America's leading philosophers, *Philosophy and Public Affairs*, appeared in the fall of 1971, with lead articles on war and abortion. Some philosophers, particularly the younger generation, turned activist, convinced that the discipline that they studied should shed light on the causes they espoused. Metaethics lost its grip over their intellectual curiosity.

The new interest in normative questions, particularly those that were on the agenda of public debate, was invigorating but not philosophically easy to realize. The era of metaethics had debilitated the old normative ethics. Yet, the new "ethicists" (for that is what they soon came to be called) had to be more than social critics; they had to be philosophical critics, using intellectual tools that were recognizably philosophical. Every well-educated philosopher should carry one set of tools: a sharp eye for logical validity of arguments and a tuned ear for subtle differences in the meaning and use of terms. The metaethical debates had refined these intellectual tools for the moral philosophers, who worked habitually in the notoriously amorphous language of moral discourse. R. M. Hare, in one of his first contacts with bioethics, asked what moral philosophy could do for bioethics. He answered:

> Philosophers spend a lot of time talking about words . . . the thing is to get the words straight—to decide what you are going to mean by . . . moral words such as "wrong." Philosophy is a training in the study of such tricky words and their logical properties in order to establish canons of valid argument or reasoning, and so enable people who have mastered it to avoid errors in reasoning (confusions or fallacies), and so answer their moral questions with their eyes open . . . the philosophical problems having been removed, we can get on with discussing the practical difficulties, which are likely to remain serious."[48]

Clarification of "tricky words" and establishing "canons of valid argument" are not unworthy contributions to discourse; many moral philosophers have greatly clarified bioethical debate in this way. Logical clarification, however, is only a philosophical instrument. Could moral philosophy bring anything more substantive to the debates? Could it establish some fundamental views, visions, theories, or principles on which to build an ethics? As the recent history of moral philosophy reveals, few moral philosophers found this a congenial task. A rare philosopher propounded a fully rounded approach to practical ethics[49] but, for the most part, a profound skepticism about doing such a task prevailed. That skepticism about conventional philosophical approaches was fueled by a brilliant moral philosopher who appeared frequently on the bioethics agenda in the early years, Alasdair MacIntyre. He had long been interested in the social and cultural context of moral argument and had come to the conclusion that moral argument was in general fruitless because "what we are confronted with is the inheritance from a variety of sources of a variety of fragmentary moral views torn from the contexts in which they were originally at home. As a result in moral debate incommensurable premise confronts incommensurable premise. . . . we have no neutral court of appeal or testing place where these rival claims may be weighed against one common standard."[50] MacIntyre continued to develop the theme of fragmented moral concepts torn from their cultural roots, yet many of his colleagues were ready and eager to move from the metaethical to the normative, from the speculative to the practical, from a philosophy wholly academic to the public philosophy once honored in the United States.

Philosophers and the Moral Problems of the New Medicine

Hans Jonas was the first philosopher of eminence to arrive on the medical ethics scene.[51] Jonas had studied philosophy during the 1920s under the German masters, Edmund Husserl, Martin Heidegger, and Rudolf Bultmann. He had concentrated on the arcane thought of the late classical Gnostics and had achieved a considerable reputation by the time he was forced to leave Germany for Palestine in 1934. After World War II (during which he fought in the Jewish Brigade of the British Army), he came to the United States and was appointed Alvin Johnson Professor of Philosophy at The New School for Social Research. His interests turned from classical antiquity to rethinking the epistemological and metaphysical connections between mind and organism which, in his view, had been distorted by the prevalent dualism of Western philosophy. His work, *The Phenomenon of Life: Toward a Philosophical Biology* explicated his "philosophy of organism."[52]

Jonas reflected on the ethical implications of his metaphysical position in *The Imperative of Responsibility: In Search of an Ethics for the Technological Age*, in which he related the notion of human responsibility to the world of technology, which flows from human creativity and surrounds humans with danger.[53] He reframed the Kantian categorical imperative as "act so that the effects of your action are compatible with the permanence of genuine human life," or "act so that the effects of your action are not destructive of the future possibility of such life."[54] This imperative was grounded in an ontology of human and physical nature which supplies both the objectivity of moral norms and the a priori motivating force for responsibility. Jonas saw this ethic as a *Versuch*, or a search, meaning that even with powerful ontological grounding for responsibility, its extension to the range of problems faced by humans in nature and technology must be continually rethought.

Professor Jonas had not yet elaborated his ethic of responsibility in 1966. Still, his reputation as a thinker and his concentration on the deeper questions raised by biology and technology made him an appropriate invitee to participate in a study of the ethics of experimentation that the American Academy of Arts and Sciences had initiated. He produced an essay entitled "Philosophical reflections on experimenting with human subjects," which he presented at the first meeting of that project in November 1967.[55] One member of the audience, Professor William J. Curran of Harvard School of Public Health, recalled, "We all knew we were hearing something really different, really significant."[56] That essay brought together a profound philosophical mind and an appreciation of the nature of biomedical research. This landmark in the history of bioethics will be discussed in Chapter 5.

When Jonas published *Philosophical Essays: From Ancient Creed to Technological Man*, he included two bioethical chapters: a previously unpublished paper, "Against the stream," in which he criticized the revision of the definition of death, and an essay on genetic engineering.[57] In the preface, Jonas acknowledges "the many debts of gratitude I owe my colleagues of the Institute of Society, Ethics and the Life Sciences."[58] Dan Callahan had enticed Jonas into his circle at Hastings, and over the next 20 years, he was an active participant in the studies and debates over genetics, euthanasia, and deeper questions about "the nature and significance of organic, animal and human life, the nature of human responsibility and our fundamental ethical obligations to the human and natural future and the practical role of the philosopher and ethicists in the public realm."[59] Although Hans Jonas's philosophical system was, perhaps, too ontological and conservative for the typical American ethicist, he provided all nascent bioethicists an exemplar of serious, disciplined, and deep philosophical reflection.

Jonas's essays were groundbreaking philosophical contributions to bioethics. Another philosopher, Samuel Gorovitz, determined to educate philosophers about the questions raised in science and medicine and thereby entice them to contribute their philosophical acumen to the search for answers. Gorovitz won his doctorate in philosophy at the University of California, Los Angeles, where logical positivism and philosophy of science reigned supreme. In 1966, Gorovitz, who was an assistant professor of philosophy at Western Reserve University and Case Institute of Technology (later Case-Western Reserve University), published "Ethics and the allocation of medical resources" in *Medical Research Engineering*, a journal rarely touched by philosophical reflections. In that short essay, he noted that "medical research and clinical practice give rise to a wide variety of situations that call for decision making in the face of acute moral dilemmas."[60] He singled out the dilemma of selecting persons for a life-saving but scarce medical technology, as faced by the Seattle dialysis program, and raised several ethical questions about that dilemma, but offered no approach to their solution. Gorovitz concluded his essay with a plea for a more systematic study of medical ethics. He recommended the establishment of centers in which physicians and philosophers, physical and social scientists, lawyers and policy makers might address the emerging issues. He urged that pertinent conferences and journals receive financial support from universities, government, and foundations.

In 1966 this was merely a vision, but Gorovitz let his vision lead him. By 1970, he had organized a Project on Moral Problems in Medicine, with encouragement from the

Dean of Case-Western Reserve's innovative medical school, Nobelist Fred Robbins. The Project, supported by the National Endowment for the Humanities' first grant in medical ethics[61] and by the Exxon Educational Foundation, created just the center that Gorovitz had described in 1966. The small group of philosophers who constituted the Project produced an anthology, *Moral Problems in Medicine*, in which descriptions of the new problems were juxtaposed with the reflections of classical philosophers.[62]

Gorovitz realized that philosophical analysis of the problems of the new medicine needed a more focused approach than the rough propinquity between problems and principles that philosophers could provide. Philosophers needed to learn the exact dimensions of the new problems and to devise new ways to think about them. Gorovitz persuaded the Rockefeller Brothers Foundation to support a Council for Philosophical Studies Institute on Moral Problems in Medicine. The purpose of the Institute was to prepare faculty in philosophy, medicine and related fields to teach courses in medical ethics from a philosophical point of view. It met for six weeks, July 1–August 9, 1974, at Haverford College in Pennsylvania. Distinguished philosophers—William Frankena, Robert Nozick, Judith Jarvis Thomson, and Bernard Williams—served on the faculty, as did the new bioethicists from The Hastings Center, Dan Callahan, Willard Gaylin and Robert Veatch. The class included many students who would subsequently play a significant role in bioethics, among them, H. Tristram Engelhardt, Stuart Spicker, Ron Carson, Tom Beauchamp, William Ruddick, and Natalie Abrams. The Institute proved a model for many subsequent medical ethics institutes sponsored by the National Endowment for the Humanities.[63]

By the time the Haverford Institute was held, Gorovitz had moved from Case-Western to the University of Maryland. He left his Case-Western colleague, philosopher Ruth Macklin, in charge of the Moral Problems in Medicine Project. Dr. Macklin, who was also originally interested in the philosophy of science rather than ethics, began a career as the leading woman bioethicist in a field dominated by white (but not yet dead) males. Sam Gorovitz's involvement in bioethics was inhibited by his move to a deanship at Syracuse University (although he continued as a consultant to the World Health Organization activities in the field). Yet, he provided a notable stimulus to the development of bioethics and to the participation of professional philosophers in its work.[64]

K. Danner Clouser was the first philosopher appointed to the faculty of an American medical school in modern times. After taking his philosophy degree at Harvard, he taught at Dartmouth and Carleton colleges. In 1968, he was appointed to the Department of Medical Humanities, a novel academic locus in a new medical school, Pennsylvania State University at Hershey. The founding Dean, Dr. George Harrell, had been interested in fostering the study of humanities in medicine and had instituted a humanities program at his former school, the University of Florida at Gainesville. Clouser, who up to that time had little contact with medicine, was invited to Hershey by the Chair of the Humanities Department, Al Vastyan. Professor Clouser recalled this experience:

Now I found myself in a medical school. Had I made a bad career decision? Many professional philosophers had told me it was professional suicide. I had no mentors, no models, no guidance. Still, it was a good time to enter the field. You could catch up on all the extant literature on one weekend and contribute to it the next. Seriously, I was straining daily to discover the relevance of philosophy to medicine and I knew in my heart the relationship would not be obvious. . . . Yet, today we know that philosophy has contributed significantly to medical ethics. Twenty-five years ago, medical ethics was a mixture of religion, whimsy, exhortation, legal precedents, philosophies of life, miscellaneous moral rules and epithets, uttered by wise or witty physicians. I believe philosophy provided the push toward systematization, consistency and clarity. . . . Philosophy asks probing questions and understands how to discover and work with assumptions, implications and foundations. Conceptual analysis, which is central to the doing of philosophy, has been central also to the doing of medical ethics. On the other hand, I doubt that philosophy has brought much of substance, that is, what things to value, what goals are most meaningful, what philosophies of life are most fulfilling.[65]

Professor Clouser provided the emerging field with useful clarifications. His essays on what medical ethics was and what it was not warned physicians about what they could expect from this new study of their work. His article "Sanctity of life" was a helpful explication of that confusing term. His article "Bioethics," in the first edition of the *Encyclopedia of Bioethics*, proposed that "bioethics is not a new set of principles or maneuvers, but the same old ethics being applied to a particular realm of concern."[66] We shall examine his fuller exposition of that view in Chapter 10.

Dan Callahan is the philosopher who has dedicated himself to bringing to bioethics the philosophical questions of substance that Clouser found lacking. "What things to value, what goals are most meaningful, what philosophies of life are most fulfilling" have been the questions that Callahan has asked and worked to answer over thirty years. Like Dan Clouser, Dan Callahan studied philosophy at Harvard, concentrating on the philosophy of knowledge; his doctoral dissertation was on the conceptual idealism of the eighteenth-century Irishman, Bishop George Berkeley. Unlike Clouser, Callahan has never held an academic post. After graduating from Harvard, he served as managing editor of the respected Catholic journal of opinion, *Commonweal,* from 1961–1968. During his time there he engaged vigorously in two moral disputes agitating the church: contraception and abortion. He commented in the press on the former question when Pope Paul VI refused to liberalize the traditional doctrine. The papal decision had dismayed liberal Catholics; Callahan, being a liberal Catholic working at a liberal Catholic journal, turned that dismay into philosophical analysis. He edited a collection of essays expressing respectful dissent to the papal teaching.[67]

The abortion question drew him into deeper ethical waters. He received grants from the Population Council and the Ford Foundation to explore the sociological, legal, and philosophical dimensions of the abortion issue. The resulting book, *Abortion: Law, Choice and Morality*, is a monumental analysis of the problem and of the policies that might be crafted to deal with it. In this book, Callahan argues for a view of the sanctity of life that strongly inclines in favor of the preservation of human life; at the same time, he acknowledges situations of personal need that might justify abortion. On the basis of this "balancing of the right to life and the right to choose," he attempts to formulate a public policy that can, to the extent possible, respect both rights. Although read by many as a defense of abortion on demand, the book is a careful and sensitive effort to navigate the rough conceptual, emotional, and political waters of a most perplexing moral issue.[68]

When he succeeded in opening the Institute of Society, Ethics and the Life Sciences, Callahan became the impresario of a significant interdisciplinary enterprise in which philosophy played one, but by no means the dominant, part. Even as an interdisciplinary scholar, Callahan has persisted in asking the perennial philosophical questions about fundamental values and meaning of life and how these affect the ways we should think about medicine, health, birth, aging and death, medical technology, and health care. Beginning in 1973, his reflections on these questions of substance began to appear: *The Tyranny of Survival: And Other Pathologies of Civilized Life*, *Setting Limits: Medical Goals in an Aging Society*, and *What Kind of Life: The Limits of Medical Progress*.[69]

Stephen E. Toulmin, like Hans Jonas, was already distinguished in philosophy when the questions of the new biology lured him from pure philosophy to bioethics. He studied with Ludwig Wittgenstein at Cambridge University and had devoted himself largely to epistemological questions in science and mathematics. Although his foray into moral philosophy, *An Examination of the Place of Reason in Ethics*, had won him instant renown as a moral philosopher, ethics remained on the periphery of Toulmin's philosophical view, which continued to focus on the rhetoric and logic of scientific discourse. Yet, he saw an analogy between the nature of scientific judgments and the nature of moral judgments and felt that as he studied scientific discourse, he understood more about moral discourse: "In ethics, as in science, incorrigible but conflicting reports of personal experience (sensible or emotional) are replaced by judgments aiming at universality and impartiality."[70] This parallel interest in ethics and in science drew him to the doorstep of the new bioethics.

Toulmin crossed the threshold when he accepted an invitation to serve as philosophical consultant to the National Commission for the Protection of Human Subjects of Biomedical and Behavioral Research. He was then on the faculty of the Committee for Social Thought at the University of Chicago. Commissioner Donald W. Seldin and I recommended Toulmin for the position because we knew him to be well versed both in moral philosophy and in the philosophy of science. Toulmin was able to arrange a leave from his professorial duties for the first year of the Commission's activities and to continue on a part-time basis for the entire life of the Commission. He brought his conceptual skills to the formulation of the problems posed to the Commission. He shaped the agenda of the philosophical discussions and edited the texts of testimony and debate. He directed the Commission's Special Study, *Implications of Advances in Biomedical and Behavioral Research*.[71] Perhaps most importantly, his remarks during the course of the deliberations inevitably brought clarifying distinctions and critical arguments.

Toulmin left a mark on the Commission's work and the work left a mark on him. One day in 1973 or 1974, while Toulmin and I were flying somewhere on Commission business, he remarked that, although the commissioners argued interminably on matters of principle, they agreed quickly about the morality of cases. I mused that the Commission might be doing something like the "old fashioned casuistry" that I had learned in my Jesuit training. This conversation inspired us to ask the National Endowment for the Humanities to support a study of "old fashioned casuistry" and its application to contemporary ethical problems. The study resulted in our co-authored book, *The Abuse of Casuistry. A History of Moral Reasoning*. The importance of that book for the field of bioethics, as well as the theoretical problems it raises, has often been noted.[72]

Casuistry bridges the gap between the speculative doctrines of philosophy and theology and the practical demands of decision making in particular circumstances. From its beginnings, bioethics has worked at the practical level and struggled to bend the generalizations of philosophy and theology to its needs. Toulmin and I suggested that bioethicists, at their best, had been doing casuistry, and we attempted to explain how casuistry worked, in its traditional form and its contemporary applications. Toulmin encapsulated some of those ideas in a widely appreciated essay, "How medicine saved the life of ethics."[73] After the Commission closed its doors in 1978, Stephen Toulmin continued to collaborate with the medical ethics activities at the University of Chicago's Pritzker School of Medicine and to contribute to the practical and theoretical literature in the growing field.

Gradually, the intrinsically interesting questions of the new medicine lured other philosophers into the debates and many of them stayed to become bioethicists.[74] Several young men took bioethics seriously enough to combine training in medicine with education in philosophy. H. Tristram Engelhardt, Jr. is a philosophical spirit who took time out from his studies of Kant and Hegel, with John Silber at the University of Texas, to take a medical degree at Tulane Medical School. Although originally interested in the philosophy of medicine, he soon was drawn into bioethics. He was invited by medical historian Chester Burns to join the faculty at Texas Medical Branch, Galveston, where he initiated ethics courses for medical students and consultation on the wards. He left Galveston to take the Joseph P. Kennedy, Sr. Chair at Georgetown in 1977; he returned to Texas to join Baruch Brody in the Program in Medical Humanities at Houston's Rice University in 1983. He made a major contribution to the intellectual quality of bioethics by founding, with Edmund Pellegrino, the *Journal of Medicine and Philosophy*, the first issue of which appeared in 1976. With another philosopher-bioethicist, Stuart F. Spicker of the University of Connecticut, he initiated a long-lasting series of conferences on medicine and philosophy, which has produced an impressive series of volumes.[75] Engelhardt has been the *enfant terrible* of bioethics: irrepressible, irreverent, unpredictable, but ever insightful and brilliant. His contribution to theory in bioethics will be discussed in Chapter 10.

A second physician, Howard Brody, completed a dual degree program in medicine and philosophy at Michigan State University in 1976 and 1977. Unlike Engelhardt, who never practiced medicine, Brody has continued to practice family medicine, giving his writing the flavor of clinical reality. His doctoral dissertation was a critical dissection of an ancient problem of medical ethics: the use of placebos—inert substances deceptively prescribed as genuine medications. Brody authored the first ethics textbook expressly designed for medical students.[76] From his position at Michigan State University School of Human Medicine, he issued a stream of philosophically astute and clinically realistic essays and books that have won the respect of ethicists and physicians alike.

Philosophy and Theology in Dialogue

Many persons who studied and took degrees in academic philosophy were pioneers in bioethics. Their philosophical studies, however, did not mold their minds in any uniform way. Apart from the European-educated Jonas, the young American philosophers were introduced to the Anglo-American philosophical fashions, which included logic and epistemology and the application of both these subjects to the philosophy of science. Moral philosophy was generally out of fashion. The heritage of the American philosophers of previous generations was neglected. No overarching philosophical theory, such as idealism or empiricism, dominated. Logical positivism was widely favored, less as an overarching theory than as a method of analysis to be applied to other disciplines and activities. The philosophers who immigrated into bioethics, then, were unlikely to bring an orthodoxy or a common methodology. They would bring, however, two characteristics of mind that philosophical study has always fostered: a desire for clarity in definition of terms and in logic of argument, and a desire to work down to the foundations of knowledge and experience. This talent was a valuable addition to the emerging bioethics, for it started to give articulate shape to the thoughtful but random conversations of the conferences. The philosophers, almost unknowingly, brought another contribution: as they plunged into practical problems, they shed the metaethical speculation that was so unsuited to the resolution of moral quandaries. They reinvented, in an unconscious atavism, the style of public philosophy that William James and John Dewey had invented decades before. The bioethics that was to come engaged the facts of the case, explored alternative solutions, tested these against the opinions of many participants and worked to turn principles into practice.

The philosophers joined the theologians as shapers of the field of bioethics. The merger was not a facile one. The two disciplines had lived apart for many years, and each had developed different methods and vocabulary. Above all, they differed profoundly in their purposes: theologians studied ethics in order to educate their congregations in the moral life; philosophers pondered ethics in order to unravel conceptual puzzles and probe theoretical foundations. They did not easily learn to converse. Dan Callahan recalls, "One of my toughest problems during the Hastings Center's first twenty years was persuading the philosophers to sit down with the theologians and to take them seriously. The secular philosophers could not give a damn for what the theologians were saying and were even scornful."[77] Indeed, some philosophers not only scorned theologians but the whole enterprise of bioethics, considering it a cheap purveying of proper philosophy.[78] Still, a dialogue was opened, and in the settings of The Hastings Center and The Kennedy Institute, the government Commissions and the medical school programs, the theologians and the philosophers began to find a common language and slowly merged into bioethicists.

Just as a trinity of theologians—Fletcher, Ramsey and McCormick—presided over the birth of bioethics, so a quintet of philosophers—Jonas, Gorovitz, Clouser, Callahan, and Toulmin—were also present. Each brought a distinct tradition and perspective, together with analytic skills sharpened by their disciplines. Together they produced an amalgam of ideas, methods, and educational structures that became bioethics. In their wake, others came from theology and philosophy into a field that had been plowed and partially planted. But, as often noted, the field was interdisciplinary. Callahan, Gustafson, and Gorovitz, in particular, insisted that the questions of the new biology be studied across disciplinary and professional lines. Physicians, such as André Hellegers, Jay Katz, Willard Gaylin, Eric Cassell, Bernard Towers, Leon Kass, and Edmund Pellegrino, became active colleagues of the philosophers and theologians. Sociologists such as Renée Fox and Bernard Barber, recognizing the social dimensions of these issues, added their voices. Lawyers, such as Paul Freund, Angela Holder, William Curran, John Robertson, and Charles Fried, brought law and jurisprudence into the discussions. Two lawyers, George Annas and Alexander Morgan Capron, were not loath to be called bioethicists. By the early 1970s, a genuine interdisciplinary conversation had blossomed, with its fruit a growing literature in which philosophy, theology, law, and other disciplines melded to describe, analyze, and advise on the questions of the new biology and the new medicine. By 1972, the conversation was mature enough that Warren Reich could conceive the epitome of interdisciplinarity, *The Encyclopedia of Bioethics*, and execute it by soliciting contributions from a rich mix of scholars.

Notes for Chapter 3

1. Dan Callahan, "Why America accepted bioethics," (paper read at the Birth of Bioethics Conference, Seattle, Wa., Sept. 23–24, 1992), transcript p. 354.

2. Vernon J. Bourke, *History of Ethics* (Garden City, New York: Doubleday, 1968); Alasdair MacIntyre, *A Short History of Ethics* (New York: Macmillan, 1966); Henry Sidgwick, *Outline of the History of Ethics* (London: Macmillan, 1886). On the transition of late scholasticism, see Bonnie Kent, *Virtues of the Will. The Transformation of Ethics in the Late Thirteenth Century* (Washington, D.C.: Catholic University of America Press, 1995).

3. Cotton Mather, *Manductio ad Ministerium* (1726), ed. Thomas J. Holmes and Kenneth Murdock (New York: Columbia University Press, 1939), p. 39; cited in Norman Fiering, *Moral Philosophy at Seventeenth Century Harvard: A Discipline in Transition* (Chapel Hill: University of North Carolina Press, 1981), p. 40.

4. Norman Fiering, *Jonathan Edwards' Moral Thought and Its British Context* (Chapel Hill:

University of North Carolina Press, 1981); Paul Ramsey (ed.), *Jonathan Edwards: Ethical Writings* (New Haven: Yale University Press, 1989).

5. Richard Price, *Observations on the Nature of Civil Liberty, the Principles of Government, and the Justice and Policy of the War with America* (London: T. Cadell and J. Johnson, 1776), I, p. 3.

6. Fiering, *Jonathan Edwards' Moral Thought*, p. 299.

7. Bruce Kuklick, *The Rise of American Philosophy: Cambridge, Massachusetts 1860–1930* (New Haven: Yale University Press, 1977), p. 9.

8. Wilson Smith, *Professors and Public Ethics: Studies of Northern Moral Philosophers Before the Civil War* (Ithaca: Cornell University Press, 1956). I have not found any concern over the "Indian question" expressed by the presidents, although Dartmouth's presiding officers must have spoken out, since it was founded for the education of Native Americans.

9. Francis Wayland, *Elements of Moral Science* (Boston: Gould and Lincoln, 1835) was the most widely used text in moral philosophy and was translated into many languages (including Hawaiian). A tour through the *Elements* reveals what college-educated Americans were taught about their moral duties. The textbook is divided into "Theoretical Ethics" and "Practical Ethics." "Theoretical Ethics" comprises an exposition on moral law, conscience, and virtues that draws heavily on the Scottish common-sense philosophy of Dugald Stewart, Thomas Reid, and Sir William Hamilton. Conscience is defined as a constituent power of the mind that distinguishes right from wrong by judging the intention of actions; moral law itself, which conscience grasps intuitively, is implanted in human nature by God and becomes evident as the human mind apprehends the relations between created beings. In light of this moral sense, principles are ascertained with certainty and the purported relativism of utilitarianism is refuted. Practical ethics, deduced from moral law, comprises obedience and reverence toward God, and reciprocity and benevolence toward humans. These principles command veracity, justice, chastity, and familial and social order. Wayland's book presents a bland picture of moral character: honest, obedient, monogamous. Wayland, however, was less than bland as a public philosopher. He vigorously opposed the Mexican war. His increasing conviction of the evil of slavery led to a reluctant approval of military action to suppress succession in 1861. So, a moral philosopher whose academic persona fostered conventional virtues displayed a vigorous engagement in the political affairs of the nation which were, in his eyes, moral questions.

10. Henry Thoreau, "Resistance to civil government," in Wendell Glick (ed.), *Reform Papers* (Princeton: Princeton University Press, 1973), pp. 63–90. This essay, written in 1846 after Thoreau's brief stay in the Concord jail for failure to pay his poll tax, was a refutation of William Paley, "The duty of submission to civil government explained," in *The Principles of Moral and Political Philosophy*, VI, iii. Thoreau's essay was required reading in the ethics course I taught at University of San Francisco in the 1960s.

11. Robert Richardson, *Henry Thoreau: A Life of the Mind* (Berkeley: University of California Press, 1986), p. 175.

12. John Edwin Smith, *The Spirit of American Philosophy* (New York and Oxford: Oxford University Press, 1963), pp. 196–210.

13. William James, "The moral philosopher and the moral life," *International Journal of Ethics* (April 1891); reprinted in John J. McDermott (ed.), *The Writings of William James* (New York: Random House, 1967), pp. 610–628.

14. James, "The moral philosopher and the moral life," p. 623.

15. James, "The moral philosopher and the moral life," pp. 611, 621, 623–625, 627. James illustrated his thesis about the strenuous ethical life nowhere more fully than in his essay, "The moral equivalent of war," a title that President John F. Kennedy appropriated to describe the Peace Corps. He proposed that "our gilded youth" be conscripted into a corps to do strenuous

public labor so that "the military ideals of hardihood and discipline would be wrought into the growing fibre of the people; no one would remain blind as the luxurious classes now are blind, to man's relations to the globe he lives on." *McClure's Magazine* (August 1910) and *Popular Science Monthly* (October 1910); reprinted in McDermott, *The Writings of William James*, pp. 660–671. See Kim Townsend, *Manhood at Harvard. William James and Others* (New York: W. W. Norton, 1996).

16. Gerald E. Myers, *William James: His Life and Thought* (Yale University Press, 1986), p. 429; John J. McDermott, "The renascence of classical American philosophy," in *Streams of Experience: Reflections on the History and Philosophy of American Culture* (Amherst: University of Massachusetts Press, 1986), pp. 223–234.

17. Henry Steele Commager, *The American Mind: An Interpretation of American Thought and Character Since the 1880s* (New Haven: Yale University Press, 1950), p. 100.

18. John Dewey and James H. Tufts, *Ethics* (New York: H. Holt and Company, 1908), pp. 393, 396.

19. Dewey and Tufts, *Ethics*, p. 334.

20. John Dewey, *Human Nature and Conduct: An Introduction to Social Psychology* (New York: Henry Holt, 1922), p. 239.

21. Dewey, *Human Nature and Conduct*, p. 296.

22. John Edwin Smith, *The Spirit of American Philosophy* (New York and Oxford: Oxford University Press, 1963), p. 140. See John J. McDermott (ed.), *The Philosophy of John Dewey* (New York: Putnam Sons, 1973); James Campbell, *Understanding John Dewey: Nature and Co-operative Intelligence* (Chicago: Open Court Press, 1995); Alan Ryan, *John Dewey and the High Tide of American Liberalism* (New York: W. W. Norton, 1995); and Franklin G. Miller, Joseph Fins, and Matthew D. Bachetta, "Clinical pragmatism: John Dewey and clinical ethics." *Journal of Contemporary Health Law and Policy* 13 (1) (1996): 27–52. Dewey made a strong plea for philosophers to turn from speculation about logic and epistemology to practical reflection on politics, morals, economics, and education in *Reconstruction in Philosophy* (New York: Henry Holt, 1920).

23. Ryan, *John Dewery and the High Tide of American Liberalism*.

24. Smith, *The Spirit of American Philosophy*, p. 188.

25. G. E. Moore, *Principia Ethica* (Cambridge: Cambridge University Press, 1903; reprinted in 1960); John Dewey, *Quest for Certainty: A Study of the Relation of Knowledge and Action* (New York: Minton, Balch, 1929).

26. Alfred Jules Ayer, *Language, Logic and Truth* (New York: Dover Publications, 1936).

27. Charles L. Stevenson, "The emotive meaning of ethical terms," *Mind* 46 (1937): 10–31; "Persuasive definitions," *Mind* 47 (1938): 331–350; *Ethics and Language* (New Haven: Yale University Press, 1944).

28. John Dewey, "Ethical subject matter and language," *Journal of Philosophy* 42 (1945): 703.

29. A. J. Ayer, "On analysis of moral judgments," *Horizon* 20 (1949): 117; L. W. Sumner, "Normative ethics and meta-ethics," *Ethics* 77 (January 1967): 95–105, p. 95; W. D. Hudson, *Modern Moral Philosophy* (Garden City, New York: Anchor Books, 1970), p. 1; Patrick H. Nowell-Smith, *Ethics* (London: Penguin, 1954).

30. William K. Frankena, "Moral philosophy at mid-century," *The Philosophical Review* 60 (1951), pp. 44–55, quotes on pp. 50, 54.

31. Mary Warnock, *Ethics Since 1900* (London: Oxford University Press, 1960), pp. 203–204.

32. William Frankena, "Moral philosophy at mid-century," *The Philosophical Review* 60 (1951): 44–55; Richard B. Brandt, *Moral Philosophy and the Analysis of Language. The Lindley Lecture* (Lawrence: University of Kansas Press, 1963); Henry Aiken, *Reason and Conduct: New*

Bearings in Moral Philosophy (New York: Knopf, 1962); Marcus George Singer, *Generalization in Ethics: An Essay in the Logic of Ethics* (New York: Knopf, 1961).

33. John Rawls, "Outline of decision procedure for ethics," *The Philosophical Review* 60 (1951): 177–198, quote on p. 177.

34. John Rawls, *A Theory of Justice* (Cambridge: Belknap Press of Harvard University Press, 1971).

35. Roderick Firth, "Ethical absolutism and the ideal observer," *Philosophy and Phenomenological Research* 13 (1952): 317–345, p. 320; Richard B. Brandt, "The definition of an 'Ideal Observer' in ethics," *Philosophy and Phenomenological Research* 16 (1955): 407–423; Richard B. Brandt, *Ethical Theory* (Englewood Cliffs: Prentice-Hall, 1959), pp. 244–259; William Frankena, "The principles of morality," in Curtis L. Carter (ed.), *Skepticism and Moral Principles: Modern Ethics in Review* (Evanston, Illinois: New University Press, 1973), pp. 43–76; Henry D. Aiken, "The concept of moral objectivity," in Hector-Neri Casteñeda and George Nakhnikian (eds.), *Morality and the Language of Conduct* (Detroit: Wayne State University Press, 1963), pp. 69–106; reprinted in Aiken, *Reason and Conduct*, pp. 134–170.

36. Patrick H. Nowell-Smith, *Ethics* (London: Penguin, 1954); Stuart Hampshire, *Thought and Action* (London: Chatto and Windus, 1959); Kurt Baier, *The Moral Point of View* (Ithaca: Cornell University Press, 1958).

37. Stephen E. Toulmin, *An Examination of the Place of Reason in Ethics* (Cambridge: Cambridge University Press, 1950). See Frankena's review in *The Philosophical Review* 60 (1951): 44–55 and Hare's review in *Philosophical Quarterly* 1 (1950): 372–375. Also see George C. Kerner, *The Revolution in Ethical Theory* (New York: Oxford University Press, 1966), chapter 3.

38. Richard M. Hare, *The Language of Morals* (Oxford: Clarendon Press, 1952); *Freedom and Reason* (Oxford: Clarendon Press, 1963).

39. Frankena, "Moral philosophy at mid-century," p. 55.

40. Ronald M. Green, "Health care and justice in contract theory perspective," in Robert H. Veatch, (ed.), *Ethics and Health Policy* (Cambridge, Mass.: Ballinger, 1976), pp. 111–126; Norman Daniels, *Just Health Care* (New York: Cambridge University Press, 1985).

41. This division was, I believe, first proposed by C. D. Broad, *Five Types of Ethical Theory* (New York: Harcourt Brace, 1930). He did not, however, intend it to cover all normative discourse but only theories of obligation.

42. Harlan B. Miller and William H. Williams (eds.), *The Limits of Utilitarianism* (Minneapolis: University of Minnesota Press, 1982); Curtis Carter (ed.), *Skepticism and Moral Principles: Modern Ethics in Review* (Evanston: New University Press, 1973).

43. Jonsen and Toulmin, *Abuse of Casuistry*, p. 394.

44. G. E. Moore, *Principia Ethica*, pp. 4–5.

45. See, for example, Hannah Arendt, *Eichmann in Jerusalem: A Report on the Banality of Evil* (New York: Penguin, 1964); *Antisemitism: Part One of the Origins of Totalitarianism* (New York: Harcourt, Brace and World, 1951); *Imperialism: Part Two of the Origins of Totalitarianism* (New York: Harcourt, Brace and World, 1951); Sidney Hook, *Revolution, Reform, and Social Justice: Studies in the Theory and Practice of Marxism* (New York: New York University Press, 1975); *Common Sense and the Fifth Amendment* (New York: Criterion Books, 1957).

46. Warnock, *Ethics Since 1900*, p. 204.

47. The lectures and discussions of the meeting are published in *Ethics* 79 (1968); Noam Chomsky, "Philosophers and public policy," pp. 1–9, quote on p. 9; John Silber, "Soul politics and political morality," pp. 14–23, quote on p. 14.

48. Richard M. Hare, "Medical ethics: can the moral philosopher help?" in Stuart Spicker and H. Tristram Engelhardt, Jr. (eds.), *Philosophical Medical Ethics: Its Nature and Significance* (Dordrecht and Boston: D. Reidel Publishing Company, 1977), p. 52. Professor John Ladd re-

minded me that "In the late 1950s, progressive philosophers became interested in philosophy of law. . . . This emancipated ethics. H. L. A. Hart was, of course, very influential." Personal communication, April 28, 1997. See H. L. A. Hart, *The Concept of Law* (Oxford: The Clarendon Press, 1961).

49. Bernard Gert, *The Moral Rules: A New Rational Foundation for Morality* (New York: Harper and Row, 1970); see also Gert with Charles M. Culver, *Philosophy in Medicine: Conceptual and Ethical Issues in Medicine and Psychiatry* (New York: Oxford University Press, 1982).

50. MacIntyre, "Patients as agents," in Spicker and Engelhardt, *Philosophical Medical Ethics*, pp. 197–212, quote on p. 198.

51. The first philosophical contribution to medical ethics, to my knowledge, came from Samuel E. Stumpf who, although educated as a theologian, was chairman of the Philosophy Department at Vanderbilt University and had worked with the physicians at Vanderbilt's Clinical Research Center. He was invited to lecture at the annual meeting of the American College of Physicians in 1965 and again at the ACP Colloquium on Ethical Dilemmas in 1967. He did not continue his interest in medical ethics, but became a college president. See Stumpf, "Some moral dimensions of medicine," *Annals of Internal Medicine* 64 (1966): 460–470; "Momentum and morality in medicine," in J. R. Elkington (ed.), "The Changing Mores of Biomedical Research," *Annals of Internal Medicine* 67, suppl. 7 (1967): 10–14.

52. Hans Jonas, *The Phenomenon of Life: Toward a Philosophical Biology* (New York: Harper and Row, 1966); Leon Kass, "Appreciating the phenomenon of life," *Hastings Center Report* 25, no. 7 (1995): 3–12.

53. Hans Jonas, *The Imperative of Responsibility: In Search of an Ethics for the Technological Age* (Chicago: University of Chicago Press, 1984, published in German in 1979); Richard Bernstein, "Rethinking responsibility," *Hastings Center Report* 25, no. 7 (1995): 13–20.

54. Jonas, *The Imperative of Responsibility* p. 11.

55. Hans Jonas, "Philosophical reflections on experimenting with human subjects," (Lecture presented at American Academy of Arts and Sciences, November 1967), *Daedalus* 98, no. 2 (1969): 219–247.

56. Interview with William Curran, March 15, 1997.

57. Hans Jonas, *Philosophical Essays: From Ancient Creed to Technological Man* (Englewood Cliffs, N.J.: Prentice-Hall, 1974).

58. Jonas, *Philosophical Essays*, p. vi.

59. Strachan Donnelley, "The legacy of Hans Jonas," *Hastings Center Report* 25, no. 7 (1995): 2; Hans Jonas, "The right to die," *Hastings Center Report* 8, no. 4 (1978): 31–36; Marion Donhoff and Reinhard Merel, "Not compassion alone: on euthanasia and ethics" (interview with Jonas, 1989), *Hastings Center Report* 25, no. 7 (1995): 44–50; Jonas, "Straddling the boundaries of theory and practice: recombinant DNA research as a case of action in the process of inquiry," in John Richards (ed.), *Recombinant DNA: Science, Ethics and Politics* (New York: Academic Press, 1978), 253–271.

60. Samuel Gorovitz, "Ethics and the allocation of medical resources," *Medical Research Engineering* 5, no. 4 (1966): 5–7, quote on p. 5.

61. National Endowment for the Humanities, grant EH-6028-72-111.

62. Samuel Gorovitz, Andrew L. Jameton, Ruth Macklin, et al. (eds.), *Moral Problems in Medicine* (Englewood Cliffs: Prentice-Hall, 1976). Gorovitz claimed that this volume was the first textbook in bioethics but Richard W. Wertz had produced *Readings on Ethical and Social Issues in Biomedicine* three years earlier from the same publisher.

63. William Ruddick, a graduate of the Institute, established the Philosophers in Medical Centers Program, which, from 1976 to 1980, situated philosophers in several leading medical centers in New York. The program was supported by the National Endowment for the Humanities and

the New York Council for the Humanities. It resulted in several permanent medical ethics programs and produced some competent bioethicists. See Ruddick, *Philosophers in Medical Centers* (New York: The Society for Philosophy and Public Affairs, 1980); Ruddick and W. Finn, "Objections to hospital philosophers," *Journal of Medical Ethics* 11 (1985): 42–46.

64. Samuel Gorovitz, *The Doctor's Dilemma: Moral Conflicts and Medical Care* (New York: Macmillan, 1982).

65. K. Danner Clouser, "What bioethics brought to philosophy," (a paper read at the Birth of Bioethics Conference, Seattle, Wa., Sept. 23–24, 1992), transcript pp. 532–542.

66. K. Danner Clouser, "Bioethics," in Warren Reich (ed.), *The Encyclopedia of Bioethics*, 1st ed. (New York: The Free Press, 1978), vol. 1, p. 116; "Medical ethics: some uses, abuses, and limitations," *New England Journal of Medicine* 293 (1975): 384; "What is medical ethics?" *Annals of Internal Medicine* 80 (1974): 657; " 'The sanctity of life': an analysis of a concept," *Annals of Internal Medicine* 78 (1973): 119–25.

67. Daniel Callahan, *The Catholic Case for Contraception* (New York: Macmillan, 1969).

68. Daniel Callahan, *Abortion: Law, Choice and Morality* (New York: Macmillan, 1970); "Abortion: Thinking and experiencing," *Christianity and Crisis* 32 (1973): 295–298; in criticism, see Paul Ramsey, "Abortion: a review article," *The Thomist* 37 (1973): 174–226.

69. Daniel Callahan, *The Tyranny of Survival: And Other Pathologies of Civilized Life* (New York: Macmillan, 1973); *Setting Limits: Medical Goals in an Aging Society* (New York: Simon and Schuster, 1987); *What Kind of Life: The Limits of Medical Progress* (New York: Simon and Schuster, 1990).

70. Toulmin, *Place of Reason in Ethics*, p. 125.

71. National Commission for the Protection of Human Subjects of Biomedical and Behavioral Research, *Implications of Advances in Biomedical and Behavioral Research* (Washington, D.C.: U.S. Government Printing Office, 1978).

72. Albert R. Jonsen and Stephen E. Toulmin, *The Abuse of Casuistry. A History of Moral Reasoning* (Berkeley and Los Angeles: University of California Press, 1988). See Edwin R. DuBose, Ron Hamel, and Laurence J. O'Connell (eds.), *A Matter of Principles? Ferment in American Bioethics* (Valley Forge: Trinity Press International, 1994); "Theories and Methods in Bioethics: Principlism and its Critics" (special issue), *Kennedy Institute of Ethics Journal* 5, no. 3 (1995); Eric T. Juengst, "Casuistry and the locus of certainty in ethics," *Medical Humanities Review* 3 (1989): 19–27.

73. Stephen Toulmin, "How medicine saved the life of ethics," *Perspectives in Biology and Medicine* 24 (1982): 736–750.

74. Among those philosophers were William Winslade, who also brought degrees in law and a diploma in psychoanalysis, Tom Beauchamp, Daniel Wikler, Dan Brock, Baruch Brody, Andrew Jameton, Richard Zaner, Arthur Caplan, Loretta Kopelman, Susan Sherwin, and Sissela Bok. I would have liked to chronicle the contributions of each to the field but limitations of space prohibits this.

75. Stuart F. Spicker and H. Tristram Engelhardt, Jr. (eds.), *Philosophy and Medicine Series* (Dordrecht and Boston: Kluwer Academic Publishers, 1974–present day).

76. Brody's thesis became *Placebos and the Philosophy of Medicine: Clinical, Conceptual and Ethical Issues* (Chicago: University of Chicago Press, 1980). The textbook was *Ethical Decisions in Medicine* (Boston: Little, Brown, 1976). See also *Stories of Sickness* (New Haven: Yale University Press, 1987).

77. Daniel Callahan, personal communication, December 11, 1996.

78. See K. Danner Clouser and Loretta Kopelman (eds.), "Philosophical Critiques of Bioethics" (special issue), *Journal of Medicine and Philosophy* 15 (1990).

4

Commissioning Bioethics: The Government in Bioethics, 1974–1983

The 1960s was the era of conferences, when scientists and a few other scholars gathered, as René Dubos had said, "to air" the issues. The speakers at those conferences were enthusiastic about the achievements of biomedicine and agonized over their attendant adverse effects on society. In 1968, that enthusiasm and agony moved momentarily from academic auditoria into the halls of Congress. This chapter reviews the federal government's entry into bioethics, beginning with Congressional hearings and moving to legislation establishing two federal commissions to study bioethical issues, The National Commission for the Protection of Human Subjects of Biomedical and Behavioral Research (The National Commission) and The President's Commission for the Study of Ethical Problems in Medicine and Biomedical and Behavioral Research (The President's Commission). The work of these bodies both profited from and contributed to the development of bioethics.

The Mondale Hearings of 1968

Senator Walter Mondale (D-MN) was attuned to developing issues in the biomedical sciences. He had close ties to the University of Minnesota where pioneering work, particularly in organ transplantation, was being done. He judged that the time had come for a national debate on the directions that medical science should take in American society. On February 8, 1968, Mondale introduced Senate Joint Resolution 145, calling for the establishment of a President's Commission on Health Science and Society. He cited genetic engineering and heart transplantation as areas of scientific advance that raised profound questions. On March 8–9, 21–22, 27–28, and April 2, 1968, the Subcommittee on Government Research of the Senate Committee on Government Operations heard testimony on Mondale's resolution. Chairman Fred Harris (D-OK) opened the first hearing with the remark, "the question is whether social institutions, national resources and policies can keep pace with medical advances." These hearings "were designed to stimulate a national dialogue on the implications of these advances." Mondale then spoke: "Recent medical advances raise grave and fundamental ethical and legal questions for our society. Who shall live and who shall die? how long shall life be preserved and how should it be altered? who will make decisions? how shall society be prepared." He proposed that his commission study organ transplantation, genetic engineering, behavior control, experimentation on humans, and the financing of research. The Senator noted that many scientists and the broader public concurred with his concerns.[1]

A constellation of scientists appeared before the committee. All of them praised the biomedical advances that disquieted Senator Mondale. Most witnesses were willing to admit that the advances did have some troubling aspects, but suggested that those aspects were often exaggerated. They supported the idea of a commission, but each scientist issued caveats. Transplant surgeon Adrian Kantrowitz felt that the ethical issues of transplantation did not differ from other ethical problems encountered in medical practice. If a commission were established, "physicians should predominate in its membership." He also worried that "we are stepping into areas in the development of medicine where a certain amount of boldness is necessary for success. . . . I am not sure that committees have established a reputation for courage and boldness."[2] Stanford University transplant surgeon Norman Shumway felt that a commission would educate the public about advances but did not believe that selection of patients or determination of death posed serious problems. Biochemist Arthur Kornberg supported a commission because it would signal to the public that research was a sound investment, but he, too, was reluctant to admit that there were many real problems. He did not see any immediate legal or ethical problems in the work on gene structure. Quizzed by Senator Abe Ribicoff (D) about the dangers of creating "a master race," Dr. Kornberg responded, "the problems that genetic engineering may bring are fortunately not yet upon us." More good science and sharing knowledge with the public and fellow scientists, he said, would encourage "socially responsible research." Increased funding for research was certainly desirable. Mondale remarked that Dr. Kornberg seemed reluctant "to have persons other than the people in your laboratory look at the social implications."

To this lukewarm response, the enthusiastic support of Nobelist Joshua Lederberg was a tonic. Appearing twice before the committee, he opened his first remarks with the pronouncement, "the real subject of these hearings is nothing less than the question how the human species can foresee and plan its own future. . . . transplantation and the replication of DNA are only the most visible examples of a tremendous biological revolution." His only problem with the commission was its brief term of life: "It should not make substantive prescriptions, after just one year's study, about the biological policy of the human species. . . . I favor the inquiry, but I believe it should be a continuing process, not confined to a one-year term." Its function would be to foster a con-

tinuing debate, not locking us "into contemporary values just at the time we are beginning to learn the way to a liberal or at least a pluralistic approach to many vital questions."[3] Dr. Henry Beecher also gave warm support: "there are limits which even medical science cannot go beyond, without violating higher moral rules. . . . these limits
can be spelled out, not in terms of rigid codes, but in terms of spirit . . . by study by a
multidisciplinary committee." He gave as examples the Harvard Brain Death Committee over which he had presided and the Seattle Artificial Kidney Committee.[4]

Three theologians appeared as witnesses, Dean Jerald Brauer of the University of
Chicago Divinity School, Rev. Kenneth Vaux of the Institute of Religion, University of
Texas Medical Center, and Father Albert Moraczewski. Dean Brauer spoke eloquently
about the need for public discussion. He also voiced the same concern as had Lederberg: "I hope the Commission will be free to take a fresh look and not be bound by past
investigative procedures. . . . it requires imagination and boldness . . . and should
be very broad in makeup."[5] Kenneth Vaux proclaimed, "As theologians, we have one
thing to say to the decisionmaking persons of our society. It is simply a human plea that
we get our priorities straight. If we achieve physical authority in the world by means of
military power and technical mastery of environment by our scientific ingenuity, what
good is it if human values and even man himself are eradicated in the process. In ancient and more profound words: 'what will it profit us if we gain the whole world and
forfeit our soul?' " Chairman Harris was moved to remark, "we have heard the voice of
conscience here this morning."[6]

Conscience may have spoken, but not to everyone. The scientists who spoke in the
next session were overtly hostile to Mondale's proposal. The one witness most in the
spotlight at the time, South African heart transplant surgeon Dr. Christiaan Barnard,
showed scant respect for the American senators sitting before him; he was not, after all,
dependent upon them for financial support. He opened his testimony boldly: "If you
mean by commission that you should have a qualified group of doctors belonging to the
institution where the transplant is done, then I have nothing further to say. . . . But if
you are trying to set up a commission which is different, I must say that you are seeing
ghosts where there are no ghosts. If I am in competition with my colleagues of this
country, which I am not, and were I completely selfish, then I would welcome such a
commission, because it would put the doctors who embark on this type of treatment so
far behind me, and hamper the doctors so much that I will go so far ahead that they will
never catch up with me." He denied that anything was new about the issues doctors
faced. When Senator Ribicoff suggested that what was new was the public paying the
costs, Barnard responded sharply, "Who pays the costs of war? The public! Who decides where the general should attack? The public? The public is not qualified to make
the decision. The general makes the decision. He is qualified to spend the public's
money the best way he thinks fit." The committee would be "an insult to your
doctors."[7]

Barnard was followed by his mentor and the mentor of many surgeons, the revered
Owen Wangensteen, Professor Emeritus of Surgery at Walter Mondale's own Univer-

sity of Minnesota. Dr. Wangensteen was even more skeptical than his pupil. He reminded his listeners that many controversies had raged over new developments that are now mundane: "When looked at in prospect, there is often a frenzied, frantic, even maniacal pitch of reaction. . . . If we are to retain a place of eminence in medicine, let us take care not to shackle the investigator with unnecessary strictures, which will dry up untapped resources of creativity." When Mondale asked whether non-physicians might offer valuable insights, Wangensteen replied, "If you are thinking of theologians, lawyers, philosophers and others to give some direction . . . I cannot see how they could help. . . . the fellow who holds the apple can peel it best."[8]

A representative of the American Heart Association, Dr. Jesse Edwards, carried a similar negative message. He had come from a meeting of the American College of Cardiology in San Francisco, where, as *Time* magazine reported, "in some surgeons' minds, Mondale's proposal has blurred into the fearsome specter of having a commission decide on each individual transplant." At the San Francisco meeting, another of Barnard's teachers, Dr. C. Walton Lillehei, said, "Decisions regarding transplantation are better left to those who are doing the work rather than to self-appointed critics who are better versed in the art of criticism than in the field under study. . . . they are people who are frustrated by their own inability to create."[9] Dr. Edwards told the senators that legislation would hamper progress. Ethical problems, if there were any, should be dealt with by "such highly qualified groups as the American Hospital Association Committee on Ethics." "We do not believe," said Edwards, "that the time is ripe for a full-dress government inquiry into these complicated technical questions."[10]

The Mondale Hearings opened a door on the melange of ideas and emotions that were in play in 1968: expression of concern about biomedical advances was countered by concern about interference in the progress of science. These hearings, interesting as they were, represented little progress over the many conferences produced by colleges and professional societies, where the issues were "aired." The mandate of the proposed commission was so broad that its *modus operandi* was likely to be more airing of the issues and, indeed, some of the witnesses, such as surgeon John Najarian, so warned the committee. Despite the politic politeness of most of the scientific witnesses, Walter Mondale came away discouraged. He later commented that "I was frankly taken aback by the spirited opposition expressed by several prominent men in the health sciences. Considering that I had merely proposed the establishment of a Presidential study commission, it was difficult to understand the opposition. . . . there were those who testified that there were really no new issues presented by the latest developments. . . . some did condescend to admit that they would appreciate continued—or increased—financial support from the government for their endeavors. But please don't distract us with any questions. Because of such opposition to the proposal in the 1968 hearings, and, in the absence of any substantial pressure for its approval, no action was taken on the bill."[11]

Senator Mondale persisted, reintroducing S.J. 145 as S.J. 71 in 1971. The skepticism also persisted. At the hearings on his reintroduced resolution, on November 9, 1971,

Assistant Secretary for Health, Dr. Merlin Duval, was the naysayer. He commended the NIH efforts to regulate research and several other activities, such as the Fogerty-Hastings Conference on Genetics. Senators Kennedy, Mondale, and Dominick were frustrated; they pushed Duval for a direct response on the administration's views. Dr. Duval answered, "we are taking the position at this time that legislation is not necessary." Mondale commented with exasperation, "all we are proposing here is to create a measly little study commission to look at some very profound issues. . . . I sense an almost psychopathic objection to the public process, a fear that if the public gets involved, it is going to be anti-science, hostile and unsupportive."[12] The Senator would not give up, reintroducing his legislation in 1973, when it passed as S.J. 71, calling for the establishment of an Advisory Commission on Health Science and Society to perform "a comprehensive study of the ethical, social and legal implications of advances in biomedical research and technology." These words were incorporated in the legislation that established the National Commission for the Protection of Human Subjects.

The Kennedy Hearings of 1973

Georgetown University students and faculty frequent "The Tombs," a basement pub in "The 1789," a popular Georgetown restaurant. Dr. André Hellegers lunched and held office hours in a corner booth, dispensing wit, wisdom, scientific knowledge, and political acumen to all who sought it. Having recently been appointed professor in the fledgling field of bioethics, I went there to consult him on April 10, 1973. As we were eating lunch, a waiter called him to the phone. After ten minutes, Dr. Hellegers returned, saying in his British-tinged Dutch accent, "That was Eunice Shriver. She wanted to discuss what should be done to stop the fetal research that was reported in this morning's *Post*."

I had read the story: the NIH had released a recommendation from one of its advisory panels, the Human Embryology and Development Study Section, that "encouraged the use of newly delivered live fetuses for medical research before they died." These fetuses, delivered intact as the result of a late abortion, could be briefly maintained alive while studies were done that might improve the care of future mothers and children. One scientist commented, "I don't think it is unethical. It's not possible to make this fetus into a child, therefore, we can consider it as nothing more than a piece of tissue." Dr. Hellegers, himself a member of the Study Section, was cited in opposition to the recommendation. Referring to the philosophy behind the Nazi experiments, he said ironically, "If it's going to die, you might as well use it." An NIH official was quoted stating that the NIH did not support such work.[13] In the following days, other articles appeared, casting doubt on the NIH official's denial. Several specific projects were reported, each performed by NIH-funded American scientists in Finland, Denmark, and Japan, where intact fetuses were more readily available than in the United States.[14]

The oddest article appeared on April 13, with the headline, "NIH Vows Not to Fund Fetus Work." The article reported that the "NIH will not fund research on live aborted fetuses anywhere in the world, it promised yesterday in a policy statement that is likely to become government-wide practice." Dr. Robert Berliner, Deputy Director for Science, made that promise before "an audience of nearly 200 Roman Catholic high school students gathered in an NIH auditorium. . . . The students were organized by a group from Stone Ridge Country Day School of the Sacred Heart, led by Renée Mier, Theo Toomey, and Maria Shriver, age 17, daughter of Sargent Shriver."[15] It is unusual for public officials to make vows and announce policy before an ad hoc audience of protesting high school girls. One of the young women embarrassed an the NIH official who said that the panel recommendations were not policy but that the NIH was debating the advisability of issuing federal guidelines. "Why are they drawing up guidelines if they don't intend to use them?" asked the skeptical questioner.

I don't know whether that occasion in Masur Auditorium was inspired by the phone conversation between the wily Dr. Hellegers and the mother of Maria Shriver. I do know that it was a momentous event for bioethics and an auspicious one for me. It was momentous for bioethics because it incited the federal legislation that led to the creation of the National Commission for the Protection of Human Subjects of Biomedical and Behavioral Research. It was auspicious for me because, as I sat in Dr. Helleger's booth, I could never have imagined that twenty-one months later I would be sworn in as a member of that Commission.

One month after the newspaper articles, a bill to authorize federal support of medical research grants (H.R. 7724) was debated in the U.S. House of Representatives. The bill contained a provision prohibiting federal funding of any research in the United States or abroad that would "violate any ethical standards adopted by NIH." The provision had been added in the House Interstate and Foreign Commerce Committee, which had reported the bill, in order to support the "policy" announced by Dr. Berliner to the Catholic schoolgirls. That provision was not strong enough for Congressman Angelo Roncollo (R-NY), who offered an amendment prohibiting any research on a fetus "with a beating heart." A highly emotional debate ensued, with strong pro-life overtones. Over the protests of the bill's sponsor, Representative Paul Rogers (D-FL), the House accepted the Roncollo amendment (354 to 9) and passed the National Research Act.

On the Senate side, the responsible committee, Labor and Public Welfare, had held public hearings during February and March under the chairmanship of Senator Ted Kennedy (D-MA). Those hearings opened with the following dramatic words from Senator Kennedy: "Scientists may stand on the threshold of being able to recreate man." He cited heart and kidney transplantation, the breaking of the genetic code, and brain research, and then asked, "Under what conditions should genetic manipulation of our population be allowed or neurological or pharmacological modification of behavior permitted? what constitutes death? who should have access to life-saving equipment in short supply? should society expose some to harm for the benefit of others?" Senator Jacob Javits (R-NY), ranking Republican member of the committee, also wished to hear testimony on two of his own bills: S. 878, which required the NIH to ensure the protection of human subjects of research by establishing review committees and requiring informed consent procedures, and S. 974, which would provide grants to medical schools for improved teaching of medical ethics.[16]

On February 21, 22, and 23, and on March 6, 1973, a parade of witnesses from the world of science and medicine appeared before the committee to comment on the senators' concerns. Drs. Louis Thomas, Michael DeBakey, James Watson, and B. F. Skinner spoke of the possibilities generated by research in their respective areas. Daniel Callahan, Willard Gaylin, and Robert Veatch from The Hastings Center articulated the ethical questions they saw in those possibilities. Veatch noted twelve examples of questionable scientific research and called for more rigorous procedures for informed consent.[17] Gaylin spoke of the dangers in psychosurgery due to the physician's inherent power to coerce. Callahan reviewed the problems attendant upon genetic and reproductive research and called for more public education and debate on these issues; "We simply cannot afford as a species to stumble about blindly in a thicket which may produce more thorns than flowers." Senator Javits commented after Callahan's presentation, "Many of the techniques you have described sound as if they come out of 1984. . . . is it possible that techniques such as cloning can be used to control the characteristics of our population?"[18]

In March, the hearings focused on human experimentation. Jessica Mitford described research using incarcerated persons, the subject of her book, *Kind and Unusual Punishment: The Prison Business*.[19] Alexander Morgan Capron, Professor of Law at the University of Pennsylvania, proposed a moratorium on prison research pending a careful study. Sociologist Bernard Barber discussed his study that showed most medical experimentation was conducted with little or no social control.[20] Henry Beecher reported on unethical medical research.[21]

The next session of the hearings, held on April 30, 1973, focused on the Tuskegee Syphilis Study. As we shall see in Chapter 5, the story of a Public Health Service experiment that deprived a group of rural, African-American men of treatment for syphilis over a 30-year period, had broken into the news. A federal panel that had examined that event had submitted its initial report in the fall of 1972. At the March hearings, Dr. Jay Katz, a member of the panel, had criticized the government's lethargic response to the report's recommendations.[22] In April, the Senate called the government to task for that lethargy. Dr. Henry Simmons, Deputy Assistant Secretary for Health, attempted to explain, much to Senator Kennedy's dissatisfaction, the government's problems in implementing the recommendations of the Tuskegee Report. In June, two bills, S. 2071, dealing with the funding of research grants and health manpower, and S. 2072, devoted to the protection of human subjects, were the subject of a hearing. The latter bill provided for the appointment of an eleven-person National Commission for the Protection of Human Subjects of Biomedical and Behavioral Research, and it included Senator Javits's proposals requiring review boards and informed consent as conditions for federally funded research.

Dr. Eugene Braunwald, a distinguished medical scientist, appeared before the committee to testify in favor of the training bill. Senator Kennedy interrogated him on the protection of human subjects of research. Dr. Braunwald admitted that guidelines were needed but warned of the danger of inflexibility. Kennedy asked, "Will this deter research?" Braunwald answered, "I do not believe so." Kennedy then asked, "Do you think it is a necessary measure?" Braunwald responded, "I think it is a helpful measure." Dr. Jay Katz, appearing for the third time, was considerably more enthusiastic: "The bill is so well drafted that it allows for a tremendous amount of latitude and thoughtful input."[23]

The Kennedy hearings were not the sole venue for the airing of concern about the problems raised by scientific advances. Congressman Paul Rogers (D-FL) also held hearings of the Subcommittee on Health and Environment of the Committee on Interstate and Foreign Commerce to consider some fifteen bills submitted by House members on the ethical, legal, and social issues associated with biomedical advances. Among them were bills to establish a National Commission on Transplantation and Artificial Organs, a Commission on Medical Technology and the Dignity of Dying, a Psychosurgery Commission, and a National Human Experimentation Standards Board. Although none of these bills left committee, they demonstrated the breadth of concern that the public had conveyed to its representatives.

The Labor and Public Welfare Committee reported the two Kennedy bills, S. 2071 and S. 2072, to the Senate floor, instead of their amended version of H.R. 7724, which had been sent to the Committee months before. When these bills reached floor debate on September 11, Senator J. Glenn Beall (R-MD) added an amendment for a two-year ban on psychosurgery pending further study and Senator James Buckley (I-NY) proposed a permanent ban on support of research using voluntarily aborted fetuses. The Beall amendment was accepted by voice vote but the Buckley amendment aroused strong debate. Senator Buckley defended his amendment: "Where the mother has already consented to the killing of her unborn offspring, it seems to me that she has abrogated any right that she might otherwise have to consent to any medical procedure on her child. . . . these children should not become guinea pigs. Let them, I say, die in peace, unmolested by prying hands, electrodes and chemicals of those who would play God in the laboratory."[24]

Senator Kennedy remarked that Buckley's amendment applied only to voluntarily aborted fetuses and not to spontaneous abortions. He then suggested that many similar distinctions needed to be made, and that the Senate floor was no place to make them. It would be preferable, he said, to ban fetal research until the anticipated commission could draw up guidelines. To Buckley's protest that commissions take forever, Kennedy suggested that the study should be concluded within four months, and moved to amend Buckley's amendment to this effect. The Kennedy amendment provided "senators unwilling to accept the abortion tinged rationale offered by Buckley, but similarly reluctant to alienate anti-abortion forces, an opportunity to base their vote on an argument of reason rather than emotion."[25] Kennedy's amendment to the Buckley amendment passed 53 to 35 and the Buckley amendment passed 88 to 0. The legislation establishing the National Commission then passed the Senate.

The Senate and House versions did not go to conference until March 28, 1974. Conference changed the proposed national commission from the permanent body envisioned in the Senate bill to a temporary one with a three-year life (although to be followed by an advisory council). The Senate received the conference report on June 27. Senator Buckley was still unhappy: "I frankly question whether a subject as sensitive, as controversial and as important (as fetal research) can be coped with, can be adequately analyzed, within four months."[26] Kennedy answered that the four-month limit was a response to the urgency of the question. The Senate then accepted the report, 72 to 14. The House adopted the conference report on June 28 with a vote of 311 to 10, with Mr. Roncollo still insisting on a permanent ban on fetal research.

Although many examples of unethical research had been noted during the Kennedy hearings, fetal research was not mentioned, even though the high school march on the NIH, led by Senator Kennedy's niece, had occurred while those hearings were being held. The battle over fetal research was fought on the floors of the House and Senate. Mr. Roncollo and Senator Buckley both advocated a total ban on federal funding. NIH officials, with their jerry-built policy slapped together to meet the high school protest, were terrified of a ban. The officials and the scientists whose work the NIH sponsored knew that "fetal research," even "research with a live fetus," meant many different things. To ban it *tout court* would be to abolish a wide range of valuable and, on careful inspection, ethical research. The creation of legislation by floor amendments also worried many legislators who did not want to be caught in an abortion debate. The Kennedy solution, which placed the problem in the proposed commission's mandate, guaranteed passage of a bill that might have otherwise been halted or hampered by the abortion issue.

Fetal research, then, while not the major issue that prompted the creation of the National Commission, was clearly a stimulus. It might be said that the bipartisan support for the legislation was motivated by the two prominent cases of the moment. The Tuskegee scandal cried out to liberals as a blatant violation of civil rights and an example of racism. The fetal research question, with its abortion implications, aroused conservatives in the pro-life camp. Had not both issues been in the news, would Congress have been so interested in human experimentation? Members on both sides of the aisle could conscientiously vote for a commission that would be charged to remedy both abuses and, at the same time, preserve the public interest in scientific progress. Before the Senate voted on the bill, Senator Langdon Hughes (D-IA) "praised the purposes of the bill but expressed concern over how a Commission would be able to translate complex philosophical and religious principles into effective federal regulations."[27] Senator Hughes's question is a thoughtful preface to the story of the National Commission. No legislation had ever before charged a government body "to identify basic ethical principles," as did Public Law 93-348.

The National Commission for the Protection of Human Subjects of Biomedical and Behavioral Research, 1974–1978

The emotional issue of research involving human subjects, with its political magnets, Tuskegee and fetal research, propelled the legislation sponsored by Senator Kennedy through the Congress and onto the President's desk. President Nixon signed the National Research Act into Public Law 93-348 on July 12, 1974. Senator Kennedy's insistent sponsorship and Senator Mondale's persistent concern had come together in legislation that focused rather tightly on the one ethical issue over which the federal government had direct control, namely, the manner in which the rights and welfare of human subjects of federally funded research should be protected. In this area, ethical principles could be translated into actual regulations that could control and sanction behavior. The legislation contained an unusual provision, requiring the Secretary of the Department of Health, Education and Welfare (DHEW) to respond to the Commission's recommendations within a stated time by issuing regulations, or to explain why he or she would chose not to do so. The regulations were to cover all biomedical researchers who received federal funds for their work (and later all research done in institutions that received federal funds). This was ethics with a bite.

Secretary Casper Weinberger of DHEW swore in the eleven members of the National Commission on December 3, 1974. I stood with my ten colleagues, of whom I knew only one, Professor David Louisell of the University of California School of Law. I suspect that I was chosen to serve on the Commission because I was one of those composites that choosers of committees rejoice to find: I was, at that time, a Jesuit priest, and could serve as the "Catholic theologian" member, but I was a faculty member of a state medical school and could be considered somewhat independent of the church. Although I did have formal education in philosophical and in theological ethics, both Catholic and Protestant, my choice was probably less due to these characteristics than to the judgment of Dr. Hellegers. He would never admit to me that he had any hand in my selection but, as a close advisor to the Kennedy family, he must have counselled them on the choice of a dependable Catholic who would not generate as much opposition as might a more prominent theologian. Also, I was not formally associated with either The Kennedy Institute or The Hastings Center and Hellegers, judging it prudent to avoid the nepotism of a Kennedy representative, also felt that Hastings should not be represented; I was a neutral party.[28]

Standing with me on that December day were three physicians, two biomedical researchers, three lawyers, one public member, and one other ethicist, Karen Lebacqz, who taught at the Pacific School of Religion in Berkeley, California. Senator Kennedy had stated in testimony before the House Subcommittee on Public Health and Environment, "The Commission will focus the most creative minds in the nation on complex moral, ethical and religious problems and will help clarify them both for society as a whole and for the individual investigator. The Commission is designed to help us find the critical balance required to satisfy society's demands for advancement of knowledge while abiding by (the rights) of its individual members."[29] We did not know who had decided that we eleven were "the most creative minds in the nation," but we were at least ready to help in the search for that "critical balance."

After the swearing-in ceremony, we met the civil servants who would administer our Commission: Executive Director, Dr. Charles U. Lowe of NIH, and Mr. Michael Yesley, a lawyer from the Commerce Department, who was staff director.[30] A small staff had been assembled to advise on medical and legal issues. We spent the rest of the meeting discussing how to meet the stringent time limits on the fetal research mandate and, at the end of the meeting, elected as our chair Dr. Kenneth J. Ryan, Professor and Chairman, Department of Obstetrics and Gynecology, Harvard University. Given the mutual ignorance we had about each other, he was a remarkably apt choice. Chosen, perhaps, because the commissioners thought that an obstetrician might be the best guide through the imminent task of the fetal research study, he proved a competent leader throughout the entire work of the Commission.

Apart from the fetal research mandate, the law directed the Commission to recommend to the Secretary of DHEW regulations that would protect the rights and welfare of human subjects of research, particularly with regard to informed consent and institutional review of research. The Commission was to study the ethical questions raised by addressing the use of several particular populations in research: children, the institutionalized mentally infirm, and prisoners. A study of psychosurgery was to recommend the conditions, if any, under which that procedure could be performed with federal funds. Congress instructed the Commission "to identify the basic ethical principles that should underlie the conduct of biomedical and behavioral research involving human subjects and develop guidelines that should be followed in such research." Finally, the Special Study, derived from Senator Mondale's S.J. 71, was to make a "comprehensive study of the ethical, legal and social implications of advances in biomedical research."[31]

The commissioners decided to meet for two days each month during its entire life. The pressure of the Congressional deadline for the fetal-research study required an even more intense schedule for the first four months, during which we met seven times. By the second meeting, work on the fetal research mandate was under way. Two scientific projects were commissioned: Dr. Maurice Mahoney of Yale was asked to survey the world's medical literature to ascertain how much and what sort of research involved the human fetus; Dr. Richard Behrman of Columbia University College of Physicians and Surgeons was directed to ascertain the medical limits of fetal viability. Alexander Capron was to prepare a paper on the legal issues involved in fetal research. Finally, eleven philosophers and theologians were invited to prepare essays on various ethical aspects of using the fetus as a research subject: Paul Ramsey, Joseph Fletcher, Richard McCormick, Arthur Dyck, Sissela Bok, Seymour Siegel, Leon Kass, Richard Wasserstrom, and Stephen Toulmin, LeRoy Walters, and Marc Lappé. At the third meeting, a public hearing was held at which twenty-five interested parties presented their views on fetal research. At the fourth meeting, March 4, 1974, Dr. Mahoney's comprehensive report was presented and the ethicists who had written papers appeared as a panel for discussion with the commissioners.

By the fifth meeting, a staff draft on "The Nature and Extent of Fetal Research" was ready for the commissioners' critique. Commissioner Lebacqz proposed that six principles govern fetal research: do no harm, proportionality between risk and benefit, informed consent by proxies, equality, equity, and proximity (subjects should be chosen in relation to their connection to the problem under investigation). At that meeting, I distributed a memorandum on the ethical difference between a fetus that was intended to go to term and a fetus intended for abortion, with reference to the definition of harm. The question was whether harm could come to a being that would not survive long enough to experience the harmful effects. That question was hotly discussed at the April meeting. This intense activity issued in a report that was approved at the seventh meeting on May 9. All commissioners concurred with the report's recommendations, with the exception of Commissioner Louisell, who submitted a dissenting opinion insisting on the equality between fetuses intended to be aborted and fetuses that were to go to term.[32]

The Commission had met the congressional deadline, delivering its recommendations on fetal research in four months. Those four months were seminal ones for bioethics. A group of strangers, all but two from the academic world and most of them from diverse disciplines, had been set a problem and told to analyze it, debate it, and come up with recommendations that could be applied to government practice and policy. The question was, on the face of it, distressing: should a living fetus be used for research. It was also perplexing because the research done on fetuses was aimed at the health of future fetuses. This group had to explore the conceptual and factual aspects of that question and bring to it a critical appreciation of some moral values. Specialists in moral philosophy and theology were recruited to assist the Commission, and the specialists, with few exceptions, had not previously reflected on these distressing and perplexing questions, but they bent their analytic skills to the task. They sought to make distinctions, to construct arguments, to find within different traditions glimmerings of guidance. Their papers are as a unique effort to comprehend a novel moral problem.

The commissioners listened to their advisors, and to the public which addressed them by word and letter; they listened to each other and, in so doing, became colleagues. The debates were long, tortuous, and often contentious, but the duty to formulate recommendations pushed debate toward closure. This was a new way of "doing ethics"—going beyond the often chaotic debate that rages around moral issues and beyond the private ruminations of scholars. In this new way, a public moral discourse began to evolve, in which a group of citizens seeks the facts of the case, asks for scholarly advice, and enters a debate with a view to resolution. Some people would hardly consider this ethics, which, in their view, should be a definitive deduction of rules from clear principles. Other people might contend that reaching ethical conclusions is impossible; ethics has no answers and debate is interminable. Yet many participants in this new way of doing ethics, even if troubled by theoretical problems, found it intellectually satisfying.

After the intense activity of the first four months, the Commission had no respite. It had a long agenda to complete before its expiration date in two years. The Commission approached each subsequent topic in the same fashion as it had the fetal research study. The commissioners first decided what sort of information and analysis they needed; they chose consultants and commissioned studies; they heard public and expert testimony; and, above all, they argued the issues around the table. The staff drafted versions of the reports, but commissioners often wrote large sections themselves and rewrote extensively the staff's contributions. Director Yesley organized meetings and hearings, contracted for studies, and oversaw drafting efficiently and equitably. One after another, reports appeared: *Research Involving Prisoners* (1976), *Research Involving Children* (1977), *Psychosurgery* (1977), *Disclosure of Research Information* (1977), *Research Involving Those Institutionalized as Mentally Infirm* (1978), *Institutional Review Boards* (1978), *Delivery of Health Services* (1978), and the *Special Study* (1978).[33] The Congress twice extended the Commission's life. The original commissioners remained on the Commission to the end, with the exception of Professor Louisell, who died on August 21, 1977, and Commissioner Robert Turtle, who died shortly before the final meeting in summer, 1978. Neither commissioner was replaced.

One congressional mandate required a special process: "identify the ethical principles which should underlie the conduct of biomedical and behavioral research with human subjects and develop guidelines that should be followed in such research." Some principles already existed. The Nuremberg Code, devised in 1947 by the prosecuting team in the International War Crimes Trial, and the Declaration of Helsinki, issued by the World Medical Association in 1962, were prominent examples. The commissioners judged that they were being asked to explore the ethical foundations for human research more deeply than had any extant statements. They decided that a closed retreat be held (meetings were usually open to the public by law) so that a freewheeling discussion could explore the nature and role of ethical principles for human research. That retreat was held at Belmont House, a conference center of the Smithsonian Institution at Elkridge, Maryland, February 13–16, 1976.

The commissioners, along with a cadre of advisors, repaired to that pleasant eighteenth-century country house for a very twentieth-century debate. They had in hand a small library of commissioned essays on the nature and role of moral principles in general and for research in particular. Other than a paper on research design from Alvin Feinstein, all the essays were by ethicists: Kurt Baier, Alasdair MacIntyre, James Childress, H. Tristram Engelhardt, and LeRoy Walters. Stephen Toulmin had prepared a meta-analysis of these essays, which he presented at the opening session. He stated that "in summary, the central question is how to reconcile protection of individual rights with fruitful pursuit of the collective enterprise."[34] After discussing Toulmin's presentation, the commissioners self-selected into small groups to discuss the principal elements of the congressional mandate: principles, risk-benefit, informed consent, and the boundaries between research and practice. After some six hours of discussion, the groups reported back and the general session reconvened.

The report of the ethical-principles group proved most significant for the future of bioethics. It was delivered by Commissioner Karen Lebacqz. That group had selected seven principles: respect self-determination, benefit individual research subjects, benefit other individuals and groups present and future, minimize harm to individual subjects, minimize consequential harm to others, and attend to distributive justice and to compensating justice. Toulmin suggested that "protect the weak and powerless" be added. Guidelines for research based on these principles were good design, identification of consequences, informed consent, compensation, and selection of subjects. Early in the discussion, Commissioner Joseph V. Brady (a behavioral psychologist who consistently, and incorrectly, denied having any philosophical acumen) objected that the group had selected "too many principles and some of them, such as compensation, are not universal" (as Baier's essay had contended any true ethical principle must be). Brady claimed that the list was not "crisp enough." He professed that he was attracted to three principles only: beneficence, freedom, and justice.

I seconded Brady's point because these three principles seemed to do what ethical principles should do—namely, serve as rational justification for decisions and policies. We also had in our dossier of philosophical essays H. Tristram Engelhardt's paper which had suggested three basic principles: "respect for persons as free moral agents, concern to support the best interests of human subjects in research, intent in assuring that the use of human subjects of experimentation will on the sum redound to the benefit of society." Tom Beauchamp had also contributed a paper entitled "Distributive justice and morally relevant differences." After much discussion, the commissioners took Engelhardt's first two principles and Beauchamp's principle of distributive justice and crafted "crisp" principles: respect for persons, beneficence, and justice. Stephen Toulmin was directed to redraft the report for presentation at the March meeting.[35]

The Belmont Report, as the document came to be known, was the subject of long rumination after the Belmont meeting. Toulmin had drafted a version for the March 1976 meeting and had slightly modified it on June 6, 1976. Chairman Ryan described the draft as "a synthesis by Dr. Toulmin of the deliberations of Belmont."[36] Although these drafts were circulated for study and comment, they were not on the agenda for discussion until one year later, at the twenty-seventh meeting on February 11–13, 1977. Sometime during the next few months, a small gathering convened at my home in San Francisco to revise the June 1976 draft in light of the February 1977 deliberations. Although the date is uncertain, the occasion is vivid in my memory. Commissioners Brady, Lebacqz, and I, together with Stephen Toulmin and Michael Yesley, spent two days in my rooftop study revising the text to produce the crisp document that Brady had called for. Three basic principles, "among those generally accepted in our cultural tradition, that are particularly relevant to the ethics of research involving human subjects: the principles of respect for persons, beneficence and justice," are defined. The application of these general principles leads to the three requirements of informed consent, risk/benefit assessment, and just selection of the subjects for research.

The revised draft was next discussed at the January 13–14, 1978, meeting: the text, dated December 2, 1977, is basically the same as the final version, with some refinements in the section on justice and, as Toulmin said, "with the fat cut out." The discussion at that meeting made no substantial changes to the draft, but refinements and more "cutting of fat" were done at a conference among myself, Toulmin, and the Commission's new philosophy consultant, Tom Beauchamp of Georgetown, who was charged with writing the polished final version. *The Belmont Report* was approved by the commissioners at their forty-second meeting, June 10, 1978. This short document, which was published in the *Federal Register* on April 18, 1979, had a major impact on the development of bioethics.[37] Its principles found their way into the general literature of the field, and, in the process, grew from the principles underlying the conduct of research into the basic principles of bioethics.[38]

The Commission delivered its reports to the Secretary of the Department of Health, Education and Welfare. They were published for public comment in the *Federal Register*, carefully crafted into regulatory language, and became public law governing the research activities of federally funded scientists. Many of the commissioned papers were eventually published in journals and became important contributions to the growing literature of careful philosophical and legal analysis of issues. The National Commission ceased to exist on October 11, 1978.

One report, *Report and Recommendations: Research Involving Those Institutionalized as Mentally Infirm,* failed to reach regulation. Another commission report, on psychosurgery, went relatively unnoticed. The fate of these two reports deserves comment. The title of the report on the institutionalized as mentally infirm was convoluted. "Mentally infirm" is not a diagnostic category recognized in psychiatry; it was a term invented by the drafters of legislation to cover the broad population of " individuals who are mentally ill, mentally retarded, emotionally disturbed, psychotic, senile, or who have other impairments of a similar nature."[39] This language is so imprecise that it impedes a clear view of the problem, since each category of mental illness poses its own difficulties for consent and competency and has its own social disadvantages. The term "institutionalized" limited the study to persons that reside in institutions such as psychiatric hospitals where they are subject to institutional constraints. Persons who suffer from mental illness but who are not institutionalized were excluded from the scope of the Commission's study. Certainly, the focus on institutionalized persons was justified: much of the reprehensible research that had come to the public's attention had been done in state institutions for the mentally disabled and little of that research was done for their benefit. Also, institutionalized persons live in a highly depersonalized setting and lack the protection of family and friends.

The Commission recommended elaborate arrangements for the protection of this vulnerable population, requiring particularly strong justification for their involvement in research. Investigators were required to make the case that there was good reason to involve institutionalized persons and the IRB was required to determine that their involvement was not expoitive. The Commission recognized that neither mental infirmity nor institutionalization eliminated the possibility of consent and set stringent requirements for the obtaining of consent when possible and for oversight of research when consent was compromised. These strict requirements were apparently too elaborate. In November 1978, the DHEW issued proposed regulations that followed the Commission's recommendations but, four years later, no regulations had been issued. The President's Commission for the Study of Ethical Problems in Medicine and Biomedical and Behavioral Research, which succeeded the National Commission, noted this failure to respond and twice requested that the Department finalize the regulations, but the commissioners were informed that the proposed regulations had generated no consensus among commentators.[40] The Secretary also suggested that the general rules for protection of research subjects provided adequate coverage for "the institutionally mentally infirm." This was, of course, quite contrary to the Commission's beliefs. No regulations have ever been issued. *Istitutionalized as Mentally Infirm* remains the only study of the National Commission to be ignored.

Psychosurgery, or creating lesions in the brain to treat mental disease, was added to the Commission's agenda by Senator J. Glenn Beall of Maryland. It was inconsistent with the general mandate because it aimed at surgical procedures that were in common but limited use rather than at research. Very little, if any, federal funds were involved. A book by a leading neurosurgeon, Elliott S. Valenstein, had charged that most of the procedures were ineffective and little more than updated versions of the discredited frontal lobotomies of the 1930s.[41] Also, Congressman Louis Stokes, one of the few African-American legislators, had introduced a bill to establish a psychosurgery commission to examine whether minority persons were improperly subjected to these procedures. The National Commission surveyed the practice of psychosurgery, examined the published results of the procedures, and concluded that only one, amygdolotomy, had any discernible effect on one mental condition, obsessive-compulsive disorders. It recommended that this procedure be considered experimental and its outcomes closely studied. Much to the commissioners' astonishment, this recommendation, which we considered quite conservative, aroused the ire of a California group of activist mental patients, the Network Against Psychiatric Assault (NAPA—Napa was the name of California's major mental hospital). The meeting at which this report was to be discussed was inadvertently scheduled in San Francisco where NAPA was headquartered. NAPA members mounted a genuine 1970s demonstration in the meeting room and succeeded in forcing adjournment. As a college president in the tumultuous San Francisco of the late 1960s, I had seen a demonstration or two, but never expected to see one at a bioethics meeting![42]

The National Commission was generally considered a success. The distinguished editor of the *New England Journal of Medicine*, Dr. Franz Ingelfinger, had been skeptical about the Commission. At its inception he wrote, "One may wonder if the diverse elements of the Commission really can reach a consensus. Or will eternal ethical verities be decided by 6 to 5 votes?" Later, he recalled his words and wrote, "Now, two years later, the skeptics have had to swallow most of their doubts. In the context of the formidability of its assignments, the Commission has been remarkably successful. . . . The members deserve gratitude for their steadfast determination to arrive at some reasonable, specific, if perhaps temporary, guidelines."[43] A few commentators were less enthusiastic. Professor George Annas, referring to Joseph Heller's satirical account of a government commission, called the National Commission "Good as Gold": it endorsed the status quo, he said, because it left unexamined three basic premises: research is good, experimentation is almost never harmful, and researcher-dominated independent review boards (IRBs) can adequately protect research subjects. Michael Yesley and I responded to Annas' rhetorical critique by arguing that we had quite carefully examined the premises he said we had ignored.[44] Still, the overall judgment of the Commission's work was favorable. Commission Chairman Kenneth Ryan commented on this success, "The Commission's success depended on ideal commissioners who were academic, experienced, nonideological, willing to take the time and do the work; on a mature, experienced staff who listened to but also collaborated with the commissioners in drafting useful and readable documents; on a political climate that did not frustrate the deliberative process and, finally, on a process that placed priority on obtaining facts, listening to the scientists and the public and taking a pragmatic approach."[45]

The Ethics Advisory Board, DHEW, 1978–1980

In several of its reports, the National Commission suggested that certain kinds of research with the fetus and with children be submitted to a "National Ethics Advisory Board" that would be permanently established within the Department of Health, Education, and Welfare. Such a board could also take on other problems as they arose. Secretary Califano chartered the Ethics Advisory Board (EAB), pursuant to Public Law 92–463, in 1977.[46] He appointed as chair James C. Gaither, a San Francisco lawyer with no experience in the arena of health and ethics, but surrounded him with a stellar cast: two bioethicists, Richard A. McCormick and Sissela Bok, and six physicians, Drs. David A. Hamburg, Donald A. Henderson, Daniel C. Tosteson, Henry W. Foster, Robert F. Murray, and Mitchell W. Spellman, the last three of whom were African-American. There were also several lawyers and lay members. Its charter specified that the EAB be available for consultation on all DHEW programs and policies and it was to review all research proposals that had been indicated by the National Commission, as well as any others submitted to them by the Secretary. Mr. Califano envisioned a broad role for the EAB. At the first meeting, February 3–4, 1978, he said, "In the time I have been Secretary, the most difficult problems with ethical ramifications have come in the health care area." He specifically mentioned the allocation of health care dollars and of renal dialysis, the competence of children and incarcerated persons to consent to research, sterilization regulations, release of health risks information about DNA research, and, a favorite subject of his, personal responsibility for health, especially responsibility for diseases caused by smoking tobacco.[47]

During the next two years, the EAB took up one problem related to fetal research—namely, research regarding the new procedure of fetoscopy, and one task given by the Secretary, "whether federal funds should support research on *in vitro* fertilization." Both studies were assiduously pursued, using the methods of the National Commission: papers were commissioned, public hearings were held, experts consulted, and vigorous and open argument cultivated. The report, *HEW Support of Research Involving Human* in Vitro *Fertilization and Embryo Transfer*, which we shall review in Chapter 9, favored federal support of research in that rapidly developing sector of reproductive medicine and suggested guidelines for its ethical conduct. The report was met with stony silence: neither Mr. Califano nor any subsequent Secretary responded negatively or positively to it. The protocol on fetoscopy, submitted by Dr. Ezra Davidson of Drew Medical School, won approval and became the first and only fetal research protocol to pass the rigors of federal regulation for such research.[48]

The EAB was about to take up another issue, compensation for injuries sustained in the course of research, when it was summarily disbanded by Secretary Patricia R. Harris on September 30, 1980. It was the victim of an argument between the Department and the White House over the funding of the newly legislated President's Commission, and its meager resources were diverted to the new panel. The two Presidential commissioners who knew the history of the EAB, Patricia King and I, protested and the President's Commission appealed to the White House to save the EAB, which had quite different functions than those assigned to the President's Commission. The appeal was to no avail. The Ethics Advisory Board still hovers as a ghostly presence in the Federal Regulations, charged with mandatory review of certain types of research, but it exists nowhere in reality. Due to its nonexistence, the Reagan and Bush administrations could avoid politically embarrassing decisions about the funding of research with human embryos or fetal tissues between 1981 and 1992.

The President's Commission for the Study of Ethical Problems in Medicine and Biomedical and Behavioral Research, 1980–1983

Several months before the National Commission was to expire, the Senate had passed S. 2579, sponsored by Senator Edward Kennedy. This bill authorized $24 million for a four-year President's Commission for the Study of Ethical Problems in Medicine and Biomedical and Behavioral Research. It "reestablished and upgraded the status of the existing National Commission, required Presidential appointments and Senate confirmation of the chairperson, extended authority beyond HEW to all federal agencies doing human research (including classified information in the Department of Defense and the Central Intelligence Agency) and added other ethical and legal studies related to health." In the floor debate, Senator Jesse Helms objected that a non-elected body "should not make life and death decisions"; he invoked the specter of euthanasia and suggested that "at least certain influential members of the medical profession were insensitive to the right to life." He sought unsuccessfully to eliminate the provisions to conduct studies on genetic screening and the definition of death. The Senate did agree by voice vote that the genetic study should "evidence concern for the essential equality of all human beings, born and unborn," but in the end, S. 2579 was passed, 68 to 10. The House passed the bill by voice vote on October 15, 1978, ten days before the expiration of the National Commission. President Carter signed PL 95-622 on November 9, 1978, but did not issue an Executive Order chartering the Commission until December 17, 1979.[49]

Several days before Christmas, I was leaving my UCSF office and was halfway down steep Third Avenue when my secretary shouted that the White House was calling. Breathless from the pull back up the hill, I picked up the phone and was astonished to be asked whether I would serve on the President's Commission. Two appointees, I was told, were to come from the National Commission to provide continuity: Professor Patricia A. King of Georgetown Law School (who had to resign within several months because she became Deputy Assistant Attorney General) and I. Although I had the uneasy feeling that there were many qualified bioethicists who could serve as well or better than I, I accepted the appointment.

The twelve commissioners were sworn in at the White House on January 14, 1980. This time, in addition to Pat King, there five were acquaintances of mine on the Commission: Professor Renée C. Fox, sociologist, of the University of Pennsylvania,; Dr. Arno G. Motulsky, medical geneticist from the University of Washington; Dr. Fritz C. Redlich, former Dean of Yale Medical School; Rabbi Seymour Siegel of Jewish Theological Seminary; and Anne A. Scitovsky, economist from Palo Alto Medical Clinic. I had not previously met Drs. Mario Garcia-Palmieri, Donald N. Medearis, Charles J. Walker, and Mathilde Krim. The chairman, Morris Abram, a New York lawyer and former president of Brandeis University, was appointed by President Carter. The executive director, Alexander Morgan Capron, who was well known in bioethics circles, left his position at University of Pennsylvania Law School to direct the Commission. Barbara Mishkin, who had ably served the National Commission, was deputy director. A very competent staff had already been hired, most of whom subsequently continued to work in bioethics: Joanne Lynn in medicine, Alan Meisel and Alan Weisbard in law, and Dan Wikler, Dan Brock, Allen Buchanan, and Dorothy Vawter in philosophy.

The first working meeting, on May 13, 1980, opened with Dan Wikler's presentation of the conceptual issues involved in the Commission's first mandate, the advisability of a uniform legal definition of death. Wikler sorted out three distinct arguments: loss of an essential characteristic of personhood, such as rationality, loss of personal identity, and loss of the value of being alive. Robert Veatch then presented the policy issues involved in particular definitions of death. Director Capron announced that he would meet representatives of the American Medical Association, the American Bar Association, and the National Conference of Uniform State Law Commissioners. Each of these organizations had drafted model statutes on the determination of death. Capron believed that common ground could be found and that the Commission could win the support of these organizations for a uniform statute. Chairman Abram rashly remarked that the task seemed a straightforward and simple one. Patricia King and I disagreed with that opinion and suggested that, while the definition of death might be relatively straightforward, it opened a multitude of questions of much greater complexity and about which there was considerable public concern. We could not fulfill the congressional mandate to find a uniform legal definition of death and leave untouched the painful issues about discontinuing life support, which had been dramatized in such cases as that of Karen Ann Quinlan in 1976 (described in Chapter 8). After vigorous discussion, our colleagues agreed that we should undertake a distinct study of the latter issue, even though such a study would add to an already loaded agenda. This was the beginning of what was to become the Commission's most notable work, the report *Deciding to Forego Life-Sustaining Treatment*.

On the next day, Pat King and I reviewed the National Commission's experience. I noted that *The Belmont Report* had matured during a long process of reflection and debate; Pat King commented that the Belmont retreat itself was for her a turning point because "after that time, it seemed to me that even though we disagreed, I understood what my fellow commissioners were saying and I understood what we wanted to focus on." A long discussion initiated by Renée Fox ensued on the role of the Commission in society. I suggested that, since the National Commission's primary task was to protect human subjects of research, the rights of individuals were always in prominent focus. I wondered whether the President's Commission might explicitly shift this focus and take as its theme and analytic framework the problem of how the common good of society could be promoted, with the protection of individual rights as a moral constraint on this goal. The staff took this suggestion seriously and produced for the next meeting, on May 17–18, an elegant essay running that theme through the various mandates of the Commission. Some of us hoped that we could begin the President's Commission in the way the National Commission had concluded: with a general statement of a moral stance. The essay, although it stimulated a rich discussion, was never seen again and the President's Commission never formulated a general statement of its principles that matched *The Belmont Report*.

Director Capron drew up a plan of action that was not merely a schedule but a concept paper that reviewed the mandates in terms of leading ideas and problems. Woven into this paper were quotations from many prominent individuals in science, policy, and ethics whose views Capron had solicited about the Commission's work. Most eloquent of these comments was a long letter from Robert Morison, professor emeritus of biology at Cornell. Professor Morison sketched his views on the relation between ethics, law, and religion and reviewed the brief history of "the infelicitously named bioethics," the results of which he "was reasonably happy [with], but I fear for the future." The future he feared was one in which ethics and religion were turned into law and regulation: "What one fears is that the Commission may become the mechanism whereby the speculations of the ethicists become the law of the land. It is already far too easy for abstract notions of right and wrong to emerge as deontological rules which begin their public life as 'guidelines' but culminate in the force of law."[50] Morison's letter was a sobering reminder of the anomalous role of an "ethics commission" in a pluralistic, secular society.

During the next meeting, July 12, 1980, a roundtable on the legal, ethical, and medical issues in the definition of death was held. Because orthodox Judaism objected to the concept of brain death, two distinguished rabbis, J. David Bleich and Moses Tendler, were invited to present their positions. They engaged in a spirited Talmudic debate, citing texts in Hebrew, much to the dismay of the recording stenographer. Other religious scholars, lawyers, and neuroscientists also presented their views. To our surprise, most of these experts found the redefinition of death relatively unproblematic. Their presentations made clear the weaknesses of earlier efforts to redefine death, such as the Harvard criteria, which had been devised twelve years before, and the several state statutes that had been enacted during the 1970s. In general, a confusion between permanent coma and total organic death had plagued those efforts. The Commission had the benefit of an extant literature in which the complex questions had been perceptively analyzed.[51] With this literature on the shelf, it was possible to produce a comprehensive report, *Defining Death,* in a relatively short period of time. The report recommended a succinct model statute: "Death is the irreversible cessation of cardiorespiratory functions or the irreversible cessation of all functions of the brain, including the brain stem."[52]

This definition, which we shall discuss in Chapter 8, garnered wide support in the medical and legal worlds. The report was approved by the Commission on July 9, 1981. The Uniform Statute was accepted by the American Bar Association, the American Medical Association, and the National Conference of Commissioners of Uniform State Laws and over the next few years, was adopted by the majority of state legislatures. Many philosophical questions were left unanswered, but a practical resolution, useful in clinical and legal settings, had been attained. A study of the ethical implications of permanent coma or persistent vegetative state, from which total brain death had been distinguished, was left to the anticipated report on termination of life support. The commissioners were encouraged by the facility and efficiency with which the first mandate had been accomplished. More difficult tasks awaited them.

At the third meeting, July 12, Frank Press, science advisor to President Carter, transmitted to the Commission a letter that the President had received from three leaders of the Protestant, Catholic, and Jewish faith communities. They expressed the concern that "genetic engineering" posed serious ethical problems and hoped that the President would find a way to address these problems. Thus the Commission added a study of genetic engineering, which would be called *Splicing Life*, to the agenda. Fortunately, this study fit nicely with an already mandated study, *Screening and Counseling for Genetic Conditions*.[53] Both of these will be discussed in Chapter 6.

The decision to prepare a distinct report on termination of life support, which the

Commission had voluntarily added to its agenda, led to extensive hearings, testimony, philosophical and legal analysis, and long debates. There was wide public interest in this issue and a number of cases had been publicized in the four years since Karen Ann Quinlan's well-known case. The Commission decided to investigate these cases in order to mix the reality of clinical tragedy with philosophical and theological wisdom; the result was the study, *Deciding to Forego Life-Sustaining Treatment*.[54] (Director Capron chose the word "forego" to cover both "withholding and withdrawing," and admits that "forgo" would have been lexically more correct.)

On April 9, 1981, the Commission convened in Miami to hear testimony in the case of Mr. Abe Perlmutter. Mr. Perlmutter, who suffered from amytrophic lateral sclerosis, had requested that his ventilator be discontinued. His doctor refused, believing that it was his duty to preserve life; the hospital also refused his request, fearing liability for "assisting in self-murder." Mr. Perlmutter sought legal remedies and received an order to remove the ventilator from the Florida State Court of Appeals. He died 41 hours later. Various participants in the case testified; many other interested parties, including representatives of religious denominations, also presented testimony, most of whom supported Mr. Perlmutter's decision. On June 4, the Commission moved to Boston, where it heard testimony on one of the best known of the "withholding cases," that of Joseph Saikewicz, a 67-year-old retarded man who was not treated for acute leukemia. The Commission also reviewed two other leading cases of foregoing life-sustaining treatment, *In the Matter of Dinnerstein* and *In the Matter of Spring*, both of which had been decided in Massachusetts. It also heard from the physicians who had devised the non-resuscitation policies of two leading Boston hospitals.[55]

On September 12, the Commission met in Los Angeles where it listened to presentations on the California Natural Death Act, passed by the state legislature in 1976, and on the practices of the burn unit of Los Angeles General Hospital, where a policy on refraining from treatment of seriously burned patients had been initiated.[56] Throughout the next six months, the Commission heard experts from medicine, law, religion, and philosophy discuss the various aspects of the problems arising in the care of the dying. Particularly informative and poignant hearings were held in January and February of 1982 on the care of infants in neonatal intensive care. During all this time, the staff drafted sections of the report and submitted them to the commissioners for criticism and to experts for technical correction.

The second chapter of *Deciding to Forego* reviewed the classical distinctions that had long been invoked by ethicists and by physicians as they faced the moral perplexity of allowing a patient to die. These distinctions included "ordinary versus extraordinary treatment," "acting versus refraining from action," "omission versus commission," "direct versus indirect killing." A certain skepticism about the relevance of such distinctions had appeared among physicians and ethicists alike. Competent philosophers, such as James Rachels and Jonathan Glover, aimed to demolish the moral relevance of the distinction between omission and commission.[57] On June 10, 1982, three of the country's leading ethicists, philosophers Joel Feinberg and Daniel Callahan and theologian

Richard McCormick, articulated their criticisms of the classical distinctions before the Commission.

The Commission realized that its report could not uncritically rely on the classical distinctions and instructed the staff philosophers, Dan Brock and Allen Buchanan, to provide a thorough analysis. They prepared a philosophically elegant draft, "Possible Constraints on Acceptable Decisions," which was discussed at the June 10–11, 1982, meeting. Chairman Abram anticipated an easy discussion, remarking that "the chief criticisms or chief suggestions (of the draft) are stylistic and some of us felt it would be very helpful to have more examples to illustrate and clarify some of the rather difficult conceptual principles." It was the latter suggestion that opened a lengthy and profound debate about the draft that went far beyond its style.[58]

My major concern was that the philosophers' analysis, acute though it was, went too far. They had written, "In sum, of all the distinctions that have been proposed to demarcate acceptable from unacceptable actions, only the voluntary–involuntary one is clearly morally relevant in itself and usually capable of unambiguous application in actual cases. . . . the other distinctions are not nearly so helpful. Each fails both to distinguish clearly between classes of action and to be in themselves morally relevant. . . . Generally distinctions of uncertain character and importance are very difficult to use in a society dedicated, as is American society, to a profound respect for pluralism."[59] I did not object to the logical critique of the distinctions but rather to the implied suggestion that almost nothing of analytic usefulness could be salvaged from the common distinctions. I doubted that language so firmly embedded in thinking and practice could be expunged, even when demolished by sharp dialectic. I expressed the opinion that the chapter both criticize and rehabilitate the classical distinctions. An afternoon of energetic debate ensued. Commissioners Scitovsky and Siegel took my side. Brock and Buchanan defended their draft, while Director Capron and Assistant Director Lynn mediated. We reached what I considered acceptable language for the revision but which the philosophers found frustrating. Underlying the debate was a differing view of how professional philosophy functions within the world of public policy.[60]

The results of that afternoon's debate appeared in a major revision of the draft, retitled "Elements of Good Decision-Making." The classical distinctions are still subjected to acute criticism, but pieces of useful meaning are mined from them. The distinction between "acting and omitting," for example, "provides a useful rule-of-thumb by separating cases that probably deserve more scrutiny from those that are not likely to need it." It does roughly distinguish between the sorts of cases that are more likely to be legally and socially problematic ("active killing") and those that have won broad social acceptance (allowing to die). "Nevertheless," according to the draft, "the difference between acts and omissions—which is hard to draw in any case—never by itself determines what is morally acceptable. Rather, the acceptability of particular actions or omissions turns on other morally significant considerations, such as the balance of harms and benefits likely to be achieved, the duties owed by others to a dying person, the risks imposed on others in acting or refraining, and the certainty of outcome."[61] After working through the relevance of the other classical distinctions, the Commission reached the conclusion that, "a decision to forego treatment is ethically acceptable when it has been made by suitable qualified decisionmakers who have found the risk of death to be justified in the light of all the circumstances."[62] A footnote on this page of the report alludes to the suggestion found in a 1980 Vatican *Declaration on Euthanasia* that the terms "proportionate" and "disproportionate" be substituted for the more traditional, but outmoded, "extraordinary" and "ordinary." That language has become common coinage in modern bioethics.

The Commission's discussion of the classical distinctions provides a fine overview of ethical argumentation about foregoing life support and has set the general tone of the subsequent discussion. Only in the matter of "active killing" is the report less than adequate. Relying on the familiar argument that "weakening the legal prohibition to allow a deliberate taking of life in extreme circumstances would risk allowing wholly unjustified taking of life in less extreme circumstances. . . . the Commission concludes that the current interpretation of the legal prohibition of active killing should be sustained."[63] Although there had been ongoing discussion of active euthanasia during the previous decade, the Commission did not take up that problem.[64] Indeed, under Rabbi Siegel's admonitions about the ravages of euthanasia, all commissioners seemed to take the conclusion for granted. We did not anticipate the vigorous, even rancorous, debate over assisted suicide that would emerge in the 1990s.

Deciding To Forego, then, endorses the competent patient as the most "suitably qualified decisionmaker," elaborates on various forms of proxy decision-making for the incompetent (stressing, for the first time, the value of "durable power of attorney" arrangements), and sets out the considerations for resuscitation policy, for care of the permanently unconscious patient, and the ill newborn. Its appendices contain sample policies and statutes and an excellent treatise on supportive care for the dying. *Deciding to Forego* is a rich compendium of information, thoughtful argumentation, and useful advice. It became the most successful of the Commission's reports and had a significant impact on practice, policy, and the field of bioethics. According to one commentator, it was "an unambiguous success in terms of having both 'critical impact on public policy' and 'significant impact on bioethics'. . . . [It] filled a tremendous need in a sensible and thoughtful way, . . . crystallized the most progressive mainstream thinking . . . and is an authoritative text even today [1993]."[65]

Other reports did not fare so well. The study of access to health care ran on the rocks. The first rock was a philosophical one. For some years, the idea of a right to health care had been popular. President Truman's Commission on the Health Needs of the Nation had proclaimed that "access to the means for attainment and preservation of health is a basic human right."[66] The 1960s political debate over Medicare and Medicaid had framed the issue in terms of a right to health care. It would have been reasonable for the Commission to deepen and broaden that concept as the basis for its treatment of access to health care. However, the ethical literature on the topic was sparse and the existing literature favored a broader philosophical approach than the doctrine of rights provided.[67] Our own staff philosopher, Allen Buchanan, felt that the language of rights was problematic, because it confused negative and positive rights and laid unfulfillable obligations on those who had the duty to respect that right. I shared these concerns and did not fight to retain the rights language as the center of our argument. Without much debate, we discarded rights doctrine as the basis of our ethical analysis and chose instead to articulate arguments in support of a social obligation to assure access to health care. Some commentators considered this move a mistake, both philosophically and politically.[68] Yet, it may have saved the report from total philosophical and political disaster.

That potential disaster came from the second rock, a large political one. When the Commission first discussed the ethical issues involved in access to health care, most of the commissioners and the staff were of a liberal bent. We had no fundamental objections to the idea that government has an obligation to remedy social problems and to help those in need. We were dismayed at the extent of the need for access to health care when Professor Karen Davis presented us with the number of Americans who lacked health insurance coverage (1978 data showed that twenty-two to twenty-five million or 11–12.6% of Americans were uninsured).[69] Like many Americans, most of us had assumed that Medicare and Medicaid had solved the problem of the uninsured. That presentation was reinforced by remarks from Commissioner Scitovsky, who was the most expert among us on health policy and economics. That presentation galvanized interest in the complex questions that called for much more than merely framing a sound philosophical argument. Political and economic problems loomed large.

By the time a draft of *Securing Access to Health Care* was ready for deliberation in 1982, the Commission's membership had changed. Ten original members, including myself, had completed our terms and President Reagan had appointed new members congenial to conservative Republican views.[70] The new members were displeased with right-to-health-care language for very different reasons than those of Buchanan and myself. It implied to them a call for socialized medicine. At the twenty-seventh meeting of the Commission, on November 13, 1982, Chairman Abram summarized the draft report. It was already a mild proposal: that society had an obligation to provide access to health care; persons are generally not responsible for the diseases they suffer; health care enables persons to help themselves; compassion obliges us to help the suffering; and inequities in health care should be remedied. Along with these modest proposals, the draft described in frank terms the difficulties faced by many Americans in obtaining health care (which many witnesses had confirmed in our hearings), and the growing number of persons uncovered by insurance.

After Chairman Abram's summary, several health-policy figures endorsed the draft. Then the Reagan commissioners attacked in force. Commissioner John J. Moran argued that individuals are responsible for themselves and that society has no obligation to care for them when they do not care for themselves. Most people get ill through their own fault, he contended, and should be left to take care of themselves. Commissioner Daher B. Rahi argued that government has an obligation to help only when other resources are exhausted; Moran conceded this point. Commissioners Thomas H. Ballantine, George R. Dunlop, Kay Toma, and Bruce K. Jacobson contended that the draft report appeared to advocate national health insurance. Commissioner Moran not only wished that any suggestion in that direction be erased; he wanted a strong warning against it. Jacobson, Ballantine, and Moran stated that they could not accept the draft. Although Dr. Ballantine doubted that it could ever be made satisfactory, the commissioners instructed staff to revise and incorporate as many of their comments as possible.[71]

The redrafting was agonizing. Commissioner Moran insisted on 219 specific modifications. The staff, which remained sympathetic with the liberal view, spent hours inserting qualifying words in every strong statement, eliminating important evidence and argument, and crafting language to express ideas with which they disagreed. When the revised draft was produced at the Commission's last business meeting on December 14, 1982, it had been cleansed of anecdotes of failure in the system and of any language that implied that government should be the primary provider or payer for health care. The Reagan commissioners, prompted by Dr. Dunlop, who had become the voice of moderation among that group, had to admit that their principal objections had been met. The Commission approved a report that was decidedly bland but retained the basic principles contained in the earliest drafts: society has an obligation to ensure equitable access for all; individuals have an obligation to pay a fair share of costs; all should receive adequate care without excessive burden; government need not intervene unless private forces fail to provide access; cost containment should not disadvantage those persons least well served. It said nothing to arouse the ire of conservatives and nothing against which liberals, unhappy though they might be at its inadequacy, could argue. Commissioner Moran voted in favor. Commissioner Ballantine dissented: his statement is a succinct summary of the essence of the dispute, "I do not agree that the failures of the market, of charity, and of activities at the local and state levels have been so severe as to warrant at this time increased intrusion of the Federal government into the health care sector."[72]

The Commissions Compared

Both the National Commission and the President's Commission are generally considered successful governmental ventures into bioethics.[73] The National Commission broke new ground. It was the first federal body to be charged specifically to "do ethics." It had no precedents to guide it. None of its members had a clear idea how, in a pluralistic society and within the bureaucratic maze, one might "determine the ethical principles underlying research with human subjects." They had no time to meander through the issues, since Congress opened the starting gate and set the term of their first task. The commissioners began to do public ethics almost by an American instinct that was inherited from James and Dewey: try to get the facts as fully as possible, talk with well-informed persons, invite all interested persons to have their say, argue in public about what you have learned, and then try to find where each member agrees and disagrees. Formal ethical theories and principles were not conspicuous, although sharp thinking by educated ethicists, working their way through the arguments, was indispensable. The President's Commission benefited from the pattern set by the National Commission and followed it closely.

The two Commissions differed in important respects. The National Commission was given a focused task: to recommend policies and procedures to protect the rights and welfare of human subjects of research. It was able to concentrate on that issue. The few tasks that fell outside that focus, such as the mandate to study psychosurgery, the ethics of delivery of care by DHEW, and the Special Study, were not done particularly well. The President's Commission was given a larger, vaguer mandate and had to regroup its resources and refocus its thinking as it moved from medical care of the dying to genetics, informed consent, and health care access. Its work was facilitated by the bioethics literature that had accumulated during the 1970s, which offered concepts and arguments that had already been formulated. The Commissions also differed in a major way in their organizational structure. Sociologist Bradford Gray in comparing the Commissions characterized the National Commission as "commissioner driven" and the President's Commission as "staff driven." The National Commissioners, all of whom served during the entire life of the Commission, came to know each other well. According to Gray, "The pattern was established of taking each other's views very seriously and seeking common ground on which to base recommendations. (Also contributing to the working relationships among commissioners and staff was a practice, established at the very beginning, of a social occasion or dinner on the Friday night of the Commission's two-day meeting. Bonds and a group history developed that would be hard to match)."[74] Director Michael Yesley dedicated himself to assuring that the commissioners' discussions were accurately drafted into text. The staff prepared the drafts, but the commissioners themselves wrote and rewrote much of the material.

The President's Commission was differently organized. Its members had limited terms; several commissioners left after only one year and over the panel's three-year life span, twenty-one persons served on the eleven-member Commission. Some of these members came on in the last year, as the result of appointments by newly elected President Reagan. They brought an unusual level of political ideology to the proceedings (I had not had a clue about the political allegiances of my National Commission colleagues). Director Capron, unlike Director Yesley, came with a deep background in bioethics and he hired a highly qualified staff, who worked intensely on particular projects. The staff did most of the writing and rewriting of reports.

The President's Commission has been faulted for not going far enough. Alan J. Weisbard, legal staff to the President's Commission, summarized the criticisms:

> To an important degree, these [critics] challenge the implicit conception and self-definition of the Commission as a body intended to forge consensus and to provide pragmatic guidance susceptible to ready adoption and implementation. They suggest that the Com-

mission should have used its stature and visibility to educate the public to a new level of awareness and sophistication, by giving voice to a greater diversity of powerfully stated alternative views, by raising new questions and providing stimulus to further discussion and debate.[75]

Other critics have charged that the President's Commission failed to be philosophical enough.[76] Still others found the Commission's almost single-minded focus on autonomy and self-determination, although in conformity with current American opinion, too limited and too lacking in moral content.[77] These are understandable criticisms. However, they are due less to the faults of the commissioners, staffs and processes than to the intrinsic difficulty of doing ethics in public.

The products of the two Commissions also had a mixed reception. As previously mentioned, *Deciding to Forego Life-Sustaining Treatment* was the unquestioned success of the President's Commission. Together with *Defining Death*, it had a significant impact on public policy and on bioethics. According to Gray's survey of the impact of the various reports, both rank high in the number of citations in the medical and ethical literature. Gray also asked a number of persons familiar with the work of both Commissions to comment on the impact of the reports. *Splicing Life* was "seen as a clear, careful and thoughtful report . . . that helped lead to the establishment of the Human Gene Therapy Subcommittee of the NIH Recombinant DNA Advisory Committee." *Screening and Counseling for Genetic Conditions* was "praised for its characterization of the issues, a good overview and for its farsightedness and comprehensiveness" although it had little policy impact. Most disappointing was *Securing Access to Health Care*. As I noted earlier, *Securing Access* clashed with the ideology of the Reagan appointees and was stripped of any powerful appeal. It may also have been too simplistic an analysis of an extremely complex problem. *Making Health Care Decisions*, which was the Commission's reframing of the mandate on informed consent, contained "lucid, constructive analysis" but had no specific audience and thus, little impact on professional practice.[78]

The National Commission had the advantage of being directed toward the recommendation of government regulations and thus almost all of its products saw their way into the policy process. Its most appreciated and influential publication, *The Belmont Report*, was its most theoretical. Although *The Belmont Report* did not have direct regulatory effect, it provided guidance to the burgeoning institutional review boards and flowed into the broad stream of bioethics. According to Gray, "the impact of *Belmont* was so substantial that some respondents were actually troubled that the three basic principles identified in the report had become an uncritically used 'mantra.' "[79] The reports on research with the fetus and with children, as well as that on institutional review boards, were deemed very successful in their analyses of the problems and in their impact on policy.

Both commissions also produced, in Gray's term, "dustcatchers." The National Commission's *Disclosure of Research Information* and *Ethical Guidelines for Health Services*, and the *Special Study* went unnoticed. The President's Commission's *Com-*

pensating for Research Injuries was the result of a serious study and energetic debate but it attracted no attention at the time. Its argument might have been relevant a decade later, at the time of the inquiry into abuses in radiation research.[80] Two reports resulted from the legislative requirement that the President's Commission report biennially to the President, Congress, and other federal agencies on the implementation of the re-search regulations. Both were duly delivered and occupied their shelf space.

Regardless of their success or failure in the world of policy or bioethics, all these re-ports resulted from a group of people—some professionals, others lay people—putting their minds to work on an ethical problem and arguing about it in a sustained, public fashion. At times, professionals in philosophy, law, theology, and the social sciences were put to work on these problems and told to produce not only speculative consid-erations but also analyses that could be translated into decisions, policies, and actions (and, unlike the invitations that usually came to scholars in those days, they were paid well for the work). This stimulation of a public, practical ethics was the finest achieve-ment of both commissions. That stimulus has inspired some state panels charged with similar tasks, such as the New York State Task Force on Life and the Law (1985 to the present) and the New Jersey Commission on Legal and Ethical Problems in the Deliv-ery of Health Care (1985–1991). The federal commissions provided these groups with models of process, and even competent staff. The federal government has continued to create ethics panels for particular tasks, but their stories lie largely beyond the bound-aries of this history.[81]

Notes for Chapter 4

1. U.S. Senate Subcommittee on Government Research, Committee on Government Opera-tions, *Hearings on S.J. Resolution 145*, 90th Congress, 2nd session, March 8–9, 21–22, 27–28, April 2, 1968, pp. 1, 3; see David J. Rothman, *Strangers at the Bedside: A History of How Law and Bioethics Transformed Medical Decision Making* (New York: Basic Books, 1991), chapter 9.
   2. Senate Committee, *Hearings on S.J.R. 145*, p. 36.
   3. Senate Committee, *Hearings on S.J.R. 145*, pp. 57, 282.
   4. Senate Committee, *Hearings on S.J.R. 145*, pp. 103–118.
   5. Senate Committee, *Hearings on S.J.R. 145*, p. 123.
   6. Senate Committee, *Hearings on S.J.R. 145*, p. 139.
   7. Senate Committee, *Hearings on S.J.R. 145*, pp. 70, 82.
   8. Senate Committee, *Hearings on S.J.R. 145*, p. 100.
   9. "Were transplants premature?" *Time*, March 15, 1968, p. 66.
   10. Senate Committee, *Hearings on S.J.R. 145*, p. 310.
   11. "Johns Hopkins case study—public policy aspects: a statement prepared by Senator Wal-ter F. Mondale for the International Symposium on Human Rights, Retardation and Research," unpublished paper, Washington, D.C., Oct. 16, 1971, pp. 4–5.
   12. Senate Committee, *Hearings on S.J.R. 145*, p. 47.
   13. Victor Cohen, "Live fetal research debated," *Washington Post*, April 10, 1973: A1, A9.
   14. Cohen, "Scientists and fetal research," *Washington Post*, April 15, 1973: A1.
   15. Cohen, "NIH vows not to fund fetus work," *Washington Post*, April 13, 1973: A1, A8.
   16. U.S. Senate Subcommittee on Health, Committee on Labor and Public Welfare, *Quality of*

Health Care—Human Experimentation (Washington, D.C.: U.S. Government Printing Office, 1973), pp. 1–2.

17. Veatch had been invited by Senator Kennedy's staff to help plan the hearings (personal communication); see his subsequent article, "Human experimentation—ethical questions persist," *Hastings Center Report* 3, no. 3 (1973): 1–3.

18. U.S. Senate Subcommittee on Health, Committee on Labor and Public Welfare, *Quality of Health Care—Human Experimentation*, pp. 1, 486.

19. Jessica Mitford, *Kind and Usual Punishment: The Prison Business* (New York: Vintage Press, 1974).

20. Bernard Barber, J. Lally, J. Makarushka, and D. Sullivan, *Research on Human Subjects: Problems of Social Control in Medical Experimentation* (New York: Russell Sage Foundation, 1973).

21. Henry K. Beecher, "Ethics and clinical research," *New England Journal of Medicine* 274 (1966): 1354–1360.

22. Jay Katz, "Reservations about the Panel Report on Charge I," *Final Report of the Tuskegee Syphilis Study Ad Hoc Advisory Panel*, reprinted in Stanley J. Reiser, Arthur J. Dyck, and William J. Curran (eds.), *Ethics in Medicine* (Cambridge, Mass.: MIT Press, 1977), p. 320. The details of the Tuskegee study will be found in Chapter 5 of this book.

23. U.S. Senate Committee on Labor and Public Welfare, "National Research Act," *Hearings*, 92nd Congress, 1st session, May 1973, p. 1326.

24. *Congressional Quarterly Almanac* 1973, xxix, Sept. 11, p. 512.

25. *Congressional Quarterly Almanac* 1973, xxix, Sept. 11, p. 512.

26. *Congressional Quarterly* 1974, xxx, June 25, p. 381.

27. *Congressional Quarterly Almanac* 1973, xxix, p. 512.

28. Personal communication from Warren Reich, October 20, 1996.

29. "Memo on the legislative background from legal staff to Dr. Lowe, November 29, 1974," National Commission for the Protection of Human Subjects of Biomedical and Behavioral Research Archive, Box 1. The papers and records of the National Commission and the President's Commission are maintained at the National Reference Center for Bioethics Literature, Georgetown University, Washington, D.C., and will be referenced below as National Commission and President's Commission Archive Box.

30. Dr. Lowe left the Commission after a year and Mr. Yesley assumed his duties.

31. Public Law 93-348, 93rd Congress, 2nd session (July 12, 1974); 88 STAT 342.

32. National Commission for the Protection of Human Subjects of Biomedical and Behavioral Research, *Research on the Fetus* (Washington, D.C.: Government Printing Office, 1975), *Federal Register* vol. 40, no. 154 (1975): 33526–33551. LeRoy Walters' essay written for the Commission makes the same point; see Appendix I of *Research on the Fetus*. The entire text of the Report and the Regulations, including Louisell's dissent, is reprinted in Reiser et al., *Ethics in Medicine*, pp. 450–486 and also in *The Hastings Center Report* (1975), 5(3), pp. 11–48.

33. National Commission for the Protection of Human Subjects of Biomedical and Behavioral Research, *Research Involving Prisoners* (1976), *Research Involving Children* (1977), *Research Involving Those Institutionalized as Mentally Infirm* (1978), *Psychosurgery* (1977), *Institutional Review Boards* (1978), *Disclosure of Research Information* (1977), *Delivery of Health Services* (1978) and the *Special Study* (1978), *The Belmont Report* (1979).

34. Transcript, 15th meeting, February 13–15, 1976, Meeting files, p. 4, National Commission Archive Box 26.

35. Transcript, 15th meeting, February 13–15, 1976, Meeting files, pp. 109–149, National Commission Archive Box 26.

36. Transcript, 27th meeting, February 11–13, 1977, Meeting Files, p. 7, National Commission Archive Box 30.

37. *The Belmont Report: Ethical Principles and Guidelines for the Protection of Human Subjects of Research* (Washington, D.C.: Government Printing Office, 1979).

38. See Tom L. Beauchamp and James F. Childress, *Principles of Biomedical Ethics* (New York: Oxford University Press, 1979, 4th ed., 1994). Tom Beauchamp began to work with the Commission staff at the beginning of 1977. He was present at the February 1977 meeting and was invited to comment on the draft of *The Belmont Report*. He became a full staff member in July 1977, working with Toulmin on subsequent drafts of that document. In the previous year, Beauchamp had begun to collaborate on a textbook with his Georgetown colleague, James Childress, which was organized around four principles that were superficially similar to those of *The Belmont Report*. They were writing at approximately the same time that they were involved with the Commission, and a mutual influence was inevitable. The role of their text is discussed in Chapter Ten of this book.

39. National Commission for the Protection of Human Subjects of Biomedical and Behavioral Research, *Report and Recommendations: Research Involving Those Institutionalized as Mentally Infirm* (Washington, D.C.: DHEW Publication (OS) 78-0006, 1978), p. xvii.

40. President's Commission, *Protecting Research Subjects: The Adequacy and Uniformity of Federal Rules and their Implementation*, (Washington, D.C.: Government Printing Office, 1981); pp. 74–76; President's Commission, *Implementing Human Research Regulations* (Washington, D.C.: Government Printing Office, 1983); pp. 23–29; see Levine, *Ethics and Regulation of Clinical Research*, chapter 11.

41. Elliot S. Valenstein, *Brain Control: A Critical Examination of Brain Stimulation and Psychosurgery* (New York and London: Wiley-Interscience, 1973); Valenstein, *Great and Desperate Cures: The Rise and Decline of Psychosurgery and Other Radical Treatments for Mental Illness* (New York: Basic Books, 1986).

42. The failure of the two reports on psychiatric issues prompts reflection on a general failure of bioethics to deal with the ethics of psychiatry. Apart from Charles Culver and Bernard Gert, *Philosophy and Medicine: Conceptual and Ethical Issues in Psychiatry* (New York: Oxford University Press, 1982), very little attention has been paid to the ethics of psychiatry. One might speculate that the rationalistic bias of bioethicists inhibits their inability to look squarely at ethical problems raised by those with impaired rationality. See Albert Jonsen and Burr Eichelman, "Ethical issues in psychopharmacological treatment," in Donald M. Gallant and Robert Force (eds.), *Legal and Ethical Issues in Human Research and Treatment* (New York: Spectrum Publications, 1977), pp. 143–176.

43. Franz J. Ingelfinger, "The unethical in medical ethics," *Annals of Internal Medicine* 83 (1975): 264–269; *New England Journal of Medicine* 296 (1977): 44–45; Bradford Gray, "Bioethics commissions: What can we learn from past successes and failures?" in Ruth Ellen Bulger, Elizabeth Meyer Bobby, and Harvey V. Fineberg (eds.), *Society's Choices: Social and Ethical Decision Making in Biomedicine* (Washington, D.C.: National Academy Press, 1995), pp. 261–306.

44. George Annas, "Report on the National Commission: good as gold," *Medicolegal News* 8, no. 6 (1980): 4–7; Albert Jonsen and Michael Yesley, "Rhetoric and research ethics: a reply to George Annas," *Medicolegal News* 8, no. 6 (1980): 8–13. See Michael Yesley, "The uses of an advisory commission," *University of Southern California Law Review* 51 (1978): 1451–1469.

45. Jay Katz, "Unethical experiments," (paper read at the Birth of Bioethics Conference, Seattle, Wa, Sept. 23–24, 1992), transcripts pp. 119–133.

46. Public Law 92–463 "Federal Advisory Committee Act," [45CFR46, 46.204], 92nd Congress, 2nd session; 86 STAT 770 (Oct. 6, 1972).

47. National Ethics Advisory Board, transcript of first meeting, February 3, 1978, pp. 10–13, National Reference Center for Bioethics Literature, EAB Archive Box 1.

48. Ethics Advisory Board DHEW, "Report and recommendations: HEW support of fetoscopy," *Federal Register* vol. 44, no. 158 (August 14, 1979): 47732–47734.

49. *Congressional Quarterly Almanac* 1978, xxxiv, pp. 605–606.

50. President's Commission for the Study of Ethical Problems in Medicine and Biomedical and Behavioral Research, Briefing book, 2nd meeting, Meeting files, President's Commission Archive Box 25.

51. Alexander M. Capron and Leon Kass, "A statutory definition of the standards for determining human death: an appraisal and a proposal," *University of Pennsylvania Law Review* 121 (1972): 87, 102–104; Dan Wikler and Michael B. Green, "Brain death and personal identity," *Philosophy and Public Affairs* 9 (1980): 105–133; Robert Veatch, *Death, Dying and the Biological Revolution: Our Last Quest for Responsibility* (New Haven: Yale University Press, 1977); "Refinements for the determination of death: an appraisal," *Journal of the American Medical Association* 221 (1972): 48–52.

52. President's Commission for the Study of Ethical Problems in Medicine and Biomedical and Behavioral Research, *Defining Death: Medical, Legal and Ethical Issues in the Determination of Death* (Washington: D.C.: U.S. Government Printing Office, 1981), p. 2.

53. President's Commission for the Study of Ethical Problems in Medicine and Biomedical and Behavioral Research, *Splicing Life: The Social and Ethical Issues of Genetic Engineering with Human Beings* (Washington, D.C.: Government Printing Office, 1982); *Screening and Counseling for Genetic Conditions: The Ethical, Social, and Legal Implications of Genetic Screening, Counseling, and Education Programs* (Washington, D.C.: Government Printing Office, 1983).

54. President's Commission for the Study of Ethical Problems in Medicine and Biomedical and Behavioral Research, *Deciding to Forego Life-Sustaining Treatment* (Washington, D.C.: Government Printing Office, 1983).

55. *Superintendent of Belchertown State School v Saikewicz* (Mass Supreme Ct 1977); *In the Matter of Shirley Dinnerstein* (Mass Appellate Ct 1978); *In the Matter of Spring* (Mass Supreme Jud Ct 1980).

56. Sharon R. Imbus and Bruce E. Zawecki, "Autonomy for burned patients when survival is unprecedented," *New England Journal of Medicine* 297 (1977): 308–309.

57. James Rachels, "Active and passive euthanasia," *New England Journal of Medicine* 292 (1975): 78–79.

58. Briefing book, 21st Meeting, June 10–11, 1982, Meeting files, p. 4, President's Commission Archive Box 32. Chairman Abram's comment is recorded in the transcript of Day 2, Box 41, p. 4.

59. President's Commission, *Deciding To Forego*, chapter 2 (draft), briefing book, 21st Meeting, June 10–11, 1982, Meeting files, President's Commission Archive Box 32, pp. II–31; the Commission's discussion is recorded in the transcript of the Meeting files, pp. 4–117, President's Commission Archive Box 41.

60. Dan W. Brock, "Public moral discourse," in Ruth Bulger, Elizabeth Bobby, and Harvey Fineberg (eds.), *Society's Choices: Social and Ethical Decision Making in Biomedicine* (Washington, D.C.: The National Academy Press, 1995) pp. 215–240; Baruch Brody, "The President's Commission: the need to be more philosophical," *Journal of Medicine and Philosophy* 14 (1989): 369–383; "Symposium: the role of philosophers in the public policy process: a view from the President's Commission," *Ethics* 97 (1987): 775–795.

61. *Deciding To Forego*, p. 61.

62. *Deciding To Forego*, p. 89.

63. *Deciding To Forego*, p. 72.

64. John A Behnke and Sissela Bok (eds.), *The Dilemmas of Euthanasia* (Garden City, N.Y.: Anchor Press, 1975); Marvin Kohl (ed.), *Beneficient Euthanasia* (Buffalo, N.Y.: Prometheus Books, 1975); Daniel C. Maguire, *Death by Choice* (New York: Schocken Books, 1973).

65. Bradford Gray, "Bioethics commissions: what can we learn from past successes and failures," in Bulger et al., *Society's Choices*, p. 286.

66. President Truman's Commission on the Health Needs of the Nation (1953), quoted in President's Commission for the Study of Ethical Problems in Medicine and Biomedical and Behavioral Research, *Securing Access to Health Care* (U.S. Government Printing Office, 1983) p. 11. The term "right to health" first appears in 1796 Congressional debates over quarantine laws. See Carleton B. Chapman and John M. Talmadge, "The evolution of the right to health concept in the United States," *Pharos* 34 (1971), 30–51.

67. Gene Outka, "Social justice and equal access to health care," *Journal of Religion and Ethics*, 2 (1974): 11–32; Ronald M. Green, "Health care and justice in contract theory perspective," in Robert M. Veatch (ed.), *Ethics and Health Policy* (Cambridge, Mass: Ballinger, 1976), pp. 111–126.

68. John D. Arras, "Retreat from the right to health care: the President's Commission and access to health care," *Cardozo Law Review* 6 (1984): 321–346.

69. *Securing Access to Health Care*, p. 93.

70. At the 23rd meeting, August 12, 1982, only four months before the statutory expiration, H. Thomas Ballantine, Bruce K. Jacobson, John J. Moran, and Kay Toma were sworn in to replace Albert R. Jonsen, Anne A. Scitovsky, Mario García-Palmieri, and Carolyn Williams, whose terms had ended on July, 1982.

71. Minutes, 26th meeting, Nov. 13, 1982, Meeting files, President's Commission Archive Box 36. Unfortunately, the transcript of this contentious meeting is missing from the National Reference Center for Bioethics Literature archives; my history relies on the minutes only.

72. *Securing Access to Health Care*, p. 203; Transcript, 27th Meeting, Dec. 12–14, 1982, Meeting files, President's Commission Archive Box 42; Dr. Dunlop's remarks are recorded on pp. 7–9 and 219–221. See Ronald Bayer, "Ethics, politics, and access to health care: a critical analysis of the President's Commission," *Cardozo Law Review* 6 (1984): 303–320; Bayer contends that there was a "staff revolt" over the Commissioners' demands for revision.

73. There is no comprehensive summary of the National Commission Reports. The President's Commission's work is gathered in *Summing Up: Final Report on Studies on the Ethical and Legal Problems in Medicine and Biomedical and Behavioral Research* (Washington, D.C.: Government Printing Office, 1983). For an assessment of the Commission's work, see Morris B. Abram and Susan M. Wolf, "Public involvement in medical ethics: a model for government action," *New England Journal of Medicine* 310 (1984): 627–632.

74. Bradford Gray, "Bioethics commissions," in Bulger et al., *Society's Choices*, p. 267.

75. Allan J. Weisbard and John D. Arras, "Commissioning morality: an introduction to the symposium," *Cardozo Law Review* 6 (1984): pp. 223–242, quote on p. 231.

76. Brody, "The President's Commission," pp. 369–383.

77. Daniel Callahan, "Morality and contemporary culture: the President's Commission and beyond," *Cardozo Law Review*, 6 (1984): 347–356.

78. Gray, "Bioethics commissions," p. 289.

79. Gray, "Bioethics commissions," p. 283.

80. Allan J. Weisbard and John D. Arras, *"Commissioning morality"; Advisory Committee on Human Radiation Experiments, Final Report* (Washington, D.C.: Government Printing Office, 1995).

81. Bulger et al., *Society's Choices*. In 1997, President Clinton established by Executive Order 12975 the National Bioethics Advisory Commission, charging it with review of issues regarding protection of human subjects of research and issues in the management and use of genetic information.

II

BIOETHICAL BEGINNINGS:
THE PROBLEMS

5

Experiments Perilous: The Ethics of Research with Human Subjects

The conferences of the 1960s discussed ethical and moral issues (rarely defining these two terms) in lengthy agendas. Speakers touched on many topics, often only to express concern, seldom to define, analyze, or resolve them. The more structured discourse of the centers and commissions brought sharper definition to the issues. The lengthy agenda was abbreviated to five topics that received extensive and concentrated attention during the first decades of bioethics. The next five chapters survey these five topics: research with human subjects, genetics, organ transplantation, death and dying, and reproduction. We shall situate each topic in its historical context and review its treatment in bioethical discourse.

Experiments Perilous

From the beginnings of medicine physicians knew that, as Hippocrates wrote, "experience is uncertain"; treatments successful in prior cases might fail in the present case.[1] In desperate moments of illness, previously untried remedies were attempted, sometimes with unexpected success. Further, Hippocratic physicians devised treatments to fit the particular needs and conditions of individual patients; they were wary of generalizations from patient to patient. In the midst of this uncertainty and variety, the Hippocratic maxim, "benefit and do no harm," urged physicians to maintain a constant intent to cure.[2] The untried and the unusual always had to be placed within a therapeutic attempt. For most of medical history, the experimental (which in Latin means "putting to the test of experience") was folded into the therapeutic; patients were experimental subjects only as their doctors worked to heal them.

Occasionally, history hints at another sort of *experimentum*. The Roman medical encylopedist, Celsus, records that the Ptolemies permitted certain Alexandrian physicians to perform vivisection on criminals. Celsus disapproved, calling the experimenters "medical murderers . . . who, instead of presiding over human health, preside over death."[3] Avicenna and Maimonides allude to "experiments on the human body," warning that patients should not be treated as mere means for learning.[4] These and other passing comments hint at experiments performed without therapeutic intent, purely for the sake of enhancing knowledge. Generally, however, from Hippocratic times until recently, medical practice was not clearly distinguished from experimentation. Medical research, such as it was, consisted primarily of observing the course of disease and the effects of treatments, be they traditional or innovative. By careful observation, the great researchers of early modern medicine, such as Thomas Sydenham and Marcello Malpighi, learned the efficacy, futility, or dangers of what they had done or failed to do. When competent practitioners introduced new treatments, they did so cautiously, observing the consequences and sharing their conclusions with colleagues. This was the "perilous experimentation" of which even the common law warned, "he who experiments does so at his peril."[5]

In 1703, Dr. Zabdiel Boylston inoculated Boston's children against smallpox; his son and two of his slaves were the first subjects. He was comforted in conscience by Boston's leading divine, Cotton Mather. Eighty-six years later, in 1789, Edward Jenner vaccinated his own son with cowpox, then a "healthy boy, about eight years old." Queen Caroline then requested that several orphan children be vaccinated before the new and frightening procedure was tried on the royal scions. These experiments hovered on the edge of therapeutic (or rather, preventive) intent. There was no other way to test the efficacy of vaccination. No concern was evinced that the subjects were unconsenting children.[6]

Two decades after Jenner's innovation, Thomas Percival's *Medical Ethics* makes but one allusion to experimentation:

> Whenever cases occur, attended with circumstances not heretofore observed, or in which the ordinary modes of practice have been attempted without success, it is for the public good, and in a special degree advantageous for the poor (who, being the most numerous class of society, are the greatest beneficiaries of the healing art), that new remedies and new methods of chirurgical treatment should be devised. But in the accomplishment of this salutary purpose, the gentlemen of the faculty should be scrupulously and conscientiously governed by sound reason, just analogy, or well authenticated facts. And no such trials should be instituted without a previous consultation of the physicians or surgeons according to the nature of the case.[7]

It is difficult to know whether this advice represents the opinion of the contemporary profession or the wishful admonition of one of its most high-minded members. Little is heard of such "peer review" over the next century and a half.

Scientific Medicine and Experimentation

During the first half of the nineteenth century, medicine began to reap the fruits of the previous century of scientific advances in chemistry and physics. The cellular basis of physiology and pathology, the germ theory of disease, the invention of instruments for investigation, such as the stethoscope and the thermometer, and the initiation of clinical teaching opened the age of experimental medicine. "The Paris School" exemplified the new scientific spirit. One of its leaders, Pierre Louis, devised the "numerical method," a primitive form of statistics, to record and analyze data. In 1835, he published research showing that in a population divided into treatment and nontreatment groups, the common practices of venesection and blistering provided no therapeutic benefit.[8]

In 1865, the French physiologist, Claude Bernard, published his groundbreaking work, *Introduction to the Study of Experimental Medicine,* arguing that medicine must be placed on a solid scientific basis by rigorously logical observations of the physiological conditions of health and disease. Bernard proposed methods to reach this goal, illustrating them with his own pioneering research. Reflecting on the morality of his work, he asks, "Have we a right to perform experiments and vivisections on man?" His answer: "It is our duty and right to perform an experiment on man whenever it can save his life, cure him or gain him some personal benefit. The principle of medical and surgical morality, therefore, consists in never performing on man an experiment which might be harmful to him to any extent, even though the result might be highly advantageous to science, that is, to the health of others." Bernard's principle remains within the Hippocratic tradition: experiments must be therapeutic in intent. He does not mention the consent of experimental subjects and even commends one experiment in which a physician "had a condemned woman without her knowledge swallow the larvae of intestinal worms, so as to see whether the worms developed in the intestines after her death." This experiment, he believed, "involved no suffering or harm (and) . . . Christian morals forbid only one thing, doing ill to one's neighbor."[9] This remark takes Bernard beyond the Hippocratic ethic. The condemned woman was not a patient whom the physician was obliged to benefit and not to harm; she was a pure experimental subject. Behavior toward her was dictated not by Hippocrates but by general Christian standards, in particular, avoidance of harm. When death by disease or execution was imminent, no harm would eventuate. Using this reasoning, some nineteenth-century experimenters, especially those interested in the behavior of bacteria, did not hesitate to infect dying patients, and some twentieth-century doctors administered radiation and radioactive substances to unsuspecting dying persons.

Several decades before Bernard's pioneering work on the function of pancreatic juice in digestion, William Beaumont, a U.S. Army physician, published the results of a decade-long experiment with a quondam patient, Alexis St. Martin, whose partly healed gunshot wound opened a window into his stomach. Beaumont had engaged St. Martin under an indenture, providing room and board and a small salary; in return, St.

Martin allowed Dr. Beaumont to drop various items into the hydrochloric acid of his stomach. The indentured research subject, while compliant, was not entirely content with his lot; he ran away several times. Beaumont's subsequent book was praised as a significant contribution to science. Dr. Beaumont wrote, "I consider myself but a humble inquirer after truth—a simple experimenter."[10]

Enthusiasm for experimentation grew during the nineteenth century. Although science was advanced, horrendous stories of abuse were told. In 1901, a Russian physician, V. V. Smidovich, using the pseudonym Vikenty Veressayev, published a memoir in which he recalled scientific work done during the preceding century. The field of venerology was a particular target of Veressayev's ire. Physicians, he asserted, often deliberately infected their patients with gonococcus and the syphilitic spirochete. Many of the patients were "hopelessly ill" or "not expected to live," although some were patients suffering from chronic diseases and others merely unfortunate enough to find themselves confined to a medical institution. The experimenters published their studies in respected scientific journals. Veressayev concluded:

> This martyrology of the unhappy patients offered up as victims to science was not compiled by any underhanded means—the culprits publicly blazoned their own infamy in black and white. One would suppose that the mere fact of publication of such experiments would make their repetition utterly impossible . . . but, unfortunately, this is not so. With heads proudly erect, these bizarre disciples of science proceed upon their way without encountering any effective opposition, either from their colleagues or the medical press.[11]

Veressayev found most of his examples in Europe, although he cited several British and American cases, including Dr. Robert Barthelow's electrical exploration of the brain of a feeble-minded woman dying of cancer that resulted in her paralysis and death. American physicians often asserted that such work would be done only in European countries, where there was little respect for patients of the lower classes.[12] Some leaders of the American profession, however, were not at all indifferent. Barthelow's experiment met severe criticism in the medical press, and even Veressayev admits in a footnote that it "aroused the indignation of the entire profession."[13] One scientific report gained special notoriety—the work of Guiseppe Sanarelli, an Italian bacteriologist working in Montevideo, Uruguay. Seeking the causative agent of yellow fever, Sanarelli injected his candidate bacillus into five hospital patients without their knowledge or consent, producing "typical yellow fever [as indicated by] a fever, congestions, hemorrhages, vomiting, steatosis of the liver, cephalalgia, rachialgia, nephritis, anuria, uremia, icterus, delirium, collapse." The patients, reported Sanarelli, recovered and the experiment provided "striking evidence in favor of the specific nature of the bacillus *icteroides*."[14]

In 1898, the Surgeon General of the United States, Dr. George Sternberg, who was an expert on yellow fever, criticized Sanarelli's work before the leaders of American medicine. Dr. Victor Vaughn called the experiment "ridiculous." Dr. William Osler was even more censorious: "Even granting that every dose of medicine we give is an experiment, to deliberately utilize a human being for the purpose of experiment without the sanction of the individual is not ridiculous, it is criminal."[15] Two years later, Osler repeated this sanction before a U.S. Senate hearing. Senator Jacob Gallinger (R-NH), who had been trained as a physician, became a champion for the anti-vivisection movement. In 1896, he had introduced *A Bill for the Further Prevention of Cruelty to Animals in the District of Columbia.*[16] The bill failed twice to reach the floor but, in the spring of 1900, Gallinger reintroduced it with broader scope and a new title, *A Bill for the Regulation of Scientific Experiments upon Human Beings in the District of Columbia.*[17]

The bill's broader scope reflected the vivisectionists' conviction that tolerance of animal research would lead inevitably to human research. The term vivisection was used to cover all animal and human research. This bill prohibited "the crime of human vivisection, [that is,] performing upon the body of any human being, in any hospital, asylum, retreat or infirmary . . . any scientific experiment involving pain, distress or risk to life and health, whether by administration of poisonous drugs for the purpose of ascertaining their toxicity, by inoculating the germs of disease, by grafting cancerous tumors into healthy tissues, or by performance of any surgical operation for any other object than the amelioration of the patient." Such procedures might be permitted only if the experimenter were granted a special license by the commissioners of the District, sought specific permission in advance, and filed a report of results. The subject of the experiment had to be at least "twenty years of age and in full and complete possession of all his or her reasoning faculties" and sign a notarized and witnessed written permission, submitted to the commissioners together with the experimenter's request. "No scientific experiment of any kind liable to cause pain or distress shall be permissible upon any newborn babe, infant, child, or youth; nor upon any woman during pregnancy nor within a year after her confinement, nor upon any aged, infirm, epileptic, insane, or feeble minded person under any circumstances."[18]

In preparation for the hearings, Senator Gallinger had collected a gallery of "human vivisection horrors," including Sanarelli's experiments, in order to verify that the offenses mentioned in the bill had actually taken place in the halls of scientific medicine. Leaders of American medicine appeared to testify against the bill. Dr. William Welch of Johns Hopkins, who had for several years headed the scientific world's opposition to the anti-vivisection movement, began by lauding the scientific progress of the previous quarter century, stating that its main cause was "the fruitful application of the experimental method of research." Dr. Osler entered into his testimony a footnote from his magisterial volume, *Principles and Practice of Medicine.* The footnote was a compendium of Osler's ethics of research. He approved physician self-experimentation, patients' voluntary acceptance of research, and the experimental use only of drugs proven harmless in animals. Citing Sanarelli's "unjustifiable experiments . . . which should receive the unqualified condemnation of the profession," he condemned as criminal "deliberate experiments with cultures of known and tested virulence, followed by nearly fatal illness."[19] Despite his disapproval of unethical experiments, Osler abruptly answered Gallinger's question whether he would oppose legislation preventing human vivisection: "Yes, sir: as a piece of unnecessary legislation."[20] The medical establishment rallied sufficient support in the Senate that the bill was not reported out of committee.

Three months after the Senate hearings, Surgeon General George Sternberg established the Yellow Fever Commission, under the direction of Major Walter Reed of the U.S. Army Medical Corps. Yellow fever had ravished tropical climes and had long been a deadly scourge of the American South. Extremely high mortality and morbidity from yellow fever contributed notably to the failure of the French endeavor to build *La Grande Tranchée* through the Isthmus of Panama in the 1880s. Thousands of American soldiers had died of the disease during the Spanish-American War. For several decades, a number of medical men had proposed that the disease was probably mosquito borne.[21]

Dr. Reed and three colleagues, Drs. James Carroll, Jesse Lazear, and Aristide Agramonte, set out for Quemados, Cuba, to verify the mosquito hypothesis. The investigators designed an experiment to specify the mode of transmission by allowing mosquitoes that had fed on yellow-fever patients to bite humans. They decided, probably at Carroll's suggestion, to make themselves the first subjects. While Major Reed was on a trip to Washington, D.C., Carroll and Lazear initiated the experiment. Both became severely ill. Carroll recovered but Lazear died. On his return, Reed was dismayed but undaunted; the scientists moved to the next phase, which involved separating research subjects into groups of those who would be bitten and those who would be exposed to soiled bedding from patients. Given the depletion of his scientific staff by one-fourth, Dr. Reed decided to omit further self-experimentation and to seek volunteers. The first volunteer was rather casually recruited. A curious soldier wandered by and was asked, "Will you take a bite?" He answered, "Sure, I ain't scared of 'em." Soon a more formal recruitment was devised. A contract was drawn up, stating the purpose of the experiment and its risks (somewhat understating the risks and overstating the likelihood of contracting yellow fever by merely living in Cuba). The volunteer, "being in the enjoyment and exercise of his own free will, consents to submit himself to experiments for the purpose of determining the methods of transmission of yellow fever." One hundred dollars would be given at the conclusion of the experiment to surviving subjects ($200 if they became sick) or to their designees in case of death. Both American soldiers and locals were enrolled (the contract was translated into Spanish for the locals). Twenty-five volunteers became ill but no one died.

The results of Reed's experiment were extremely valuable. They identified the source and the mode of infection of a tropical disease that killed and disabled untold numbers in the countries where it was endemic. This scientific information became the basis for a public hygiene program in Cuba and contributed to the success of the American Panama Canal project. It was a socially and scientifically important experiment and was recognized as such by the public and even the Congress of the United

States. Walter Reed's reputation as an intrepid researcher and the bravery of his colleagues were celebrated for decades afterwards.[22]

Eight years after Reed's experiments, on November 20, 1907, Dr. Osler, who was now Regius Professor of Medicine at Oxford University, was invited to appear before a Royal Commission on Vivisection. Osler's biographer comments, "It was not his first experience, for he has already been seen giving somewhat heated testimony before a U.S. Senator, when a similar inquiry was being held, although on that occasion ignorance and prejudice presided, whereas a British Parliamentary hearing is of a different caliber."[23] Osler's dialogue with the commissioners articulates the view of the enlightened profession about research.

> *Commissioner:* I understand that in the case of yellow fever the recent experiments have been on man.
> *Osler:* Yes, definitely with the specific consent of these individuals who went into this camp voluntarily. . . .
> *Commissioner:* We were told by a witness yesterday that, in his opinion, to experiment upon man with possible ill result was immoral. Would that be your view?
> *Osler:* It is always immoral, without a definite, specific statement from the individual himself, with a full knowledge of the circumstances. Under these circumstances, any man, I think, is at liberty to submit himself to experiments.
> *Commissioner:* Given voluntary consent, you think that entirely changes the question of morality or otherwise?
> *Osler:* Entirely.[24]

Walter Reed's experiments dramatically illustrated the arrival of a new actor in medical research, namely, the healthy volunteer. Osler's testimony suggests that by the first decade of the century volunteers had become familiar enough that an addition to the Hippocratic ethic was needed—the principle of voluntary consent. However, the hospital, with its available patients, remained the home for most medical research. In the last decades of the nineteenth century, hospitals in the United States not only multiplied (from 178 in 1873 to 4,359 in 1909), but were transformed from poorhouses for the dying into doctors' workshops in which the best medicine was practiced. Among the physicians who cared for patients, some were intrigued by the new sciences and the best of them had been trained in places like Berlin and Vienna. The innovative therapies they had learned abroad and read about in the medical literature could be applied to their patients. This experimentation remained largely within the scope of therapeutic intent, but the temptation to go beyond that was sometimes compelling.

In an 1886 dissertation that won Harvard's Boylston Prize, *The Relation of Hospitals to Medical Education*, Dr. Charles Francis Withington recognized that "the occupants of hospital wards are something more than merely so much clinical material during their lives and so much pathological material after their death." While it may be true that patients are often treated in a new way or with a new drug, they "have a right to immunity from experiments merely as such," even if those experiments entail no particular harm or discomfort. Should an investigator ask patients to submit to these "as a favor . . . few, if any would refuse him." But should discomfort or harm result from interventions that serve no therapeutic purpose, it is "an egregious usurpation. . . . If experimenters wish to investigate the physiological action of a drug, they should call for volunteers; they have no right to make any man the unwilling victim of such experiments." Dr. Withington advocated "a Bill of Rights which shall secure patients against any injustice from the votaries of science."[25]

As the experimental spirit took hold, a roughly defined ethic accompanied it. A physician might use new treatments as he sought to cure the patient. While clearly experimental, the new treatments fell within the scope of the physician's duty to benefit the patient. Patients, however, were not to be used to test methods or drugs that had no relation to the patient's illness or condition. As for dangerous experiments, volunteers, not patients, were to be recruited. In this case, the free consent of the subject had to be solicited. Finally, the researcher was to make himself the first volunteer, as Lazear and Carroll had done.[26]

Despite these general understandings, the research enterprise was neither immune from interior scandals nor from external criticism. The Anti-Vivisection Society continued its attack on "scientific assassination" up to the eve of World War I, and riveted public attention with outrageous (but not always accurate) examples of the abuse of research subjects. Stories of the use of children in orphanages for infectious disease research were particularly offensive and were propagated by the Hearst newspapers, which promoted the anti-vivisectionist cause.[27] In 1912, the work of a leading microbiologist, Dr. Hideyo Noguchi of the Rockefeller Institute, came under public scrutiny. He had injected "luetin," a solution of inactivated *Treponema pallidum,* the spirochete that causes syphilis, into 400 persons without consent; half of these subjects were syphilitic inhabitants of mental hospitals and the other half were healthy orphan children and patients in public hospitals. His report, published in the *Journal of Experimental Medicine,* prompted a feature story in *Life* magazine, which supported the anti-vivisectionist cause, and a public outcry ensued. Criminal charges were filed but not pursued and several state legislatures attempted to regulate research. Dr. Noguchi (who had tested luetin on himself and on his fellow researchers before applying it to research subjects) continued his work on infectious disease and died in 1928 while in Africa studying yellow fever.[28]

Leading medical scientists defended research, repudiating its worst cases and attempting to inculcate a sense of responsibility in investigators. Harvard physiologist Walter Cannon led the defense. As chairman of the Council on the Defense of Medical Research, he championed the notion that patients and families be "fully aware of and consenting to the plan" of using any novel diagnostic or therapeutic procedure, and that journals insist that articles attest to that fact. In 1916, Dr. Cannon urged the American Medical Association to adopt a formal resolution in which the conditions for acceptable experimentation be spelled out, including formal, prior consent of patients. Other leading medical scientists, such as Simon Flexner and Cannon's Harvard colleague, Francis

Peabody, were reluctant to support this measure. Dr. Peabody was particularly uneasy with the idea of patient consent which, while necessary in risky experiments, would detract from the physician's responsibility to act always for the patient's welfare. The character of the researcher was the principal issue and, said Dr. Peabody, those who pursued a career in scientific medicine were generally "among the more high minded of the profession."[29] Cannon's proposal came to naught: The AMA House of Delegates did not consider it at the 1916 meeting and the issue disappeared from the agenda until after World War II.

After World War I, the anti-vivisection movement lost some of its momentum and the virulent attacks on animal and human research abated. Problems in human research continued, however, and occasionally reached public attention. The testing of vaccines remained as problematic as it was in the days of Boylston and Jenner, since the only suitable research subjects were children who were still susceptible to infection. In 1935, nine children who had been vaccinated with an experimental live polio vaccine died. This tragic incident retarded polio vaccine research for two decades.[30]

It is one of history's ironies that the first clear ethical standards for modern medical research came from the German government. As early as 1900, the Prussian Ministry of Religious, Educational and Medical Affairs had established rules that forbade all nontherapeutic experimentation unless "the person concerned has . . . declared unequivocally that he consents to the intervention . . . on the basis of a proper explanation of the adverse consequences that may result from the intervention."[31] (The Prussian rules are not dissimilar from those in Senator Gallinger's bill of the same year.) On February 28, 1931, two years before Adolf Hitler became Chancellor of Germany, the Reich Minister of the Interior issued even stronger "Regulations on New Therapy and Experimentation." These regulations "enumerate clear directives concerning the general, technical, and ethical standards of medicine, informed consent, documented justification of any deviation from protocol, a risk-benefit analysis, justification for the study of especially vulnerable populations, such as children, and the necessity to maintain written records. In many ways, these guidelines are more extensive than either the subsequent Nuremberg Code or the later Declaration of Helsinki."[32] Only ten years later, German physicians initiated the most blatantly unethical and inhumane experimentation.

The Doctors' Trial at the Nuremberg Tribunal

After the Allies defeated the Axis Powers in 1945, the victors decided that the behavior of certain German, Italian, and Japanese leaders went beyond the harsh politics of planning and executing a war and into the realm of crimes against humanity. Courts were set up to try these leaders as war criminals. The major trials were held over several years in Nuremberg, Germany. On August 19, 1947, one of these trials, called The Doctors' Trial, concluded after seven months of testimony. Twenty physicians and three medical administrators, charged with "murders, tortures and other atrocities committed in the name of medical science," stood to hear the verdict delivered by Judge Walter Beals. The defendants had been charged with subjecting unwilling victims to medical procedures that were loosely called "scientific experiments," thereby having caused their death, disfigurement, or disability. Nine of the defendants were sentenced to long prison terms and seven were sentenced to death by hanging. The defendants were judged against standards that their prosecutors had devised precisely to try them. Although *ex post facto* norms are ordinarily a legal impropriety, the prosecutors and the judges believed that, far from being *ex post facto,* these standards expressed moral imperatives that should be known to all civilized humans. These standards were, they thought, contemporary expressions of natural law and of the long tradition of medical ethics.

Never before or since has medicine's major moral mandate, "do no harm," been so flagrantly, unambiguously, and indefensibly violated than by the Nazi crime. Yet it was more than a horrifying transgression; it opened a worldwide discussion about one feature indispensable to modern medicine as a scientific enterprise: experimentation using living humans. Even apart from the brutality, racism, and tyranny that corrupted the condemned experiments, medical experimentation using human beings is morally problematic. While the problematic nature of human experimentation had long been recognized, the Nuremberg trial and the Nuremberg Code drew unprecedented attention from the public, from the medical and scientific professions, and from public authorities. That attention marks a new beginning in the moral traditions of medicine, a beginning that would become bioethics.[33]

The Tribunal asserted that the evidence had shown that "with the outbreak of World War II, criminal medical experiments on non-German nationals, both prisoners of war and civilians, including Jews and 'asocial' persons, were carried out on a large scale in Germany and the occupied countries." The Tribunal acknowledged that "certain types of medical experiments . . . conform to the ethics of the medical profession generally" and went on to delineate ten "basic principles that must be observed in order to satisfy moral, ethical and legal concepts." These ten points have become known as the Nuremberg Code.[34]

The Code first states, "The voluntary consent of the human subject is absolutely essential. This means that the person involved . . . should be so situated as to be able to exercise free power of choice without the intervention of any element of force, fraud, deceit, duress, overreaching or any other ulterior form of constraint or coercion." These formal, legal words veil the horror of the concentration camps in which these "experimental subjects," totally stripped of their freedom and dignity, were mutilated and murdered under the guise of scientific research. The second norm, "the experiment should be such as to yield fruitful results for the good of society," directs the research to a human good rather than to the goals of an ideology. Subsequent principles require prior experiments with animals, the avoidance of unnecessary physical and mental suffering and injury, the a priori assurance that no death or disabling injury will result, the scientific qualifications of the researchers, and the subject's right and researcher's duty to terminate harmful experiments.

The "crimes committed in the guise of scientific research," as the prosecution's brief described the Nazi experiments, violated all of those principles. High-altitude research deprived victims of oxygen until they died. Persons were slowly frozen to death. More than one thousand persons were infected with malaria and treated with various experimental drugs; many died from the disease and many from drug complications. Persons were infected with jaundice, typhus, cholera, smallpox, and diphtheria in studies to develop vaccines. Battle wounds were simulated and infected, and then subjects were randomized between non-treatment and sulfanilamide treatment. People were also randomized in a study in which some drank desalinated water and others salt water until symptoms of iodine poisoning appeared. Various poisons were administered to observe lethal effects. Men and women were sterilized in various ways to determine the most efficient methods for widespread population sterilization. The most notorious of the Nazi doctors, Josef Mengele, who escaped capture, was particularly interested in the genetic study of twins. He had collected twin children from the camps, measured their physical features, performed cross-transfusions, transplanted genitals and other organs, and even created artificial Siamese twins. He also used his twin collection for comparative studies, infecting one child and then killing both for autopsy.[35] Although most of the experiments were designed to resolve urgent problems in military medicine, some research, particularly that of Dr. Mengele, was inspired by the racist and pseudoscientific eugenics that we shall discuss in the next chapter.

An American physician, Dr. Andrew C. Ivy, who had been chosen by the American Medical Association to serve as the prosecution's medical expert, was largely responsible for the language of the Code. The judges drew much of that language from Dr. Ivy's report to the AMA Board of Trustees after his initial visit to Germany in the late summer of 1946. In that document, Dr. Ivy stated that "the rules of human experimentation had been well established by custom, social usage and the ethics of medical conduct." His list of the established rules became the provisions that appeared in the judges' version of the Code. When he mentioned that there should be no a priori reason to suspect that death or disabling injury might result from an experiment, he recalled the most famous exemption from this rule: "such experiments as those on Yellow Fever where the experimenters serve as subjects along with non-scientific personnel."[36]

The other American physician associated with the Tribunal, Dr. Leo Alexander, a Tufts Medical School psychiatrist, published a long, horrifying article in *The New England Journal* on July 14, 1949. He detailed the gradual degradation of German medicine under the Nazi regime, beginning with sterilization of retarded persons, proceeding to "euthanasia of the chronically ill (275,000 victims over ten years), and ending in murderous medical research and genocide." He wrote, "An important feature of the experiments performed in concentration camps is the fact that they not only represented a ruthless and callous pursuit of legitimate scientific goals but also were motivated by rather sinister practical ulterior political and personal purposes, arising out of the requirements and problems of the administration of totalitarian rule." He believed that medicine was able to be captured by ideology because of a "subtle shift in emphasis in the basic attitude of physicians . . . toward the nonrehabilitable sick."[37] Alexander concluded his long article with a warning to American physicians, whom he worried were being infected by "the Hegelian, cold blooded, utilitarian philosophy . . . 'what is useful is right.'" American physicians, he said, "have become dangerously close to being mere technicians of rehabilitation . . . in an increasingly utilitarian society, they (incurable patients) are being looked down upon . . . as unwanted ballast."[38]

The horrors of the Nazi experiments shocked medicine worldwide. The World Medical Association, founded soon after World War II, approved "Principles for Those in Research and Experimentation" at its General Assembly held in Rome in 1954. An expanded version of these principles was issued at the WMA's eighteenth assembly, held in Helsinki in June 1964 and, although amended at Tokyo, 1975, Venice, 1983, and Hong Kong, 1989, remains known as the Helsinki Declaration. The Declaration stresses even more strongly than the Nuremberg Code the scientific standards that should govern good research. A distinction appears in the Helsinki Declaration that is not found in the Nuremberg Code but that was consonant with the contemporary understanding of medical research: research in which the aim is primarily diagnostic or therapeutic for a particular patient (called clinical research) is distinguished from research that is purely scientific, without expected benefit for the patient (nonclinical research).

This distinction allows the Helsinki document to weaken the Nuremberg Code's strong requirement for consent. It implies that the investigator who is also the treating physician is judge of the best course of treatment and is permitted to omit informed consent under special circumstances. Also, the Declaration modifies the Code's consent requirement by authorizing consent from guardians and relatives of incompetents, "according to national legislation."[39] It is noteworthy that in the Declaration, the provisions relating to the consent of subjects do not hold primacy of place, as in the Code, but appear in the middle of the text, surrounded by exhortations to the physician to be a responsible and scientific researcher. This stylistic form mirrors the approach taken toward research ethics by many responsible researchers of that day: the essence of research ethics is the integrity and vigilance of the investigator.

The Second World War produced not only the most horrendous examples of research malpractice and the first international ethical code for research but also an intensification of scientific research. In 1941, President Roosevelt's Committee on Medical Research (CMR) began to coordinate researchers in universities, hospitals, research institutes, and industrial firms for the rapid improvement of military medicine. Some 600 protocols at 135 universities, costing $25 million, were sponsored and supervised by the CMR. Much of that research, especially the study of infectious diseases, was done in prisons, mental hospitals, and military camps, often with little regard for the rights of the subjects. When the press reported malaria research done on prisoners at Michigan's Joliet prison, the tone was laudatory, praising the prisoner's contribution to the war effort.[40] Historian David Rothman suggests that for the researchers of the time (as well as for the public who might learn of their work), the nation was at war and "a sense of urgency pervaded the laboratories. . . . the rules of the battlefield seemed to apply to the laboratory. Researchers were no more obliged to obtain the permission of their subjects than the Selective Service was to obtain the permission of civilians to become soldiers." Only when there was risk of public outrage did the Committee on Medical Research impose the safeguard of consent.[41]

After the war, the CMR's sponsorship of medical research was passed to the National Institutes of Health (NIH). Federal support of scientific research, now of proven public value, grew apace, and Congress bestowed largess upon the NIH. Its intramural research expanded and its grant program began to fund not only laboratory scientists but also clinical researchers in every medical school throughout the nation. University hospitals became major research centers, making available thousands of patients as subjects for their physicians' scientific investigations. As the money flowed out of the NIH into the nation's hospitals and laboratories, little attention to the rights and welfare of human research subjects was attached to the dollars.

The problems raised by human experimentation were not unknown to the American medical profession. Articles about the Nuremberg trials appeared in major medical journals. A 1946 editorial in the *Journal of the American Medical Association* condemned the Nazi research and laid down three conditions for ethical research: the consent of the subject, the prerequisite of animal experiments, and proper medical supervision. These three conditions were endorsed by the AMA House of Delegates on December 28, 1947.[42] In 1951, a symposium called "The Problem of Experimentation on Human Beings" was held at an important research center, the University of California School of Medicine, San Francisco; the lectures were published in *Science*.[43] A 1963 anthology, *Clinical Investigation in Medicine: Legal, Ethical and Moral Aspects,* collected seventy-three articles written in the preceding decade and added a bibliography of five hundred more articles, all published in English-language professional journals.[44]

It can hardly be said, then, that the problem of research with human subjects was ignored or that the general outlines for ethical research were unknown. The most vivid description of research activities in that era, sociologist Renée Fox's *Experiment Perilous,* showed researchers concerned about the essential questions, particularly the uncertainty of the risks of research to their volunteers.[45] Despite all this, the lesson of Nuremberg seems to have made little impression on the American world of medical research. Rothman states, "The prevailing view was that [the Nuremberg medical defendants] were Nazis first and last; by definition nothing they did and no code drawn up in response to them was relevant to the United States."[46] Dr. Jay Katz puts it even more bluntly, "It was a good code for barbarians but an unnecessary code for ordinary physicians."[47]

A few physicians saw it differently and were outspoken very early in the debate. Drs. Ivy and Alexander had already articulated their concerns in the strongest terms. Dr. Otto Guttentag of the University of California School of Medicine, San Francisco, was among the boldest of the concerned physicians. His concern was understandable. Born, educated, and certified in medicine in Germany, Otto Guttentag immigrated to the United States in 1935. After World War II, he returned to his homeland as an American Army doctor and met some of his erstwhile medical colleagues. Guttentag returned to America as a crusader for the ethics of research. Speaking at the 1951 UCSF symposium, which he had conceived and organized, he made a crucial point that had not often been noted about research: "The relationship between the experimenter and the experimented on, entered upon not to help but to confirm or disprove some . . . biological generalization, is impersonal and objective. The original, basic patient–physician relationship implies the concept of solidarity, of life's finiteness. . . . Experimentation as just described is foreign to it." A distinction had to be made, he said, between, "the physician–friend . . . a fellow partner with his patient to conquer a common enemy who has overwhelmed one of them, [and] the physician experimenter . . . research and care should not be pursued by the same person."[48]

A later federal committee would note that "among physicians, Dr. Guttentag was nearly unique . . . in raising such problems in print."[49] When I joined the faculty at UCSF, Dr. Guttentag, who was Hahneman Professor Emeritus of Medical Philosophy, confided to me that his encounters with the German physicians had shocked him profoundly. They seemed little disturbed by the revelations of the concentration-camp experiments; indeed, they even sought to justify them. In my first days at UCSF, Dr. Guttentag lent me his copy of Mitscherlich and Mielke's *Doctors of Infamy*,[50] the first book to describe the abominations of the Nazi doctors, and introduced me to Fr. Charles Carroll, an Episcopal chaplain at UCSF hospital who had been on the legal staff of the Nuremberg Tribunal. While Guttentag's distinction between physician-friend and physician-researcher was never elevated to regulation, it had repercussions within the research world. Many medical scientists of that era recalled Guttentag's thesis as a key concept in their appreciation of the nature of medical research.[51] The distinction captured an essential conflict between research and practice that had not always been apparent to medical researchers.

On August 6, 1945, an atomic bomb was dropped on Hiroshima and the world entered the atomic century. As the enormous power of plutonium and uranium became visible to the world, and as nations began to explore peaceful and military uses of these elements, it became imperative to understand the effects of nuclear radiation upon the human body. The terrible lesions inflicted on the unprepared citizens of Hiroshima and Nagasaki, the more subtle effects on researchers and others in regular contact with radiation sources, and the general effects upon the environment were not well understood. The prospect of a war fought with nuclear weapons demanded that medicine learn how to care for the myriad patients, military and civilian, who might need medical attention. Even the progeny of survivors could be seriously affected. This ignorance of the health consequences of ionizing radiation had to be overcome by research. The Atomic Energy Commission (AEC) organized the Atomic Bomb Casualty Commission, which undertook an extensive study of the survivors of the two bombings (and continues under the supervision of the Radiation Effects Research Foundation). During the three decades following the war, biomedical research on the physiological effects of radiation was sponsored by the Atomic Energy Commission and the Department of Defense.

One peculiar feature marked this scientific endeavor: almost all the research was conducted in secret. In the past, medical research was performed to be published; researchers shared knowledge with each other in open communication. The radiation research, however, dealt with matters of national security in a Cold War atmosphere. It was deliberately kept under close guard. This led to the greatest of ironies: the official order of Secretary of Defense Charles Wilson, which was issued on February 26, 1953, and intended to govern all research conducted under Armed Forces auspices, was kept "Top Secret" until August 22, 1975! Wilson's directive, issued after considerable discussion at various governmental levels, made the Nuremberg Code the ruling policy for all "use of human volunteers . . . in experimental research in the fields of atomic, biological and/or chemical warfare."[52] Yet, for years after its issuance, only the highest authorities were privy to it. The military services, particularly the Army, which honored the memory of Major Reed's experiments, did have policies that required consent of volunteers, but these policies were not communicated in any systematic way to civilian researchers working under contracts or grants from the services. The AEC also developed policies requiring the consent of volunteers, but it made little effort to communicate them to researchers.[53] An absence of clear policy marred the entire era of radiation research. Researchers worked either with the ragged concepts of research that were prevalent in the profession or with very little consciousness of their responsibilities to human subjects.

When the story of these experiments began to leak out in November 1993, President Bill Clinton appointed a committee to investigate their history. Bioethicist Ruth R. Faden of Johns Hopkins School of Public Health and the Kennedy Institute of Ethics at Georgetown was appointed chair. The final report of the President's Advisory Committee on Human Radiation Experiments (ACHRE) summarizes the accepted conditions for human experimental research during the 1940s and 1950s.

> Of particular importance in this picture are the practical and moral distinctions that many researchers made between investigations with healthy subjects and those with sick patients. Those working with healthy subjects could cite a tradition of consent that dated, at least, to Walter Reed's turn-of-the-century experiments; those working with sick patients were in a clinical context that was conditioned by a tradition of faith in the wisdom and beneficence of physicians, a tradition that was dominant until at least the 1970s. . . . Obtaining consent from patients within the normal clinical relationship was not a common practice in late 1946. At that time, and for many years to come, patient trust and medical beneficence were viewed as the unshakable moral foundations on which meaningful interactions between professional healers and the sick should be built.[54]

Even with these principles relatively clear in the minds of researchers, there is evidence that "many physicians during the period let themselves slide into nontherapeutic research with patients."[55] Patients, because of their abject condition, might often be convenient subjects for research not related to their disease, particularly when their doctors did not consider the research maneuvers particularly dangerous. "It is most often subjects in this category to whom disclosure is not made," said one researcher at a meeting of the Boston University Law-Medicine Research Institute on April 29, 1961.[56] When interviewed by the ACHRE, many prominent researchers of that era recalled with chagrin the practices of their youth.[57] Still, thorough review of the more than 4,000 radiation experiments between 1944 and 1974 revealed little harm: "most of these tracer studies involved adult subjects and are unlikely to have caused physical harm . . . in some nontherapeutic tracer studies involving children, radioisotope exposures were associated with increases in the potential lifetime risk of developing cancer that would be considered unacceptable today."[58]

In general, despite the awareness of the problem evidenced in the literature of the post-war era, many researchers had little interest in the ethics of research, which they must have considered (if they considered it at all) as an obstacle to social progress and personal success. Those researchers who were sensitive to the problems abided by the concepts prevalent at the time. The few medical men who spoke out publicly, such as Dr. Otto Guttentag, were listened to with respect, but no institutional changes resulted.

The Thalidomide Story

The story of radiation research was a Cold War secret. Few members of the public knew anything about it. But another story about the problems inherent in developing new medicines captured public attention. On July 15, 1962, *The Washington Post* reported that a sleeping pill compounded with the new drug thalidomide was suspected of causing serious limb deformities in the human fetus. The drug had been widely prescribed in Europe and thousands of babies had been born missing one or several limbs. The babies' mothers had taken the drug in early pregnancy not only as a hypnotic but also for morning sickness during pregnancy. The *Post* announced that the drug had been kept off the American market by an officer of the U.S. Food and Drug Administration (FDA), Dr. Frances O. Kelsey. Dr. Kelsey made that decision despite the insistent pressure of the American company that wished to market the drug, Merrell Pharmaceuticals, and also in face of noncooperative, even hostile superiors in the FDA.[59] Dr. Kelsey's stubborn courage earned her the Distinguished Federal Civilian Service Medal, bestowed on her by President Kennedy only one month after the *Post* article appeared. She had been nominated for the award by Senator Estes Kefauver, who was sponsoring Congressional hearings into the antiquated and even corrupt practices of the FDA, which was in complicity with drug manufacturers.

Dr. Kelsey had kept thalidomide (called "Kevedon" by Merrell Pharmaceuticals) off the American market, but she had been unable to prevent its use as an experimental drug. In 1960, Merrell began a premarketing campaign "in the guise of a clinical investigation program . . . to introduce Kevedon to those of the nation's most influential physicians who were likely to prescribe the drug once it was put on the market."[60] Merrell salesmen targeted senior faculty in the academic departments of medicine, surgery, anesthesia, and obstetrics-gynecology who would be invited to test Kevedon on their patients. When Merrell's application for FDA approval reached Dr. Kelsey, she was skeptical about the scientific data, even before suspecting the fetal deformity problem. She concluded that "Merrell had compiled an interesting collection of meaningless pseudoscientific jargon apparently intended to impress chemically unsophisticated readers."[61] Several months later, Kelsey noticed a report in the *British Medical Journal* that some users of the drug had experienced peripheral neuropathy. She began to wonder about the possibility of fetal effects. By this time, however, the drug had spilled into doctors' offices and pharmacies. Merrell's assiduous "detail men" had enlisted some 1,200 "influential physicians" who prescribed the drug for some 20,000 women. During this time, America's most distinguished woman physician, Dr. Helen Taussig of The Johns Hopkins School of Medicine, undertook a personal investigation of the European and British "epidemic of infant monsterism" and added her prestige to Dr. Kelsey's lonely fight.[62]

Merrell Pharmaceuticals reluctantly began to inform physicians of the danger and finally withdrew its New Drug Application on March 8, 1962. The company, however, had never ceased to harass Dr. Kelsey. Her fight had consequences beyond the protection of women and their babies from a dangerous drug. It served as the centerpiece of Senator Kefauver's investigation of the FDA, which had begun in December 1959 and which resulted in amendments to the Federal Food, Drug and Cosmetic Act three years later[63] The 1962 Kefauver-Harris amendments strengthened the government's control over the approval of new drugs, demanding "substantial evidence of efficacy" and requiring for the first time full and free consent of all subjects of drug trials conducted within the United States. This provision was added during floor debate by Senator Jacob K. Javits (R-NY) and was at first stated only permissively. It emerged from conference as a mandatory requirement. Even in its mandatory form, however, the provision was a far cry from later versions of informed consent. It required only that the physician inform the subject that the new drug is "being used for investigational purposes and will obtain the consent of such human beings or their representatives, except where they deem it not feasible or, in their professional judgment, contrary to the best interest of such human beings."[64]

The FDA rapidly implemented the new law, issuing regulations on February 7 and June 20, 1963. However, the regulations did nothing to clarify the ambiguous and open language of the law's consent requirement. Again, Dr. Kelsey made a valuable contribution, writing an article in which she narrowed the broad understanding of the "investigator's discretion" and the meaning of "feasibility" and "best interests."[65] Dr. Kelsey's interpretation, while personal, was somewhat reluctantly ratified as "cleared by the FDA prior to publication."[66] Not until 1966, under the aegis of a new commissioner, Dr. James Goddard, did the FDA issue clearer regulations regarding the consent requirement. The new version was heavily dependent on the language and concepts of the Nuremberg Code and the Helsinki Declarations.

The thalidomide story is not often told as part of the history of bioethics. It is, of course, a story of moral courage but it does not, in the strict sense, pose an ethical problem. It is, rather, a story of commercial greed and political collusion, leading to a tragedy. Still, the thalidomide story is an opening event in the federal government's direct involvement in the ethics of experimentation with human subjects. The FDA assumed more vigilant oversight of clinical investigations; the 1962 consent requirement was an important moment in the evolution of a central theme in bioethics, medical practice, and public policy—the concept of informed consent.

The National Institutes of Health and Regulation of Research

In 1953, the Clinical Center of the National Institutes of Health opened and, in addition to its research subject-patients, welcomed "normal volunteers." These persons, often coming from the traditional "peace" churches and from colleges, offered themselves as healthy controls in drug studies. Investigators realized that these healthy volunteers, not being patients, fell outside the fiduciary responsibilities between physicians and their patients; thus, they deserved special protection from risks and full information about these risks. Even those who were admitted to the Clinical Center with a particular disease were not being admitted to a regular hospital: they were there not only to be treated but also to be studied. Otto Guttentag's distinction between "physician-friend" and "physician-investigator" aptly described the situation at the Clinical Center, where many of the physicians either had no physician-friend relation at all with those whose bodies they manipulated or had to move awkwardly between the two roles.

This difference in the moral quality of the relationship became clear at the NIH over the next decade. Slowly, the leadership realized that attention had to be paid to the rights and welfare of all experimental subjects and that the good will of the investigator was not enough. In 1960, the U.S. Public Health Service made a grant of $97,000 to the Boston University's Law-Medicine Research Institute, which Professor William J. Curran had established in 1958, to study the ethical and legal aspects of clinical investigations, with particular reference to use of children, prisoners, and informed consent. During the course of that study, Professor Irving Ladimer compiled his anthology, *Clinical Investigations in Medicine: Legal, Ethical and Moral Aspects,*[67] which revealed that the major questions attending research with human subjects had been aired in the literature by the early 1960s; these included the importance of informed consent and elimination of coercion, expectation of social benefit, and competent research design. However, the paradox of consent relative to children and incompetents and the prospect of some sort of community oversight over research remained unexplored.

The NIH sponsored a survey of its grantee institutions in 1962 and discovered that only nine of fifty-two departments of medicine had any policy regarding rights of research subjects; sixteen stated that they used written consent forms. Thirty-four departments did not bother to answer the survey questionnaire.[68] In 1964, NIH Director James Shannon appointed an internal committee chaired by Associate Director Robert Livingston to review the issues in human experimentation. The Livingston committee came to a remarkable conclusion: "in the setting in which the patient is involved in an experimental effort, the judgment of the investigator is not sufficient as a basis for reaching a conclusion concerning the ethical and moral set of questions in that relationship."[69]

The event that brought about this conclusion was an incident at the Jewish Chronic Disease Hospital in Brooklyn during 1963. Dr. Chester Southam of Sloan-Kettering Institute for Cancer Research had approached Dr. Emanuel Mandel, Medical Director of the Jewish Chronic Disease Hospital, with a proposal to study the immunological effects of injecting cancer cells under the skin of elderly, debilitated patients. Dr. Mandel was interested in collaborating on this project. No effort was made to obtain consent of the subjects. Several of the hospital's doctors learned of the research and objected strongly. A member of the hospital's board of directors, Mr. William Hyman, was outraged and compared the research to what had happened at Dachau. He complained that the directors' approval for the research had not been sought and sued to obtain the patients' records. In addition, the medical disciplinary board of New York State brought disciplinary charges against Drs. Southam and Mandel. They were judged to have acted fraudulently and deceitfully in failing to obtain the informed consent of the experimental subjects. The doctors' licenses were suspended for one year, but the suspension was stayed. (Dr. Southam was elected President of the American Association for Cancer Research four years later.) All these events were widely publicized during 1964. Dr. Southam's study had been funded by the National Institutes of Health, thus the adverse publicity about the case caught the attention of NIH officials.[70]

The conclusion of the Livingston committee is remarkable because it repudiates the axiom that the conscience of the investigator is an adequate judge of the ethics of an experiment, an axiom on which research ethics had been firmly based for a century. Although Thomas Percival had suggested that "no such trials [of new remedies] should be instituted without a previous consultation of physicians or surgeons," and although an occasional voice had called for "a consultative body" to review proposed experimentation, it had been the custom to leave this judgment to the researcher alone.[71] The Helsinki Declaration espoused the principles of voluntary consent and risk–benefit evaluation, but it placed the responsibility for ascertaining these on the investigator alone. (Not until the revision of 1975 does the requirement of "a specially appointed independent committee for consideration, comment and guidance" appear in the Declaration.)[72] After receiving the Livingston report, Director Shannon decided that the investigator's judgment must be subject to prior peer review to ensure an independent determination of risks and benefits and to assure the voluntary informed consent of the subject. His position was endorsed by the National Advisory Council of the NIH on

December 3, 1965, and a Policy and Procedure Order was issued to research institutions in early 1966, requiring that they establish such an independent review
body. Thus the institutional review committee became an official instrument of public
policy.[73]

The same year, "Ethics and clinical research" was published in the *New England
Journal of Medicine.*[74] The prominence of its author, Dr. Henry Beecher, Dorr Professor of Research in Anesthesia at Harvard Medical School, and the prestige of the *Journal* combined to cast disconcerting light on the practice of human experimentation in
the highest realms of American medical science. Beecher's earlier article, "Experimentation in man," had distinguished the motives and practices of research from those of
therapy, and the researcher-physician from the treating physician, as Otto Guttentag
had done.[75] That article received little notice; "Ethics and clinical research," however,
was very much noticed. The earlier article was written at a level of broad generalization; the new article was very concrete. Dr. Beecher presented twenty-two examples of
unethical experimentation, drawn from published articles by leading research scientists
(some were his colleagues at Harvard Medical School). He showed that they exposed
patients to excessive risks, ignored the need for consent, used poor, mentally incapaci-
tated persons, and withheld therapies of known efficacy.

Valuable as the exposé was, Beecher did not transcend the conventional research
ethic—namely, "the more reliable safeguard (is) provided by the presence of an intelligent, informed, conscientious, compassionate, responsible investigator."[76] In his 1970
Research and the Individual, Beecher gave only the briefest mention to external review, "whenever even remote hazard is a possibility, group decision supported by a
proper consultative body should be employed."[77] David Rothman writes, "Without
[Beecher's] courage, the movement to set new rules for human experimentation would
have proceeded on a much slower track. Few others had the scientific knowledge and
ethical sensibilities to call into question researchers' ethics."[78] The truth of Rothman's
comment is supported by the quite different reaction to another criticism of research
ethics, published by the English physician Maurice H. Pappworth. His book, *Human
Guinea Pigs,* which is equally if not more detailed and much more caustic than
Beecher's critique, was scarcely noted. When it did receive attention, it was vilified.[79]
Dr. Pappworth was not a renown scientist, nor was his critique published in a leading
medical journal.

During these decades, there was a quantitative increase in medical research; there
was also qualitative improvement in the methods whereby research results could be obtained and evaluated. The methods of controlled clinical trials and their statistical
analysis, introduced in the 1940s, gradually became familiar to researchers and soon
became standard practice. These methods, which employed such techniques as randomization of subjects between treatments and the "blinding" of researcher and subject
to the nature of the intervention, raised significant ethical problems. Those problems
were clearly stated by one of the pioneers of research design, the British statistician Sir
Bradford Hill, in 1951 and again in 1963.[80] Hill detailed the main ethical problems of

the controlled clinical trial: determination of the safety of the proposed intervention, the relative values of old and new treatment, the random allocation of patients to different arms of the trial, the patient's consent, placebos, and blinding of the physician to the treatment being administered. These were new problems raised by new methods of clinical research. Medical research was no longer simply doing something unusual in order to observe the results; it incorporated doctor and patient in a carefully designed program to produce valid knowledge by methods that put the subjects at risk. Sir Bradford concluded, much like Beecher, with the hope that these new tools of research would be rightly applied "by the ethical perception and the code of honor that is the second nature of those qualified in medicine."[81]

The initiation of peer review by an institutional review board, however, was the beginning of the end of the naive reliance on investigator integrity. Even those who recognized the importance of "ethical perception and the code of honor" began to realize the intrinsic conflict of interest and difference of roles between the physician as caregiver and the physician as researcher. Still, even as the old ideal was fading, it lingered in the hearts of many investigators. In 1968, at Senator Mondale's hearing, medical researchers expressed their dismay that public or governmental oversight might be initiated. One witness stated that medical innovators "would be manacled by well-intentioned but meddlesome intruders. . . . I would urge you with all the strength I can muster, to leave this subject to conscionable people in the profession who are struggling valiantly to advance medicine."[82]

Seven years later, at a 1975 conference sponsored by the National Academy of Science entitled "Experiments and Research with Humans: Values in Conflict," the same sentiment prevailed. Dr. Walsh McDermott asserted that "human experimentation committees and all the rest, I think are fine . . . but there is no one who can relieve the investigator from assuming that responsibility and making the decision to put another person at risk." Dr. Francis Moore spoke even more strongly against peer review by an institutional review board: "Nothing could be more unethical than critical judgment in this field made by persons who have not studied the biology of the field or the patient." Dr. Jay Katz was the sole voice to challenge the prevailing opinion. He objected, "Sorting out this value conflict cannot be left to the individual conscience of investigators."[83] Dr. Katz's lecture at that conference had done little more than suggest that investigators sit down and talk with subjects until they are fully satisfied that subjects understand the research and appreciate its risks. Dr. Katz recalled the occasion: "There was nothing inflammatory in what I said. I was to speak in the afternoon and, as I listened to the morning's speakers, I realized that my comments would not sit well with many of the participants. Al Jonsen was sitting next to me in the audience. I asked him whether he would be willing to administer the last rites to me when I was finished. He whispered into my ear, 'But, Jay, I can't do it in Hebrew.' I whispered back, 'Latin will suffice.'"[84]

Dr. Katz's premonitions were verified. He did not need last rites, but he was rebuffed by a noted scientist, Dr. Albert Sabin: "While Dr. Katz was talking, I was looking around the audience to see how many of my colleagues whom I know to be engaged

. . . in human medical research had horns sticking out of their foreheads."[85] Jay Katz was hardly a crank: he was a psychiatrist who was professor of family law at Yale Law School and had taken an interest in the ethics of human experimentation in the early 1960s, when he read the transcripts of the Nuremberg Trials. Having lost relatives in the Holocaust, he wondered whether any of them had been condemned to those experiments. Dr. Katz then reflected on his own research on dreams under hypnotic suggestion. He and his fellow researchers were aware that there might be detrimental effects on the subjects, but it did not occur to them to disclose these concerns to their subjects.

> We did not raise questions that deserved searching inquiry. . . . The unique responsibilities which physicians confront in the conduct of research had not been discussed in my medical education even though we were encouraged to do research. Thus, I was unprepared to consider them when I invited research subjects to join in my projects. Once I appreciated what I had done, I became disturbed by my thoughtlessness and the lacunae in my education. I began to immerse myself in the then scant literature on human experimentation. These preliminary explorations made me appreciate that the moral, medical and legal dilemmas posed by such research could not be adequately resolved, as generations of doctors had assumed, by a pledge of allegiance to such undefined principles as "do no harm" or to vague aspirational codes.[86]

Dr. Katz initiated a seminar on human experimentation at Yale Law School in 1966, the same year in which Henry Beecher's article "Ethics and clinical research" appeared. He invited Dr. Beecher, who had been his teacher at Harvard Medical School, to join the seminar: "His presence deepened my students' appreciation of the seriousness and importance of the studies they were pursuing with me." In the same year, Katz lectured at Yale Medical School on the ethics of research and, to his dismay, was not well received. It was Katz's emphasis on disclosure and consent of subjects, and particularly his suggestion that the medical school establish a forum for scholarly inquiry into the problems of medical research, that offended his medical colleagues.

Katz's law school seminar was more successful; it produced a compendious casebook, *Experimentation with Human Beings*.[87] Working with Alexander Capron, Katz compiled a multitude of cases and articles on the subject of human experimentation, within a structure of inquiry that raised systematic questions. The many issues are condensed into sections with significant titles: "The Authority of the Investigator as Guardian of Science, Subject and Society" and "The Authority of the Subject as Guardian of His Own Fate." Behind these general themes stands Katz's fundamental concern with consent. When the National Commission for the Protection of Human Subjects first convened, each commissioner was given a copy of Dr. Katz's volume.

The Tuskegee Revelations

The July 26, 1972 edition of *The New York Times* carried a shocking story: "For forty years, the United States Public Health Service has conducted a study in which human beings with syphilis, who were induced to serve as guinea pigs, have gone without treatment for the disease. . . . the study was conducted to determine from autopsies what the disease does to the human body." The article announced that the subjects of the study were "about 600 black men, mostly poor and uneducated, from Tuskegee, Alabama."[88] The men had been promised free transportation to and from hospitals, free hot lunches, free medical care for any disease other than syphilis and free burial after autopsies were performed. In the next days and weeks, details of the Tuskegee study were revealed in the press. Of the six-hundred research subjects, four hundred had diagnosed syphilis, but they were never told of their disease and never treated for it. They were also never informed that they were research subjects or that treatment for their condition could have been provided. The other two hundred who did not have syphilis were controls. Patients and controls alike were told that they had "bad blood" and should have periodic medical examinations, including occasional spinal taps. When national conscription began in 1941, an arrangement was made between the Public Health Service (PHS) and the local draft board to keep the subjects off the list of draftees needing treatment. When the story broke in 1972, seventy-four of the untreated subjects were still living.

The syphilis study began in 1932, after a Public Health Service venereal disease treatment program initiated several years before in Macon County, Alabama, lost its funding. It occurred to the Public Health Service officer in charge of the treatment program, Dr. Taliaferro Clark, that the population of Macon County, which had one of the highest rates of syphilis in the country, offered an unparalleled opportunity to study the natural history of syphilis in the untreated patient. At that time, the standard treatment with arsenical and mercurial medications was arduous and of dubious efficacy. The collaboration of the hospital at one of the nation's premier African-American educational establishments, Tuskegee Institute, was secured. The study, initially planned for one year, persisted for forty years, even after effective treatment with penicillin became available. On a number of occasions, officials of the Public Health Service had evaluated the study and decided that its scientific value justified its continuance.

The story of the Tuskegee Study had not been kept a secret within the Public Health Service nor within the wider scientific and medical community, since many articles reporting its data were published in medical journals. However, until a employee of the PHS in San Francisco, Peter Buxtun, accidentally learned of it and began to explore further, the story was hardly known to the public. Beginning in 1966, Buxtun tried unsuccessfully to press the PHS to examine the moral implications of the study. Finally, his letter that associated the study with the racial politics of the day caught the attention of officials at the PHS Center for Disease Control, which was responsible for the conduct of the research. They called a high-level meeting to review the study. The participants in that meeting, all experts in infectious disease, determined that the research required scientific upgrading and should continue. Frustrated by this response Buxtun told the story to an Associated Press journalist, Edith Lederer, who passed it to another reporter, Jean Heller, and the *New York Times* story appeared.

Dr. Merlin Duval, Assistant Secretary for Health, whose jurisdiction covered the Public Health Service, announced that he was "shocked and horrified." On August 24, 1972, he appointed the Tuskegee Syphilis Study Ad Hoc Panel of nine citizens, headed by the distinguished African-American educator, Dr. Broadus Butler. The panel was fortunate to have Dr. Jay Katz among its members. Its charge was to determine whether the Tuskegee Study was justified at its inception and after penicillin became available, to recommend whether it should be continued or, if not, how it should be terminated "in a way consistent with the rights and health needs of its remaining participants," and to determine whether the rights of patients participating in research sponsored by the Department of Health, Education and Welfare were adequately protected. The panel presented its initial recommendations on October 25, 1972, and its final report on April 28, 1973. The report judged the study unethical both at its inception and in its continuation and recommended its immediate termination and compensation for surviving victims. The report called for establishment of a national human investigation board with authority to regulate all federally supported research with human subjects.[89]

The Tuskegee story propelled the ethics of experimentation into public view. Other events that had taken place in the latter half of the 1960s also cast suspicion on the probity of scientific researchers, including the incident at the Jewish Chronic Disease Hospital mentioned previously; the story of Willowbrook State Hospital will be related later in this chapter. Both these events, when publicized in the media, shocked the public, but no event had more impact on the public conscience than the Tuskegee Study. Its revelation appeared at a time of heightened concern and anger about racial discrimination and of heightened sensitivity to the abuse of the poor and powerless. The study had been perpetrated by the government through officials of the Public Health Service, whose sworn duty it was to protect the health of Americans, not to exploit them, even for science's sake. The revelations seemed to bring the horrors of the Nazi medical experiments, which many had judged impossible in the United States, into our benign scientific and medical world. The ethics of research, which had been under quiet scrutiny for a decade, now broke into public view.

Ethicists and Experimentation

Until the late 1960s no philosophers and few theologians had considered the moral problems associated with medical research. Philosophers did not generally comment on practical ethics, as we have seen, and they lived mentally remote from the world of biomedical research. In 1929, a Jesuit priest who was close to that world, Father Alphonse Schwitalla, Regent (a sort of Jesuit supervisor) of the Medical School of St. Louis University, praised the ethos of the modern research hospital, where new knowledge was assiduously sought for the future welfare of humankind. It is important in such a setting, he wrote, "not to lose sight of the patient . . . whose life, health and safety are foremost." In his paean to the use of medical science in the hospital he admitted that "the sick human being is, to be sure, not a laboratory animal but neither is he so isolated in his human glory that he must be regarded as completely outside the possibilities of sane, carefully controlled, watchfully supervised experimentation, which may bring health to himself and health to countless other beings."[90]

Another Jesuit, moral theologian John Ford, was more cautious. Writing immediately after World War II, he recognized the fundamental moral dilemmas of medical research. His analysis stressed the importance of consent by patients to treatments administered "not to cure this patient, but to discover experimentally what the effects of the new treatment will be." To do so without consent "is not only immoral, but is unethical from the physician's standpoint, and is illegal as well." He also mentioned prior animal experimentation and an acceptable risk–benefit ratio as moral prerequisites for research.[91] Ford cited the teaching of Pope Pius XII who, in a 1952 address to the International Conference on the Histopathology of the Nervous System, recalled the Nuremberg Doctors' Trial, endorsed the necessity of consent from all research subjects, sick or healthy, and stressed a favorite theme of his own theology: "Man, in his personal being, is not ordained to the utility of society; rather, the community is ordained to the good of man."[92]

The scientific researchers did not see this principle as clearly as the Pope did. Dr. Walsh McDermott posed a counterthesis at the American College of Physicians Colloquium on Ethical Dilemmas in 1967: "The core of this ethical issue [is] to ensure the rights of society, even if an arbitrary judgment must be made against an individual." Society gains its right over individuals "from the demonstration that knowledge gained by studies in a few humans can show us how to operate programs of great practical benefit to the group." According to McDermott, peer review was of little value, and it should not be allowed to dilute the responsibility of the clinical investigator. Dr. McDermott delivered a provocative defense of the clinical researcher.

> Society may not have given us a clear blueprint for clinical investigation, but it has long given us immense trust to handle moral dilemmas of other sorts, including many in which, in effect, we have to play God. . . . The hard core of our moral dilemma will not yield to Declarations or Regulations for, as things stand today, such statements must completely ignore the fact that society, too, has rights in human experimentation. We will have to learn how to institutionalize "playing god," while maintaining the key elements of a free society.[93]

The apparent paradox between the papal principle and the scientist's thesis bothered many thoughtful persons. Through 1966–1968, a study of human experimentation was organized under the aegis of the American Academy of Arts and Sciences. The study had its genesis in a working party appointed by the president of the academy, Harvard law professor Paul A. Freund, probably at the urging of Henry Beecher.[94] This working party chose scholars to research and analyze the issues and planned two conferences— the first (November 3–4, 1967) to review memoranda prepared by the working party; the second (September, 26–28, 1968) to discuss the penultimate drafts of the papers that would appear as the final product of the study. These papers are models of thoughtful, interdisciplinary analysis of the broad issue of human experimentation. The conference participants were from more disciplines than in any previous conference: medicine and law, of course, were represented, but anthropology, sociology, history of science, and theology were also present. The collected essays of the conference provided the first profound and comprehensive study of the ethics of human experimentation.

Stephen R. Graubard, the Academy's editor, prefaced the conference report with the remark that the Academy's project was a response to the "articulate demand . . . for assurance that the experimentation for which these public monies were being used would bear public screening . . . how can the interests [of investigators, subjects, and the larger society] be defined, protected and controlled? The 'regulation' of research, particularly that significant segment involving human subjects, has become a matter of the greatest moment." Graubard also noted that "the uniquely tragic European experience" which transpired during the Nazi terror had instigated "substantial inquiry of jurists and physicians . . . to reflect on that activity and to establish codes that would make such bestial activity impossible."[95]

Hans Jonas's contribution to the Academy study, "Philosophical reflections on experimenting with human subjects," is a landmark in the ethics of experimentation and in bioethics in general.[96] It is a philosophical *tour de force,* revealing how a mind imbued with the philosophical tradition is able to dissect concepts and construct arguments. Jonas took as his theme the provocative words of Dr. McDermott (who was present). Jonas acknowledged that the most common way to conceptualize the moral problem of research was to see a polarity between the good of individuals and the common good. He denied that this is the proper way to frame the problem. Rights and obligations arise in the quite different context of protecting society from disintegration and individuals from harm. It is claimed, he noted, that experimentation is justified by the common good of society or by the social contract. But experimentation, by its very nature, produces the good—not of preservation of social life, but of progress and enhancement. These goals are "melioristic," and are, as such, gratuitous, not obligatory: "Our descendants have a right to be left an unplundered planet; they do not have a right to new miracle cures." The pursuit of melioristic goals cannot generate any right of society over against the right of the individual. Melioristic goals, while not obligatory, are noble; they call humans to a free, even sacrificial, engagement of self. The social enterprise of experimentation must be seen within "an ethical dimension [that] far exceeds that of the moral law and reaches into the sublime solitude of dedication and ultimate commitment." Jonas's perceptive arguments reveal a philosophical mind informed by Kantian teachings on obligation, freedom, and the nature of perfect and imperfect duties, as well as his own philosophical perspective that persons are agents in responsible engagement with their own purposes and in voluntary participation with the purposes of others.

Jonas brought this vision to medical experimentation. Mere "consent," often seen as the justification that converts the use of others as means into honoring others as ends in themselves, is not enough. True volunteering, that is, active engagement in the purposes of another and identifying them with one's own purposes, is the proper justification for research. On the basis of this argument, an order of research participants can be established. Those most identified with the melioristic goal, the researchers themselves, should be the first volunteers. Those poorer in knowledge, motivation, and freedom of decision should be last. These latter candidates are not apodictically excluded but, as they are approached, the justification must become more compelling. While Jonas's essay dwelt in the rare air of philosophical reflections, its principle proposition was a powerfully compelling one that had not yet been clearly made: participation in research must be seen, in all its aspects and for all participants, as an exercise in freedom. Society cannot infringe on individual rights for the production of its future goods. Individuals have not a duty but a calling to which they may respond in freedom, to aid in the production of those goods. Hans Jonas gave to the ethics of research a solid philosophical foundation.

The National Commission

The national human investigation board was not created in the form recommended by the Tuskegee Panel. However, in the following year, Congress passed the National Research Act, establishing the National Commission for the Protection of Human Subjects of Biomedical and Behavioral Research.[97] Congress charged that body with the task of recommending to the Department of Health, Education and Welfare regulations to protect the rights and welfare of human subjects of research, especially those with certain disabilities, and developing principles to govern the ethical conduct of research. The Commission's makeup and process have already been described in Chapter 4. Here we recall its influence on the ethics of research with human subjects. The Commission's deliberations, as well as the literature that surrounded its work, made at least four major contributions to understanding the ethics of research: it clarified the definition of research, promoted consent to prominence, unraveled the paradoxes of research with persons of diminished capacity to consent, and moved the debate about research into the public sphere.

First, the Commission formulated a definition of research that captured its essential features. There are many ways to define experimentation: trial of an unfamiliar intervention, the testing of a hypothesis, a departure from standard practice, the first use of a medical technique, adventure into the unknown, or, in more polemical terms, using people as guinea pigs or as means rather than ends. In the early days of the discussion, no clear definition was in common use. As the methods of clinical research became more formal, the definition of research became clearer, and the delineation of the ethical issues became more definitive. The particular methodological feature of research is formulation of an intellectual strategy to guide interventions in a way that will produce information that can be validated. Thus, research is done according to a protocol. The protocol designates techniques, such as randomization and blinding, that reduce the variables and the biases that impede validity, and it states the statistical requirements that produce confidence in the results. The protocol itself puts the human subject at risk, just as much as the unknown toxicity of an untried drug or uncertain outcome of a novel surgical maneuver does. In the course of applying these methods, all subjects become "means," regardless of whether they experience any therapeutic benefit. The protocol allows external observers to judge the hypothesis of the investigator as well as the risks of the procedure and locates the experiment in the context of previous knowledge. In light of this understanding of research, the National Commission, after much debate, framed a definition: "'research' designates an activity designed to test an hypothesis, permit conclusions to be drawn, and thereby to develop or contribute to generalizable knowledge (expressed, for example, in theories, principles and statements of relationships). Research is usually described in a formal protocol that sets forth an objective and a set of procedures to reach that objective."[98]

This definition implicitly abolishes the long-cherished but misleading distinction between therapeutic and nontherapeutic research. The Commission had already accepted that distinction, drawn from the Helsinki Declaration, in its first report on *Research on the Fetus*. It then deliberately discarded it, realizing that any "systematic investigation," whether done in a sick person or a healthy volunteer, poses the risks of the protocol—for example, the risk of being randomized into the ineffective arm of the trial. Consequently, the requirement for consent pertains not only to the healthy volunteer but also to the sick who are under the care of a physician-investigator, a point that had not been clearly appreciated in prior discussions. Four long essays on the nature of research, and its distinction from practice, authored by the Commission's medical advisor, Dr. Robert Levine of Yale, were seminal in generating this new definition of research.[99]

The Commission's second contribution to the ethics of research was the elevation of consent from a *pro forma* practice to an implication of a fundamental moral principle, respect for persons. This move placed the ethics of research in stark opposition to a utilitarian view. To many advocates of research, the utilitarian maxim, "for the greater good of the greater number," had sanctioned the use of subjects, even without consent and even in dangerous experiments. Dr. Leo Alexander had already condemned this "utilitarianism" in his article, "Medical science under dictatorship." Although few American researchers would have subscribed to the extreme forms of this principle, the utilitarian attitude survived as an undertone. As philosophers entered the debate, the utilitarian principle as a fundamental maxim of research ethics was subjected to critique. Philosophers espoused the hegemony of personal autonomy or sought guidance in other ethical theories that demonstrated greater respect for the freedom of individuals.[100]

Hans Jonas's "Some reflections" laid the groundwork for this move. Paul Ramsey's opening chapter in *Patient as Person* argued that "informed consent alone exhibits and establishes medical practice and investigation as a voluntary association of free men in a common cause."[101] Charles Fried's *Medical Experimentation: Personal Integrity and*

Social Policy espoused the primacy of personal autonomy over social benefit.[102] H. Tristram Engelhardt's essay for the National Commission articulated this principle in language that would in turn influence *The Belmont Report*: "Respect for persons [is] a logical condition for morality. . . . one should respect human subjects as free agents. . . . [this] first principle is a deontological one in the sense of focusing on a consideration of rights and duties independently of any issue of goods and values."[103] Engelhardt regarded "free and informed consent of the human subject . . . [and] proxy consent . . . to protect the best interests of individuals unable to consent, and avoiding coercion," as procedural issues that reflect respect for persons. This view of respect for persons as deontological and immune from balance with other goods repudiates philosophical utilitarianism as an ethical justification for research. The Commission unequivocally espoused respect for persons as the first of the basic principles relevant to the conduct of research. This principle, it says, "incorporates at least two ethical convictions: first, that individuals should be treated as autonomous agents and, second, that persons with diminished autonomy are entitled to protection."[104]

Research with Children

The Commission's third major contribution to the ethics of research was the clarification of the paradoxical place of persons with diminished autonomy as subjects of research. On the one hand, such persons—children, the mentally disabled, the very sick—belong to classes of persons in need of improved care; on the other hand, they have often been abused when corralled into sometimes dangerous research simply because they were institutionally available. Attempts to regulate research by codes and laws, such as the 1900 proposed Senate Bill 3432 and the Nuremberg Code, sought to eliminate the abuse by totally ruling out these persons as research subjects. The Helsinki Declaration allowed "consent of the legal guardian" for incompetents, but it did not explain how legal guardians had the authority to expose their wards to risk. The National Commission was instructed to investigate "under what conditions, if any," research could involve persons unable to consent for themselves.

An episode at New York's Willowbrook State Hospital vividly demonstrated the paradox of how to improve the care of children and protect them from disease and, at the same time, not abuse their impotence. Beginning in 1956, Drs. Saul Krugman and Joan Giles began to study the natural history of infectious hepatitis, a disease that was endemic in populations of institutionalized children. They approached the authorities at Willowbrook, New York's largest institution for retarded persons, with a proposal to infect a cohort of newly admitted children with hepatitis and watch carefully the progress of their illness, which in children is a mild, flu-like condition. This seemed not unreasonable, since almost all children eventually contracted hepatitis in the conditions of the institution and, in addition, the induced infection would subsequently immunize them. Krugman and Giles aimed to understand more clearly the natural history of hepatitis and eventually to develop a vaccine.

When the first results of their research were published in 1958, controversy exploded. Newspapers reported it in outraged tones, parents of children at Willowbrook protested, and some in the medical community were dismayed. Drs. Krugman and Giles defended their research as ethical, but few heard their defense; they were even branded as Nazis.[105] Krugman and Giles, however, succeeded in developing a vaccine. The editors of the *Journal of the American Medical Association* (JAMA) then chastised the critics. Referring to a series of censorious letters published in the British journal *Lancet, JAMA*'s editors wrote, "Letters to the editor of *Lancet* harshly criticized Krugman and his colleagues for their studies. . . . One writer [Goldby] was 'amazed that the work was published and that it has been actively supported editorially by the *JAMA*.' In pious tone, *Lancet*'s editor supported Goldby's view. . . . This issue of the *Journal* carries the most recent report from Krugman's group and, as it turns out, *Lancet*'s editor would have been well advised to keep his pen away from paper. The evidence is now in: viral hepatitis, type B, can be prevented by active immunization induced by inoculation of an inactivated preparation of MS-2 serum."[106] This retrospective elation, however, does not solve the problem of consent. As Henry Beecher stated previously, "An experiment is ethical or not at its inception; it does not become ethical *post hoc*—ends do not justify the means."[107] The paradox remains: should persons incapable of consent ever be research subjects, even if the harm is minimal and there is prospective benefit? Willowbrook was a complex and controversial case, caught in this paradox.

Paul Ramsey took research with children as a "prismatic case" for the new ethics of medicine that he would later explore in the Beecher Lectures. Ramsey proffered an unyielding thesis: children, who cannot consent and thus cannot enter into covenants of loyalty, can never be used as research subjects. Only when the child is a prospective beneficiary of an investigative procedure may research be joined to that child's care. This thesis poses many problems, the most serious being that restricting research with children forgoes the medical progress that might benefit many future children. Paul Ramsey was not moved: "To experiment on children in ways that are not related to them as patients is already a sanitized form of barbarism [which] pays no attention to the faithfulness-claims which a child, simply by being a normal or a sick or a dying child, places upon us and medical care. We should expect no significant exceptions to this canon of faithfulness to the child."[108] Ramsey, in pointing to the centrality of consent in the covenant between researcher and patient, rejected the moral legitimacy of proxy consent for nontherapeutic research. He drew this fixed line just as the National Institutes of Health was attempting to reformulate its policy governing research. His position would have abolished much of pediatric research.

The National Commission for the Protection of Human Subjects invited Ramsey to present his position and asked Fr. Richard McCormick to provide an alternative ethical opinion. The two theologians debated before the commissioners. McCormick argued that parents' proxy consent for their children to participate in research could be ethically valid on the presumption that it was based not on what the child would wish for himself or herself (the usual justification for proxy consent), but, more deeply, on what the child *ought* to wish. All humans, regardless of maturity, have an orientation to certain goods, including health; thus, all humans have an obligation to seek the means to reserve those goods. Also, all humans have an obligation to seek those goods for others, "for we are social beings and the goods that define our growth . . . are goods that reside also in others."[109] These are themes drawn from the natural law vision at the center of McCormick's theological ethic. His unique twist on the argument consists in revising the usual basis for proxy consent from "would" to "ought." His thesis, however, had to answer certain immediate objections, one of which derived indirectly from Jonas and directly from Ramsey: participation in research is supererogatory rather than obligatory. McCormick countered with an argument that introduces levels of risk, discomfort, and inconvenience and then claimed that when risks are not excessive, the obligation to contribute to others derives not from charity but from justice.

The commissioners argued over many months and through many drafts. In the end, their deliberations resulted in a complex document that accepted in principle the legitimacy of proxy consent for nontherapeutic research with children, provided that the research involved nothing more than minimal risk to the child. The document defined levels of risk and associated those levels of risk with levels of protection for the child and with the importance of the research. Richard McCormick's general perspective, if not his precise argument, had prevailed. The report included a long chapter that summarized the theses of Ramsey and McCormick, as well as the positions of several other ethicists who had analyzed the issue.[110]

Paul Ramsey later wrote that McCormick's writings, "together with those of his colleague, LeRoy Walters, had considerable influence on the deliberations of the National Commission."[111] McCormick responded, "Walters and I would be happy to think that is the case, but the matter of influence remains speculative."[112] As one commissioner, I can affirm that McCormick's influence on my thinking about this perplexing topic was not at all speculative. His argument drew attention to the child as an inchoate participant in a social reality, rather than as an isolated and vulnerable entity. This perspective allowed me and the other commissioners to reset the questions raised by research in a larger context in which both protection of vulnerability and contribution to the goods of children and society could be considered. The Commission's report did not settle all questions about research with children, but it provided the basis for a sound ethic and allowed regulations to be issued that were both carefully restrictive and sensibly permissive.[113]

Research Involving Prisoners

The ability to consent can be compromised not only by mental or maturational capacity; it can also be vitiated by coercion. Clearly, the first rule of the Nuremberg Code envisions the extreme coercion brought on concentration camp prisoners. Prison inmates in the United States had also been the subjects of experimentation. During World War II, research on infectious diseases was often carried out among prison populations. The Governor of Illinois permitted such research in the state prisons without any prior promise of parole or reduction of sentence. Several years after the war ended, the question whether participation in research should count as "good time" toward reduction of sentence was raised, perhaps by some of those who had been research subjects. Governor Dwight Green appointed a committee to study the problem. It was chaired by Dr. Ivy of Nuremberg fame; Dr. Morris Fishbein, Editor of *JAMA,* several other physicians, a rabbi, a priest, and two businessmen served as the committee's members. The committee's report endorsed the recently adopted principles of the American Medical Association, raised the question of undue influence and coercion, and concluded that research participation could count toward reduction of sentence unless the expected reduction was excessive. They considered that their conclusion was consistent with the general principles of the parole system.[114]

Research continued in American prisons, and medical school researchers gained access to incarcerated persons. The Institutional Review Board at the University of California, San Francisco, on which I served, regularly reviewed protocols for studies at California's Vacaville prison, the state's major medical facility for the incarcerated. Many pharmaceutical companies established research centers within prison walls. Little protest was heard until Jessica Mitford published her *Kind and Usual Punishment: The Prison Business.*[115] Mitford relayed stories of dangerous research behind bars and claimed that the prisoners' situation was inherently coercive. As the National Commission turned to prison research, it encountered a peculiar problem. When the commissioners and staff visited half a dozen prisons, they went with the presumption that prison research could not be conducted with free and informed consent; they returned with the belief that prisoners, almost unanimously, understood the research projects and wanted to participate in them. Prisoners claimed that they had a right to do so, which had not been curtailed by their sentence (as had their right to liberty and to vote), that research provided an interesting diversion, and that it gave some of them the opportunity to expiate their crimes. We were greeted by one inmate at Michigan's Jackson State Prison where The Upjohn Company maintained a large research center. He said, "Ladies and Gentlemen: You are in a place where death at random is a way of life. We have noticed that the only place in this prison that prisoners don't die is in the research unit. Just what is it that you think you are protecting us from?"[116] At the same time, we learned that access into desired research had often been surreptitiously commandeered by prisoners who used it as reward and punishment and that in some places, research centers had become desirable alternatives for sick inmates to the shabby prison infirmaries. Prison research presented much more of a paradox than the commissioners had anticipated.

The Commission crafted a complex report that tolerated prison research under stringent conditions, such as assurance of equal access to research for all who wished to volunteer and improvement of prison health care. When *Research Involving Prisoners* was delivered to DHEW Secretary Joseph Califano, he recognized that our recommendations amounted to a program of prison reform. He rejected the report on the grounds that he had no authority over the prison system. Instead, the department issued regulations that limited prison research to those physical, psychological, and social conditions affecting the lives of incarcerated persons.[117] The Justice Department, which did have authority over federal prisons, took the simpler step, in March 1976, of abolishing medical experimentation in those institutions. State prisons generally followed that lead. Where research was allowed, it was surrounded by an array of safeguards against co-optation and coercion. Prison research has, for practical purposes, ceased to exist. The modern prison, infected with drugs, disorder, and disease, is no longer the ideal of a clean, orderly place for science that it was once thought to be.

Human Experimentation and Public Discourse

The fourth major contribution of the National Commission was the transformation of debate on the ethics of experimentation from a private argument within the world of medicine into broad, public discourse. The commissioners invited scientists to educate them about research, and scholars, particularly from philosophy and religion, to educate them about moral and social matters. These scholars, often themselves novices in this area, produced thoughtful reflections, widening the appreciation of the problems of research beyond the researchers themselves. By endorsing the NIH policy of institutional review boards, the Commission created local forums where research was discussed—not in the abstract, but in the concrete particulars of specific protocols. Institutional review boards (IRBs) do not debate protocols without guidance: definitions and rules are conveyed to them through federal regulations, supplemented by guidebooks, and enhanced by the past experiences of the reviewers. The IRB system, while not perfect in conception or realization, has succeeded in preventing abusive research for over two decades and, more importantly, has introduced the ethical problems into the realm of public discourse.[118] Thousands of persons, from health professionals to hospital chaplains, have served on IRBs and become familiar with the language and the topics of clinical research. Protocols are reviewed, sent back to researchers for correction, revised, and once approved, become public property. Public Responsibility in Medicine and Research (PRIM&R) was founded in 1974 to foster communication and education for IRBs across the country. The Hastings Center initiated the publication of *IRB,* a newsletter for IRB members, edited by Dr. Robert Levine.

At the National Institutes of Health, Dr. Don Chalkley was appointed to oversee the implementation of the policy guidelines in the late 1960s. In 1974, that position was enhanced. A new office was established, called the Office for Protection from Research Risks (OPRR). OPRR interprets regulations, prepares educational materials, sponsors education, and above all, monitors the compliance of institutions with the regulations. In 1979, Dr. Charles McCarthy became director of OPRR. As a professor at Catholic

University, he had become an expert in the canon law of the Catholic Church and after moving to the NIH, applied some of his canonical skills to the framing of regulations and their acute interpretation. He was, in a sense, an *eminence grise* of the emerging bioethics, always ready behind the scenes with advice, information, and political arcana. In 1975, the Director of the Clinical Center, NIH, Dr. Morton Lipsett, lured Dr. John C. Fletcher from the world of theological education to the Clinical Center, where he had studied informed consent as a graduate student a decade before. Fletcher was given the title Associate to the Director for Bioethics and charged with developing a program for internal review of research and for clinical consultation.[119] The closed world of research had been opened to many eyes and it became familiar to many people who understand its problems and its principles. The Commission's work and the resulting regulations significantly changed the climate of research in the United States.[120]

Conclusion

During the 1970s, many activities in bioethics shaped the ethics of research with human subjects into a coherent topic with its own discourse of new, usable definitions, sets of questions, and an array of arguments that allowed individuals to frame rational views and communities to adopt reasonable policies. This bioethical discourse was sustained by the concentrated attention of scholars who were suited by their disciplines to perform moral, legal, and social analysis, the collaboration of scientists, and the debate that took place on a variety of issues in such focused forums as the National Commission, congressional hearings, offices of various federal agencies, committees, and symposia of professional groups. This discourse differed from that of previous eras: the anti-vivisection era was confrontational and contentious, fueled by passionate ideology; the discourse over research during World War II and early postwar eras was secretive and sporadic. During the 1970s, with the National Commission established to sustain the discussion of research in medicine, discourse became collaborative, scholarly, and public. Above all, the discourse over research could be directed toward resolutions that would be widely accepted in American society.

Notes to Chapter 5

1. Hippocrates, *Aphorisms I*, in W. H. S. Jones (trans.), *Hippocrates with an English Translation* (Cambridge, Mass.: Harvard University Press, 1959), vol. 4, p. 99. The Hippocratic maxim "experience is uncertain" can also be translated "experiment is perilous."

2. Hippocrates, *Epidemics I*, xi in Jones, *Hippocrates*, vol. 1, p. 165.

3. Celsus, *De Medicina*, proemium, 23–27, 40–44, in W. G. Spencer, *Celsus De Medicina with an English Translation* (Cambridge: Harvard University Press, 1960), vol. I, pp. 15, 23; John Scarborough, "Celsus and human vivisection at Ptolomaic Alexandria," *Clio Medica* 11 (1976): 25–38.

4. J. P. Bull, "The historical development of clinical therapeutic trials," *Journal of Chronic Disease* 10 (1959): 218–248.

5. An interesting account of an experiment perilous appears in William Withering, *An Account of the Foxglove and Some of Its Medical Uses* (London: G. G. J. and J. Robinson, 1785), cited in Ralph H. Major, *Classic Descriptions of Disease*, 4th ed. (Springfield: Charles Thomas, 1949), pp. 442, 439. The legal principle is stated first in *Slater v Baker and Stapelton* 95 Eng Rep 860 KB (1767); *Carpenter v Blake* 60 Bart 448 (NY Sup Ct 1871); *Jackson v Burnham* 20 Colo 532; 39 Pac 577 (1895).

6. Norman Howard-Jones, "Human experimentation in historical and ethical perspective," *Social Science and Medicine* 16 (1982): 1429–1448; Cotton Mather, "Variolae triumphatae," in Gordon W. Jones, (ed.), *The Angel of Bethesda* (Barre, MA: Barre Publishers, 1972), pp. 93–116; Genevieve Miller, *The Adoption of Inoculation for Small Pox in England and France* (Philadelphia: University of Pennsylvania Press, 1957); Derrick Baxby, *Jenner's Smallpox Vaccine. The Riddle of Vaccinia Virus and Its Origins* (London: Heinemann, 1981).

7. Percival, *Medical Ethics*, I, xii. In Chauncey Leake (ed.), *Percival's Medical Ethics* (Baltimore: The Williams and Wilkens Company, 1927), p. 76.

8. Pierre-Charles-Alexandre Louis, *Recherches sur les effets de la saignée* (Paris, 1835).

9. Claude Bernard, *Introduction to the Study of Experimental Medicine*, trans. H. Greene (New York: Dover, 1957), chapter II, section iii, pp. 101–102 (original publication in French, 1865).

10. William Beaumont, *Experiments and Observations on the Gastric Juice and the Physiology of Digestion* (Plattsburgh: F. P. Allen, 1833), p. 31; Ronald L. Numbers, "William Beaumont and the ethics of human experimentation," *Journal of the History of Biology* 12 (1979): 113–135.

11. Vikenty Veressayev [V. V. Smidovich], *Memoirs of a Physician*, trans. Simeon Linden (New York: Alfred Knopf, 1916), reprinted in Jay Katz, *Experimentation with Human Beings* (New York: Russell Sage Foundation, 1972), pp. 284–291.

12. "In the older European countries, where the life and happiness of the so-called lower classes are perhaps held more cheaply than with us, enthusiastic devotees of science are very apt to encroach upon the rights of the individual patient in a manner which cannot be justified. In this country we are less likely to fall into this error." Charles Francis Withington, *The Relation of Hospitals to Medical Education* (Boston: Cupples, Uphman and Co.), quoted in Stanley Reiser, Arthur J. Dyck, and William J. Curran, *Ethics in Medicine* (Cambridge, Mass.: MIT Press, 1977), p. 260.

13. Katz, *Experimentation with Human Beings*, p. 291; Susan E. Lederer, *Subjected to Science: Human Experimentation in America before the Second World War* (Baltimore: Johns Hopkins University Press, 1995), p. 9.

14. Giuseppe Sanarelli, "Etiologia e pathgenesi della febbra gialla," *Annales d'Igiene Sperimentale* (1897) new series 7: 345, quoted in W. Bean, "Walter Reed and the ordeal of human experiments," *Bulletin of History and Medicine* 51 (1977): 75–92, pp. 81–82. Sanarelli was wrong; icteroides lost out to a virus, discovered in 1927 by Adrian Stokes, who was lethally infected in the course of his own experiments.

15. Harvey Cushing, *The Life of Sir William Osler* (Oxford: Clarendon Press, 1925), Vol. I, p. 486.

16. U.S. *A Bill for the Further Prevention of Cruelty to Animals in the District of Columbia* (1896) 54th Congress, S. 34.

17. *A Bill for the Regulation of Scientific Experiments upon Human Beings in the District of Columbia* (1896) 54th Congress, S. 3424.

18. S.R. 3424; Senate Document No. 337 (Washington, D.C.: Government Printing Office, 1896); cited in Lederer, *Subjected To Science*, Appendix I, p. 143.

19. Sir William Osler, *Principles and Practice of Medicine*, 3rd ed. (New York: Appleton, 1898), p. 18.

20. Cushing, *The Life of Sir William Osler*, Vol. I, p. 522.

21. In the 1880s, Carlos Juan Finlay, a Scottish physician trained at Jefferson Medical College in Philadelphia and a long-time practitioner in Havana, correctly indicated the mosquito *Stegomyia fasciata*, a subspecies of *Aedes aegypti*, as the carrier of the disease. His experiments, which won him great honor, were not unlike those of Sanarelli. See David G. McCullough, *The Path Between the Seas: The Creation of the Panama Canal 1870–1914* (New York: Simon and Schuster, 1977), pp. 413–415.

22. Lederer, *Subjected to Science*, chapter 6.

23. Cushing, *The Life of Sir William Osler*, Vol. II, p. 108.

24. Cushing, *The Life of Sir William Osler*, Vol. II, p. 109.

25. Charles Francis Withington, *The Relation of Hospitals to Medical Education* (Boston: Cupples, Uphman and Co., 1886), quoted in Reiser et al., *Ethics in Medicine*, p. 260.

26. Lawrence K. Altman, *Who Goes First? The Story of Self-Experimentation in Medicine* (New York: Random House, 1987).

27. Lederer, *Subjected to Science*, chapter 4.

28. Lederer, *Subjected to Science*, chapter 4.

29. Cited in Lederer, *Subjected to Science*, p. 99. In 1909, Dr. Cannon became exasperated with his Harvard colleague, William James, who, in a published letter that had affirmed the essential morality of vivisection, criticized experimenters for their insensitivity to the suffering of animals. In a letter to James, Cannon upbraided his friend for giving too much to the anti-vivisectionists and complained, "I get very much discouraged at times about this fight. We are all too prone to misinterpretation." Gerald E. Myers, *William James: His Life and Thought* (New Haven: Yale University Press, 1986), p. 434.

30. John R. Paul, *A History of Poliomyelitis* (New Haven: Yale University Press, 1971), pp. 252–262.

31. Prussian Ministry of Health, *Centralblatt der gesamten Unterrichtsverwaltung in Preussen* (1901), 188–189, quoted in George J. Annas and Michael A. Grodin, *The Nazi Doctors and the Nuremburg Code. Human Rights in Human Experimentation* (New York and Oxford: Oxford University Press, 1992), p. 127.

32. Annas and Grodin, *The Nazi Doctors and the Nuremburg Code*, pp. 131–132.

33. "Biomedical ethics and the shadow of Nazism. A Conference on the proper use of the Nazi analogy in ethical debate, April 8, 1976," *Hastings Center Report* special supplement 6, no. 4 (1976).

34. *Trials of War Criminals before the Nuremberg Military Tribunals under Control Council Law No. 10* (Washington, D.C.: U.S. Government Printing Office, 1949), Vol. 2, p. 181.

35. Eva Moses-Kor, "The Mengele twins and human experimentation: a personal account," and Telford Taylor, "The opening statement of the prosecution, Dec. 9, 1946," in Annas and Grodin, *The Nazi Doctors and the Nuremberg Code*, pp. 53–59, 67–93; see also Gerald L. Poser and John Ware, *Mengele: The Complete Story* (New York: McGraw-Hill, 1986); Lucette Matalon Lagnado and Sheila Cohn Dekel, *Children of the Flames: The Untold Story of the Twins of Auschwitz* (New York: Morrow, 1991); Robert J. Lifton, *The Nazi Doctors: Medical Killing and the Psychology of Genocide* (New York: Basic Books, 1986); Alexander Mitscherlich and Fred Mielke, *Doctors of Infamy: The Story of the Nazi Medical Crimes* (New York: H. Schuman, 1949).

36. "Report on war crimes of a medical nature committed in Germany and elsewhere on German nationals and the nationals of occupied countries by the Nazi regime during World War II," *AMA Archives*, quoted from Advisory Committee on Human Radiation Experiments, *Final Report* (Washington, D.C.: U.S. Government Printing Office, 1995), pp. 133–134.

37. Leo Alexander, "Medical science under dictatorship," *New England Journal of Medicine* 241 (1949): 39–47, quote on p. 44; see Annas and Grodin, *The Nazi Doctors and the Nuremberg Code;* Arthur L. Caplan (ed.), *When Medicine Went Mad: Bioethics and the Holocaust* (Totawa, N.J.: Humana Press, 1952).

38. Alexander, "Medical science under dictatorship," p. 45.

39. World Medical Association, *Declaration of Helsinki* in W. Reich (ed.), *Encyclopedia of Bioethics* (New York: Simon & Schuster Macmillan), Vol. 5, pp. 2765–2766.

40. David J. Rothman, "Research, human: historical aspects," in Warren Reich (ed.), *The Encyclopedia of Bioethics*, Vol. 4, p. 2252.

41. David J. Rothman, *Strangers at the Bedside: A History of How Law and Bioethics Transformed Medical Decision Making* (New York: Basic Books, 1991), pp. 48–49.

42. "German experiments at Auschwitz Camp," *Journal of the American Medical Association* 130 (1946): 892–893; Andrew C. Ivy, "History and ethics of the use of human subjects in medical experiments," *Science* 108 (1948): 1–5; Willard L. Sperry, "Moral problems in the practice of medicine: with analogies drawn from the profession of the ministry," *New England Journal of Medicine* 239 (1946): 985–990; W. B. Bean, "Testament of duty: some strictures on moral responsibility in clinical research," *Journal of Laboratory and Clinical Medicine* 39 (1952): 3; Otto E. Guttentag, "On the clinical entity," *Annals of Internal Medicine* 31 (1949): 484–496; Leo Alexander, "Medical science under dictatorship," *New England Journal of Medicine* 24 (1949): 39–47.

43. Otto E. Guttentag, "The problem of experimentation on human beings," *Science* 117 (1953): 205–214; "Ethical problems in human experimentation," in E. Torrey Fuller (ed.), *Ethical Issues in Medicine: The Role of the Physician in Today's Society* (Boston: Little, Brown and Company, 1968).

44. Irving Ladimer and Roger W. Newman (eds.), *Clinical Investigation in Medicine: Legal, Ethical and Moral Aspects* (Boston: Boston University Law and Medicine Institute, 1963).

45. Renée C. Fox, *Experiment Perilous: Physicians and Patients Facing the Unknown* (Philadelphia: University of Pennsylvania Press, 1959).

46. Rothman, *Strangers at the Bedside*, pp. 62–63.

47. Jay Katz, "The consent principle of the Nuremberg Code," in Annas and Grodin, *The Nazi Doctors and the Nuremberg Code*, p. 228.

48. Otto E. Guttentag, "The physician's point of view," *Science*, 117 (1953): 205–214, quote on p. 209.

49. Advisory Committee on Human Radiation Experiments, *Final Report* (Washington, D.C.: U.S. Government Publications Office, 1995), p. 141.

50. Mitscherlich and Mielke, *Doctors of Infamy*.

51. These were scientists interviewed during 1995 for the Advisory Committee on Radiation Experiments. Ruth Faden, chair, ACHRE, personal communication.

52. Advisory Committee on Human Radiation Experiments, *Final Report*, p. 105.

53. Advisory Committee on Human Radiation Experiments, *Final Report*, pp. 91, 781–782.

54. Ruth R. Faden (ed.), *The Human Radiation Experiments: Final Report of the President's Advisory Committee* (New York: Oxford University Press, 1996), pp. 131, 149.

55. Advisory Committee on Human Radiation Experiments, *Final Report*, p. 143.

56. Irving Ladimer and Roger W. Newman (eds.) *A Study of the Legal, Ethical, and Administrative Aspects of Clinical Research Involving Human Subjects: Final Report of Administrative Practices in Clinical Research* (Boston: Law-Medicine Research Institute, 1963), pp. 43–44, quoted in Advisory Committee on Human Radiation Experiments, *Final Report*, p. 143.

57. Advisory Committee on Human Radiation Experiments, *Final Report*, pp. 143–150.

58. Advisory Committee on Human Radiation Experiments, *Final Report*, pp. 777–778. A 1994 newspaper story about one such experiment sponsored in the 1940s, not by the government

but by a commercial food producer, catches the essence of the problem. Retarded children at the Fernald School in Waltham, Massachusetts, were fed oatmeal with calcium and iron tagged with radioactive tracers to determine the absorption of those nutrients. According to the news report, in 1993, "a state panel said the small amounts of radioactive calcium and iron eaten by 74 residents of the Fernald School had no discernible effect on their health. But the panel said researchers violated the children's human rights." Even well-intentioned researchers of that era would have found it difficult to understand how this harmless research "violated . . . human rights." Associated Press, "Suit seeks millions for kids who ate radioactive cereal in postwar test," *Sacramento Bee*, December 7, 1995: A15.

59. Morton Mintz, "Heroine of FDA keeps bad drug off market," *Washington Post*, July 15, 1962: A1, A8; see also Mintz, *The Therapeutic Nightmare* (Boston: Houghton Mifflin, 1965). Merrell had bought the license for thalidomide from the German company Chevre Gruenthal, which had synthesized it in 1953.

60. Ralph A. Fine, *The Great Drug Deception: The Shocking Story of MER/29 and the Folks Who Gave You Thalidomide* (New York: Stein and Day, 1972), pp. 168–169; John Lear, "The unfinished story of thalidomide," *Saturday Review*, September 1, 1962: 38ff.

61. Fine, *The Great Drug Deception*, p. 171.

62. Helen Taussig, "A study of the German outbreak of Phocomelia," *Journal of the American Medical Association* 180 (1962): 1105–1114.

63. See Richard Harris, *The Real Voice* (New York: Macmillan, 1964). Strangely, Dr. Kelsey never appeared before Kefauver's Subcommittee on Antitrust and Monopoly but rather before Senator Hubert H. Humphrey's Subcommittee on Government Reorganization.

64. *Federal Food, Drug and Cosmetic Act of 1962*, PL 87-781, 76 STAT 780; Section 505(I), 87th Congress, 2nd session.

65. Frances Kelsey, "Patient consent provisions of the Federal Food, Drug and Cosmetic Act," in Irving Ladimer and Roger W. Newman, (eds.) *Clinical Investigation in Medicine: Legal, Ethical and Moral Aspects* (Boston: Law-Medicine Research Institute, Boston University, 1963), pp. 336–339; William J. Curran, "Governmental regulation of the use of human subjects in medical research: the approach of two federal agencies," in Paul A. Freund (ed.), *Ethical Aspects of Experimentation with Human Subjects* (Cambridge, Mass.: American Academy of Arts and Sciences, 1969), pp. 542–594; 21 CFR 50.20 *Federal Register* Vol. 46, no. 17 (January 27, 1981): 8951; National Commission for the Protection of Human Subjects, *The Belmont Report: Ethical Principles and Guidelines for the Protection of Human Subjects* (Washington, D.C.: U.S. Government Printing Office, 1979), pp. 5–6; Ruth R. Faden and Tom L. Beauchamp, *A History and Theory of Informed Consent* (New York: Oxford University Press, 1986).

66. This clearance was stated in private correspondence from Commissioner George P. Larrick to Dr. Henry Beecher. See Curran, "Governmental regulation of the use of human subjects in medical research," pp. 418–419.

67. Ladimer and Newman, *Clinical Investigation in Medicine*.

68. Mark S. Frankel, "The development of policy guidelines governing human experimentation in the United States: a case study of public policy-making for science and technology," *Ethics in Science and Medicine* 2 (1975): 48.

69. R. B. Livingston, "Progress report on survey of moral and ethical aspects of clinical investigation: Memorandum to Director, NIH," November 4, 1964; quoted in Frankel, "The development of policy guidelines governing human experimentation in the United States," p. 50.

70. *Hyman v Jewish Chronic Disease Hospital* 42 Misc.2d 427, 1963; reprinted in Katz, *Experimentation with Human Beings*, pp. 9–65.

71. Chauncey Leake (ed.), *Percival's Medical Ethics* (Huntington, NY: Krieger, 1975), chap-

ter 1, xii, p. 76; M. B. Shimkin, "The researcher's point of view," *Science* 117 (1953): 205–207, quote on p. 206.

72. World Medical Association, Declaration of Helsinki I, June 1964; Declaration of Helsinki II, October 1975; reprinted in Annas and Grodin, *The Nazi Doctors and the Nuremberg Code*, pp. 331–342.

73. The NIH issued its first comprehensive policy statement in a pamphlet, *The Institutional Guide to DHEW Policy on Protection of Human Subjects* (Washington, D.C.: U.S. Government Printing Office, 1971), commonly called The Yellow Book. The present name for such review committees (Institutional Review Boards, or IRBs) first appeared in the National Research Act of 1974 (P.L. 93-348, Section 212 (a)). The language was then adopted into the DHEW regulations for protection of human subjects (45 CFR 46, May 30, 1974). See National Commission for the Protection of Human Subjects, *Institutional Review Boards: Report and Recommendations* (Washington: D.C.: U.S. Government Printing Office, 1978), pp. 42–43.

74. Henry K. Beecher, "Ethics and clinical research," *New England Journal of Medicine* 274 (1966): 1354–1360.

75. Henry K. Beecher, "Experimentation in man," *Journal of the American Medical Association* 169 (1959): 461–478.

76. Beecher, "Ethics and clinical research," p. 1360; See Rothman, *Strangers at the Bedside*, chapter 4.

77. Beecher, *Research and the Individual* (Boston: Little, Brown and Company, 1970), p. 82.

78. Rothman, *Strangers at the Bedside*, p. 84.

79. M. H. Pappworth, *Human Guinea Pigs: Experimentation on Man* (Boston: Beacon Press, 1968); Franz J. Ingelfinger, "The unethical in medical ethics," *Annals of Internal Medicine* 83 (1975): 264–269.

80. Austin Bradford Hill, "The clinical trial," *British Medical Bulletin* 7 (1951): 278–282; "Medical ethics and controlled trials," *British Medical Journal* 1(1963): 1043–1049; reprinted in Reiser et al., *Ethics in Medicine*, pp. 278–284.

81. Hill, "Medical ethics and controlled trials," p. 1049.

82. U.S. Senate Committee on Government Operations, Hearing on the National Commission on Health Science and Society, 90th Congress, 2nd session, 1968, p. 98; see also Rothman, *Strangers at the Bedside*, p. 173.

83. Walsh McDermott, "The risks of research," Francis D. Moore, "A cultural and historical view," Jay Katz, "Individual risks vs. societal benefits: how are the risks distributed? Inquiry and commentary," in National Academy of Sciences, *Experiments and Research with Humans: Values in Conflict* (Washington D.C.: National Academy Press, 1975), pp. 42, 30, 155, respectively.

84. Jay Katz, "From experiment to clinical trials: Unethical experiment," (paper read at the Birth of Bioethics Conference, Seattle, Wa., Sept. 23–24, 1992), transcript p. 116.

85. Albert Sabin, "Individual risks vs. societal benefits: how are the risks distributed? Inquiry and commentary," in National Academy of Sciences, *Experiments and Research with Humans*, p. 164; see Jay Katz, "'Ethics and clinical research' revisited," *Hastings Center Report* 23, no. 5 (1993): 31–39.

86. Jay Katz, "From experiment to clinical trials," pp. 106–118.

87. Jay Katz with Alexander Morgan Capron and Eleanor Swift Glass, *Experimentation with Human Beings* (New York: Russell Sage, 1972).

88. Jean Heller, "Syphilis victims in US study went untreated for 40 years," *New York Times*, July 26, 1972: A1, A8.

89. James H. Jones, *Bad Blood* (New York: The Free Press, 1981); Alan Brandt, "Racism and research: the case of the Tuskegee Study," *Hastings Center Report* 8, no. 6 (1978): 21–29; *Final*

Report of the Tuskegee Syphilis Study Ad Hoc Advisory Panel (Washington, D.C.: U.S. Government Printing Office, 1973).

90. Alphonse M. Schwitalla, "The real meaning of research and why it should be encouraged," *Modern Hospital* 33(1929):77–80, reprinted in Reiser et al., *Ethics in Medicine*, pp. 264–266.

91. John Ford, "Notes on moral theology," *Theological Studies* 6 (1945): 543–544; "Human experimentation in medicine: moral aspects," Symposium on the Study of Drugs in Man, *Clinical Pharmacology and Therapeutics* 1 (1960): 396–400.

92. Allocution to the First International Congress on the Histopathology of the Nervous System, Sept. 14, 1952; *Acta Apostolicae Sedis* (1952) 44: 779; English translation reprinted in *The Linacre Quarterly: Official Journal of the Federation of Catholic Physicians' Guilds* 19 (1952): 98–107; cited in Advisory Committee on Human Radiation Experiments, *Final Report*, p. 154.

93. Walsh McDermott, "Opening comments," in J. Russell Elkington (ed.), "The changing mores of biomedical research," *Annals of Internal Medicine* 67, supplement 7(Sept. 67), pp. 41–42.

94. William Curran, personal interview, March 15, 1996.

95. Stephen R. Graubard (ed.), Preface to "Ethical Aspects of Experimentation with Human Subjects," *Daedalus* 98, no. 2 (1969): iv–v.

96. Hans Jonas, "Philosophical reflections on human experimentation," *Daedalus* 98, no. 2 (1969): 219–247, p. 230.

97. *The National Research Act*, Public Law 93-348, July 12, 1974.

98. *The Belmont Report*; 45CFR46, 45.102 (e), p. 3.

99. Robert J. Levine, "The boundaries between biomedical or behavioral research and the accepted and routine practice of medicine"; "The role of assessment of risk-benefit criteria in the determination of the appropriateness of research involving human subjects"; "The nature and definition of informed consent in various research settings"; and "Appropriate guidelines for the selection of human subjects for participation in biomedical and behavioral research," in *The Belmont Report: Ethical Principles and Guidelines for the Protection of Human Subjects of Research*, (Washington, D.C.: U.S. Government Printing Office, 1979), Appendix I.

100. Ruth Macklin and Susan Sherwin, "Experimenting on human subjects: philosophical perspectives," *Case Western Reserve Law Review* 25 (1975): 434–471.

101. Paul Ramsey, *The Patient as Person: Exploration in Medical Ethics* (New Haven: Yale University Press, 1970), p. 11.

102. Charles Fried, *Medical Experimentation: Personal Integrity and Social Policy* (New York: American Elsevier, 1974); see also "Human experimentation: philosophical aspects," in Warren T. Reich (ed.), *Encyclopedia of Bioethics*, 1st ed., (New York: The Free Press, 1978), Vol. 2, pp. 699–702.

103. H. Tristram Engelhardt, Jr., "Basic ethical principles in the conduct of biomedical and behavioral research," in *The Belmont Report*, Appendix I, p. 8–5.

104. *The Belmont Report*, p. 4.

105. Speakers at a New York University symposium hurled that ugly epithet. I recall that when Dr. Krugman came to lecture at UCSF in the 1970s, demonstrators carrying Nazi accusations marched in front of the medical school.

106. Editors, "Prevention of Viral Hepatitis—Mission Impossible?" *Journal of the American Medical Association* 217(1971):70–71; see Katz, *Experimentation with Human Beings*, pp. 1007–1111 for the *Lancet* letters; David J. Rothman and Sheila M. Rothman, *The Willowbrook Wars* (New York: Harper and Row, 1984), chapter 11.

107. Beecher, "Ethics and clinical research," p. 1360.

108. Ramsey, *The Patient as Person*, pp. 12–13.

109. Richard A. McCormick, "Proxy consent in the experimentation situation," in *How Brave a New World? Dilemmas in Bioethics* (New York: Doubleday, 1981), p. 62; originally published in *Perspectives in Biology and Medicine* 18 (1974): 12.

110. William G. Bartholome, "Proxy consent in the medical context: the infant as person," in The National Commission for the Protection of Human Subjects of Biomedical and Behavioral Research, *Research Involving Children,* (Washington, D.C.: U.S. Government Printing Office, 1977), Appendix; Richard A. McCormick, "Proxy consent in the experimental situation"; Paul Ramsey, "The enforcement of morals: nontherapeutic research on children," *Hastings Center Report* 6, no. 4 (1976): 21–30; Richard A. McCormick "Experimentation in children: sharing sociality," *Hastings Center Report* 6, no. 6 (1976): 41–46; Paul Ramsey, "Children as research subjects: a reply" *Hastings Center Report* 7, no. 2 (1977): 40.

111. Ramsey, "The enforcement of morals," p. 30, footnote 21.

112. Richard A. McCormick, "Sharing in sociality: children and experimentation," in *How Brave a New World?,* p. 87.

113. National Commission for the Protection of Human Subjects of Biomedical and Behavioral Research, *Research Involving Children*; Protection of Human Subjects, Policies and Procedures, Department of Health, Education and Welfare, *Federal Register*, Vol. 38, No. 221, Part 11, November 16, 1973.

114. "Ethics governing the service of prisoners as subjects in medical experiments," *Journal of the American Medical Association* 136 (1948): 447–458.

115. Jessica Mitford, *Kind and Usual Punishment: The Prison Business* (New York: Vintage Press, 1973); "Experiments behind bars: doctors, drug companies and prisoners," *Atlantic Monthly*, January 1973; pp. 64–73.

116. Quoted in Robert J. Levine, *Ethics and Regulation of Clinical Research*, 2nd ed. (New Haven: Yale University Press, 1988), p. 277.

117. 45CFR46, subpart C, section 46.306.

118. The President's Commission was required to report biennially on the success of the system. It did so in *Protecting Human Subjects* (Washington, D.C.: Government Printing Office, 1981) and *Implementing Human Research Regulations* (Washington, D.C.: Government Printing Office, 1983).

119. John C. Fletcher was not related to Joseph Fletcher, although both were Episcopal clergymen; both were Southerners and social activists and, coincidently, both finished their careers in bioethics as Professors at the University of Virginia.

120. Robert J. Levine, *Ethics and Regulation of Clinical Research*.

6

Splicing Life: Genetics and Ethics

Children are like their parents: common sizes and shapes, virtues and strengths, weaknesses and sufferings trail through families, and humans must always have wondered why. Four centuries ago, Michel de Montaigne reflected on the excruciating pain he and his father shared from stones in the bladder. In his essay "Of the resemblance of children to their fathers" the essayist reflected, "I was born twenty-five and more years before his illness, at a time when he enjoyed his best health. Where was the propensity to this infirmity hatching all this time? And when he was so far from the ailment, how did this slight bit of his substance, with which he made me, bear so great an impression of it? How did it remain so concealed that I began to feel it forty-five years later? . . . Will anyone enlighten me about this process?"[1] This sixteenth-century savant asked a question that only modern genetics could answer. Modern genetics flows from human curiosity about "the resemblance of children to their fathers." That curiosity could only speculate about this resemblance until a little over a century ago, when speculation turned into science. In the 1860s, Gregor Mendel, abbot of the Augustinian monastery of Brno in Austria, mathematically calculated the inherited characteristics of pea plants that he bred in his monastery garden.[2]

A little less than a century later, on April 25, 1953, a one-page paper entitled "The molecular structure of nucleic acids," by James D. Watson and Francis H. Crick, appeared in the British scientific journal *Nature*. The authors described the deoxyribonucleic acid molecule (DNA), a fragment of matter hidden in the nucleus of almost all animal cells, as "two helical chains each coiled around the same axis." The article is a lucid description of an ingenious scientific idea. It said not a word about ethics but its concluding words were, "It has not escaped our notice that the specific pairing we have postulated immediately suggests a possible copying mechanism for genetic material."[3] The same fact did not escape the notice of others. *The New York Times* promoted the authors' concluding remark to the headline of its report: "Clue to Chemistry of Heredity Found."[4] The biochemical structure and function revealed by the Watson–Crick hypothesis, and by the torrent of scientific work that followed their observation, has opened up a wide realm of ethics. The words "genetic" and "heredity" cannot be uttered without arousing profound human questions: What is it to be human? Is there a perfect form of humanity? If so, can it be achieved by human choice?

Six months after the publication of the *Nature* paper, Pope Pius XII addressed the First International Conference of Medical Genetics on the ethical issues which, then and now, swirl around genetics. Since the general purpose of genetics "is to influence the transmission of hereditary factors in such a way as to promote what is good and eliminate what is harmful," the Pope pronounced genetics "morally irreproachable." Some means toward achieving this end, however, are not irreproachable. He mentioned abortion, sterilization for eugenic purposes and state prohibition of marriage and reproduction.[5]

The devastation of World War II was but a few years in the past when the new genetics appeared in the scientific world. The war had been fought under an ideology that espoused changes in social and physical life designed to create a "master race." Genetic science, regardless of how well intentioned it was, could not totally escape that memory. As science and medicine, genetics represents extraordinary scientific progress, but that progress is haunted by the fears and worries associated with the possibilities of capricious, careless, even vicious power over human life. Although genetics is beautiful as science, it is an ethical minefield. This chapter traces the path of modern genetics through that minefield. The perilous trip begins with the eugenics of the nineteenth and early twentieth centuries.

Eugenics

Philosophical, religious, and ethical questions have accompanied the gradual articulation of the modern view of human origins and evolution. Charles Darwin anticipated the direction those questions would take after his epochal announcement of the evolutionary hypothesis that biological progress resulted from a natural selection whereby certain inheritable variations are advantageous for survival and are passed on to successive generations. Darwin reflected, "We civilized men do our utmost to check the process of elimination [of the unfit]; we build asylums for the imbecile, the maimed and the sick; we institute poor laws; and our medical men exert their utmost skill to save the life of every one to the last moment. . . . Thus, the weak members of civilized societies propagate their kind."[6]

Although Darwin did not pursue this thought further, it presaged the eugenics movement fostered by his cousin, Francis Galton. Beginning in 1865, Galton began to develop the thesis that the human race might be improved by deliberately multiplying desirable human qualities and eliminating undesirable ones through selective breeding.

Having been a Cambridge honors student, he certainly would have read Plato's proposals for such a program in the fifth book of *The Republic*.[7] Also, as a nineteenth-century English gentleman scholar, he had distinct ideas about desirable human qualities, which included "reputation," arising from "intellectual ability, eagerness to work and power to work." These qualities were innate and could be inbred through successive generations of careful breeding.[8] For the next fifty years, he promoted these ideas to a society willing to hear. Galton spoke as a scientist as well as a propagandist. He discovered the emerging science of statistics, formulated by the German mathematician Carl Friedrich Gauss, and applied its now familiar concept of a normal distribution along a bell curve to a variety of empirical observations about plant propagation and human pedigrees. He initiated the studies of twins that were to become a central technique of genetics. He promoted the career of mathematician Karl Pearson who, with Walter Weldon, created the new science of biometry, the statistical study of evolution and heredity. In his 1883 book, *Inquiries into Human Faculty,* Galton coined the word "eugenics" to describe the improvement of the human race by better breeding.[9]

While these scholarly activities were progressing in Great Britain, an attitude was forming in the United States. Historian Mark Haller describes this attitude: "Before a movement bearing the name eugenics had begun in the United States, the stage had been set. By the mid-1890s, a number of educated Americans were becoming aware of the seeming threats to the quality of the national stock. On the one hand, an increase in asylums, prisons, and poor relief revealed, as never before, the enormity of the task of caring for the dependent, delinquent, and pauper. . . . On the other hand, the stream of immigration into the country caused many Americans to feel threatened . . . that the future of their own nation might not belong to their own kind."[10] The popularity of social Darwinism, which proclaimed the "survival of the fittest" and was preached by admired intellectuals such as Herbert Spencer (who was much more popular in the United States than in his native England) and Yale's William Graham Sumner, fed the public attitude.[11] The scholarly eugenics from abroad and the populist eugenics of America began to flow together as the nineteenth century turned into the twentieth.

In the late 1880s, German biologist August Weismann proposed that the determinants of inherited traits lay in germ cells passed from generation to generation. In 1900, three biologists independently discovered the ignored experiments of Abbot Mendel with pea plants, which had first been printed in an obscure Austrian journal in 1866. Mendel demonstrated with simplicity and elegance that traits such as color and height passed from generation to generation in a lawful manner, thereby demonstrating the fundamental postulates of heredity.[12] The ideas of Weismann and of Mendel, together with the biometrics of Pearson and others, opened new routes for the scientific study of the inheritance and evolution of physical and behavioral characteristics of animals and humans. In 1906, the American Breeders Association, dedicated to the improvement of animal stock, established a committee on eugenics "to investigate and report on heredity in the human race . . . and emphasize the value of superior blood and the menace to society of inferior blood."[13] The members of the committee were all leaders of

American science, among them David Starr Jordan, President of Stanford University, Alexander Graham Bell, Luther Burbank, William Castle, and one man who would epitomize eugenics in the United States, University of Chicago biologist Charles B. Davenport.

In 1904, Davenport persuaded the Carnegie Institution to fund a research station for the experimental study of evolution at Cold Spring Harbor, Long Island. In addition to biological studies of the inheritance of traits in animals, the researchers investigated human inheritance through extended family pedigrees. This aspect of Davenport's work was lavishly financed by the personal philanthropy of several of the nation's wealthiest persons, Mrs. Edward H. Harriman and Mr. John D. Rockefeller. In 1910, their gifts enabled Davenport to open the Eugenics Record Office, which over the next thirty years collected reams of data on American families and racial groups and provided "scientific" information to individuals and organizations enthusiastic about the improvement of "the stock," by which was meant the American white middle class. Out of this vast database, Davenport and his followers claimed to be able to demonstrate that a wide variety of characteristics, from physical ones such as epilepsy to behavioral ones such as criminality and alcoholism, were inheritable. Various races, they believed, shared certain inherited characteristics.

Many Americans were concerned over the "problems" caused "by the great influx of blood from Southeastern Europe," but Charles Davenport believed that he could scientifically specify what those problems were. He proposed, for example, that "Mediterranean blood" would make the American population "darker in pigmentation, smaller in stature, more mercurial, . . . more given to crimes of larceny, kidnapping, assault, murder, rape, and sex-immorality."[14] Eugenics associations were formed in the United States and England to disseminate these supposedly scientific views about certain human groups and to educate the public about better breeding. Major public figures, such as President Theodore Roosevelt, Harvard president Charles William Eliot, and Reverend Harry Emerson Fosdick, the most popular preacher of the era, enthusiastically espoused eugenic doctrines.

The eugenics movement endorsed what later came to be called "positive eugenics," or the deliberate selection of desirable physical and behavioral traits through reproductive choices. However, "negative" eugenics was an inevitable implication: was it possible to "breed out" undesirable characteristics by preventing reproduction, either voluntarily or involuntarily? Eugenicists saw around them a vast population of "the feebleminded," a capacious term that included persons with serious mental disorders, the mentally retarded, the slow learners, the ignorant, and the "degenerate" of all sorts. Eugenicists frequently asserted that "the support of these defectives has become a veritable burden upon the taxpaying community." Even worse, these feebleminded were "afforded the opportunity to propagate their unfit kind."[15] Asylums and prisons and reformatories were full of "the feebleminded." It seemed only reasonable to prevent them from passing on their feeblemindedness by sterilization.

Castration had been sometimes employed for sterilization, but a much less invasive and more efficient procedure, vasectomy, came into use at the end of the nineteenth century (first reported by the distinguished surgeon, A. J. Ochsner).[16] The procedure quickly became standard practice, largely motivated by its utility for eugenic purposes. (The female equivalent, salpingectomy, came somewhat later; it was believed that female "degenerates" were usually sterile.)[17] The 1914 Report from the American Breeders Association's Committee, *On the Best Practical Means of Cutting Off Defective Germ-Plasm in the American Population,* stated that "society must look upon germ-plasm as belonging to society and not solely to the individual who carries it." The report recommended that the segregation, sterilization, and education of that ten percent of the population who were socially inadequate should be the chief means of reducing defective germ plasm. The report included a model statute for eugenic sterilization, authored by committee secretary Harry Laughlin, Assistant Director of the Eugenics Record Office. The statute would allow sterilization of potential parents of socially inadequate offspring: "feebleminded, insane, criminalistic, epileptic, inebriate, diseased, blind, deaf, deformed and dependent."[18]

In 1907, Indiana passed the first law authorizing compulsory sterilization of any criminal, idiot, rapist, or imbecile in a state institution whose condition was confirmed as "unimprovable" by a panel of physicians. By 1931, thirty states had such laws on the books. These laws authorized institutional superintendents to order sterilization of inmates with little or no due process. California's law, passed in 1909, and amended in 1913, provided for sterilization of mental patients on their release from the asylum.[19] From 1909 to 1927, 2,558 men and women were, in the language of the law, "asexualized." Activity in other states was considerably less: the total for all states during those years was 3,233 persons. In 1929, Drs. Paul Popenoe and Edward Gosney published *Sterilization for Human Betterment,* a report on the success of the California program. They concluded that asexualization was cost effective and without serious medical sequelae, and could reduce the number of mentally defective persons in a community by half in three or four generations. Their report was gratefully acknowledged by the German eugenicists who designed the 1933 Eugenic Sterilization Law that would effect "racial hygiene" by sterilizing all persons, institutionalized or not, who suffered from hereditary disabilities of all sorts.[20] Harry Laughlin published regularly in German journals and, in 1936, was awarded an honorary doctorate from the University of Heidelberg. The climate in Germany was ideal for eugenics: not only had there been a long scientific and medical interest but also the new Führer had written, "to prevent defective persons from reproducing equally defective offspring is an act dictated by the clearest light of reason."[21]

In America, the rush of state legislation was checked by constitutional challenges. Suits argued that sterilization laws violated either the equal protection or due process clauses of the fifth and fourteenth articles of the Bill of Rights. Several state statutes were struck down on these grounds, but in 1927, the Supreme Court upheld a Virginia statute that had been crafted to withstand legal challenge. Under that law, Virginia sterilized Carrie Buck, a seventeen-year-old girl who had been certified as a "moron," with an IQ score of less than nine years. Carrie's mother had been institutionalized as feeble-minded and Carrie had given birth to an infant judged less than normal. Thus, the state claimed that the Buck line suffered from hereditary feeblemindedness. Harry Laughlin acted as "expert" consultant to the state and, although he had never personally examined Carrie, her child, or her mother, he testified that Carrie Buck was "the potential parent of socially inadequate offspring."[22] In *Buck v Bell,* the Court affirmed Virginia's statute. Justice Oliver Wendell Holmes wrote the majority opinion: "We have seen more than once that the public welfare may call upon the best citizens for their lives. It would be strange if it could not call upon those who already sap the strength of the State for these lesser sacrifices . . . in order to prevent our being swamped with incompetence. . . . Three generations of imbeciles are enough."[23] After *Buck v Bell,* the pace of sterilization, which had been slowed by the legal doubts, "picked up and did not slacken until World War II."[24]

In addition to its support of sterilization, the eugenics movement favored limiting immigration of "inferior races." One eugenicist wrote, "The same arguments which induce us to segregate criminals and the feebleminded and thus prevent their breeding apply to excluding from our borders individuals whose multiplying here is likely to lower the average of our people."[25] Popular books, such as Madison Grant's *The Passing of the Great Race* (1911) and Lothrup Stoddard's *The Rising Tide of Color against White Supremacy* (1920), eulogized the "Nordic" physique, personality, and civilization.[26] These mythologies, together with the pseudo-science of the eugenicists, powered congressional action, first in 1921, and then in 1924. The Immigration Act of 1924 (which went into effect on July 1, 1929) strictly limited the entry of Caucasians by a formula based on racial origins and forbade entry to Orientals. A historian comments, "Most nativists believed the laws had rescued the nation from the brink and that Americans, having made the decision to keep America for Nordic stock, could begin to re-forge the bonds of social and racial unity. In immigration policy, at any rate, they believed the nation had chosen the road that eugenics had pointed out."[27]

Although the racism of the eugenicists was directed overtly toward the Oriental and "Mediterranean" people, eugenicists and most white people, whose beliefs were tainted by pervasive prejudice against Negroes, believed that the inferiority of Blacks needed no scientific proof. Nevertheless, the Stanford-Binet IQ tests, which became widespread in the first decades of the century, provided eugenicists and the public with "proof" beyond doubt that Blacks were intellectually inferior. Unable to distinguish between the better and worse educated, the wealthier and the poorer, the tests consistently showed Negro children as slow learners. Lest Negro inferiority dilute "White supremacy," over half the states passed anti-miscegenation laws forbidding marriage between "Caucasians" and persons with some admixture of Negro blood. These laws stood in some states until the Supreme Court invalidated them in 1967.[28] Other forms of racial separation—in education, in the armed services, in housing, transport, and elsewhere—assured that Nordic blood would not be contaminated. All eugenicists did not favor sterilization (some opposed it, less for civil rights reasons than because it might foster licentiousness); nor did all support the immigration restrictions. These moderate eugenicists remained convinced, however, that there was a strong moral obligation to encourage selective breeding of the best people.

Eugenics had strong opponents. Among the most vocal were leaders of the Catholic Church, many of whose communicants were of Celtic stock ("gifted with imagination and oratory, but lazy and given to the bottle") and of "Mediterranean" origin ("given to crimes of sex and violence").[29] Catholic leaders were not merely defending their flocks. They could base their objections on a foundational doctrine of their faith, the inherent dignity of each person before God. A leading theologian, Father John Ryan, wrote, "The Church counts the earthly existence of a helpless cripple, a chronic invalid, or a mental weakling intrinsically good, and she knows that all such persons are capable of a life of eternal happiness face to face with God . . . a viewpoint infinitely removed from that of those practical atheists who measure the worth of a subnormal person by the same standard that they apply to a dog or a horse."[30] Supreme Court Justice Pierce Butler, who cast the only dissenting vote in *Buck v Bell,* was a practicing Catholic. Theologians argued that sterilization was an intrinsically immoral mutilation that was not justified by any presumed civic good, "for bodily members exist for the good of the individual, but individuals do not exist for the good of the state. . . . the state exists [rather] for the good of the individual, to safeguard and defend his natural rights."[31] The English Catholic polemicist, G. K. Chesterton, devoted a book to eugenics in which, with the sharp witticisms that were his style, he accused the eugenicists of fashioning a scientific tyranny over "the most secret and sacred places of human freedom." His *Eugenics and Other Evils* furnished a stock of arguments against eugenics.[32]

The theological and polemical arguments were affirmed in the papal encyclical, *Casti Connubii* (1930), in which Pope Pius XI condemned eugenics, along with other evils, such as divorce and birth control, which undermined the sanctity of marriage. He castigated those who would legally prohibit marriage to persons simply because "they consider, according to their norms and conjectures . . . that (such persons) would bring forth defective offspring." Even worse, he said, was depriving persons of their reproductive ability against their will. This power civil authority cannot arrogate to itself. While individuals may be dissuaded from procreation, "it is wrong to brand men with the stigma of crime because they contract marriage, on the ground that, despite the fact they are in every respect capable of matrimony, they will give birth only to defective children, even though they use all care and diligence."[33] The next pope, Pius XII, who reigned through the Nazi regime, repeated his predecessor's condemnations in even stronger terms.[34]

Scientific Genetics

Serious doubts about eugenics also came from within the scientific community. Those who had followed the development of genetics from Galton to Pearson to Thomas Hunt

Morgan and Herbert Jennings were beginning to appreciate the complexity of the new science. In light of this knowledge, the eugenics programs, both positive and negative, appeared simplistic. The limited ability to apply methods of quantification to human characteristics cast doubt on the eugenicists' global attribution of degeneracy or feeble-mindedness, or of any specific behavioral traits, to hereditary causes. The intricate interplay of environment and heredity, ignored if not denied by the eugenicists, was being revealed: in the 1920s, Hermann Muller demonstrated that genetic mutations could be induced by X-rays. Further, genetics was turning biochemical. During the 1930s, increasing attention was given to serological studies, which determined the genetics of the blood groups and of certain diseases known to be hereditary, such as hemophilia and the thalassemias. The biochemistry of the "inborn errors of metabolism," as British physician Archibald Edward Garrod had named conditions in which normal metabolic processes were deficient due to an inherited defect, became another focus of attention. In 1938, another British physician, Lionel Penrose, announced his observations on the genetic origins of one of these inborn errors, phenylketonuria, and J. B. S. Haldane unraveled the biochemistry of that condition. The biochemistry of hemoglobin in sickle cell anemia was described by Linus Pauling in 1949. Cytology, the study of the cell, also advanced with new techniques for observation. In the mid-1950s, the exact number of human chromosomes was finally determined and studies of the structure and function of these carriers of the genes began in earnest. In 1959, a French geneticist, Jerome Lejeune, traced the source of the mental and physical defect then called Mongolism and now called Down's syndrome to the presence of an extra twenty-first chromosome. These investigations, which combined statistical genetics, cytology, and biochemistry, marked the future of genetics and rendered the old eugenics obsolete. The simplistic science and the oversimplified policies appeared unrealistic and unrealizable in light of the emerging genetics.

The final blow to eugenics came when the Nazi's eugenics policies, initiated soon after their ascendancy to power in 1933, burgeoned into a diabolic plan to eliminate wholesale the Jewish inhabitants of Europe as well as other "inferior" groups, such as Gypsies, and "defectives," such as homosexuals. In the three years following the promulgation of the Eugenic Sterilization Law, 225,000 people were sterilized under orders of the Hereditary Health Courts. The eugenics program turned explicitly anti-Semitic with the Nuremberg Laws of 1935, which prohibited marriage between persons of different racial backgrounds and in 1939, the sterilization program was supplemented with a euthanasia program to eliminate from society the burden of "useless eaters." As historian Daniel Kevles writes, "The revelations of the Holocaust had all but buried the eugenic ideal. After the Second World War, 'eugenics' became a word to be hedged with caveats in Britain and virtually a dirty word in the United States, where it had long been identified with racism."[35]

Many leading geneticists remained eugenicists at heart but they were, according to Kevles, "reform eugenicists . . . who rejected in varying degrees the social biases of their mainline predecessors yet remained convinced that human improvement would better proceed with . . . the deployment of genetic knowledge."[36] Among these "reform eugenicists" was Nobelist Hermann Muller. In 1935, he declared that "'eugenics' . . . is a hopelessly perverted movement . . . powerless to work any change for the good and (doing) incalculable harm by lending a false appearance of scientific basis to advocates of race and class prejudice, defenders of vested interests of church and state, Fascists, Hitlerites, and reactionaries generally." At the same time, Muller insisted that it was imperative to bring about "improvement in our hereditary constitutions."[37] He offered a panoply of suggestions based, he believed, on sound genetic science. These many suggestions were gradually narrowed down to a favored one: in a 1959 article, "The guidance of human evolution," Muller argued that "it will be only natural for people to wish each new generation to represent a genetic advance, if possible, over the preceding one," and that the "most effective method presently feasible is . . . artificial insemination . . . an entering wedge of positive selection."[38] He advocated "germinal choice," the voluntary creation of sperm banks by genetically fit, that is, physically and intellectually superior persons.

The "reformed eugenics" was displayed at a conference sponsored by the American Academy of Arts and Sciences entitled "Genetics and the Direction of Human Evolution," September 30 to October 2, 1960. Hermann Muller, as the keynote speaker, asked his audience, "Should we weaken or strengthen our genetic heritage?" He noted that some of the most remarkable advances in science and social practices were, in fact, endangering the genetic health of the world's population by increasing the load of deleterious genes. He urged serious consideration of his proposal for selective breeding by eugenic sperm banks. While his colleagues offered some cautions about the ethical feasibility of his proposals, they agreed with his analysis of the problem of genetic deterioration.

At the 1962 Ciba Conference, "Man and His Future," the session devoted to reproduction and genetics stirred up a storm. Muller, whose paper was read in absentia, expressed his fears about the genetic contamination of humankind and proposed once again his "germinal choice" solution. Joshua Lederberg, who was less concerned about genetic contamination than about future development, criticized all eugenic schemes as too slow and minimal in impact. He suggested that science concentrate on euphenics, the engineering of human development, using our increasing mastery of DNA to improve brain power, control immune response, and diminish senescence. Man must accept responsibility for his future and, in so doing, "we must face the issue of a definition of man."[39] These two talks aroused vigorous debate among the participants, most of whom were willing to admit that not even they were competent to select the qualities for the future human. Jacob Bronowski exclaimed, "If we are ever to make use of our growing eugenic powers, we shall need a wisdom greater than our own."[40] Many participants feared the degree of social coercion that programs of controlled reproduction would demand.

Paul Ramsey was the first ethicist to enter the genetics debate. Invited to speak at the Gustavus Adolphus Nobel Conference in 1965, he meticulously prepared himself to discuss the moral and religious implications of genetic control. He had educated himself in genetics by requesting a list of readings from Professor Hermann Muller. Muller, hardly prescient that he was about to become the target of Ramsey's polemic, had graciously replied, noting that he too had been invited to speak at the Nobel Conference but had been unable to accept. The reading list he supplied included many of his own writings, giving Ramsey ample ammunition to turn against him.[41]

The ethical problem, as formulated by Muller and accepted by most leading geneticists of the time, was the suspected increasing genetic load of deleterious mutations in the human species due to the conditions of civilization that favor the less fit and less adaptable genotypes. Among geneticists, an attitude of "genetic pessimism" prevailed. At the same time, the science of molecular biology had moved at breathtaking speed toward a deeper understanding of genetic mechanism. This scientific advance promised multiple possibilities for intervention in genotype and phenotype that might alleviate the genetic burden on the species. The scientific discussion, therefore, was about the feasibility and consequences of these interventions. As Ramsey noted, "The crisis of our present civilization is, at least in part, genetic and one that goes to the very *humanum* of man."[42]

Ramsey considered Muller's "genetic pessimism" and his proposals to relieve the genetic load. He did not deny the geneticists' thesis about genetic deterioration, rather he attempted to make explicit what he believed are the values that underlie "the atmospheric humanism and liberal progressivism which sustains any ostensibly science-based ethics." A science-based ethic, claimed Ramsey, views man as a being whose "whole dignity consists in thought" and the genetic apocalypse that Muller saw coming consists in the deterioration of this dignity in those who follow us. Ramsey countered with a theological dissertation on the view of the biblical religions: humanity's dignity does not consist in assuring that those who come after us will be better than we are. Christians, no less than secular geneticists, expect an apocalypse in which "none like us will come after us," but Christians believe that this apocalypse is ordained by a loving God in such a form and at such time as He wills. Such a belief liberates the Christian from the moral weight of attempting to prevent the apocalypse. The Christian does not see any "absolutely imperative end of genetic control or improvement."[43] Rather, other values will validate the means that might be taken to save one's progeny from harm; among these, Ramsey chose to dwell on the value of maintaining the unitive and procreative purposes of sex and marriage. The Christian is not absolved from working to alleviate the suffering attendant on genetic deterioration by any legitimate means. Ramsey contended that the humanistic ethic, "expecting ultimate success when ultimate success is not to be reached, is particularly apt to devise extreme and morally illegitimate means for getting there."[44] He counted Muller's proposals among those means, not insofar as they are "voluntary," but because they separate what the Christian believes must be always united—the two goods of sexuality, the unitive and the procreative.

Ramsey then assessed the various means of genetic control, from voluntary restraint from procreation to genetic surgery, in light of his theology of procreation, concluding that "there is ample and well-established ground in Christian ethics for enlarging upon the theme of man's genetic responsibility," but that responsibility must be exercised only within the bounds of certain values.[45] Professor Muller's proposals for "germinal choice" did not fall within those bounds. Ramsey endorsed certain means for eugenic selection, such as voluntary sterilization and voluntary abstinence from procreation. He stated his inclination toward negative eugenics, the elimination of negative traits, rather than positive eugenics, the attempt to breed more perfect humans. Ramsey advocated "an ethics of genetic duty," in which Christians would adopt policies of restricted reproduction for the sake of future generations. He agreed with Muller's statement that "although it is a human right for people to have their infirmities cared for by every means that society can muster, they do not have the right knowingly to pass on to posterity such a load of infirmities of genetic or partly genetic origin as to cause an increase in the burden already being carried by the population."[46] Ramsey concluded his essay by raising questions about the capability of any human to select the "ideal" genotypes for eugenic purposes.

Joseph Fletcher was also not reticent during the eugenics debates. He argued in favor of eugenic sterilization. Voluntary sterilization is an act of rational freedom and compulsory sterilization is a matter of social justice: "It is impossible to see," he wrote, "how the principle of social justice . . . can be satisfied if the community may not defend itself and is forced to permit the continued procreation of feeble-minded or hereditarily diseased children"[47] As the new genetic science appeared, Fletcher was fascinated by its prospects. In 1971 he wrote, "It seems to me that laboratory reproduction is radically human compared to conception by ordinary heterosexual intercourse. It is willed, chosen, purposed, and controlled and surely these are among the traits that distinguish Homo sapiens. . . . I cannot see how humanity or morality are served by genetic roulette sexually."[48] Three years later, Fletcher used that captivating image as the title of an impassioned book, *The Ethics of Genetic Control: Ending Reproductive Roulette*.[49] "Genetics is the real frontier," he exclaimed, "revealing exciting possibilities of quality control for our children."[50] He discussed current practices, such as genetic screening, and future possibilities, such as asexual reproduction, surrogate pregnancy, gene therapy, and genetic engineering, and found them all good, since all of them enhanced human control over nature.

The book's title, *Genetic Control,* announces the ground for genetic ethics: in Fletcher's view, control was a good thing, the very essence of rationality. In the eyes of many critics of the new genetics, control was ethically problematic. Increased power to control evolution implied increased power to abuse and exploit. Even the optimistic Fletcher hinted at the problem at the end of his ethical eulogy of modern genetics: "Utopian biology in the sense of embracing a prefabricated system for prefabricated human beings according to an ideal model, no matter how humane and disinterested it might be, is exactly what we ought to avoid as pretentious and fanatical."[51] In the early years of ethical controversy over the new genetics, Ramsey and Fletcher faced off;

standing on opposite sides of the debate, they articulated the arguments firmly and clearly. No reader of those two authors could be in doubt about the ethical implications of the new genetics.

Medical Genetics

From the mid-1930s on, genetics was converted from a pseudo-scientific prop for eugenics into a biochemical science and then into a tool for medical diagnosis and treatment. Medical genetics matured slowly but steadily. By the early 1960s, a few medical genetics clinics had been established, staffed by the rare physicians who had specialized in genetics and by a new professional, the genetic counselor. Persons who suspected that they or their family carried a hereditary disease could seek diagnosis based on their family pedigree and receive advice, usually about procreation. Biochemical and chromosomal tests were soon added to the resources of these clinics. It became possible to screen populations for certain genetic conditions. Phenylketonuria, an inborn error of the metabolism of phenylalanine that causes mental retardation in early childhood, was the first serious condition open to detection and treatment. A simple diagnostic test for newborn infants was devised and the onset of the condition could be prevented by a diet low in phenylalanine. It seemed reasonable, then, to screen all newborns and, at the instigation of pediatricians across the country, many states made such screening tests mandatory. The genetics of Tay-Sachs disease, a progressive neurological degeneration that slowly kills infants, was unraveled. A blood test could reveal whether a person was a carrier of the defective gene; if such a person married another carrier, their children had a 25 percent chance of having that terrible disease. Once warned of their carrier state, persons could avoid marriage with another carrier. Similarly, screening for carriers of the mutation for sickle cell anemia, a painful, debilitating, and often lethal blood disease that affects primarily persons of African ancestry, became possible and was mandated by law in many states.

In the mid-1960s, the procedure known as amniocentesis, in which amniotic fluid is withdrawn by needle from the pregnant uterus for examination of fetal cells, was coming into use. This made possible prenatal testing, potentially enabling physicians to detect a wide range of serious fetal defects. Among the chromosomal and inborn errors of metabolism that could be detected, the most common was Down's syndrome, which occurs about once in every seven hundred births, but more frequently to women over the age of 40. Should the amniocentesis reveal a fetal abnormality, the parents could choose abortion. In the early days of the procedure, some physicians refused to perform it unless the woman agreed to abort an affected fetus. This feature of the new technology prompted the remark attributed to Dr. C. Everett Koop, later to become President Reagan's Surgeon General, that amniocentesis was "a search and destroy mission."[52]

Abortion cast its shadow over the initiation of prenatal screening programs. In 1971,

Congress passed the National Sickle Cell Anemia Control Act, which provided for research, screening, counseling, and education. In the same year, the National Cooley's
Anemia Control Act, a disease that affects persons of Mediterranean ancestry, was also
passed. In 1976, these two laws were absorbed into the National Genetic Diseases Act,
which added screening for Tay-Sachs, cystic fibrosis, Huntington's chorea, and muscular dystrophy. This laudable legislation was left unfunded for several years because of
the association between abortion and screening, although proponents of screening insisted that the overwhelming number of negative tests (showing no defect) prevented
abortions that might otherwise be sought because of uninformed fear.

   These testing and screening programs, while well-intentioned and beneficial for individuals, were not immune from ethical questions. Although far from the crude proposals of the eugenics movement, these programs were faintly redolent of their discriminatory quality. It is certainly laudable to detect disease or potential disease, but is it
equally laudable to eliminate the disease by eliminating its victim? or to mark the surviving victim as defective? or to stigmatize a group as carriers of a defect? Should a diagnosis be offered when there is no treatment for the disease? These subtle mutations
of the Hippocratic duty to benefit and do no harm troubled some practioners of the new
genetic medicine.

   The time had come for a more careful examination of these questions, and answers
were necessary if programs were to be defined and implemented. In May, 1970, the
Fogerty Center for Advanced Study in Health Sciences at the National Institutes of
Health sponsored a small conference, "Early Diagnosis of Human Genetic Defects:
Scientific and Ethical Considerations." Several associates of The Hastings Center participated, including Dan Callahan, John Fletcher, Harold Green, and Leon Kass. The
meeting was chaired by Robert Morison of Cornell University, the first chairman of the
Hastings Board. Dr. Morison opened the conference with the remark, "However uneasy the conventional moralist may be when faced by these new powers and responsibilities, there are many of us who find satisfaction in the fact that the progress of science enables us to pose the historic ethical problems with more precision and with
more knowledge of the consequences than ever before."[53] Most of the presentations
were scientific, but in the closing lecture, geneticist James Neel reviewed the ethical
questions raised by early diagnosis; these included abortion, impact on the gene pool,
the balance between risks to mother and fetus and disease prevention, as well as the
problem of uncertainty of diagnosis. He concluded with words frequently heard at
similar gatherings: "This presentation has been directed much more toward the formulation of issues than toward their solution." The Hastings participants, however, recognized an opportunity.

   After this first meeting, Fogerty Center authorities asked Dan Callahan to organize a
larger conference focused exclusively on ethical issues in human genetics. He gathered
a remarkable cast in a short time. On October 10–14, 1971, scientists Arno Motulsky,
Michael Kaback, Robert Sinsheimer, James Neel, Robert Murray, Jerome Lejeune,
Leon Kass, and Robert Morison, philosophers Henry Aiken and Dan Callahan, theolo-

gians James Gustafson, Paul Ramsey, and John Fletcher, lawyers Alexander Capron, Charles Fried, Harold Green and Clark Havighurst, and many others gathered for a wide-ranging, close examination of the issues raised by the new genetic capabilities. Although speakers alluded to genetic therapy, cloning, and noncoital reproduction, they focused on the use of genetic knowledge for decision making by individuals, with specific attention to the knowledge gained by amniocentesis. As geneticist Tracy Sonneborn said in the opening lecture, "The major ethical issue is whether abortion is justified when the child is found to have defective or abnormal genes or chromosomes."[54]

The lectures and discussions posed the ethical obligation of the genetic counselor to remain neutral and nondirective against the ethical obligation to avoid harm. Participants appreciated the ambiguities of terms such as harm and benefit when a decision might result in abortion. They were also sensitive to the discriminatory and stigmatizing effects of genetic knowledge. Paul Ramsey's "Screening: an ethicist's view" judged the screening of the unborn or newly born to be a species of "statistical morality, cost-effectiveness analysis and . . . an ethics of the 'greatest net benefit.'" This leads, claimed Ramsey, "to the vanishing of the individual into the mass."[55] Callahan was equally concerned that the eagerness to eliminate genetic disease not diminish respect for those who suffer from it. "How can we both manage to live humanely with genetic disease and yet to conquer it at the same time?" he asked.[56] Through the dense arguments of the four-day meeting, most of the issues surrounding genetics were articulately discussed. Although many cautions were offered, no effort was made to draw these arguments into a set of coherent recommendations for policy. Yet the scientists and the ethicists seemed to be listening to each other.[57]

In the following year, Canon Michael Hamilton of the National Cathedral in Washington, D.C., who had attended the 1970 Fogerty Conference, assembled many of the same cast at Airlie House, Virginia, for a conference entitled "The New Genetics and the Future of Man." The scope of this conference was wider than that of the Fogerty Conference; it included sessions on reproductive technologies and on environmental effects on the gene pool and its central session was devoted to genetic therapy. Dr. French Anderson of the NIH, then as now the leading figure in this field, explained the science that would allow a corrective gene to be inserted, via a bacterial vector, into a person whose defective genetic structure led to a serious disease. Dr. Arno Motulsky cautioned that this sort of intervention was far in the future. Alexander Capron put Anderson's explanation within a broader social context, stressing the experimental nature of the work that would have to be done and the difficulties the law might have in limiting the directions of that work. Finally, Paul Ramsey criticized the overbroad use of the term "therapy," for which "engineering" is a more proper substitute, and called for a recognition that a profound and questionable philosophy of human nature underlay the geneticists' dreams: "Geneticists are, of course, troubled humanists. Still, piece by piece, genetic science seems to be leading to an additive view of man: . . . each of us is a package of normal abnormalities or abnormal normalities, combinations of more or less weak genetic strengths and more or less strong genetic weaknesses." All of this, with enough science, could be sorted out and the weaknesses abolished or made into strengths. This was not, in Ramsey's mind, either a feasible or an ethical view of humankind.[58] These commentators on Anderson's rather sunny hopes for genetic therapy express, in varying degrees of skepticism and gloom, the concerns about the power inherent in genetic science.

Some leading scientists were admitting their own concerns. In 1974, Dr. Arno Motulsky, a pioneer medical geneticist at the University of Washington, listed a litany of ethical issues associated with each of the present and potential capabilities of genetic science. Questions surrounded the diagnosis, prevention, and treatment of birth defects, screening for inherited disease, genetic counseling, intrauterine diagnosis, sex selection, population screening, early detection of late onset genetic disease, artificial insemination, in vitro fertilization, embryo research, cloning, and gene therapy. Dr. Motulsky, who had heard Paul Ramsey's severe homilies at the Fogerty and Airlie conferences, did not share his skepticism. "Ways must be found to deal with these issues in a manner acceptable to most human beings . . . by harmonizing our scientific, cultural, and ethical capabilities, the potentially achievable results can place us at the threshold of a new era of better health and less human suffering."[59]

Thus, in the early 1970s, genetics leapt ahead and ethical questions followed in profusion. These ethical questions were often posed as comprehensive worries: Where is this science leading us? What does it mean for our human future? However, the area of genetic advance that was closest to practice, screening for genetic disease, lent itself to more precise questions and some practical recommendations. The Fogerty Conference exposed the broad concerns about screening. These broad concerns now had to be narrowed down to specific principles, policies, and practices for the ethical conduct of genetic screening.

One of the research groups of The Hastings Center was devoted to genetic engineering and counseling. Theologian James Gustafson and scientist Richard Roblin were its chairpersons and Associate Marc Lappé was staff director. The group went to work on preparing a comprehensive statement of ethical principles for the design and implementation of screening programs. John Fletcher, who was a participant, recalls:

> Two ethical principles echo throughout this document: respect for persons and for their reproductive choices and fairness. The ethical weight of the document was clearly on the side of using genetic information to improve the reproductive choices of individuals. The document also placed screening within the realm of experimentation. We did that to assure that the new Federal policy on informed consent in experimentation also should be operative in screening programs. . . . The story of human genetics in the 20th century is the reversal of a situation in which societies abuse unscientific genetic information in the name of eugenics to one in which the power to choose to use reliable genetic information is situated in the couple and finally in the pregnant woman. In my opinion, the early bioethics movement helped to bring about this situation.[60]

The group's ensuing article, "Ethical and social issues in screening for genetic disease," recommended that screening programs be designed with clear goals in view and that those goals serve the decision making of individuals about having or not having children and the welfare of affected individuals. Eleven principles were then articulated. The program should have an attainable purpose; the affected community should participate in its design and implementation; there should be equal access; adequate testing procedures; and absence of compulsion; and participants should be fully informed. Whenever screening was to be done with untried procedures, it should be defined as human experimentation. Information obtained should be fully disclosed to those screened and counseling provided to them, and the relation of screening to available therapy should be explained. Finally, methods for protecting privacy and confidentiality needed to be in place and be enforceable by law. The article concludes with a strong warning about the dangers of discrimination and stigmatization. "Ethical and social issues" was one of the first products of the emerging bioethics to appear in a major medical journal.[61] Staff director Lappé commented, "*The New England Journal* published the report as its lead article two weeks after receiving it. I do think it made a difference in what was then a flood tide of ill-considered programs in genetic screening."[62]

The Hastings group reached these conclusions by debating the relevance of ethical principles to screening, but they also profited from the first-hand experience of Drs. Robert Murray and Michael Kaback, who were deeply engaged in screening programs.[63] Dr. Kaback recognized that a screening program for those persons most likely to be carriers of the Tay-Sachs gene, persons of Ashkenazi Jewish descent, could be implemented with the collaboration of the tight-knit Jewish communities. He spent fourteen months educating the leaders of these communities, soliciting their advice and making them partners in the program. Rabbis preached in their temples about the program; marriage brokers became active participants in counseling. Kaback's approach showed the practical value of the principles of autonomy and community participation.

Programs for sickle cell screening also seemed promising. The test for carrier status could be easily done and, if carriers were identified, they could be warned about the risk of marrying another carrier (since the disease is produced only if two carriers produce a child, who has a 25 percent chance of having it). Since the disease primarily affects persons of African descent, it seemed good, in that era of sensitivity to discrimination against Black Americans, to do something about a disease that imposed significant suffering on that community. Legislation was passed in thirteen states and for the District of Columbia during 1970–1972. President Nixon called attention to the need for effective detection and control of the disease in his health message of 1971.

These positive efforts quickly turned negative. The programs were badly designed. They targeted preschool children—for whom the information is hardly beneficial and possibly damaging. They were mandatory, tied to school admission, and to marriage licensing. They were rarely accompanied by education and counseling. Confusion reigned about the difference between sickle cell trait (the presence of one mutation, which is harmless) and the actual disease. Discrimination in employment by those who misunderstood the nature of the condition and the specter of singling out the Black community as disease carriers began to appear. Black physicians, including Dr. Robert Murray, raised serious criticisms of the badly designed, badly administered programs and, one by one, states revised or abolished their laws.[64] The Hastings group drew on Dr. Murray's first-hand experience and used the infelicitous sickle cell screening programs as a paradigm of a poorly designed screening program that violated most of the ethical guidelines they recommended.

Congress ordered the President's Commission to study the ethical and legal implications of genetic screening, counseling, and education programs. When the Commission began to prepare its report in 1981, it profited from a decade of experience and reflection about genetics and ethics. The commissioners read a second report from the Hastings genetics research group on prenatal diagnosis which provided a succinct analysis of the ethical issues together with seventeen specific recommendations for the clinical application of amniocentesis.[65] They also consulted an NIH Consensus Development Conference report, *Antenatal Diagnosis,* which reviewed the ethical and legal, as well as the scientific and clinical aspects of amniocentesis and other forms of prenatal testing.[66] The commissioners read the extensive literature and heard testimony from experts and from the public. Their report, *Screening and Counseling for Genetic Conditions,* endorsed programs for genetic screening, counseling, and education "when they are established with concrete goals and specific procedural guidelines founded on sound ethical and legal principles." It then spelled out those principles: preservation of confidentiality, respect for personal autonomy, improved knowledge about genetics, provision of benefit, and equity in access. Each of these principles is explained and one chapter illustrates how they might be applied to a specific screening program which did not yet exist but appeared to be imminent—screening for cystic fibrosis. The essential message of the report is that genetic screening should serve the decisions and welfare of individuals and that "the goals of a 'healthy gene pool' or a reduction in health costs cannot justify compulsory genetic screening."[67] The eugenic ideology was clearly repudiated.

Molecular Biology

This chapter began with Watson and Crick's announcement of the double helical structure of DNA. It moved backward to the eugenics movement of the early years of this century and then forward to the preventive genetics of the seventies. We now return to the scientific world of molecular biology. That world evolved with exciting rapidity during the 1940s and 1950s. In 1943, Oswald Avery, Colin MacLeod, and Maclyn McCarty demonstrated that a molecule known as deoxyribonucleic acid (DNA) was the material of which genes were made, and ten years later, Watson and Crick described the double helical structure of DNA. In the ensuing years, biochemistry, genetics, microbiology, virology, and crystallography converged in imaginative ways to form the new field of molecular biology.[68]

In the early 1970s, Professor Paul Berg of Stanford University learned how to insert bacterial genes into the genome of a simian virus, SV40. This discovery had major implications for molecular biology, but it also had worrisome aspects. It was theoretically possible that modification of the viral genome might cause disease in humans: SV40 was known to cause cancer in some small animals and to transform human cells in culture into cancer-like forms. Berg and some of his colleagues were concerned about this problem, and at Berg's urging, a conference of scientists was convened in January 1973 at Asilomar, a conference center on California's Monterey Peninsula. That conference, later called Asilomar I, reviewed the scientific data about the carcinogenic effects of various viruses of laboratory interest. Although the available evidence was not damning, further studies were clearly required. Berg summed up the conference by saying, "Prudence demands caution and some serious efforts to define the limits of whatever potential hazards exist."[69]

Several months before Asilomar I, Drs. Herbert Boyer and Howard Goodman at the University of California, San Francisco, had discovered a restriction enzyme, *EcoRI,* that cleaved the SV40 DNA at a specific site and made possible the splicing of foreign DNA into the genome. The ability to construct genetic hybrids between DNA molecules from different sources, or "recombinant DNA," was a scientific breakthrough that enhanced the worries about risk and raised even more far-reaching questions. Scientists continued to discuss these issues, and in 1973, a group of them submitted a letter to *Science,* expressing concern that the new recombinant techniques, though scientifically exciting, "could be used to combine DNA from animal viruses with bacterial DNA, or DNAs of different viral origin might be so joined. In this way new kinds of hybrid plasmids or viruses, with biological activity of unpredictable nature, may eventually be created."[70] The writers requested the National Academy of Sciences and the Institute of Medicine to establish a committee to study the issues and to recommend guidelines to limit the possibilities of "biological activity of unpredictable nature." The National Academy accepted the request and over the next few months several meetings were held under Berg's direction to plan Asilomar II.

On February 24, 1974, some one hundred fifty scientists from the United States and twelve other countries gathered among the fog-shrouded cypresses of the Asilomar Center. They were the elite of molecular biology. A small cadre of lawyers had been selected to join the scientists, as well as a group of respected science journalists. The lawyers were well chosen, for all had experience with biomedical science, and three of the four—Harold Green, Daniel Singer, and Alexander Capron—were closely associated with The Hastings Center. After a day's review of the science, the conference developed recommendations for classifying and monitoring various kinds of experiments, with particular attention to "biological containment," or the deliberate crippling of potentially pathogenic viruses, and "physical containment," the construction of laboratory facilities and designation of procedures for risky research. The lawyers discussed various legal regulatory schemes and the potential for legal liability. As one commentator notes, "listening to the lawyers predict what might happen to the decision to be made on the morrow, the scientists stiffened their resolve to close ranks so that the world would see that the scientific community was able to finish what it had begun."[71] The conferees produced a report which, while supporting continued recombinant DNA research, urged caution and made specific recommendations about how those cautions could be made concrete. The recommendations of Asilomar II became the template for the government body that had recently been appointed to oversee federally supported research in this field, the NIH Recombinant DNA Advisory Committee (RAC).

The scientific and technical questions asked at Asilomar were preface to an ethical question; indeed, it was an ethical question in disguise. The scientists asked what the likelihood was of physically endangering people by engineering organisms in the laboratory and, to the extent that such risk can be estimated, how could it be contained or prevented? Philosophers and theologians cannot answer that question; lawyers can only suggest what might happen if the scientists fail to answer it. But philosophers and theologians can reveal how any answer to questions of risk and likelihood of harm implies a valuing of human life, both individual and social. The ethical question that has motivated bioethics from its beginnings was silently present at the Asilomar discussions: how should we evaluate risks to achieve goods? It was a particularly urgent question since, as the signers of the *Science* letter had said, here the risks were "biological activity of an unpredictable nature." Asilomar was a covert ethics conference at which science accepted the moral responsibility to answer questions that it had raised and that had important implications for public safety and welfare.

A few months after the Asilomar II Conference, I was appointed to the first Biosafety Committee at the University of California, San Francisco. Again, I found myself faced with issues of which I was ignorant: my knowledge of molecular biology was minimal, but it was clear that I would have to become, as I was becoming in medicine, an informed amateur. My first lesson came from Dr. Herb Boyer, whose work had advanced the research and who had been at Asilomar II. He addressed the first meeting of the new committee, explaining the scientific background and the policy recommendations. I was at that time involved with the ethics of human research as a commissioner on the National Commission and as a member of our UCSF Institutional Review Board (IRB). The discussions at the monthly meetings of the Biosafety Committee were not at all like the discussions at the weekly IRB meeting. The standard topics of IRB discussions fitted our usual perception of moral discourse: we debated over informed consent, best interests of incompetent persons, and coercive incentives. None of these issues surfaced in biosafety discussions. The protocols that came to the Biosafety Committee were laboratory sterile, such as describing the intimate details of organisms like *E. coli* and the specifics of metal doors and venting hoods for A or B levels of containment. Yet behind these technical questions lay a serious ethical issue: should concerns about public safety justify the inhibition of scientific research, particularly when the risks to public safety are so unspecified and uncertain?

Outside the calm discussions of the Biosafety Committee, a more heated debate raged that leaked out of the scientific community into the civic community. Asilomar's cautious science did not satisfy everyone who had heard about "biohazards." Neighborhoods where major scientific institutions were located worried that the recommended containment might be inadequate. Harvard University's plan to open a new laboratory was met with hostility by the community of Cambridge, Massachusetts. Mayor Alfred Vellucci worried aloud, "They may come up with a disease that can't be cured—even a monster. Is this the answer to Dr. Frankenstein's dream?"[72] Mayor Vellucci's comment, naive though it might seem to a scientist, alluded to the deepest concern about molecular biology, molecular genetics, and what is now called molecular medicine. The concern is less about the containment of organisms than about the ability to modify the human organism by genetic manipulation. The problems of biosafety soon faded from view. Once methods of containment had been described and mandated, and once the scientific behavior of the organisms under study had been clarified, the problems of protecting the public became technical rather than ethical. Molecular biology, however, was not absolved from ethical scrutiny. During the next decade, genetic engineering, the manipulation of the molecular structure, became a major issue of bioethical reflection.

Splicing Life

On June 20, 1980, Dr. Claire Randall, Rabbi Bernard Mandelbaum, and Bishop Thomas Kelly, the General Secretaries of the National Council of Churches, the Synagogue Council of America, and the United States Catholic Conference, signed a letter to President Jimmy Carter. The letter began:

> We are rapidly moving into a new era of fundamental danger, triggered by the rapid growth of genetic engineering. Albeit, there may be opportunity for doing good; the very term suggests the danger. Who shall determine how human good is best served when new life forms are being engineered? Who shall control genetic experimentation and its results which could have untold implications for human survival? Who will benefit and who will bear any adverse consequences, directly or indirectly? These are not ordinary questions. These are moral, ethical, and religious questions. They deal with the fundamental nature of human life and the dignity and worth of the individual human being.[73]

The religious leaders exclaimed, "Those who would play God will be tempted as never before." These words could have been the clarion for another crusade like that against the evolutionists.

President Carter, a religious man, must have pondered over the letter, but instead of responding himself, he forwarded it to the President's Commission. A covering letter from Dr. Frank Press, the President's Science Advisor, urged the Commission to respond. The Commission was already committed to a study of the ethical issues attending genetic screening and counseling. In its second meeting, on May 16, 1980, the commissioners had decided not to include the multiple issues associated with gene therapy, genetic engineering, and recombinant DNA in its projected study of genetic screening. But by its third meeting, one month later, President Carter's request arrived, and it was, of course, a request we could not refuse. We decided to prepare a separate report based on the questions of the three religious leaders, covering the issues generally comprised under the heading "genetic engineering." That phrase, coined in 1965, covered a wide range of techniques for adding and subtracting various genetic characteristics at the molecular level. The technique of gene splicing, in which a bit of one chromosome is cut and attached to another chromosome, carrying with it the DNA that controls various genetic expressions, was the primary example. A piece of human DNA, for example, that governs the production of insulin can be spliced into the DNA of a bacterium, causing the bacterium to produce human insulin.[74] This technique was still in its laboratory infancy when a physician rushed it to clinic, attempting to cure a rare disorder, hyperargininemia.[75] Many other therapeutic possibilities leapt to mind. This technical capability aroused the imagination: how far can we, or should we, go toward changing nature, mixing species, controlling evolution or, in the words of the religious leaders, "playing God"?

The three religious leaders had spoken on behalf of their denominations. They defined their questions as "moral, ethical and religious." The Commission's first step was to ask those leaders "to elaborate on any uniquely theological considerations underlying their concern about gene splicing in humans." We wished to know whether they placed any solid theological ground under the popular phrase that they invoked, "playing God." Did they perceive a divine command against creating new life forms or crossing species boundaries? Was this science infringing on a divine prerogative? The three General Secretaries appointed theological committees to respond to our question. The Commission summarized the theologians' conclusions:

> Contemporary developments in molecular biology raise issues of responsibility rather than being matters to be prohibited because they usurp powers that human beings should not possess. The Biblical religions teach that human beings are, in some sense, co-creators with the Supreme Creator. Thus . . . these major religious faiths respect and encourage the enhancement of knowledge about nature, as well as responsible use of that knowledge. Endorsement of genetic engineering, which is praised for its potential to improve the human estate, is linked with the recognition that the misuse of human freedom creates evil and that human knowledge and power can result in harm.[76]

The commissioners realized that the theologians and religious leaders had essentially the "same concerns [that] have been raised—sometimes in slightly different words—by many thoughtful secular observers of science and technology." The concerns of religious and secular observers alike focused on the potential misuse of information and powers that could do much good. The moral, ethical, and religious questions raised could also be framed in terms of radical ambiguity of human choices, an ambiguity that might be particularly telling to persons steeped in the biblical faiths, but which could also be perceived by any sensitive person. The Commission cited the words of another religious leader, Pope John Paul II, who, addressing a meeting of genetic scientists, had stated his approval of genetic science "when its aim is to ameliorate the conditions of those who are afflicted with chromosomic diseases. . . . I have no reason to be apprehensive for those experiments in biology that are performed by scientists who, like you, have a profound respect for the human person, since I am sure that they will contribute to the integral well-being of man."[77]

Ambiguity lurks even in the papal words: What does contribute "to the integral well-being of man"? What actions and limits on action does "profound respect for the human person" dictate? Does it "ameliorate the condition of those afflicted with chromosomal disease" to abort a fetus so afflicted? (Certainly the Pope would answer no to the last question, but many decent people would answer yes.) These are the broad and deep questions stimulated by the religious leaders' questions. They can be articulated in the particular language of theological discourse or in terms of secular values. They are unlikely ever to be definitively answered but they demand reflection, discussion, and clarification. One of the commissioners, Dr. Arno Motulsky, admitted to being a "nonreligious person," but reflected, "when the theologians told the Commission, 'Humans are co-creators with God, and when you engage in these co-creations, you should do right and not misuse the freedom you have been given,' I appreciated that view. I was impressed that the secular and the religious, who might use very different language, could find common grounds to discuss these questions, foresee the dangers and advance this wonderful science, which is a triumph of human creativity, with respect for human dignity."[78]

As the sole geneticist among the commissioners, Motulsky helped chart the direction of the Commission's study. He told his fellow commissioners, "The hardest thing is to articulate what we should be worried about. The fears [over genetics] seem amorphous, a vague feeling that we can do things we have never done before and that we may change the human species for the worst. These worries are important, but hard to deal with." Those words opened the Commission's eleventh meeting, held at Airlie House, Virginia, on July 9–10, 1981. That meeting was the closest the President's Commission came to the National Commission's Belmont meeting. Like Belmont, it demonstrated that an informed group in intense and focused conversation could gradually move from the "amorphous" and "vague" to a set of specific questions, posed at varying levels of generality.

We had before us at that meeting a draft report that addressed the therapeutic, diagnostic, and "other" uses of genetic engineering. Several of us considered the draft "less than lyrical"—that is, it avoided entirely the broader yet vaguer and amorphous questions about changing nature, controlling evolution, and "playing God" that most troubled the religious leaders and many other concerned persons. We were determined to deal with these questions as articulately as we could. The final report contained lucid discussion of obscure concepts such as "interference with nature," "creating new life forms," "the malleability of human nature," and "the sense of personal identity." We then addressed questions in which scientific knowledge about consequences of genetic engineering could clarify the issues and questions in which political and social mechanisms could control the application of genetic engineering. The current and future capability of preventing and curing genetic disease by gene therapy was explained. The perplexing problems surrounding germ-line therapy, that is, efforts to modify germ cells that carry DNA from one generation to another, were discussed, and the technical and ethical problems associated with this technique were judged to be "strong contraindications against [this] becoming a useful clinical option in the near future."[79]

The draft concluded with recommendations for continued oversight of developments in genetics, suggesting that the existing NIH panel called the Recombinant DNA Advisory Committee (RAC) be revised to enhance its capability to discuss the issues we had defined. This was eventually done and a bioethicist, Dr. LeRoy Walters, became its chairperson. *Splicing Life: The Social and Ethical Issues of Genetic Engineering with Human Beings* was presented to President Carter on November 16, 1982.[80] I consider *Splicing Life* the most eloquent product of both Commissions on which I served. The Commission's executive director, Alexander Capron, also held *Splicing Life* in high esteem. He wrote, "The Commission's Report quieted a great deal of the concern that had been raised about the issues of human gene therapy. . . . By carefully dissecting the complaint that gene therapy amounted to 'playing god,' the report was able to differentiate important concerns about means and consequences from rhetorical claims and the line it drew between somatic cell and germ-line therapies has shaped subsequent discussions and policy formulation."[81]

Mapping the Human Genome

The science of molecular genetics had unfolded so rapidly after the structure of DNA was elucidated that the idea of identifying the exact location of genes on chromosomes and specifying their chemical makeup—or "mapping and sequencing the human genome"—quickly leapt to the scientific mind. This idea was soon transformed into a research reality. In May 1985, Chancellor Robert Sinsheimer of the University of California, Santa Cruz, a distinguished biologist, invited an elite group of molecular biologists and geneticists to his campus to discuss the possibility of completely sequencing the genome. He hoped to establish an institute for that purpose at U.C. Santa Cruz. Sinsheimer recalled, "The achievement would be a landmark in human history and the knowledge would be the basis for all human biology and medicine of the future. Why not now?"[82] Nobel laureate Renato Delbecco also broached the idea in the March 7, 1986 issue of *Science,* suggesting that the "war on cancer" would be speeded immeasurably by the knowledge gained by sequencing the human genome.[83] On July 23, 1986, the Howard Hughes Institute presented a symposium on the NIH campus. Many leaders in genetic science were present. The purpose of the symposium was to debate the pros and cons of initiating a massive cooperative scientific project of mapping and sequencing the human genome. This meeting inserted a fresh idea directly into the National Institutes of Health, the center of scientific research. For several days, scientists debated the scientific and policy questions. It was decided that a two-step strategy would be pursued—the first step concentrating on genetic linkage mapping, physical mapping, and technologies for sequencing DNA; the second step undertaking the sequencing of part, or perhaps all, of the human genome.[84]

As scientific interest in mapping the human genome was growing, the National Research Council had assembled a committee of biological scientists "to examine the desirability and feasibility of mapping and sequencing the human genome and to suggest options for implementing the project, if it were deemed feasible."[85] The chairman of the committee, Dr. Bruce Alberts, who was a faculty colleague at UCSF, asked me to advise the group on the ethical and social implications of the project. I confessed that my knowledge of genetics and molecular biology was thin but that the UCSF Division of Medical Ethics had another faculty person, Dr. Eric T. Juengst, who was adept in those subjects. Together we drafted the final chapter of the committee's report, "Implications for Society."

Juengst and I admitted that the exciting scientific project of creating a complete biological book on humankind would raise profound philosophical and ethical questions but that "the ethical and social challenges presented by the human genome mapping and sequencing project are largely the same as those already addressed by scientists, clinicians, patients and policymakers in other settings." We noted that there was already a large literature and lively public discussion of the relevant questions, which included confidentiality, the ambiguity surrounding genetic normalcy and genetic risk, and the potential for social, employment, and insurance discrimination. We also referenced the two reports from the President's Commission, *Splicing Life* (1982) and *Screening and Counseling for Genetic Conditions* (1983). This sample of literature reflected the ethical issues that had troubled workers in genetics during its century of life and anticipated the issues that would attend the field in the next century.[86]

Dr. James Watson was designated to lead the genome mapping project. He could hardly have imagined that thirty-five years after the publication of his novel paper on the double helix, he would testify before a congressional committee that a portion of the funding for human genome research be devoted to the ethical, legal, and social implications of mapping the human genome.[87] He realized that Congress and the public saw the scientific project that he was advocating not only as a major research effort in biology but also as an ethical minefield. He knew that the word "genetics" stirred up a multitude of moral issues. He was prudent enough to see that by adding an ethics component to the scientific study, he would assuage some of those concerns. All this bubbled up, in Watsonian fashion, when, at a press conference, he spontaneously announced that he intended to set aside three to five percent of the genome project budget for research into the ethical, social, and legal implications of the scientific project. He bluntly told a doubting colleague that unless ethics was part of the genome program, "Congress will chop your head off."[88]

Robert Cook-Deegan, chronicler of the political origins of the human genome project, summarizes the concerns of Congress and the public:

> The project would unleash a flood of new information about human genetics. In an unjust society, genetic information could be harmful. In a world full of computers, intimate information could fly out of control, with only weak, incomplete, and outdated protections for confidentiality. Once debate about the genome project joined with concern about genetic testing, public reactions to the project were principally channeled through discussions of how increased genetic information would change individual choices.[89]

The project initiators were correct in their anticipation of congressional scrutiny. The House Appropriations Committee required the NIH to prepare a systematic plan to address the ethical issues and to develop public policy to deal with them, and the Ethical, Legal, Social Implications Program (ELSI) was the result. The human genome project came into existence officially on October 1, 1989, with Dr. James Watson as director and my former colleague, Dr. Eric Jeungst, in charge of ELSI. Jeungst, a graduate of Georgetown University's Ph.D. program in bioethics, was the first bioethicist to hold a major government post. ELSI developed an internal process for consideration of ethical issues, relying on a working group chaired by Professor Nancy Wexler, and an external program to fund academic research relevant to the ethical issues and the policy responses to them. The Department of Energy, which had long been involved in the genetic aspects of radiation research, mounted a parallel genome mapping project, with an ELSI component.

Conclusion

Bioethics came into being as the eugenics debates were waning and as the debates over the new molecular genetics and its personal and social implications were beginning. From concerns about cloning to worries over screening and fears about genetic engineering, the most fundamental questions of human morality have been raised and the old eugenics haunts the new genetics in more scientific guises. In the era of bioethics, those debates have been, as Robert Morison said, "posed with more precision . . . abstract questions about right and wrong [have been reduced] to a series of rather clearly defined situations in which decisions must be reached in relatively concrete terms."[90] The result of these debates has been the adoption of policies and programs in genetic research and genetic medicine that aim at the cure of disease, respect the autonomy of individuals, and repudiate utilitarian and eugenic perspectives. At the same time, new questions appear with each new technical innovation. It is a pity to walk away from these fascinating bioethical debates, but they occurred during the years beyond the bounds of this history and belong to the future of bioethics.

Notes for Chapter 6

1. Michel de Montaigne, "Of the resemblance of children to their fathers," (1579) in *The Complete Essays of Montaigne*, trans. Donald Frame (Stanford: Stanford University Press, 1957), p. 579.

2. Robert C. Olby, *The Origins of Mendelism* (New York: Shocken Books, 1966).

3. James Watson and Francis Crick, "The molecular structure of nucleic acids," *Nature* 4356 (1953): 737; see also James D. Watson, *The Double Helix: A Personal Account of the Discovery of the Structure of DNA* (New York: Atheneum, 1968).

4. "Clue to chemistry of heredity found," *New York Times* June 13, 1953: A17.

5. "Pope says Church raises no bars against quest for scientific truth," *New York Times*, September 9, 1953: A18; "Allocution to First International Conference of Medical Genetics," *Acta Apostolicae Sedis* 45 (1953): 596–611, p. 605.

6. Charles Darwin, *Descent of Man and Selection in Relation to Sex*, 2nd ed. (New York: Appleton, 1922), p. 136, quoted in Mark Haller, *Eugenics: Hereditarian Attitudes in American Thought* (New Brunswick: Rutgers University Press, 1963), p. 4. Several other excellent studies review the history of eugenics: Kenneth M. Ludmerer, *Genetics and American Society: A Historical Appraisal* (Baltimore: Johns Hopkins University Press, 1972); Daniel J. Kevles, *In the Name of Eugenics: Genetics and the Uses of Human Heredity* (New York: Knopf, 1985).

7. Plato, *The Republic*, V, 459–462.

8. Francis Galton, *Hereditary Genius: An Inquiry into Its Laws and Consequences*, 2nd ed. (London: Macmillan, 1922), p. 35.

9. Francis Galton, *Inquiries into Human Faculty* (New York: Dutton and Co., 1883), 2nd ed. n.d., footnote p. 7.

10. Mark Haller, *Eugenics*, pp. 56–57.

11. See Richard Hofstadter, *Social Darwinism in American Thought* (New York: George Braziller, 1953), pp. 31–66.

12. Olby, *The Origins of Mendelism*, chapter 6.

13. American Breeders Association, *Proceedings* 11 (1906); quoted in Haller, *Eugenics*, p. 62.

14. Charles B. Davenport, *Heredity in Relation to Eugenics* (New York: Holt, 1911), pp. 221–222, quoted in Kevles, *In the Name of Eugenics*, p. 47.

15. Kevles, *In the Name of Eugenics*, p. 72.

16. A. J. Ochsner, "Surgical treatment of habitual criminals," *Journal of the American Medical Association* 53 (1899): 867–868.

17. Philip R. Reilly, *The Surgical Solution: A History of Involuntary Sterilization in the United States* (Baltimore: Johns Hopkins Press, 1991).

18. Harry Hamilton Laughlin, *Eugenical Sterilization in the United States* (Chicago: Psychopathic Laboratory of the Municipal Court of Chicago, 1922), p. 446, cited in Haller, *Eugenics*, p. 133.

19. California law cited in Reilly, *The Surgical Solution*, p. 48.

20. E. S. Gosney and Paul Popenoe, *Sterilization for Human Betterment: A Summary of Results of 6,000 Operations in California* (New York: The Macmillan Company, 1929); Kevles, *In the Name of Eugenics*, p. 118; Robert N. Proctor, *Racial Hygiene: Medicine Under the Nazis* (Cambridge: Harvard University Press, 1988), pp. 173–175; Reilly, *The Surgical Solution*, p. 106.

21. Adolph Hitler, *Mein Kampf*, quoted in Reilly, *The Surgical Solution*, p. 106.

22. Reilly, *The Surgical Solution*, p. 68.

23. *Buck v Bell*, 274 US 201 (1927); J. David Smith and K. Ray Nelson, *The Sterilization of Carrie Buck* (Far Hills, N.J.: New Horizon Press, 1989).

24. Reilly, *The Surgical Solution*, p. 68.

25. Prescott Hall, *Reports of the Immigration Commission*, vol. 41, (Washington, D.C.: United States Government Printing Office, 1911), p. 106, quoted in Haller, *Eugenics*, p. 147.

26. Madison Grant, *The Passing of the Great Race; or The Racial Basis of European History* (New York: C. Scribner's Sons, 1911), published in German in 1925 (Der Untergang der grossen Rasse); Lothrup Stoddard, *The Rising Tide of Color Against White Supremacy* (Westport, Conn.: Negro University Press, 1920).

27. Haller, *Eugenics*, p. 157.

28. *Loving v Commonwealth of Virginia*, 87 S. Ct. 1817, 388 U.S. 1, 18 L. Ed. 2d 1010 (U.S. Va. 1967).

29. Edward Alsworth Ross, *The Old World in the New* (New York: The Century Co., 1914), cited in Haller, *Eugenics*, p. 147.

30. John Ryan, *Family Limitation and the Church and Birth Control* (New York: Paulist Press, 1916); Thomas Gerrard, *The Church and Eugenics* (New York: Herder, 1912).

31. E. J. Maloney, "The morality of sterilization," *Thought* (September 1928), reprinted in J. F. Leibell, *Readings in Ethics* (Chicago: Loyola University Press, 1926), pp. 1077–1093, quote on p. 1087.

32. G. K. Chesterton, *Eugenics and Other Evils* (London: Cassel, 1922), p. 151.

33. *Casti Connubii* in *Five Great Encyclicals* (New York: Paulist Press, 1939), pp. 96–97.

34. Allocution, Oct. 29, 1951, *Acta Apostolicae Sedis* (1951): 835–860, in particular, p. 844.

35. Kevles, *In the Name of Eugenics*, p. 251.

36. Kevles, *In the Name of Eugenics*, p. 173.

37. Hermann J. Muller, *Out of the Night. A Biologist's View of the Future* (New York: The Vanguard Press, 1935), pp. ix, 103. This book was Dr. Muller's first published treatment of the biological future of the human race, based on lectures delivered at Columbia University in 1910. He urges the separation of reproduction from personal love and suggests that, once this is done, artificial insemination would make it possible for "a vast number of children of the future generation [to] inherit the characteristics of some transcendently estimable man, without either of the parents ever having come in contact . . ." (p. 111).

38. Hermann J. Muller, "The guidance of human evolution," *Perspectives in Biology and Medicine* 3, no. 1 (1959): 1–43, pp. 19, 29; see also Muller, "Should we weaken or strengthen our genetic heritage?" in Hudson Hoagland and Ralph Burhoe (eds.), *Evolution and Man's Progress* (New York: Columbia, University Press, 1962); "Our load of mutations," *American Journal of Human Genetics* 2 (1950): 111–176; "Means and aims in human genetic betterment," in T. M. Sonneborn (ed.), *The Control of Human Heredity and Evolution* (New York: Macmillan, 1965), pp. 100–122.

39. Joshua Lederberg "The biological future of men," in G. E. W. Wolstenholme (ed.), *Man and His Future* (Boston: Little, Brown, and Co., 1963), p. 270.

40. Jacob Bronowski "Discussion: Eugenics and genetics," in Wolstenholme, *Man and His Future*, p. 286.

41. Private correspondence between Ramsey and Muller, in the possession of Dr. LeRoy Walters.

42. Paul Ramsey, *Fabricated Man: The Ethics of Genetic Control* (New Haven: Yale University Press, 1970), p. 7.

43. Paul Ramsey "Moral and religious implications of genetic control," in John D. Roslansky (ed.), *Genetics and the Future of Man* (Amsterdam: North-Holland Publishing Co., 1966) p. 139.

44. Ramsey, *Fabricated Man*, p. 31.

45. Ramsey in Roslansky, *Genetics and the Future of Man*, p. 168.

46. Ramsey, *Fabricated Man*, p. 58; Hermann J. Muller (ed.), *Man's Future Birthright: Es-*

says on Science and Humanity (Concord, NH: University of New Hampshire Press, 1958), p. 18.

47. Joseph F. Fletcher, *Morals and Medicine* (Princeton: Princeton University Press, 1954), p. 168.

48. Joseph F. Fletcher, "Ethical aspects of genetic controls," *New England Journal of Medicine* 285 (1971): 776–783; see also *Humanhood: Essays in Biomedical Ethics* (Buffalo: Prometheus Books, 1979), chapter 7, p. 88.

49. Joseph F. Fletcher, *The Ethics of Genetic Control: Ending Reproductive Roulette* (Garden City, N.Y.: Anchor Press, 1974).

50. Fletcher, *Ethics of Genetic Control*, p. 52.

51. Fletcher, *Ethics of Genetic Control*, p. 201.

52. Although this remark is widely attributed to Dr. Koop, I can find no confirming citation.

53. Maureen Harris (ed.), *Early Diagnosis of Human Genetic Defects: Scientific and Ethical Considerations, Fogerty International Center Proceedings No. 6* (Bethesda: NIH Publication, 1971), quotes on p. 228 and p. 10.

54. Tracy Sonneborn, "Ethical issues arising from the possible uses of genetic knowledge," in Bruce Hilton, Daniel Callahan, Maureen Harris, Peter Condliffe, and Burton Berkley (eds.), *Ethical Issues in Human Genetics* (New York and London: Plenum Press, 1973), p. 2.

55. Paul Ramsey, "Screening: an ethicist's view," in Hilton et al., *Ethical Issues in Human Genetics*, p. 151.

56. Daniel Callahan, "The meaning and significance of genetic disease: philosophical perspectives," in Hilton et al., *Ethical Issues in Human Genetics*, p. 89.

57. Hilton et al., *Ethical Issues in Human Genetics*.

58. Paul Ramsey, "Genetic therapy: a theologian's view," in Michael P. Hamilton (ed.), *The New Genetics and the Future of Man* (Grand Rapids, Mich.: Wm. B. Eerdman Publishing Company, 1972), p. 172. Both Canon Hamilton's conference and the Fogerty conference were held at Airlie House, Virginia; I distinguish them by calling the former the Airlie conference and the latter the Fogerty conference.

59. Arno Motulsky, "Brave new world?" *Science* 185 (1974): 653–663, quote on p. 663; see also "Impact of genetic manipulation on society and medicine," *Science* 219 (1983): 135–140.

60. John Fletcher, "From cloning to genome: genetic screening," (paper read at the Birth of Bioethics Conference, Seattle, Wa., Sept. 23–24, 1992) transcript, pp. 276–285.

61. Research Group on Ethical, Social and Legal Issues in Genetic Counseling and Genetic Engineering of the Institute of Society, Ethics and the Life Sciences, "Ethical and social issues in screening for genetic disease," *New England Journal of Medicine* 286 (1972): 1129–1132.

62. Marc Lappé, "From cloning to genome: human genome," (paper read at the Birth of Bioethics Conference, Seattle, Wa., Sept. 23–24, 1992) transcript, pp. 286–289.

63. Robert Murray, "Screening: a practitioner's view"; Michael M. Kaback, "The John F. Kennedy Institute Tay-Sachs Program: practical and ethical issues in an adult genetic screening program," in Hilton et al., *Ethical Issues in Human Genetics*, pp. 121–130, 131–146.

64. Philip Reilly, *Genetics, Law and Social Policy* (Cambridge: Harvard University Press, 1977), chapter 3; Tabitha Powledge, "Laws in question: confusion over sickle-cell testing," *Hastings Center Report* 3, no. 1 (1972): 3–4.

65. Tabitha Powledge and John Fletcher, "Guidelines for the ethical, social and legal issues in prenatal diagnosis," *New England Journal of Medicine* 300 (1979): 168–172; *Hastings Center Report* published some twenty articles on genetic testing during the decade 1971–1980.

66. *Antenatal Diagnosis. Report of a Consensus Development Conference, National Institute of Child Health and Human Development*, March 5–7, 1979, NIH Publ. No. 80-1973. Dr. Kaback was chairman of this consensus panel and I was a member.

67. President's Commission for the Study of Ethical Problems in Medicine and Biomedical

and Behavioral Research, *Screening and Counseling for Genetic Conditions* (Washington, D.C.: United States Government Printing Office, 1983), pp. 5–7.

68. Horace Freeland Judson, *The Eighth Day of Creation: Makers of the Revolution in Biology* (New York: Simon and Schuster, 1979); Robert Olby, *The Path to the Double Helix* (Seattle: University of Washington Press, 1974).

69. Donald S. Fredrickson, "Asilomar and recombinant DNA," in Kathi E. Hanna (ed.), *Biomedical Politics* (Washington, D.C.: National Academy Press, 1991), pp. 258–298.

70. Maxine Singer and Dieter Soll, "Letter: guidelines for hybrid DNA molecules," *Science*, 181 (1973): 1114.

71. Fredrickson, "Asilomar and recombinant DNA," p. 281.

72. John Kifner, "'Creation of life' experiment at Harvard stirs heated dispute," *New York Times*, June 17, 1976: A-22; Nicholas Wade, *The Ultimate Experiment* (New York: Walker, 1977). My own institution, University of California at San Francisco, was prevented from occupying a building because of similar neighborhood concerns.

73. Reprinted in President's Commission for the Study of Ethical Problems in Medicine and Biomedical and Behavioral Research, *Splicing Life: The Social and Ethical Issues of Genetic Engineering with Human Beings* (Washington, D.C.: United States Government Printing Office, 1982), Appendix B, p. 96.

74. Rollin D. Hotchkiss, "Portents for a genetic engineering," *Journal of Heredity* 56 (1965): 197–202.

75. French Anderson, "Gene therapy" in Michael Hamilton (ed.), *The New Genetics and the Future of Man* (Grand Rapids, Mich.: Wm. B. Eerdmans, 1972), p. 118. In 1969, Dr. Stanfield Rogers administered inserted Shope virus, which has a gene that produces arginase, into two German girls affected with hyperargininemia; the experiment was unsuccessful and much criticized. See Theodore Friedmann and Richard Roblin, "Gene therapy for human genetic disease?" *Science* (1975) 175: 949–955.

76. President's Commission, *Splicing Life*, pp. 53–54.

77. President's Commission, *Splicing Life*, p. 56; *Osservatore Romano*, Oct. 24, 1982: 2.

78. Arno Motulsky, "How medicine and theology learned to converse," (paper read at the Birth of Bioethics Conference, Seattle, Wa., Sept. 23–24, 1992), transcript pp. 331–335.

79. *Splicing Life*, p. 48; Eric T. Juengst, "Germ-line gene therapy: back to basics," *Journal of Medicine and Philosophy* 16 (1991): 587–592; Gregory Fowler, Eric Juengst, and Burke Zimmerman, "Germ-line gene therapy and the clinical ethos of medical genetics," *Theoretical Medicine* 10 (1989): 151–165.

80. President's Commission, *Splicing Life*; President's Commission's 11th meeting, July 9–10, 1981, President's Commission Archive, Box 25.

81. Alexander Morgan Capron, "The impact of the report, *Splicing Life*," *Human Gene Therapy*, 1 (1990): 69–71.

82. Robert Sinsheimer, "The Santa Cruz Workshop," *Genomics*, 5 (1989): 954–996, quoted in Robert Cook-Deegan, *The Gene Wars: Science, Politics and the Human Genome* (New York: W. W. Norton, 1994), p. 82.

83. Renato Delbecco, "A turning point in cancer research: sequencing the human genome," *Science* 231 (1986): 1055–1056.

84. Cook-Deegan, *The Gene Wars*, p. 122.

85. National Research Council Committee on Mapping and Sequencing the Human Genome, *Mapping and Sequencing the Human Genome* (Washington, D.C.: National Academy Press, 1988), p. vii.

86. Albert Jonsen and Eric Juengst, "Implications for society," in National Research Council, *Mapping and Sequencing the Human Genome*, pp. 100, 103. Examples of the literature are: Joan

Ablon, "Stigmatized health conditions," *Social Science and Medicine* 15 (1981): 5–9; Alexander M. Capron (ed.), *Genetic Counseling: Facts, Values and Norms* (Birth Defects: Original Article Series, vol. 15) (New York: Alan R. Liss, 1979); Eric Juengst, "Prenatal diagnosis and the ethics of uncertainty," in John F. Monagle and David C. Thomasma (eds.), *Medical Ethics: A Guide for Health Professionals* (Rockville: Aspen Press, 1988); Marc Lappé, *Genetic Politics: The Limits of Biological Control* (New York: Simon and Schuster, 1979); Ruth Macklin, "Mapping the human genome: problems of privacy and free choice," in Aubrey Milunsky and George Annas (eds.), *Genetics and the Law III* (National Symposium on Genetics and the Law) (New York: Plenum Press, 1985); and Thomas H. Murray, "Genetic screening in the workplace," *Journal of Occupational Medicine* 25 (1983): 451–454.

87. See Eric Juengst, "Self-critical federal science? The ethics experiment with the United States Human Genome Project," *Social Philosophy and Policy* 13, no. 2 (1996): 63–95, story on p. 63.

88. Cited in Cook-Deegan, *The Gene Wars*, p. 262.

89. Cook-Deegan, *The Gene Wars*, p. 263. For a comprehensive view of the ethical questions, largely from the scientists' view, see Leroy Hood and Daniel Kevles (eds.), *The Code of Codes: Scientific and Social Issues in the Human Genome Project* (Cambridge, Mass.: Harvard University Press, 1992).

90. Harris, *Fogerty International Center Proceedings No. 6*, p. 10.

7

The Miracle of Modern Medicine: The Ethics of Organ Transplantation and Artificial Organs

Medieval Catholic doctors practiced under the heavenly patronage of Saints Cosmos and Damien. According to legend, the two saints were brothers who practiced medicine in fourth-century Syria. Their reputation for skill was enhanced by their generosity in caring for the poor. One day, a certain Vincent, deacon of the local church, came to their clinic. An arrowhead was embedded in his leg, which was rotting away. The holy doctors took one look at the gangrenous limb and told the deacon that their treatments would be futile. He should, they advised, take himself to church and pray for a good death. Vincent followed their advice. While at prayer, he fell asleep (as often happens). Meanwhile, the holy doctors were visited by an angel who told them to go to the church, amputate the leg of a corpse laid out for burial, amputate the sleeping Vincent's leg, and attach the dead limb to the living man. Vincent awoke with a sound leg, and patient and doctors praised the Lord.

If Vincent walked away from his ecclesiastical surgery on two good legs, it was a real "miracle" of transplantation. A miracle, according to theologians, is an event contrary to nature, manifesting the power and benignity of God. Certainly, Vincent and his attending physicians experienced an event "contrary to nature." Who could even imagine that a corpse's leg could be stitched onto a living man and come alive? We now know how contrary to nature such an event is: the cellular capacity for physiological function had been lost, and even had it not been lost, immunological barriers would have repelled the union. And, just to confirm the miraculous nature of this event, no surgeon until Amboise Paré, in the sixteenth century, could sew blood vessels together.

Despite many efforts to replicate that miracle in one form or another, secular physicians and surgeons never succeeded. During the 1920s and 1930s, interest in transplantation revived. The great surgeon Alexis Carrel perfected microsurgical techniques that furthered the possibility of suturing organs into a new place and, collaborating with aviator Charles Lindbergh, created a "mechanical heart" that would perfuse organs out-side the body.[1] Russian surgeons fascinated the world by switching heads of dogs and watching them pant, and eat for a few hours. Scientific study of the physiological basis for tissue rejection intensified. Blood transfusion, repeatedly attempted during the nine-teenth century, became feasible with the discovery of the four "blood groups" in 1900. The often fatal transfusion reaction, in which red blood cells of the recipient are de-stroyed when mixed with a donor's blood, could usually be avoided by transfusing blood only from a group identical with that of the recipient. Skin grafting and corneal transplantation advanced with increasing but limited success; Some impassable barrier still stood between the tissue of one individual and that of another.

That barrier seemed much lower when the donor and recipient were related. The blood-group discovery suggested this hypothesis; it was confirmed in the 1930s by suc-cessful skin grafting between identical twins.[2] Sir Peter Medawar and his colleagues clarified the genetic nature of the immunological barrier when, during World War II, they sought to repair the wounds of burned soldiers. The way for organ transplantation was opening.[3]

Kidney Transplantation

In the early 1950s, a surgical group at Boston's Peter Bent Brigham Hospital began a series of experimental kidney transplants from cadavers into patients close to death from renal disease. All efforts failed (with one exceptional survival of 175 days). On December 23, 1954, Drs. Joseph Murray and John Merrill took what one commentator called "a major ethical leap."[4] They excised a healthy kidney from 24-year-old Ronald Herrick and sutured it into his twin brother Richard. The recipient not only survived the critical days after the surgery while rejection threatened, but lived eight more years, eventually dying of coronary artery disease and glomerulonephritis.[5] Murray's bold surgery inaugurated the era of major organ transplantation. His experiment succeeded because of the genetic similarity between the two twins. He performed seven more transplants on monozygotic twins before attempting a transplant between dyzygotic twins, and in 1960, he was the first to use the drug azathioprine to suppress immune re-sponse, opening the possibility of transplantation from cadavers and from donors with less than identical genetic matches.[6] During the decade 1954–1964, more than 600 re-nal transplants between living persons were performed in the United States, Great Britain, and France, with two-year survival rates hovering around fifty percent. These pioneering days of renal transplantation transformed the divine miracle of Cosmos and Damien into a human, clinical miracle—at first with halting success, then with increas-ing efficacy in prolongating life and restorating health. Renal transplantation was hailed a miracle of modern medicine.[7]

The miracle was not an unalloyed grace. Many of the identical twins who sought transplantation at the Peter Bent Brigham Hospital were minors, who are not considered capable of consent to medical procedures, particularly if the procedure offers them no personal benefit. Officials at the Brigham thought it prudent to seek judicial review of three cases. In all three cases, judges allowed the surgery under four conditions: parental consent, necessity to save the sick twin's life, informed and free consent of the donor and, most unusual of all, psychiatric evidence that the healthy twin's future welfare was promoted by the donation.[8] This last condition was the central issue in the most famous of such cases, heard in Kentucky in 1969. The problem of consent was compounded by the fact that the potential donor, Jerry Strunk, although not a minor in age, was a resident of a state mental hospital. The Kentucky court was forced to ignore the Massachusetts requirement for consent of the donor and to concentrate exclusively on the potential well-being of the donor. The court approved taking Jerry's kidney only through the tortuous reasoning that the retarded child would himself be benefited by the continued life of his brother, to whom he was devoted. In so reasoning, the court upheld, though shakily, the principle that a person should not be put at risk unknowingly and unwillingly unless a benefit would accrue to that same person.[9]

These rulings were not mere legal niceties; they ran up against a very old imperative of medical ethics. The Hippocratic maxim "do no harm" had been understood to mean that any harm that might be done should contribute to the patient's benefit. Excision of a healthy organ from a healthy donor was, under this interpretation, an impermissible harm. This medical maxim was taken for granted by jurisprudence, which would judge as a battery any intervention not intended to benefit the patient. Even the consent of the "battered" did not justify the intervention. The unprecedented medical and scientific breakthrough posed a challenge to medical ethics and jurisprudence.

The moral dimensions of the miracle were quickly recognized. In 1964, the editor of *Annals of Internal Medicine,* Dr. Russell Elkington, wrote a provocative article, pointing out the "social and moral problems inherent in . . . advances that hold great hope for many patients with organs diseased beyond any chance of healing and repair." Among these problems were the failure of the procedures to live up to expectations, the necessity of choosing among patients, and the great social investment required to "prolong for an uncertain period the lives of a relatively few people." He described these issues and deplored the absence of serious discussion. Elkington's editorial stimulated the discussion he had hoped for. An avalanche of letters descended on the *Annals,* many from the leaders of the new medicine—among them, Peter Medawar, Joseph Murray, Thomas Starzl, Belding Scribner, and Willem Kolff. All correspondents agreed with Elkington's concerns; most of them confessed that they had, as Dr. Murray said, given "a great deal of soul searching to these problems." Dr. Starzl, acknowledging the many problems, was confident that advances in the field of transplantation had been made "in a sturdy framework that is ethical, practical and efficiently policed." He announced that his own book on renal transplantation included a chapter by Dr. Chauncey Leake on the moral and ethical considerations.[10] One writer, internist Dr. William Bennett, suggested "a study of these problems by scholarly specialists of high renown from the fields of philosophy, religion, biology and the social sciences. Few physicians are sufficiently grounded in these disciplines to bring to bear the wisdom of the ages on such questions."[11]

The leading British transplanter, Sir Michael Woodruff, wrote a brief note, saying that he had thought deeply about the moral issues of transplantation. Two years later, he carried his thought into action. In 1966, he persuaded the Ciba Foundation to convene a meeting of "medical men, lawyers and others concerned in the ethical and legal problems of organ transplantation." In the preface to the published proceeding, *Law and Ethics of Transplantation,* Ciba's director, Dr. G. E. W. Wolstenholme, listed the problems associated with the topic and wondered how they could be covered in three brief days:

> In what circumstances could a volunteer donor be considered free from undue influence? for how long should life be maintained in a person with irrevocable damage of the brain? does a parent always have the right to accept or refuse treatment of his child? what special protection must be given to minors, people of low intelligence, or prisoners in regard to clinical trials or donation of tissues? when does death occur in an unconscious patient dependent on artificial aids to circulation and respiration? are there ever circumstances when death may be mercifully advanced? when may pregnancy be ended? how far is it justified to destroy an animal in order to prolong human life? does the law permit operations which mutilate the donor for the advantage of another person? what protections do medical men require from society in the extension of new life-saving techniques? to what extent must a community underwrite the cost, however great, of the latest means of sustaining life?[12]

A pantheon of renal surgeons and nephrologists—Joseph Murray, Roy Calne, Keith Reemtsma, Thomas Starzl, Michael Woodruff, George Schreiner, Hugh deWardener, Jean Hamburger and others—discussed these issues with a bench of scholarly lawyers, including David Daube, David Louisell, and Lord Kilbrandon. One clergyman represented ethics; patients and public were absent.[13] The participants acknowledged the many ethical and legal problems that rendered ambiguous this "miracle of modern medicine" (they were particularly concerned about donor death and donor coercion), but the earnest discussions made little progress in resolving the ambiguity.

The novel clinical situations created by transplantation also directly challenged the authority of the physician as sole determiner of the course of treatment. Clearly, the recipient of a kidney, heart, or lung from another human must be a fully informed participant. Yet, the precise roles of the patient and the physician in making decisions were still vague. In the early days of transplantation, one of the pioneers, Harvard's Dr. Francis Moore, stated, "It is not enough to tell the patient that 'there is no other hope'. . . . He should be given a clear picture of the hazards involved and allowed to join in the discussion. . . . Yet under no circumstances should the final decision be left in the hands of the patient; he has not the education, the background nor dispassionate view necessary to make the decision in his own best self-interest."[14] Dr. Moore asserts a paternalism that will soon come under severe attack.

An early episode in my career as a professor of bioethics illustrated this conflict between paternalism and autonomy. Several months after I joined the faculty of the UCSF

School of Medicine, a popular member of our faculty, cardiologist Chad Calland, committed suicide after undergoing five kidney transplants. In the same week that Dr. Calland died, his article "Iatrogenic problems in end-stage renal failure" appeared in *The New England Journal of Medicine*.[15] In his dying words, he complained that his physicians and surgeons failed to comprehend his feelings about life on dialysis and after transplantation. He felt he was the object of competition between his nephrologists and his surgeons: "As physician-partaker, I am distressed by the controversial dialogue that separates the nephrologist from the transplant surgeon so that, in the end, it is the patient who is given short shrift." Those nephrologists and surgeons were his dear friends, and his article aroused anguish and moral searching.

A conference to discuss the Calland case was held on April 10, 1974, two years after his death, at which the distress was still palpable. I was invited to present the moral issues in the case. I suggested that "there may be an inverse relation between scientific, technological medicine and freedom of therapeutic choice. If so, this would be the most crucial ethical problem of modern medicine." I meant that physician and patient may interpret success in very different ways: the physician sees success in maintenance of physiological state, the patient views success as the restoration of his or her previous quality of life. Freedom of therapeutic choice is compromised by a common failure, by physician and patient, to deal with scientific medicine's most adverse side effect, "iatrogenic chronic disease." I proposed that "modern medicine . . . should learn to comprehend more fully and manage more expediently the sociological and psychological environments within which it advances."[16]

Heart Transplantation

The moral dilemmas over renal transplantation came into sharp focus on December 3, 1967. On that day, at the Groote Schuur Hospital in Cape Town, South Africa, Dr. Christiaan Barnard took a still-beating heart from the chest of 22-year-old Denise Daarvall, who had been seriously injured in an automobile accident the day before, and sewed her heart into the chest of 55-year-old Louis Washkansky, whose own heart had nearly ceased to function. Washkansky lived for 18 days. The drama of heart transplantation had begun.

Media coverage of the event was incessant. *Time* dubbed it "the ultimate operation."[17] Surgeons around the world, some of whom were on the verge of leaping this therapeutic chasm, watched with some jealousy. They realized, more than did the general public, that the mechanical aspects of transplanting the heart were relatively simple, but they were also vividly conscious of the immunological barriers to success. Barnard did not report that Washkansky's death was due to immunological rejection of the transplanted heart but to respiratory failure due to bilateral pneumonia.

The South African surgeon was not discouraged by Washkansky's death. Only a few weeks later, he put a heart into Dentist Philip Blaiberg.[18] This time, the watching world was not disappointed: Blaiberg lived 594 days, during which time he was photographed sporting on the Cape Town beach. In the following year, other eager surgeons rushed to the operating theater and performed over 100 transplants. The worldwide results were not encouraging. By August 1969, only 37 of 142 patients transplanted during the previous 20 months were alive; in June 1970, 10 survivors were counted among 160 procedures. These discouraging results stimulated a crisis of conscience among transplanters. Although eager to pursue this exciting innovation, they hesitated to subject patients to its rigors while its promise was so uncertain.

Barnard's operations ushered in what *Time* hailed as "The Year of the Transplant." Yet, three years later, *Life*'s cover pictured eight men who had lived with transplanted hearts and were by then dead. The magazine announced the "heart transplant tragedy." On November 9, 1971, surgeon John Najarian argued before a U.S. Senate hearing that, in reality, "success had been achieved, even though the article in *Life* would make it difficult for anyone to do heart transplants in the present setting of public misinformation." Over the previous three years, he said, 176 transplants had been done, of whom 28 were still alive.[19] Clearly, the "Miracle of Capetown" had precipitated a storm of controversy both within and without the medical profession.

Within the profession, many surgeons believed that the science of immunology was not yet ready to guide transplantation. Although Medawar's studies had advanced immunology, one crucial technique, the typing of white blood cells, had only been suggested by French geneticist Jean Dausset in the same year as Barnard's daring operation. The critics maintained that the success of transplantation would require more exact tissue typing and more powerful anti-rejection drugs (cyclosporin was not introduced into clinical use until 1978). Other surgeons insisted that even if tissue matching was not perfected and rejection remained a major threat, the remote chance of life could not be denied to patients. The critics were victorious; initial enthusiasm subsided. Quietly and unofficially, a moratorium descended on heart transplants. The most enthusiastic transplant centers slowed down or ceased operations; the more conservative institutions decided not to initiate them. A few centers, such as the one supervised by Dr. Norman Shumway at Stanford University Hospital, continued on a careful experimental basis. The miracle was returned to the laboratory for further study. Not until the mid-1970s were surgeons confident enough to accept new patients.[20] No moratorium was called on the ethical and legal questions raised by transplantation, however, for the debates continued.

Transplantation: Mutilation or Donation?

One of the first moral quandaries quickly struck the consciences of the transplanters themselves. Dr. Murray's first transplant between identical twins was called a "major ethical leap." The leap was over the hurdle of the ancient medical maxim, "do no harm." Was it right to remove a healthy organ from a healthy person, even to save the life of another person? Dr. Murray himself noted, "As physicians motivated and educated to make sick people well, we make a basic qualitative shift in our aims when we risk the health of a well person, no matter how pure our motives." He hoped that the time would soon come when "even identical twins will not require a living donor."[21] Medical jurisprudence as well as medical ethics posed a barrier to excision of healthy organs. Lord Kilbrandon, chairing the Ciba Conference on transplantation, stated, "It is said that a person cannot consent . . . (in the law) to be maimed."[22] So it happened that the era of organ transplantation, certainly one of medicine's most innovative procedures, opened with an ethical and legal question left over from earlier medical ethics.

Do persons have the moral authority to mutilate their bodies—that is, to separate from themselves a part or organ that is a natural constitutive part? This moral question was raised long before organ transplantation was possible. Jewish religious law had from ancient times forbidden the mutilation of the human body, including mutilation of the cadaver, even for purposes of autopsy.[23] Catholic moralists also had prohibited any mutilation of a healthy body.[24] A necessary surgical amputation could be justified by "the principle of totality": only the health of the total body justifies the removal of a diseased part. Similarly, mutilation was justified if a person could save his life only by cutting off his hand (trapped, for example, under a fallen beam).[25]

The principle of totality was designed for amputation, the most common surgical operation of antiquity; organ transplantation was inconceivable to the moralists of that time. But in 1944, a moral theologian, Father Bert Cunningham, anticipated its possibility: he submitted a doctoral dissertation in theology to the Catholic University of America entitled "The Morality of Organic Transplantation."[26] He had only two actual examples: the rare attempts to transplant an ovary from one woman to another and the more common transplantation of a cornea from a seeing person to a blind one. He asked how this could be justified, since the principle of totality requires that the body and life of the one who is mutilated be restored to health by the mutilation. His answer is drawn from Catholic theology: all humans are integral parts of the Mystical Body of Christ (either actually as members of the Church or potentially as redeemed by Christ). Thus, "there exists an ordination of men to one another and as a consequence, an order of their members to one another. . . . Thus, we contend that men are ordinated to society as parts to the whole and, as such, are in some way ordinated to one another."[27] This spiritual order allows a person to mutilate himself for the good of his threatened neighbor. Only two restrictions are imposed: the donor must not be the certain or probable cause of his own death, and the mutilation must not constitute a sterilization.[28] Cunningham's thesis was not widely accepted by his Catholic colleagues. It seemed to reach too far beyond the traditional interpretation of the principle of totality. It was at odds with strongly worded ecclesiastical documents, such as the papal encyclical *Casti*

Connubii (1930), in which Pope Pius XI had written, "People are not free to destroy or mutilate their members . . . except when no other provision can be made for the good of the whole body."[29] Pope XII, speaking to the Symposium on Corneal Transplant, criticized Father Cunningham's teaching and reinforced the traditional principle of totality.[30]

The preeminent Catholic moralist, Father Gerald Kelly, added his voice to the critique of Father Cunningham's thesis; nevertheless, Kelly recognized that it was time for a "revision of the treatise" on mutilation. Although he was skeptical of extending the principle of totality to justify transplantation, he admitted that Catholic doctrine, as far back as Aquinas, had seen the sacrifice of one's life for the good of another as an act of charity. Much more so, he said, was the undertaking of a risk for a proportionate benefit to another.[31] As transplantation moved from the rare and speculative to the frequent and real, Catholic theology and Rabbinic law were pushed to reconsider old doctrine. Soon both faiths accepted that the removal of an organ for immediate and genuine benefit of another person should not be considered a reprehensible mutilation. Indeed, it is an act of virtue, and in the eyes of the rabbis, it is an observance of the law that gives highest priority to the saving of life.[32] This view reconceptualized transplantation from "mutilation" to "donation," a shift that melded with the growing public perception of the "gift of life" offered by one person to another. Father Cunningham's controversial thesis had prepared the way for a fresh analysis of mutilation.[33]

Paul Ramsey provided one of the earliest extensive moral analyses of the ethics of donation. In "The self-giving of vital organs," he worried about Father Kelly's "revision of the treatise" on mutilation, suggesting that as the revision opened the classic restriction on mutilation to the benefit of others, it became dangerously generous and could lead even to the donation of organs necessary for the donor's life. "Physicians," he wrote, (quoting Dr. Francis Moore) "are exceedingly sensitive to the fact that 'for the first time in the history of medicine a procedure is being adopted in which a perfectly healthy person is injured permanently in order to improve the well being of another.' This, at the very time theological moralists are busy entirely dissolving the protections of past teaching on self-mutilation. . . . Moralists should learn to follow the lineaments of the physicians' reasoning . . . while undertaking the unique medical procedure of impairing one patient to heal another." After all his worrying, however, Ramsey admitted a carefully circumscribed principle of reasonable self-sacrifice. He insisted that the advantage to the recipient had to be greater than the disadvantage to the donor. A strong respect for the bodily integrity and health of the donor was the only protection against the false belief that an organ belongs as much to the one as to the other, "interchangable parts between interchangeable personal embodiments."[34]

These religious views supported the widespread public view that the giving of an organ for another's life and health was a noble act. The law, however, needed to evolve as well. As Lord Kilbrandon had commented at the Ciba conference, "One cannot consent to be maimed." Two legal scholars at the conference took issue with Kilbrandon.

Professor David Daube, respected both in common law jurisprudence and Talmudic law, took a position not unlike the theological one. "I would advocate viewing the whole transaction (therapeutic transplantation), from the start with the living donor to the finish, which one hopes is some relief for the recipient, as one composite, curative transaction. . . . Undeniably, there is a very special problem in transplantation from the living, because of this terrible element that a healthy donor suffers injury. . . . This is a novel and unique feature; the role of the donor fits into no orthodox category, it needs working out and plainly very special safeguards are required." Daube suggested that more than consent is required. A medical judgment of relative risks to donor and recipient, a high degree of caution and concern for the donor, and the absence of alternatives "place on the transplanting surgeon a far greater responsibility."[35] The other legal scholar, David Louisell, was not troubled by the problem posed by Lord Kilbrandon, even as resolved by Professor Daube. He took a straightforward, American view: "When both donor and donee are competent adults who knowingly and intelligently consent to the transplantation, after full explanation, no serious legal problem normally exists." Increasingly, he noted, "American courts are requiring a knowing, educated, voluntary consent . . . to serious medical procedures."[36]

Whatever the opinion of jurisprudents, an actual statute or precedential judgment gives comfort to the law. Judicial rulings were not slow in coming; many cases in Britain and America authorized voluntary donation. In 1968, the National Conference of Commissioners on Uniform State Laws drafted a model law, called the Uniform Anatomical Gift Act, which enabled competent adults to indicate their intention to donate their bodily organs after their deaths by signing a legally valid document. In the absence of such a document, specified family members could authorize the taking of organs, unless the deceased had specifically denied the intent to donate.[37] By the end of 1970, all states had adopted the Uniform Anatomical Gift Act. Many states allowed persons to signify their willingness to donate organs by a notice on their driver's license. Although the Uniform Anatomical Gift Act applied only to organs harvested after death, it reinforced the concept that living persons had a legal right to make such a gift prior to death.

The moral theme of the era of transplantation had become donation. Both the living and the dead could freely give the "gift of life" to another desperately ill person. Kin would strengthen the bond of love; strangers would be united by a bond of flesh. Although some worried about the psychological and emotional repercussions, the "gift relationship" entered medical ethics as a new moral value. It sanctioned a formerly forbidden mutilation and provided a noble motive for offering one's organs in life or after death. The combined reflections of physicians, lawyers, and theologians converged around a central concept that carried both moral weight and public appeal. One theologians wrote: "It is surely the mark of the most profound reverence toward one's neighbor to be willing to sacrifice—for serious reasons—an organ of one's own body for him in his necessity."[38]

The Supply of Organs

The elevation of donation to the pinnacle of transplantation ethics made it possible to obtain organs during life and after death. At the same time, the ethics of donation closed certain sources that could have made more organs available. In 1985, it was estimated that approximately 200,000 persons were declared dead each year on the basis of brain-related criteria; organs were obtained from approximately 2,000. Yet the need for kidneys, hearts, and lungs was estimated to be in the range of 50,000 potential beneficiaries.[39] Two proposals to increase the supply of organs, "harvesting" organs from those who had not made the gift and "marketing of organs," or buying and selling them for compensation, both failed before the ethics of the gift relationship.

Some commentators wondered whether an ethical case could be made for harvesting, or removing organs for transplant without, or even against, the explicit wishes of the decedent or the decedent's family. Does the cadaver, in some sense, belong to the state or to society? One author closely associated with the origins of bioethics, psychiatrist Willard Gaylin, wrote an essay (with how much tongue in cheek it is difficult to discern) suggesting the routine harvesting of organs from "neomorts."[40] An occasional philosopher posed the utilitarian argument that routine harvesting of organs would contribute to the greater good of the greater number. One philosopher wrote: "With regard to organs such as kidneys—given the relatively good chances of successful transplantation—we (pragmatically) ought to be (hence, if acting rationally would be) willing to relinquish our right to be buried intact."[41] Most ethicists argued against routine harvesting. Paul Ramsey proposed that "the routine taking of organs would deprive individuals of the exercise of the virtue of generosity."[42] Robert Veatch suggested that "in a society which values personal integrity and freedom, we must be able to control our bodies not only in our lifetime but within reasonable limits after that life is gone."[43] Transplanters, despite their desire to increase the supply of organs, did not disagree; they feared that efforts to increase the organ supply by methods that seemed coercive would denigrate their endeavor. Policy makers were reluctant to adopt positions so contrary to American legal traditions.

Arthur Caplan was recruited from The Hastings Center to the University of Minnesota's School of Medicine, one of the nation's major transplant centers. From that vantage point, he became the bioethical specialist in transplantation. While accepting the donation thesis and rejecting the utilitarian one, he was dedicated to improving the supply of organs. He first attempted to craft a position that blended a "presumed consent" with a utilitarian motive.[44] He proposed that, unless a person or a family explicitly objects to the removal of organs, it can be presumed that a person is willing to donate for the good of others. A bill in the legislature of the Commonwealth of Virginia proposed to waive the consent requirement for cadaver harvesting, but it failed on account of religious and legal objections.[45] Caplan subsequently modified this concept to "required request": hospital personnel would be required by law to request permission of the family. His suggestion was enthusiastically adopted and many states and the federal government enacted legislation to this effect. Unfortunately, required-request laws had little effect on the supply of organs. Caplan regretfully surmised that this was probably due to the continued reluctance of health care providers to introduce this subject in the tragic circumstances of death.[46]

An occasional commentator suggested that the supply of organs would be enhanced by establishing an open market in which organs were bought and sold for financial consideration.[47] A market in several human tissues, blood and sperm, had long existed; why should major organs be treated differently? The first objection to an organ market arose from the belief that it would exploit the poor. From the earliest years of corneal and renal transplantation, indigent persons have occasionally offered to sell "disposable" organs. In India a thriving market flourished for kidneys, many of which were exported to the developed world.[48] In 1983, an American physician proposed a brokerage house for organs that offered to negotiate a price between sellers and buyers. Several leading transplant centers in the United States were reported to have allowed wealthy patients from abroad to bring with them their paid "donor," passed off as an altruistic relative.[49] These proposals met strong opposition. British scholar Richard Titmuss, in his book *The Gift Relationship*,[50] argued that free, noncommercial blood donation was a significant and necessary demonstration of altruism in an industrial society of strangers. Titmuss' concept, together with the life-saving drama of transplantation and the American predilection for voluntary assistance to others in need, built a strong ethos of gift around transplantation. The proposal that a market replace this gift ethos, while rational to the economic mind, shocked morally sensitive persons. Caplan summarized the majority opinion: "Allocating life saving organs by the ability of those in need to pay what the market will bear is blatantly unfair to the poor. Nor can medicine morally allow itself to be used by those who would risk their own health out of greed, desperation or ignorance."[51]

In 1984, Congress enacted the National Organ Transplant Act. The law prohibited the acquiring, receiving, or otherwise transferring of "any human organ for valuable consideration for transplantation if the transfer affects interstate commerce."[52] It made available federal grants to inaugurate a national organ-sharing system. It also established a twenty-five-member Task Force on Organ Transplantation to examine the medical, legal, ethical, social, and economic issues presented by organ procurement. Two bioethicists, James Childress and John Robertson, were members.

The task force endorsed "the position that organs are donated in a spirit of altruism and volunteerism and constitute a national resource to be used for the common good."[53] It also advocated equal access to transplantation and rejected "any element of commercialization in the distribution of organs." A section entitled "Ethical Framework" lists five values to be preserved in the world of transplantation: saving and improving quality of life, respecting individual autonomy, promoting a sense of community through acts of generosity, showing respect for the decedent, and showing respect for the wishes of the family. The task force quoted a report from The Hastings Center

Project on Organ Transplantation, issued in the previous year: "Moral considerations other than efficiency must be acknowledged and respected even in the face of the challenge posed by life threatening diseases . . . [namely] individual autonomy and privacy, the importance of the family, the dignity of the body, and the value of social practices that enhance and strengthen altruism and our sense of community."[54] The task force rejected proposals to enact presumed consent laws, which would allow harvesting of organs unless there was explicit refusal and, instead, encouraged a variety of methods to enhance the voluntary donation system and to improve the efficiency of sharing information and organs across a national network.

The critical shortage of organs continued to inspire ingenious but ethically problematic solutions. One such solution was the implantation of animal organs, known as xenografts, in humans. In the first two decades of the transplantation era, some twenty xenographs had been performed between humans and primates, all unsuccessfully. In 1964, Dr. James Hardy transplanted a chimpanzee heart into a 68-year-old man who survived for several days.[55] Twenty years later, Dr. Leonard Bailey of Loma Linda Medical School in California transplanted a baboon's heart into a newborn girl whose heart lacked a left ventricle.[56] The infant died several days later. This operation, unlike the earlier ones, was widely noted in the press and aroused much criticism, primarily because the inadequate scientific preparation for such a transplant offered the dimmest prospect for success. Questions about the propriety of exchanging organs between species and about using an animal from an endangered species were also raised. Again, the transplant community imposed an informal moratorium on xenografting.

Another proposal to alleviate the shortage of organs suggested transplantation from anencephalics into infants in need. Anencephaly is a congenital anomaly in which the higher portions of the brain and the skull do not develop during fetal life; after birth, the baby will live a few hours or at most several days. Some 2,000 anencephalic infants are born in the United States each year. Approximately the same number of infants need transplanted hearts, livers, and kidneys. The anencephalic infant, once born, is a living human being in the eyes of the law. Although missing higher brain portions, the baby has a functioning brain stem and thus is not legally dead by brain criteria. Salvaging viable organs would, under current law, constitute direct killing of the donor infant.

In the mid-1980s, Michael Harrison, a talented, imaginative pediatric surgeon at UCSF, who had invited me to be an ethics advisor for his innovative operations on fetuses,[57] suggested that the legal determination of death by brain criteria be modified to include the "brain absent," or those born without the major portion of their brains. I used to tease Dr. Harrison by describing him as "ethicogenic": he seemed to generate ethical problems with everything he did. At the same time, he was a thoughtful, concerned, and ethical innovator. I criticized Harrison's proposal and advised him against pursuing it. He persisted, however, and enlisted a California State Senator, Milton Marks, who sponsored legislation to amend the state's determination of death statute. The amendment went nowhere, largely because of the opposition of California's Catholic bishops. Dr. Harrison sought other bioethicists to defend his position.[58] In the ensuing debate, opponents countered that this proposal was the first step on the slippery slope leading to the use of many other brain-damaged, but not brain-dead, persons as donors.[59]

The Artificial Heart

The scarcity of human organs, as well as the problem of immunological rejection, stimulated researchers to explore the possibility of a mechanical heart. The heart is a relatively simple organ: it is a muscular blood pump with an intrinsic electrophysiological regulator, much less physiologically complex than the liver, lungs, or kidneys, and thus, easier to mimic with a device of metal, plastic, and fabric. Since the 1930s, scientists had hoped to create a mechanical substitute for the failing heart. On April 7, 1969, Dr. Denton Cooley implanted a mechanical heart pump in Mr. Haskell Karp, who died 32 hours later.[60] In the 1960s, the Congress provided funding for a research program to develop an artificial heart. Laboratories at the National Heart and Lung Institute, in collaboration with external contractors, initiated an intensive work plan in July 1964. The most promising device under development was a plastic flexible pump that was powered by a small capsule containing 24 grams of plutonium 238. This compact, self-contained, and radioactive machine would be totally implanted in the chest and abdominal cavity.

Dr. Theodore Cooper, Director of the National Heart and Lung Institute, realized that this extraordinary innovation had significant social implications. After all, the human heart was a symbol of life and love; its replacement by a machine would stir images that ranged from the biblical imprecation "I will take away your hearts of flesh and put in your breasts hearts of stone" to the Tin Man of *The Wizard of Oz,* who mourned that he had no heart. Further, the experimental route was a risky one and the costs of development significant. In July 1972, Dr. Cooper convened a Totally Artificial Heart Assessment Panel with the charge "to detail the economic, ethical, legal, medical, psychiatric and social implications of clinical application of a totally implantable artificial heart."

The Totally Artificial Heart Assessment Panel was the federal government's first ethics panel. Dr. Cooper invited me to join the panel. The group convened on August 21, 1972, with a Washington lawyer, Harold Green, as chair. His years of service with the Atomic Energy Commission gave him a mastery of the problems of nuclear radiation. We other panelists were only remotely familiar with these problems. I had to learn the vocabulary of rads and rems as well as the hemodynamics of heart and lung. We were thoroughly briefed on the nature of the technology and the state of the research. Through a year of meetings, we were entranced by the technology and troubled by its implications. We were concerned about how the economics of the artificial heart might affect health resources, how its availability might be skewed by its high cost, and how fairness in the selection of recipients could be assured. We were concerned about recipients' quality of life and quality of death. But, above all, the unique problem of developing a therapy for some persons that might be harmful to other persons gave us pause. The prospect of people walking about with 240 grams of radioactive plutonium in their chests was disconcerting. While the panel concluded that research on the artificial heart should proceed, it was skeptical about the nuclear power source. Its second recommendation read: "Every effort should be made to develop more satisfactory non-nuclear energy systems," and the seventh recommendation stated, "The nuclear-powered artificial heart should not be implanted in human beings until it has been scientifically determined that such a device can be used without significant risk to other persons."[61]

We learned that it was no easy task to reach such a scientific determination. A number of scientific studies had educated us about the problems of calculating radiation risk. One scientist answered our request for advice with the single sentence, "my main worry about the Plutonium-238-powered artificial heart is that one day on a Trans-Pacific flight, economy class, I will be seated between two of them." While the panel's other advisors were not so worried, those words echoed in my conscience and, I think, in that of most of my colleagues. After the panel submitted its report, research on the nuclear power source was de-emphasized in favor of other less problematic designs and the Atomic Energy Commission terminated its support.[62]

Even though the nuclear power source faded from the researchers' dreams, scientists continued to work on the artificial heart and, ten years after the Panel's report, the dream became a device implanted in the chest of Dr. Barney Clark. Dr. Clark, a Seattle dentist, age 61, was a very sick man, suffering from chronic obstructive pulmonary disease, emphysema, and cardiomyopathy. He had smoked heavily from his twenties until he turned 50, but his lung and heart problems worsened, forcing him to retire from practice at age 55. In March 1982, Clark's cardiologist recommended him for a heart transplant at Norman Shumway's program at Stanford University Hospital, but he was rejected because he was over 50 years of age. Clark then entered an experimental drug study at the University of Utah Hospital. There he learned that one of the surgical faculty, Dr. William C. DeVries, was seeking an appropriate candidate for the first implantation of a mechanical heart devised by his colleague Robert Jarvik under the tutelage of one of the geniuses of artificial organs, Dr. Willem Kolff. Clark's diagnosis of idiopathic cardiomyopathy with class IV congestive failure met DeVries' requirements and after signing a lengthy consent form, he agreed to be the first patient. He was scheduled for surgery on December 2, but his condition deteriorated rapidly and he was rushed into surgery just before midnight on December 1, 1982. A Jarvik 7 mechanical heart replaced his own heart, a thick hose connecting it through his chest to a pneumatic pump by his bedside. Clark's post-operative course was difficult: air leaks in the chest, blood clots, seizures, a ruptured valve on the mechanical heart and only intermittent lucidity made the next few weeks a horror. Yet, by February, he was out of intensive care, taking exercise, seeing visitors and preparing for transfer to an extended-care facility. Within a few weeks, however, his condition worsened, and on March 23, 1983, Barney Clark died of circulatory collapse due to multi-organ system failure.

During those 112 days, Barney Clark was the lead player in what *New York Times* medical reporter Lawrence K. Altman called "one of the most dramatic stories in medical history."[63] The University of Utah had decided to allow open media coverage of the operation. An army of reporters invaded the hospital and settled for days in its corridors. Regular news releases were issued. DeVries and Jarvik appeared constantly on television and in the press. Dr. DeVries was undaunted by Clark's death. In the next three years, five more patients were implanted. The longest survivor was William Shroeder, who lived 620 days, suffering one medical crisis after another. Despite years of testing in dogs, sheep, and calves, unanticipated physical and physiological problems plagued the human patients. Each patient's stormy course was followed closely by the media and persistent debates occurred about the utility of this device, which promised (and cost) so much, but delivered so little.[64]

Dr. DeVries moved to Humana Hospital in Louisville, Kentucky, where he was given munificent resources for an artificial heart program. All of the Humana patients died after short and difficult courses. The surgeons, the engineers, and the administrators decided to re-evaluate this dramatic therapy. In 1987, Humana administrators invited me, University of Virginia law professor Walter Wadlington, and Harvard cardiac surgeon Dwight Harkin to review the program. We issued a critical report to the Humana management, emphasizing that the artificial heart must be considered an experimental device and that the time was not here for its regular clinical use. The Humana program was closed and the artificial heart returned to the laboratory.

In 1983, Dr. Claude Lenfant, Director of the National Heart, Lung and Blood Institute (the new name of the National Heart and Lung Institute) appointed the Working Group on Mechanical Circulatory Support "to examine the broad medical, societal, ethical and economic aspects of the developments in this area." I was again asked to serve. We were able to review the disappointing clinical experience and the lessons learned scientifically and clinically. We performed a cost-benefit calculation that compared probable survival of patients who might receive an artificial heart with costs incurred by patients under conventional care. We estimated that the costs to society would fall in the range of 2.5 to 5 billion dollars annually, which one of our members, Dr. David Eddy, contrasted with the cost-effectiveness of equivalent efforts to reduce cigarette smoking. Since the risk to others posed by the nuclear device no longer threatened, this evaluation was dominated by the risks to others created by high-cost technology. The working group insisted, "Cost-effectiveness should be an essential ingredient in decisions on appropriate medical care. . . . Even life-saving technologies should be accepted for public funding only if they fall within the accepted cost-effectiveness boundary." Dr. Lenfant announced in May 1988 that he was going to cancel contracts for further research on the artificial heart. He may have considered carefully the ethical, economic, and social concerns, but he had not, as science writer Barbara Culliton said, considered the "politics of the heart." Under pressure from research institutions that already held contracts and from Senators Ted Kennedy and Orrin Hatch, Dr. Lenfant reversed his decision.[65]

The two artificial heart reports exemplified a style of doing ethics that would become common in bioethics. In neither was a rigorous ethical analysis performed, in accord with ethical theory. Rather, a group of informed persons encountered each other around a broad, rather undefined problem. Each person brought to the discussion not a theory of ethics, but a set of personal values crafted through education, experience, and acculturation. They learned about the factual features of the problem posed to them. They argued; they imagined; they offered examples; they tested new insights against familiar personal and social standards. Out of this discourse came conclusions that drew the vague ethical problem toward some definition that was useful for setting a course of action.

At one moment during the artificial heart panel's discussions, Clark Havighurst, Professor of Law at Duke University, asked me whether I had read John Rawls's *Theory of Justice,* then two years in print. I had to answer that I had not. Havighurst suggested that the panel needed a theory like that of Rawls, as he wrote in an appendix, "to come to some principled judgment on why we should, or should not, as a society, provide expensive life saving technology to all who want it."[66] I went home and read Rawls. The panel did not use Rawlsian theory, and as the ethicist, I did not know quite how it might have been used. This was my first intimation of a methodological question that has persisted in bioethics: how is ethical theory to be fitted to practical deliberations—or should it be fitted at all? That question would come to center stage in the bioethics of the 1990s.

Selection of Patients for a Scarce Resource

In Seattle, Washington, on March 9, 1960, a small loop of plastic was sutured into a vein and an artery in the forearm of Clyde Shields, a 39-year-old machinist dying of renal failure. This plastic arteriovenous shunt and cannula allowed Mr. Shields to be connected to a hemodialysis machine, which cleansed his blood of metabolically accumulated poisons that his diseased kidneys could not eliminate. The shunt had been invented during the previous month by Dr. Belding H. Scribner, a nephrologist on the faculty of the University of Washington School of Medicine, assisted by a biochemical engineer, Wayne Quentin. Although Dr. Willem Kolff built the first dialysis machine in The Netherlands during Nazi occupation, it served only persons afflicted with acute kidney failure from trauma or poisoning, whose blood could be cleansed in a few treatments. It could not be used for patients with chronic kidney failure because the required surgical "hook-up" could be performed only several times. Dr. Scribner's invention made chronic dialysis possible: patients could be connected to and disconnected from the machine with ease, sustaining their lives for indefinite periods and, even better, returning them to active daily life. Twenty-two-year-old Harvey Gentry was the second patient, followed quickly by four others.

The success of chronic dialysis treatment created a practical problem. Dr. John Hogness, Medical Director of the University of Washington Hospital, had provided funds for the care of the first patients. He felt that, since a moral obligation required that patients once admitted to dialysis could not be denied it, a problem of resources was looming as more and more patients were admitted. He informed Dr. Scribner that no more patients be accepted until funding could be assured for this expensive treatment, which cost between $10,000 and $20,000 per patient per year. Scribner acquired a $100,000 grant from the John A. Hartford Foundation and began negotiations with the King County Medical Society to establish a clinic. On January 1, 1962, the Seattle Artificial Kidney Center opened at Swedish Hospital. The Center, stated Dr. James W. Haviland, first chairman of the Center's Board of Trustees, was "a medical school conceived, medical society sponsored, community effort."[67]

In the months before the Center's opening, its planners saw difficulty in the offing. They estimated that between five and twenty candidates for chronic dialysis existed among every one million people. The nine-bed capacity of the center would be stressed after its first year, since patients would need treatment indefinitely. In addition, the costs would be staggering and would fall largely on parties other than the patients. "We could see the handwriting on the wall," recalls Dr. Scribner.[68]

The Board of Trustees of the King County Medical Society devised a procedural solution to this potential problem of resource allocation. Two committees were established: a Medical Advisory Committee, composed of physicians, would select patients who were medically and psychiatrically suitable, and an Admissions and Policy Committee would then choose, out of those medically suitable, patients who would be offered dialysis. The Admissions and Policy Committee was composed of seven anonymous members from varied backgrounds—initially, a minister, lawyer, homemaker, businessman, labor leader, and two physicians from specialties other than nephrology. Rather than creating abstract criteria for selection, the committee members began to work case by case, reviewing extensive personal, social, psychological, and economic information on the candidates, none of whom they knew by name or in person. The first selection criterion on which the members agreed was residency in Washington State since, they reasoned, Washington taxpayers had funded the initial research. Gradually they drew up a list of considerations that they judged relevant: age, gender, marital status and number of dependents, income, educational background, occupation, past performance, and future potential. For the next four years, the committee used these rough criteria, which came to be designated "social worth criteria," to perform their agonizing task of choosing "who shall live and who shall die."

Journalist Shana Alexander selected those words from an ancient Hebrew prayer as the title of her *Life* magazine article on the Seattle committee, "They decide who lives, who dies. Medical miracle puts moral burden on small committee."[69] Alexander called the article "the most awesome and disturbing story that I have ever worked on." One of *Life*'s few women writers, she was in Portland, covering the birth of a baby elephant, when her editors ordered her to Seattle. They had seen a front page story in the *The New York Times*: "Panel holds life or death vote in allotting artificial kidney."[70] The story reported a ten-minute talk that Dr. Scribner had given at the American Society of Clinical Investigations in Atlantic City, during which he mentioned casually the existence of the Admissions and Policy Committee. Alexander spent six months in Seattle, interviewing the doctors, the patients, and the members of the Committee. "It was a heavy burden," she recalls, "something I will never forget. . . . I wrote 10,000 words, the longest article ever published in *Life*. It sparked national interest in what is today called bioethics."[71]

Spark national interest it did. The National Broadcasting Corporation prepared a documentary, "Who Lives? Who Dies?," hosted by Edwin Newman, which aired in the fall of 1965. *Redbook* told the story as "The rest are simply left to die."[72] Sociologists Renée C. Fox and Judith P. Swazey visited Seattle in 1968 to study the dialysis program, and they published *The Courage to Fail,* which vividly tells the most complete story of the Committee.[73] Professional reaction was cool; Dr. George E. Schreiner criticized fellow nephrologist Scribner: "We have never had such a committee in Washington D.C. [at Schreiner's dialysis program at Georgetown University Hospital] and never will have. We feel that this is a device to spread the responsibility to people who by experience and education are really less equipped to take responsibility than the physicians in charge of the case."[74] Philosophers and theologians considered the selection process a serious ethical problem in need of analysis.[75]

Dr. Scribner was taken aback by the publicity. He told Fox and Swazey,

> All of us who were involved felt that we had found a fairly reasonable and simple solution to an impossibly difficult problem by letting a committee of responsible members of the community choose what patients [should receive treatment] among those who were medically ideal. . . . In retrospect, of course, we were terribly naive. We did not realize the full impact that the existence of the committee would have on the world. We simply could not understand why everyone was more interested in the existence and operation of the lay selection committee than in the fact that in two years we had taken a disease and converted it from a 100 percent fatal prognosis to a two-year survival. Nor were any of us prepared for the very severe storm of criticism that was to be forthcoming at the annual medical meetings and in the scholarly literature.[76]

Dr. Scribner was not so naive that he was unable to present, as his 1964 presidential address to the Society for Artificial Internal Organs, a candid review of the ethical problems created by his own invention. He began, "After long reflection and much soul-searching, I have decided to tackle for my presidential address a subject that wiser and more mature persons might steer clear of. I have decided to discuss this subject at risk of making both you, my audience, and myself uncomfortable, because I feel with great sincerity and urgency that we must bring these problems out in the open and face them squarely." He outlined the problems that he and his colleagues had faced over the last four years. These problems were patient selection, overt termination of dialysis, "dialysis suicide," "death with dignity," and donor selection for transplantation. He offered no solutions but hoped for some. He concluded, "There are those who argue that we scientists should have no concern for the effects that our discoveries will have on society. My answer is simply that we too are members of society and as such have an obligation."[77]

The Seattle dialysis program, with its unusual selection process, was a dramatic instance of the new medicine meeting traditional medical ethics: one of the first genuinely life-sustaining therapeutics challenged the loyalty of the physician to the single patient for whom he or she is caring. The idea of turning over this responsibility to a lay committee was, as Dr. Schreiner had noted, shocking. The idea of choosing for life or for death, although familiar to medicine in emergency triage, seemed appalling when it came to the common use of a life-saving treatment. The problem of selecting patients for dialysis was generalizable to the whole field of transplantation and other scarce resources. The public attention that this event aroused, and the scholarly debate that it stimulated, were unprecedented. The public attention was strong enough to effect a legislative change to the Social Security Act providing federal funding for patients with end-stage renal disease. After the passage of the End-Stage Renal Disease Amendment in 1972, the need for the Selection Committee diminished. Although never formally disbanded, it ceased to meet about that time.

Dr. Judith Swazey summed up the impact of the Seattle Artificial Kidney debate:

> The Seattle group was struggling in a much more forthright manner than most medical groups at the time with a number of issues that at once were medical, moral and social, and would become the major foci of those who . . . became known as bioethicists. These topics included the appropriate ways of financing a costly medical technology, the prolongation and quality of life, and the termination of treatment by a physician or by a patient.[78]

James Childress had just begun his career as a professor of religious ethics at the University of Virginia when he was invited to participate in a panel discussion of the selection for renal dialysis and, shortly afterwards, in a faculty seminar on the ethical issues posed by artificial and transplanted organs. He shaped his considerations into an article, "Who shall live when all cannot live?" Childress contrasted egalitarian with utilitarian criteria for selection. Egalitarians commend some system of random selection as the only mechanism consonant with the dignity and equality of all candidates. Utilitarians demand a choice that selects those whose lives contribute to society. Egalitarians appeal to values such as equal respect for personal dignity by avoiding judgments of comparative social worth and by providing equality of opportunity for individuals apart from the social roles they occupied. These two positions rest on two distinct foundations for moral judgment: social utility—that is, the achievement of the greater good for the greater number in a society, or the absolute moral claims of each person to basic human goods, such as life and liberty. Childress also argued that society would more readily accept a random selection mechanism as fair. He defended a random selection procedure by analogy with the jurisprudence of *United States v Holmes,* an 1842 case in which the court ruled that a lottery was the most equitable way of choosing which passengers should be pushed out of an overloaded lifeboat to enhance the chances of the others.[79]

Childress contrasted his egalitarian approach with the approach of Nicholas Rescher, a philosopher at the University of Pittsburgh. Rescher's essay, "The allocation of exotic medical lifesaving therapy," appeared in the staid philosophical journal *Ethics.* Along with Hans Jonas's essay on human experimentation, Rescher's essay was arguably one of the first genuinely philosophical contributions to bioethics.[80] Rescher delineated an argument for utilitarian selection, asserting, "Society 'invests' a scarce resource in one person as against another and is thus entitled to look to the probable prospective 're-turn' on its investment." This statement implicitly endorses the principle of social util-ity and suggests certain criteria for selecting (or excluding) entire groups for a scarce resource—criteria that will maximize society's return on its investment. The inclusion criteria are: (*1*) the constituency of the selecting institution, (*2*) the needs of medical re-search, and (*3*) the prospect of success. Once a group has been designated on the basis of these criteria, a second set of criteria are applied: (*1*) relative likelihood of success, (*2*) life-expectancy, (*3*) family role, (*4*) potential future contribution to society, and (*5*) past services rendered to society. If the selection produces more candidates than can be accommodated, a random method of choosing the finalists can be employed. It is clear that Rescher's selection criteria involve valuing each candidate for their "social worth." Future contributions and past service are particularly valued. Rescher acknowledged that such judgments are difficult, yet affirmed that "such distasteful problems must be faced, since a failure to choose some is tantamount to sentencing all. Unpleasant choices are intrinsic to the problem of selection." The essay endorses the approach of the Seattle Selection Committee, as he saw Shana Alexander describe it, in which "so-cial worth" seemed to play so large a role.

Childress disagreed with Rescher by criticizing the feasibility and justifiability of the utilitarian approach. It was not feasible because it is impossible to quantify and com-pare the values that Rescher believed should be counted in assessing social worth. It was not justifiable because "the utilitarian approach would, in effect, reduce the person to his social role. . . . A person's transcendence, his dignity as a person . . . cannot be reduced to his past or future contribution to society." That dignity and transcendence "can be protected and witnessed to by a recognition of his equal right to be saved."[81] Childress saw the "equal right to be saved" as requiring random selection: a lottery in which each person has an equal opportunity to be saved.

Paul Ramsey came to the same conclusion in his final Beecher lecture, "Choosing how to choose," which, coincidentally, he was preparing just as Childress was writing his analysis.[82] The two theologians offer remarkably similar arguments favoring an egalitarian principle of selection and a random process. Both refer to the "life boat" analyses. Ramsey added a theological argument: "When the ultimate of life is at stake, and when not all lives can be saved . . . men should then 'play God' in the correct way: he makes his sun rise upon the good and evil and sends rain upon the just and the unjust alike." A third theologian, Helmut Thielicke, had reached similar conclusions, which he presented in his Houston lecture, delivered one month before Ramsey gave his Beecher lectures. Thielicke also repudiated the utilitarian view; "There is an alternative to this view of man in terms of his 'utility.' One can speak instead of his 'infinite worth'. . . . The basis of human dignity is seen to reside not in any immanent quality of man whatsoever, but in the fact that God created him." Thielicke differs from Childress and Ramsey only in one respect. Rather than opting for a random selection, such as a lottery, he urged those who must decide to accept the radical ambiguity and "metaphysical guilt" of any way they choose to choose.[83] Perhaps as a European, Dr. Thielicke could not appreciate the American proclivity to flip a coin.

The theologians' insistence on the equality of all persons was seconded by secular critics of the utilitarian approach. The first serious criticism of the Seattle selection technique came from a lawyer and a psychiatrist, David Sanders and Jesse Dukeminier. In "Medical advance and legal lag: hemodialysis and kidney transplantation," they criticized mercilessly the "prejudices and mindless clichés that pollute the committee's deliberations . . . the bourgeoisie sparing the bourgeoisie . . . [ruling out] the creative non-conformists, who rub the bourgeoisie the wrong way but who historically have contributed so much to the making of America. The Pacific Northwest is no place for a Henry David Thoreau with bad kidneys." In their less splenetic moments, Sanders and Dukeminier provide a rational critique of social worth, using the same lifeboat analogy that had inspired Ramsey and Childress. They admited that society does evaluate persons in many, and often biased, ways, and in the matter at hand—the provision of a life-saving resource—evaluation approaches the impossible. The only way to avoid evaluation is by lottery or by the first-come, first-serve rule.[84] Another legal commentator, Paul Freund, expressed the problem as follows: "The more nearly total is the estimate to be made of an individual, and the more nearly the consequences determine life or death, the more unfit the judgment becomes for human reckoning. . . . Randomness as a moral principle deserves serious study."[85]

Randomness did get serious study; however, it did not please everyone. It was certainly a stranger to the world of medical care, in which the situation of critical shortage was resolved by triage rules of long standing.[86] Far from seeing a human lottery as appropriate to human dignity, some authors were repelled by the idea. Even Edmund Cahn, to whom both Ramsey and Childress appealed, considered "the stakes too high for gambling and the responsibilities too deep for destiny." He would rather see all die than some saved by any imperfect technique.[87] Joseph Fletcher, the frank utilitarian, called a lottery "literally irresponsible, a rejection of the burden, refusal to be rational."[88] Even Jay Katz and Alex Capron, who ultimately favored a lottery, considered it a necessary but deficient way to protect the moral and legal value of equality of persons: "The Lottery is more blind than fair, for an evenhanded approach is desirable only insofar as it deals with like classes of individuals."[89]

Other authors noted the practical problem of a lottery. It requires that a group gather before lots can be drawn, a situation that is unrealistic since patients appear serially with an urgent need for help. Lotteries can be rigged, and in matters of such import, they are likely to be so. Even a queue can be "jumped" by those who have knowledge and power. Some authors doubted that random selection would alleviate anxiety, and several authors distinguished between the "natural" sorts of random selection, such as the first-come, first-serve rule, and artificial ones, such as lotteries. All systems of random selection make it possible for certain socially disreputable and dangerous persons to receive the gift of life, a prospect that critics of the lottery find unpalatable but proponents consider the price of fairness.[90]

The 1986 Department of Health & Human Services (DHHS) Task Force on Organ Transplantation recommended public policy that mitigated the urgency of the debate over selection. Scientific techniques for identifying histocompatability (the biological properties that allow the immune system to accept foreign tissue) improved greatly during the 1970s. Transplant centers began to share data about the availability of organs and to match appropriate organs to suitable recipients. The United Network for Organ Sharing (UNOS), a private, nonprofit corporation that operates a registry of transplant recipients and a system of organ procurement and distribution, was established in the early 1980s. The (DHHS) task force commended this approach and proposed a "Model Organ Procurement and Transplantation Network"; UNOS received a DHHS contract to implement the model. By the mid-1980s, a national system had been established: all patients are entered in a single coordinated waiting list for all organs, in which each patient is given priority in terms of time on list, histocompatibility, urgency, age, etc. The original ethical crisis faced by doctors and advisory committees who were forced to choose patients one by one for life or for death has been mitigated, although internal debates over equity and efficiency continue.[91]

Access to Transplantation and Other Health Services

Organ transplantation and renal dialysis saved the lives of identifiable persons in a highly visible way. The procedures were also very expensive. The cost and the relative paucity of trained professionals and elaborate equipment made these services difficult to obtain. The question arose in the professional and the public mind: should any individual be allowed to die because he or she could not afford the high costs of transplantation or dialysis? From its inception in 1962, The Northwest Kidney Center (as the Seattle Artificial Kidney Center was called after 1970) attempted to help its patients pay the annual bill to stay alive. While some costs were assumed by NIH research grants, incessant fund drives supplemented patients' often inadequate insurance coverage. *The Seattle Times* announced one of those drives with a front page picture of nine dialysis patients under the banner, "Will These People Have to Die?"[92]

The National Kidney Foundation and the National Association of Patients on Hemodialysis determined to obtain sound government funding for patient care. They lobbied Congress successfully—a patient was dialyzed in front of the House Ways and Means Committee. The case was not difficult to make before the Congress of that era:

these salvageable citizens would be left to die when they could be saved by a technology that had been perfected by the research funds provided by that very Congress.
An amendment, Section 299I, was added to the Medicaid Bill, H.R.1, with the strong
support of influential members of Congress, principally Congressman Wilbur Mills and
Senators Vance Hartke and Russell Long. The Congress passed HR1 with the end-stage
renal disease amendment (ESRD) and President Nixon signed it on October 30, 1972.
Senator Long reflected, "We are the greatest nation in the world, the wealthiest per
capita. Are we so hard pressed that we cannot pay for . . . a life extended for ten to
fifteen years."[93]

Section 299I provided financial support for kidney dialysis and transplantation to all
persons eligible for Social Security coverage. In its first phase, the costs appeared modest: 11,000 patients were supported at a cost of $280 million but numbers and costs
rapidly escalated. In the 1990s, the program supports approximately 50,000 patients at a
cost of over one billion dollars. The end-stage renal disease amendment was an
anomalous form of health insurance. Only patients with a specific diagnosis—renal disease—were covered; patients with cardiac, liver, or bowel disease could ask, "why not
us?" Persons with hemophilia, in fact, did ask, without success. Gradually, as cardiac,
liver, and other transplants emerged from experimental status, Medicaid paid for these
transplants in a fragmentary way. The availability of this insurance relieved the pressure on dialysis centers, which increased in number around the nation. Since the payment mechanisms of the ESRDA encouraged dialysis of marginal utility, some entrepreneurial providers developed profitable companies. Still, even with these problems,
the federal funding reduced the ethical crisis of selecting patients for a scarce life-saving
resource. Much of the urgency of the debate over egalitarian and utilitarian principles
dissipated; the government had opted for the egalitarian way and had chosen to pay for
it.[94]

In the quarter century after the enactment of the end-stage renal disease amendments, concern about access to all medical treatment, not only to the expensive and
"exotic" forms, became a national issue. The cost of medical care and the proportion of
the national product devoted to its financing have become a major public concern. Although two national health insurance programs—Medicare for citizens over 65 and the
federal–state joint Medicaid for the indigent—became law in 1967, large gaps in coverage remained. The primary source of health insurance through employment could be
lost when workers lost their jobs and many persons were employed in low-paying jobs
that lacked health benefits. In addition, the costs of health care were increasing faster
than costs in the general economy. The burden of the public programs began to be felt
by government and taxpayers. As costs were rising, access was diminishing.

The problem of inadequate access to health care is an economic and political problem; it is equally an ethical problem. During the 1970s, as health policy scholars began
to articulate the growing problem of the costs of care that would catch political fire in
the 1980s, a few ethicists attempted a parallel articulation of the ethics of the problem.
One of the first commentators, Paul Ramsey, was skeptical: he concluded the Beecher

lectures with a meditation on the problem of ordering health care priorities among themselves and in relation to other national needs. With uncharacteristic humility, he admitted, "I do not know the answer to these questions, nor how to go about finding the answer."[95] In 1973, André Hellegers and I argued that the agenda of bioethics should include "a theory of the common good . . . consisting of a comprehensive description of the exigencies of medical care and the institutional forms that serve these exigencies at present. It must propose criteria whereby these institutional forms can be analyzed and criticized." These criteria are found in the theories of justice long familiar to ethics, "which . . . have not been fully mined for their relevance to the moral problems of medicine." We did not mine them and Paul Ramsey, the commentator on our lecture, criticized us for our timidity.[96]

Other ethicists did initiate a deeper exploration. Gene Outka, while spending a semester at the Kennedy Institute, wrote "Social justice and equal access to health care,"[97] in which he examined the concept of social justice for its relevance to health care. Justice, in its traditional definition, requires that social burdens and benefits be distributed (*1*) according to merit, (*2*) according to contribution, (*3*) according to market supply and demand, (*4*) according to need, and (*5*) by similar treatment of similar cases. The first three criteria, Outka argued, do not suit the nature of the social good that health and health care are; the latter two criteria are the proper ones to analyze justice in health care. Several institutions of health care, such as health insurance and the fee-for-service system, are subjected to criticism in light of these criteria of justice. Outka offered a conceptual scheme for analysis of justice in health care, but he hardly opened the door on the complex questions of public policy. Other authors—Robert Veatch, Charles Fried, and Ronald Green—also contributed to the conceptual formulation of the problems. For these authors, the general moral concepts of justice, equality, equity, and rights urged an improvement in the institutions of health care that would render them more accessible and more affordable. Their essays did not merely claim that this was so; they offered careful arguments in support of their theses.[98]

In the late 1970s, growing concern that the health care system was broken could be heard. In its scientific, technical, and educational aspects, in its buildings, equipment, and finance, American medicine was clearly the best in the world, yet millions of Americans could not afford it or gain access to it and often, when they did obtain care, they came away dissatisfied. The title of a 1977 issue of *Daedalus*, "Doing Better and Feeling Worse: Health in the United States," captured the sense of concern. Contributions to that issue by a number of America's leading physicians explored the problems of health care in the United States. Remarkably, the two initial essays came from nonphysicians closely associated with bioethics. Professor Renée Fox brilliantly analyzed the "medicalization and demedicalization of American society," the extension of medical concepts and definitions over a wide range of cultural and social phenomenon. In passing, she noted the interest in bioethical issues: "a bioethics 'subculture' with certain characteristics of a social movement has crystallized around such issues."[99] One of that subculture's denizens, Dan Callahan, contributed "Health and society: some ethical imperatives" to the issue. He critically reflected on the meaning of health and on the right to health and health care, concluding with a note that would be heard more loudly in subsequent years:

> Scarcity—restraint—limit: these are rapidly becoming the slogans of the times. . . . Curiously enough [I would hold] these are precisely the conditions under which it becomes possible effectively to examine ethical goals. Medicine is in part a moral enterprise, one that seeks the human good. But excessive affluence combined with excessive individualism discourages our asking just what constitutes this human good . . . now we can ask again about that good which medicine is said to serve, and about what its role in the quest for a larger human good might reasonably be.[100]

Conditions of scarcity sharply focused the ethics of social justice on the problem of availability of health services. Some philosophers who were dedicated to equity and fairness in health care worried that the strong endorsement of a positive right to health care would require dedication of unlimited resources to the health benefits of individuals. Such a right would rule out comparisons between various health goods and between health goods and other social goods, such as education, environmental protection, and defense. Even when these thinkers gave cautious approval to the idea of a right, they denied that any particular health care intervention, such as cardiac transplantation or artificial heart implantation, must be provided as a matter of right to every individual needing such an intervention, even if it is life saving.[101] However, the life-saving nature of many medical interventions seems to obstruct all efforts to implement restrictive policy. The rational judgment that expensive life-saving interventions should be rationed encounters a strong psychological and social imperative to save those threatened by death, which I later named "rule of rescue."[102]

In 1978, the Congress ordered the President's Commission for the Study of Ethical Problems in Medicine to study the question of access to health care from an ethical viewpoint. The story of the writing of *Securing Access to Health Care* has been told in Chapter 4. Despite the difficulties experienced in producing it, the report was a useful exposition of the problem of justice in health care. Many scholars in philosophy, economics, social policy, and health sciences contributed to its formulation. The report concluded that "society has an ethical obligation to ensure equitable access to an adequate level of health care without the imposition of excessive burdens."[103] "Adequate" is defined as the level of care that will enable individuals to achieve sufficient welfare, opportunity, information, and evidence of interpersonal concern to facilitate a reasonably full and satisfying life. The Commission refrained from attempting to specify what adequate care should include. Instead, it suggested characteristics of adequacy that deserve attention in any discussion of an equitable health policy: the relationship between various forms of care and the health needs of individuals, and the relationship between the benefits of care and its costs, including diversions of resources from other socially desirable endeavors. The Commission concluded:

> Consequently, the level of care deemed adequate should reflect a reasoned judgment not only about impact of the condition on the welfare and opportunity of the individual but also about the efficacy and the costs of the care itself in relation to other conditions and the efficacy and cost of the care that is available for them . . . and the cost of each proposed option in terms of foregone opportunities to apply the same resources to social goals other than that of ensuring access [to health care].[104]

The Commonwealth of Massachusetts attempted to translate the Commission's general principles into practical policy. The Secretary of Human Services and the Commissioner of Public Health appointed a Task Force on Organ Transplantation on September 26, 1983. Bioethicist George Annas was named chairperson. The Task Force was asked to study how two major transplant procedures, heart and liver transplantation, should be introduced into Massachusetts. The Commonwealth had many premier medical institutions eager to initiate these services, although several years before, the prime candidate among these institutions, Massachusetts General Hospital, had decided not to engage in heart transplantation for the time. Now some were asking if the time had come to reverse that decision. Also, the appointment of the Task Force was stimulated by a dramatic public event. In 1982, Mr. and Mrs. Charles Fiske of Bridgewater, Massachusetts, had been unable to obtain a liver transplant for their eleven-month-old daughter, Jamie. Mr. Fiske made a dramatic public appeal before the annual meeting of the Academy of Pediatrics, which attracted nationwide media attention. Jamie was transplanted several days later at the University of Minnesota Hospital.[105] Public sympathy for patients needing transplants had been generated. The overarching problem was how the state should finance these costly procedures. The Task Force report, issued after a year's study, concurred with the conclusion of the President's Commission that society has an ethical obligation to ensure equitable access to health care for all and that the cost of achieving equitable access ought to be shared fairly.

The Task Force affirmed that "the primary values at stake in organ transplantation are human life, equity, and fairness," and applied those principles in a concrete way to the introduction of high-cost services. The report recommended that transplant services be introduced in a controlled, phased manner and that hospitals be granted a certificate of need that would permit them to initiate transplant programs only when reliable data about need, costs, and outcomes justify expansion. Patient screening criteria should be public, fair, and equitable, based primarily on medical need and then on a first-come basis. The rationale for the Task Force's decision to endorse transplantation services was, "It believes that it can be done without decreasing services in other medical sectors, and that the total demand can be met without additional capital expenditure . . . if it turns out that liver and heart transplantations take resources away from higher priority health care services, and decreases their accessibility to the public, these transplantation procedures should not be performed."[106] The Task Force believed that control of costs and equity in access could be managed together but, should they conflict, the principles of equity and fairness had priority over the saving of life.

As the Task Force was completing its mission, another Bostonian, Tufts University's philosophy professor Norman Daniels, was about to publish the study that was—and perhaps still is—the most thorough analysis of justice in health care. Daniels did what my Artificial Heart Panel colleague, Clark Havighurst, had suggested to me, and what I did not know how to do: he adapted the theory of justice elaborated by his teacher John Rawls to health care. In Rawls's contractarian theory of justice, the individuals who contract to create a society and its institutions do so behind "a veil of ignorance" which hides from their view the social status and class, intelligence, strength, and talents that they might enjoy once the society based upon their contract comes into being. They must determine the principles that will govern their institutions and the distributions of social goods without knowing whether they will be among the better or worse off members of the society. Their contract will, then, specify two principles: "first, each person is to have an equal right to the most extensive liberty compatible with a similar liberty for others and, second, social and economic inequalities are to be arranged so that they are both (a) reasonably expected to be to everyone's advantage, and (b) attached to positions and offices open to all."[107] This latter principle is called the equal-opportunity principle.

Daniels imports that principle into social institutions that provide the social good of health care. He seeks philosophically sound answers to such questions as: "What sort of a social good is health care? Are there social obligations to provide health care? What inequalities in its distribution are morally acceptable? What limits do provider autonomy and individual liberties of physicians and patients place on just distribution of care?"[108] After extended arguments about the nature of health and the status of health care as a social good, Daniels ventures into applications of his theoretical exposition to various health care situations, such as care of the elderly and workplace safety.

Health care is an enormously complex enterprise, ranging from recommending aspirin for headaches to transplanting hearts, from nursing care to neurosurgery, and from health education to accident prevention. Daniels sees in that complexity one fundamental aim, the preservation of normal species functioning that is impaired by illness and disability. When normal species functioning at the biological and social levels is impaired, individuals are hindered from pursuing their "plans of life" and thus denied equal opportunity to enjoy the benefits of social life. Health and health care are linked to the primary social good of opportunity. The institutions that deliver health care and the social policies that structure those institutions are judged to be just and fair when they are designed to provide to each individual "a fair share of the normal opportunity range for their society at each stage of their life."[109]

That opportunity range, Daniels insists, extends over the full lifetime of individuals. Rational persons choosing the principles of fair health care, he believes, would assure that they had available to themselves the kind of health care that would support their opportunities at various stages of life. They would not judge it unfair to be denied heart transplants or renal dialysis as elderly persons if they had enjoyed the full range of services that supported health during their youth and middle age. Daniels' key to the allocation problem is not rationing of specific technologies or services but their distribution through those ranges of opportunity in which they can most effectively sustain normal species functioning. He rejects the accusation that this distribution constitutes an invidious rationing by age. Daniels' account of justice in health care was not without its critics.[110] Still, it was theoretically sophisticated enough to serve as a basis for the escalating debate over access to health care during the 1990s.

Conclusion

By the end of the 1980s, organ transplantation had become a common and accepted medical practice. Thousands of patients had benefited from improved transplantation techniques and anti-rejection drugs; many others had been disappointed, dying before being transplanted or in the immediate aftermath of the operation or after a short life of diminished quality. The transplanters moved into new fields—pancreas, bowel, segmental lung, block transplantation of multiple organs—and each move raised questions about experimentation, efficacy, cost, and consent. Some unique proposals, such as fetal tissue transplantation for Parkinson's disease and for diabetes, aroused strong emotions. In 1987 I participated in a symposium on the ethics of fetal tissue transplantation, organized by bioethicist Mary Mahowald, at which researchers and bioethicists reviewed the ethical and legal implications of this innovation.[111] The Director of the National Institutes of Health established the Human Fetal Tissue Transplantation Research Panel in March 1988: the panel was deeply divided and the Secretary of the Department of Health and Human Services declined to accept its conclusions.[112]

The world of transplantation would remain ethically contentious. The ethics of personal autonomy and fairness in selection had prevailed over utilitarianism and social worth.[113] The contention over fair selection had been relaxed by the establishment of UNOS, but debates erupted about particular problems, such as giving liver transplants to alcoholics.[114] The problem of access had been ameliorated by the passage of the end-stage renal disease amendments for persons with renal disease, but sufferers from other conditions that could benefit from transplantation still faced enormous costs that were sometimes covered only partially, if at all, by the various sources of health insurance. This, of course, was symptomatic of the entire American health care system. The problem of access to high-technology interventions was folded into the overall ethical question of justice in health care. Justice in health care became one of the central questions of bioethics in the 1990s, during which bioethicists participated vigorously in the debates about health reform and about the transformation of American medicine into for-profit managed care.[115]

Notes for Chapter 7

1. Alexis Carrel and Charles A. Lindbergh, *The Culture of Organs* (New York: Paul B. Hoeber, 1938). See also Theodore J. Malinin, *Surgery and Life: The Extraordinary Career of Alexis Carrel* (New York: Harcourt Brace Jovanovich, 1979).

2. E. C. Padgett, "Is iso-skin grafting practicable?" *Southern Medical Journal* 25 (1932): 895; J. B. Brown, "Homografting of skin: with report of success in identical twins," *Surgery* 1 (1937): 558.

3. Peter B. Medawar, "The behavior and fate of skin autografts and skin homografts in rabbits," *Journal of Anatomy* 78 (1944): 176, and *Journal of Anatomy* 79 (1945): 157.

4. Gerald Leach, *The Biocrats* (London: Cape, 1970), p. 286.

5. J. P. Merrill, J. E. Murray, J. H. Harrison, and W. R. Guild, "Successful homotransplantation of the human kidney between identical twins," *Journal of the American Medical Association* 160 (1956): 277–282.

6. J. E. Murray, J. P. Merrill, and J. H. Harrison. "Kidney transplantation between seven pairs of identical twins," *Annals of Surgery* 148 (1958): 343; J. E. Murray, J. P. Merrill, G. J. Dammin, et al., "Study of transplantation immunity after total body irradiation; clinical and experimental investigation," *Surgery* 48 (1960): 272; J. E. Murray, J. P. Merrill, J. H. Harrison, et al., "Prolonged survival of human kidney homografts by immunosuppressive drug therapy," *New England Journal of Medicine* 268 (1963): 1315.

7. For a general overview of the early years of tissue transplantation, see Francis D. Moore, *Give and Take. The Development of Tissue Transplantation* (Philadelphia and London: W. B. Saunders, 1964).

8. *Masden v Harrison*, Mass Sup Jud Ct, June 12, 1957; *Huskey v Harrison*, Mass Sup Jud Ct, Aug 30, 1957; *Foster v Harrison*, Mass Sup Jud Ct, Nov 20, 1957; see William J. Curran, "A problem of consent: kidney transplantation in minors," *New York University Law Review* 34 (1959): 891–898.

9. *Strunk v Strunk*, 445 S. W. 2d 145 (Ky 1969). In a parallel case, a Louisiana court refused to authorize a transplant from an institutionalized sibling, apparently because he and his sister had little or no contact. *In re Richardson*. La. App., 284 So. 2d 185, 1973.

10. Thomas E. Starzl, "Ethical problems in organ transplantation: a clinician's point of view," in J. Russell Elkington (ed.), *The Changing Mores of Biomedical Research, Annals of Internal Medicine* 67, Suppl. 7 (Sept. 67), p. 36.

11. J. Russell Elkington, "Moral problems in the use of borrowed organs, artificial and transplanted," *Annals of Internal Medicine* 60 (1964): 309–313, p. 309; "Letters and comments," *Annals of Internal Medicine* (1964): 355–363, pp. 355, 362.

12. G. E. W. Wolstenholme, "Preface," in Wolstenholme and Maeve O'Connor (eds.), *Law and Ethics of Transplantation* (London: J & A Churchill, Ltd. 1966), pp. vii–viii. First titled *Ethics in Medical Progress with Special Reference to Transplantation* (1966).

13. One prominent clergyman was present *in distans*, Pope Pius XII, whose 1957 "Allocution to anesthesiologists" is included as an appendix (in French). The papal statement may have been appended at the suggestion of the Italian participant, Dr. Raffaello Cortesini of Rome, whose conference remarks had referred to it, as well as to another papal pronouncement on the legitimacy of removing cadaver organs for transplantation. Wolstenholme and O'Conner, Cortesini "Discussion of Transplantation," and "Outlines of a legislation on transplantation" in Wolstenholme and O'Conner, *Law and Ethics of Transplantation*, pp. 97, 175. I do not know of any other papal commentary on transplantation other than the Pope's allocution to the Symposium on Corneal Transplants, May 9, 1956, where he endorsed, with some cautions about respect for the

cadaver, organ removal for transplant. F. Angelini (ed.), *Discorsi ai Mediei* (Rome: Orizzanti, 1959), p. 446.

14. Quoted in Leach, *The Biocrats*, p. 303.

15. Chad Calland, "Iatrogenic problems in end-stage renal failure," *New England Journal of Medicine* 287 (1972): 334–336.

16. Albert R. Jonsen, "Scientific medicine and therapeutic choice," *New England Journal of Medicine* 292 (1975): 126–127.

17. "The ultimate operation," *Time*, Dec. 15, 1967, pp. 64–72, quote on p. 65.

18. The transplanted heart for Blaiberg was taken from a 24-year-old black man (in the argot of apartheid, a 'cape-colored'), Clive Haupt; in the miracle story of Cosmos and Damien, the cadaver from which the limb was taken was a Moor! "Second heart transplant performed in Capetown," *New York Times* January 3, 1968: A1, 32; "Heart transplant surgery performed on west coast," *New York Times* January 7, 1968: A1, 50. Barnard said on February 2, 1975, that he would no longer use hearts from black persons because of the controversies. "The impression has been created that we just sit here and wait for some poor black person to be brought into the hospital so we can use his organs." "Barnard to stop transplanting hearts of blacks," *New York Times* February 3, 1975: A3.

19. Subcommittee on Health, Committee on Labor and Public Welfare, U.S. Senate, November 9, 1971, p. 103.

20. Renée C. Fox and Judith P. Swazey, *The Courage to Fail: A Social View of Organ Transplants and Dialysis* (Chicago: University of Chicago Press, 1974), chapter 6.

21. John E. Murray, "Organ transplantation: the practical possibilities," in Wostenholme and O'Conner, *Law and Ethics of Transplantation* pp. 54–64, quote on p. 59; see also Francis Moore, "New problems in surgery," *Science* 144 (1964): 391.

22. Lord Kilbrandon, "Chairman's opening remarks," in Wostenholme and O'Conner, *Law and Ethics of Transplantation*, p. 3.

23. See Fred Rosner, *Modern Medicine and Jewish Ethics* (New York: Ktav Publishing House, and Yeshiva University Press, 1986), chapter 3; and J. D. Bleich, "Organ transplants," in *Judaism and Healing* (New York: Ktav, 1981), pp. 129–133.

24. Gerald Kelly, "The morality of mutilation: towards a revision of the treatise," *Theological Studies* 17, no. 3 (1956): 322–344.

25. Thomas Aquinas, *Summa Theologiae II–II*, q. 65, a. 1; Martin Nolan, "The principle of totality in moral theology," in Charles E. Curran (ed.), *Absolutes in Moral Theology* (Washington, D.C.: Corpus Books, 1968), pp. 232–248.

26. Bert Cunningham, "The morality of organic transplantation," *Studies in Sacred Theology*, no. 86 (1944): On Cunningham's work, see David F. Kelly, *The Emergence of Roman Catholic Medical Ethics in North America: An Historical-Methodological-Bibliographical Study* (New York and Toronto: The Edwin Mellin Press, 1979), pp. 332–341.

27. Cunningham, "The morality of organic transplantation," p. 63.

28. Cunningham, "The morality of organic transplantation," p. 101.

29. Cited in Gerald Kelly, "Moral notes," *Theological Studies* 8 (1947): 99.

30. *Discorsi ai Medici*, p. 446.

31. Gerald Kelly, "The morality of mutilation: toward a revision of the treatise"; Kelly cites Thomas Aquinas, *In III Sententiae*, d. 29, a. 5: "when one gives one's life for one's friend, he does not love the friend more than himself, but rather prefers one's own 'good of virtue' to a physical good."

32. David Daube, "Limitation on self-sacrifice in Jewish law and tradition," *Theology* 72 (1969): 291–299; see also Immanuel Jacobovits, *Jewish Medical Ethics* (New York: Bloch Publishing, 1959), pp. 96–97, 290–291. Not only the Jewish but also the Buddhist and the Muslim

traditions have ancient prohibitions against dissection and, it would appear, this prohibition cannot be overridden by the choice of the decedent. It is interesting to note, however, how these religious traditions have responded to the novel situation of transplantation. Islamic beliefs about resurrection require bodily integrity at the time of death. Buddhism also abhors mutilation of the body, and transplantation has been viewed skeptically. Nevertheless, in most Islamic and Buddhist countries, donation after death has been permitted if the explicit consent of the donor has been obtained before death (Muhammad Abdul-Rauf, "Medical ethics, history of: contemporary Muslim perspectives," and Hajime Nakamura, "Buddhism," in Warren T. Reich (ed.), *Encyclopedia of Bioethics* (New York: The Free Press, 1978). In Japan, however, a persistent public reluctance, particularly over the question of brain death, has prevented the medical profession from instituting heart, liver, and lung transplantation, although kidneys and corneas can be legally transplanted. See M. Brannigan, "A chronicle of organ transplant progress in Japan," *Transplant International* 5 (1992): 180–186.

33. Professor Warren Reich recalls that his first venture into bioethics was a lecture entitled "Medico-moral problems and the principle of totality: a Catholic viewpoint," given in a 1967 Veteran's Administration series on "Moral Questions in Medicine," (Washington, D.C.: Veterans Hospital Administration, 1967). He recalls that he was able to offer moral approbation of transplantation and, at the same time, place moral limits around it (interview, December 13, 1995). Dr. Edmund Pellegrino also recalls that his first contact with a medico-moral problem occurred when his philosophy professor at St. John's University presented him with a copy of Cunningham's thesis (interview, December 12, 1995). Dr. John Fletcher dates the beginnings of modern bioethics from Father Cunningham's novel thesis, since it opened the scope of medical morality to a wider population than patients alone (interview, October 15, 1995).

34. Paul Ramsey, *The Patient as Person: Explorations in Medical Ethics* (New Haven: Yale University Press, 1970), pp. 173, 197, citing Francis Moore, "New problems for surgery," *Science* 144 (1964): 391.

35. David Daube, "Transplantation: acceptability of procedures and the required legal sanctions," in Wolstenholme and O'Conner, *Law and Ethics of Transplantation*, p. 194.

36. David Louisell, "Transplantation: existing legal constraints," in Wolstenholme and O'Conner, *Law and Ethics of Transplantation*, p. 80.

37. Uniform Anatomical Gift Act, *Uniform Laws Ann* 15 (1983); Alfred Sadler and Blair Sadler, "Transplantation and the law," *Georgetown Law Review* 57, no. 4 (1968): 31; A. M. Sadler, B. L. Sadler, and E. Blythe Stason, "The Uniform Anatomical Gift Act," *Journal of American Medical Association* 206 (1968): 2501–2506.

38. Bernard Häring, *The Law of Christ: Moral Theology for Priests and Laity* Vol. III, trans. Edwin G. Kaiser (Westminster: Newman Press, 1964), p. 242; see also Roberta G. Simmons, Susan D. Klein, and Richard L. Simmons, *The Gift of Life: The Social and Psychological Impact of Organ Transplantation* (New York: Wiley, 1977); Harmon L. Smith, "Organ transplantation and experimentation," in *Ethics and the New Medicine* (Nashville: Abingdon Press, 1970), chapter 3. The charitable and donative principle of transplantation was reinforced by the law's adamant refusal to lower the barrier of bodily inviolability. In one case, the plea of a person who needed bone marrow transplantation was rejected by his cousin, the most compatible donor: the judge thought this morally reprehensible, but legally defensible. *McFall v Shimp* no. 78–17711 in Equity (Allegheny County, PA, July 26, 1978).

39. Harry S. Schwartz, "Bioethical and legal considerations in increasing the supply of transplantable organs: from UAGA to 'Baby Fae,'" *American Journal of Law and Medicine* 10 (1985): 397–438.

40. Willard Gaylin, "Harvesting the dead," *Harpers* 249 (September 1974): 23–30.

41. James L. Muyskens, "An alternative policy for obtaining cadaver organs," *Philosophy and Public Affairs* 8 (1978): 88–99, quote on p. 97.

42. Ramsey, *The Patient as Person*, p. 210.

43. Robert M. Veatch, *Death, Dying and the Biological Revolution: Our Last Quest for Responsibility* (New Haven: Yale University Press, 1976).

44. Arthur L. Caplan, "Organ transplants: the costs of success," *Hastings Center Report* 13, no. 6 (1983): 23–32.

45. "'Harvest of dead' bill advances in Richmond," *Washington Post*, January 23, 1981: C1; P. Lombardo, "Consent and 'donations' from the dead," *Hastings Center Report*, 11, no. 6 (1981): 9–10. Many European and Asian nations have laws that authorize procurement of organs without consent, as long as no objection from the patient, before death, or the patient's family is evidenced. For example, see Alain Raymond, "France: the automatic transplant," *Washington Post* August 16, 1978: A15. See Robert Veatch, "The Myth of presumed consent: ethical problems in new organ procurement strategies," *Transplantation Proceedings* 27 (1995): 1888–1892.

46. Arthur L. Caplan, "Ethical and policy issues in the procurement of cadaver organs for transplantation," *New England Journal of Medicine* 311 (1984): 981–983, "Obtaining and allocating organs for transplantation," in Dale H. Cowan, Jo Ann Kantorowitz, Jay Moskowitz, and Peter H. Rheinstein (eds.), *Human Organ Transplantation: Societal, Medical-Legal, Regulatory, and Reimbursement Issues* (Ann Arbor: Health Administration Press, 1987), pp. 5–17. Although Caplan was the first to publish the required request proposal, it had already been conceived and debated in the Hastings Project on Organ Transplantation (Robert Veatch, private communication).

47. James F. Blumstein and Frank A. Sloan (eds.), *Organ Transplantation Policy: Issues and Prospects* (Durham: Duke University Press, 1989).

48. A. K. Salahudeen, "High morality among recipients of bought living-unrelated donor kidneys," *Lancet* 336 (1990): 725–728.

49. Robert M. Veatch, "Medical ethics," *Journal of the American Medical Association* 252 (1984): 2296; Benjamin Freedman, "The ethical continuity of transplantation," *Transplant Proceedings* 17, Suppl. 4 (1985): 17–23.

50. Richard M. Titmuss, *The Gift Relationship: From Human Blood to Social Policy* (London: George Allen and Unwin, 1971).

51. Arthur L. Caplan, "Organ transplants: the costs of success," *Hastings Center Report* 13, no. 6 (1983): 23–32.

52. *1984 National Organ Transplantation Act*, Public Law, 98-507.

53. Task Force on Organ Transplantation, *Organ Transplantation: Issues and Recommendations* (Rockville, Md.: (DHHS), 1986), p. xxi.

54. The Hastings Center, "Ethical, legal and policy issues pertaining to solid organ procurement," *A Report of the Project on Organ Transplantation* (October 1985): 2, cited in the Task Force Report on Organ transplantation, *Organ Transplantation*, p. 28.

55. James Hardy, Carlos Chavez, Fred Kurrus, et al., "Heart transplantation in man: developmental studies and report of a case," *Journal of the American Medical Association* 188 (1969): 1132–1140.

56. Leonard L. Bailey, Sandra L. Nehlsen-Cannarella, Waldo Conception, and Weldon B. Jolley, "Baboon to human cardiac xenographic transplantation in a neonate," *Journal of the American Medical Association* 254 (1985): 3321–3329; Lawrence K. Altman, "Learning from Baby Fae," *New York Times* November 18, 1984: A1, 30.

57. Michael R. Harrison, Michael Golbus, Roy A. Filly (eds.), *The Unborn Patient: Prenatal Diagnosis and Treatment* (Philadelphia: W. B. Saunders, 1984); M. R. Harrison, M. S. Golbus,

R. A. Filly, A. R. Jonsen, et al., "Fetal surgery for congenital hydronephrosis," *New England Journal of Medicine* 306 (1982): 591–593.

58. Michael R. Harrison and Gilbert Meilaender, "The anencephalic newborn as organ donor," *Hastings Center Report* 16, no. 2 (1986): 21–23; John C. Fletcher, John A. Robertson, and Michael R. Harrison, "Primates and anencephalics as sources for pediatric organ transplants," *Fetal Therapy* 1 (1986): 150–164.

59. Alexander Morgan Capron, "Anencephalic donors: separate the dead from the dying," *Hastings Center Report* 17, no. 1 (1987): 5–9; John D. Arras and Shlomo Shinnar, "Anencephalic newborns as organ donors: a critique," *Journal of the American Medical Association* 259 (1988): 2284–2285; Larry R. Churchill and Rosa Lynn B. Pinkus, "The use of anencephalic organs: historical and ethical dimensions," *The Milbank Quarterly* 68, no. 2 (1990): 147–169. Physicians at Loma Linda medical school, acknowledging that anencephalics did not meet the legal definition of death, instituted an experimental protocol in which anencephalic infants were ventilated for two weeks and, if they met traditional cardiorespiratory death criteria, would be used as donors. The experiment failed to produce a single donor and was discontinued. Joyce L. Peabody, Janet R. Emery, and Stephen Ashwal, "Experience with anencephalic infants as prospective organ donors," *New England Journal of Medicine* 321 (1989): 344–350. See Joyce L. Peabody and Albert R. Jonsen, "Organ transplantation," in Ammon Goldworth, William Silverman, David K. Stevenson, Ernle W. D. Young (eds.), *Ethics and Perinatology* (New York: Oxford University Press, 1995), pp. 184–213.

60. Fox and Swazey, *The Courage to Fail*, chapter 7.

61. Artificial Heart Assessment Panel, *The Totally Implantable Artificial Heart: Economic, Ethical, Legal, Medical, Psychiatric, and Social Implications* (Bethesda, Md.: DHEW Publication No. (NIH)74-191, 1973), pp. 1, 197, 199–200.

62. Artificial Heart Assessment Panel, pp. 197, 199, 132; John R. Hogness and Malin VanAntwerp (eds.), *The Artificial Heart: Prototypes, Policies and Patients* (Institute of Medicine: Washington, D.C.: National Academy Press, 1991), 207; Albert R. Jonsen, "The totally implantable artificial heart," *Hastings Center Report* 3, no. 5 (1973): 1–4.

63. Lawrence K. Altman, "Dr. Clark's death laid to failure of all organs but artificial heart," *New York Times* March 25, 1983: A1; see also "Reflections of a reporter on unresolved issues," in Margery W. Shaw (ed.), *After Barney Clark: Reflections on the Utah Artificial Heart Program* (Austin: University of Texas Press, 1984), pp. 113–128.

64. T. A. Preston, "Who benefits from the artificial heart?" *Hastings Center Report* 15, no. 1 (1985): 5–7; Renée C. Fox and Judith P. Swazey, *Spare Parts: Organ Replacement in American Society* (New York: Oxford University Press, 1992), chapters 5 and 6; Albert R. Jonsen, "The artificial heart's threat to others," *Hastings Center Reports* 16, no. 1 (1986): 9–11.

65. *Artificial Heart and Assist Devices: Directions, Needs, Costs, Societal and Ethical Issues* (Rockville, Md.: DHHS, 1985), p. 35; Barbara J. Culliton, "The politics of the heart," *Science* 241 (1988): 283.

66. Artificial Heart Assessment Panel, *The Totally Implantable Artificial Heart*, Discussion I, p. 243.

67. James W. Haviland "Experience in establishing a community artificial kidney center," *Transaction of the American Clinical Climatics Association* 77 (1965): 130.

68. Personal communication to Albert Jonsen. I thank Dr. Scribner, Dr. Haviland, Dr. Charles Odegaard, president emeritus of the University of Washington, and Rev. John Darrah, last surviving member of the Committee, for their reminiscences which are recorded in John J. Quinn, "Who's Worth Saving: Social Worth and Selection for Scarce, Life-Saving, Medical Resources" (M.A. thesis, Department of Medical History and Ethics, University of Washington, 1995).

69. Shana Alexander, "They decide who lives, who dies," *Life* 53 (1962): 102–125.

70. Harold Schmeck, "Panel holds life or death vote in allotting of artificial kidney," *New York Times* May 6, 1962: A1.

71. Shana Alexander, "Covering the God committee," (paper read at the Birth of Bioethics Conference, Seattle, Wa., Sept. 23–24, 1992), transcript, pp. 24–26.

72. Jhan Robbins and June Robbins, "The rest are simply left to die," *Redbook*, November 1967, pp. 80–81.

73. Fox and Swazey, *The Courage to Fail*.

74. G. E. Schreiner, "Problems of ethics in relation to hemodialysis," in Wolstenholme and O'Connor, *Ethics in Medical Progress*, p. 128.

75. Paul Ramsey, *The Patient as Person*, chapter 7; James Childress, "Who shall live when not all can live?" *Soundings* 53 (1970): 339–355.

76. Fox and Swazey, *The Courage to Fail*, p. 241.

77. Belding Scribner, "Ethical problems of using artificial organs to sustain human life," *Transactions of the American Society of Artificial Internal Organs* 10 (1964): 209–212.

78. Judith Swazey, "Discovering the ethical dilemma," (paper read at the Birth of Bioethics Conference, Seattle, Wa., Sept. 23–24, 1992), transcript pp. 47–48.

79. Childress, "Who shall live when not all can live?" pp. 339–335; Edmond Cahn, *The Moral Decision. Right and Wrong in the Light of American Law* (Bloomington, Ind.: University of Indiana Press, 1955).

80. Nicholas Rescher, "The allocation of exotic medical lifesaving therapy," *Ethics* 79 (1969): 173–186.

81. Childress, "Who shall live when not all can live?," p. 343.

82. Ramsey, *The Patient as Person*, chapter 7.

83. Helmut Thielicke, "The doctor as judge of who shall live and who shall die," in Kenneth Vaux (ed.), *Who Shall Live: Medicine, Technology, and Ethics* (Philadelphia: Fortress Press, 1970), pp. 171–173.

84. David Sanders and Jesse Dukeminier, "Medical advance and legal lag: hemodialysis and kidney transplantation," *UCLA Law Review* 15 (1968): 366–380.

85. Paul Freund, "Introduction to the ethical aspects of experimentation with human subjects," *Daedalus* 98 (1969): xiii.

86. Gerald Winslow, *Justice and Triage* (Berkeley: University of California Press, 1982); Paul Ramsey, *The Patient as Person*, pp. 117–118, 253–255.

87. Cahn, *The Moral Decision*, p. 71.

88. Joseph F. Fletcher, "The Greater Good" (unpublished lecture, 1969).

89. Jay Katz and Alexander M. Capron, *Catastrophic Diseases: Who Decides What?: A Psychosocial and Legal Analysis of the Problems Posed by Hemodialysis and Organ Transplantation* (New York: Russell Sage Foundation, 1975), p. 193.

90. Charles Fried, *Medical Experimentation: Personal Integrity and Social Policy* (New York: Elsevier, 1974); John Harris, "The survival lottery," *Philosophy* 50 (1975): 81–87; L. Duane Willard, "Scarce medical resources and the right to refuse selection by artificial chance," *Journal of Medicine and Philosophy* 5 (1980): 225–229.

91. Arthur L. Caplan, *If I Were a Rich Man, Could I Buy a Pancreas?* (Bloomington: Indiana University Press, 1992); James F. Burdick, Jeremiah G. Turcotte, and Robert Veatch, "General principles for allocating human organs and tissues," *Transplantation Proceedings* (1992) 24: 2226–2235; M. Benjamin, C. Cohen, and E. Grochowski, for the Ethics and Social Impact Committee, "What transplantation can teach us about health care reform," *New England Journal of Medicine* 330 (1994): 858–860.

92. Fox and Swazey, *Courage to Fail*, chapter 8; H. Williams, "The first artificial kidney patient," *Seattle Times Magazine* July 11, 1971, pp. 8–9.

93. Richard A. Rettig, "Origins of the Medicare kidney disease entitlement: the Social Security Amendments of 1972," in Kathi E. Hanna (ed.), *Biomedical Politics* (Washington, D.C.: National Academy Press, 1991), pp. 176–206, 204; Rettig, "The policy debate on patient care financing for victims of end-stage renal disease," *Law and Contemporary Problems* 40 (1976): 196–206; Richard A. Rettig and Norman G. Levinsky (eds.), *Kidney Failure and the Federal Government* (Washington, D.C.: National Academy Press, 1991); Rettig, "The politics of health cost containment: end-stage renal disease," *Bulletin of the New York Academy of Medicine* 56 (1980): 115–137.

94. See Guido Calebresi and Philip Bobbitt, *Tragic Choices* (New York: Norton, 1978) for a provocative analysis of how public policy is made when life is at stake; many early bioethicists were impressed with this book.

95. Ramsey, *The Patient as Person*, p. 272.

96. Albert R. Jonsen and André E. Hellegers, "Conceptual foundations for an ethics of medical care," in Laurence R. Tancredi (ed.), *Ethics of Health Care* (Washington, D.C.: National Academy of Sciences, 1974), pp. 3–20; Paul Ramsey, "Commentary," in *Ethics of Health Care*, pp. 21–29.

97. Gene Outka, "Social justice and equal access to health care," *Journal of Religious Ethics* 2, no. 1 (1974): 11–32.

98. Robert M. Veatch, "What is a 'just' health care delivery?" and Ronald M. Green, "Health care and justice in contract theory perspective," in Veatch and Roy Branson (eds.), *Ethics and Health Policy* (Cambridge, Mass.: Ballinger Publishing Company, 1976), pp. 127–153; 111–126. Charles Fried, "Equality and rights in health care," *Hastings Center Report* 6, no. 1 (1976): 30–32. Dr. Robert Sade became the *bête noir* of all who favored a right to health are. It was a fallacy, he claimed, to suggest that there was a right to medical care. There certainly were natural rights: the rights to life and to freedom of action. Beyond these, people create products and property by their work and ingenuity and offer them to others in the marketplace. Medical care is just such a property, provided by doctors to those who wish to purchase it. Sade traces the fallacy that anyone other than the producers of care has a "right" to it through several government health-policy proposals, seeing in them unjust impositions on the doctor's freedom and on "the most fundamental professional commitment, that of using his best judgment at all times for the greatest benefit of his patient. . . . Any physician can say to those who would shackle his judgment and control his profession: I do not recognize your right to my life and my mind which belongs to me alone; I will not participate in legislated solutions to any health problems." Robert Sade, "Medical care as a right: a refutation," *New England Journal of Medicine* 285 (1971): 1288–1292, p. 1292. Dr. Sade's Ayn Randesque argument was met by a spate of furious letters in a subsequent issue of *The New England Journal*; Letters, *New England Journal of Medicine* (1972): 286: 488–493.

99. Renée Fox, "The medicalization and demedicalization of American society," (special issue, "Doing Better and Feeling Worse: Health in the United States") *Daedalus* 105 no. 1 (1977): 9–22, p. 13.

100. Dan Callahan, "Health and society: some ethical imperatives," *Daedalus* 105 no. 1 (1977): 33.

101. Charles Fried, "Equality and rights in health care," *Hastings Center Report* 6, no. 1 (1976): 30–32; Ronald Green, "The priority of health care," *Journal of Medicine and Philosophy* 8 (1983): 373–380; Laurence B. McCullough, "Justice and health care: historical perspectives and precedents," in Earl E. Shelp (ed.), *Justice and Health* (Dordrecht and Boston: D. Reidel, 1981), pp. 51–71. H. Tristram Engelhardt took a contrarian position, denying that ethical reasoning could devise a just pattern of resource allocation. There will be persons, he advised, who unfortunately need expensive health resources, but he found no solid argument to justify the claim

that such persons are treated unfairly, should society not provide them with those resources. "Differences in need, both medical and financial, must be recognized as unfortunate. . . . However, it must be understood that though unfortunate circumstances are always grounds for praiseworthy charity, they do not always provide grounds, by that fact, for redrawing the line between the circumstances we will count as unfortunate but not unfair and those we will count as unfortunate and unfair." H. Tristram Engelhardt, Jr., "Shattuck lecture: allocating scarce medical resources and the availability of organ transplantation: some moral presuppositions," *New England Journal of Medicine* 311 (1984): 66–71, pp. 67, 71.

102. K. D. C. Hadorn, "Setting health care priorities in Oregon: cost-effectiveness meets the rule of rescue," *New England Journal of Medicine* 265 (1991): 2218–2285; Albert R. Jonsen, "Bentham in a box: technology assessment and health care allocation," *Law, Medicine and Health Care* 14 (1986): 172–174.

103. President's Commission for the Study of Ethical Problems in Medicine and Biomedical and Behavioral Research, *Securing Access to Health Care: A Report on the Ethical Implications of Difference in the Availability of Health Services* (Washington, D.C.: Government Printing Office, 1983), p. 4.

104. President's Commission, *Securing Access to Health Care*, pp. 36–37.

105. Deirdre Carmody and Laurie Johnston, "Appeal for a child," *New York Times* October 29, 1982: B2; "Infant girl undergoes a liver transplant," *New York Times* November 6, 1982: B6.

106. "Report of the Massachusetts Task Force on Organ Transplantation," *Law, Medicine and Health Care* 13 (1) (1985): 8–27, pp. 9, 10–11. See Clark C. Havighurst and Nancy M. P. King, "Liver transplantation in Massachusetts: public policymaking as morality play," in James F. Blumstein and Frank A. Sloan (eds.), *Organ Transplantation Policy. Issues and Prospects* (Durham: Duke University Press, 1989), pp. 229–260.

107. John Rawls, *A Theory of Justice* (Cambridge: Belknap Press of Harvard University Press, 1971), p. 60.

108. Norman Daniels, *Just Health Care* (New York: Cambridge University Press, 1985), p. ix.

109. Norman Daniels, *Am I My Parents Keeper?: An Essay on Justice Between the Young and the Old* (New York: Oxford University Press, 1988), p. 82.

110. For example, see Nancy Jecker, "Toward a theory of age-group justice," *Journal of Medicine and Philosophy* 14 (1989): 655–676.

111. Mary B. Mahowald, "Neural fetal tissue transplantation: scientific, legal and ethical aspects," *Clinical Research* 36 no. 3 (1988): 187–188.

112. Advisory Committee to the Director, National Institutes of Health, *Report of the Human Fetal Tissue Transplantation Research Panel* (Washington, D.C.: National Institutes of Health, 1988); Dorothy Vawter, Warren Kearney, Karen Gervais, Arthur Caplan, Daniel Garry, and Carol Tauer, *The Use of Human Fetal Tissue: Scientific, Ethical and Policy Concerns* (Minneapolis: Center for Biomedical Ethics, University of Minnesota, 1990). A ban on federal funding of research using human fetal tissue was issued by the Assistant Secretary of Health in 1988, and remained intact until it was revoked by President Bill Clinton on January 22, 1993 (*Federal Register* 58: 7457).

113. Two of the early, sympathetic observers of the field of transplantation, Renée Fox and Judith Swazey, offered a severe criticism of its current state in *Spare Parts: Organ Replacement in American Society* (New York: Oxford University Press, 1992).

114. Alvin H. Moss and Mark Siegler, "Should alcoholics compete equally for liver transplantation?" *Journal of the American Medical Association* 265 (1991): 1295–1298.

115. Norman Daniels, *Seeking Fair Treatment: From the AIDS Epidemic to National Health Care Reform* (New York: Oxford University Press, 1995); Daniel W. Brock and Norman Daniels, "Ethical foundations of the Clinton administration's proposed health care system," *Journal of the*

American Medical Association 271 (1994): 1189–1196; E. Haavi Morreim, *Balancing Act: The New Medical Ethics of Medicine's New Economics* (Dordrecht/Boston: Kluwer Academic Publishers, 1991); Charles J. Dougherty, *American Health Care: Realities, Rights, and Reforms* (New York: Oxford University Press, 1988); Larry R. Churchill, *Rationing Health Care in America: Perceptions and Principles of Justice* (Notre Dame: University of Notre Dame Press, 1987).

8

Who Should Live? Who Should Die? The Ethics of Death and Dying

"Death, as the Psalmist says, is certain to all; all shall die," Justice Shallow tells Justice Silence in Shakespeare's *Henry IV*.[1] Justice Shallow's pious platitude is the one indubitable truth. Death has always been the expected and feared result of serious illness or severe injury, as well as the anticipated end of a long life. Human efforts to fend it off have been frail and futile. The manner in which humans meet death has been a constant theme of meditation and literature in every culture. During the Christian Middle Ages, writers and preachers expounded an "art of dying" (*ars moriendi*), preparation to encounter one's creator and redeemer. Physicians had relatively little part to play in the drama of human death. Greek physicians were admonished to refrain from applying their art to those who were "overmastered by their disease."[2] While this admonition lingered through the tradition of medical ethics, it was gradually mollified: even though physicians should not attempt to cure the incurable, they should remain with the dying to comfort them and relieve their pain. Thomas Percival eloquently urged his colleagues to be "the minister of hope and comfort to the sick; that by such cordials to the drooping spirit, he may smooth the bed of death, revive expiring life, and counteract the depressing influence of those maladies which rob the philosopher of fortitude and the Christian of consolation."[3]

German physician Carl F. H. Marx, writing in 1826, spoke of "that science, euthanasia, which checks oppressing features of illness, relieves pain and renders the supreme and inescapable hour a most peaceful one . . . [but never] should the physician be permitted, prompted either by other people's requests or by his own sense of mercy, to end the patient's pitiful condition by purposely and deliberately hastening death."[4] In this passage, the word "euthanasia," coined by Francis Bacon in the sixteenth century, appears in its etymological meaning, "a good or easy death." Dr. Marx, it appears, must have known some physicians who would consider another form of euthanasia—"deliberately hastening death"—although he, like most physicians in the Judeo-Christian tradition of medicine, would recoil in horror at the thought.

From the beginnings of medicine, apparent victory over impending death has resulted, often unknowingly, from the benign course of disease rather than from an applied treatment. During the nineteenth century, an improved science of pathology began to sharpen diagnostic skills and to anticipate therapeutic interventions that could reverse or impede the course of fatal disease. In the latter half of that century, surgical removal of tumors saved persons otherwise doomed to quick death (leaving them, often enough, to die of recurrent disease). In the 1930s, insulin stopped diabetes in its course to early death. At the end of the 1940s, the first antibiotics repelled lethal infection. After World War II, medicine was equipped with drugs to control hypertension, metabolic disorders, and cancer. Tuberculosis, "captain of the legions of death," in William Osler's words, almost disappeared from the fray. Devastating epidemic diseases, such as polio, yielded to perfected immunization. Surgery moved boldly into the heart and the brain. Anesthesia and respiratory support were also the beneficiaries of wartime research. During the 1950s and 1960s, medicine became what it had never been before: a science and an art of life saving.

One might think that such human progress against the ancient enemy would be cause only for rejoicing. Yet there were doubts that the progress was entirely pure. As the ability to detect cancer became sharper at the end of the nineteenth century, strenuous therapies, particularly surgical ones, promised prolonged life, but they gave instead a miserable, prolonged dying.[5] Pensive reflections about euthanasia appeared in the lay and medical press. Physicians wondered whether Dr. Marx's admonition that the physician should never hasten death was outdated. Perhaps "smoothing the bed of death," under the new conditions of medical treatment, should include hastening death.[6] Most authors were cautious; still, the notion grew that physicians might ethically back away from strenuous efforts to save life. An 1884 editorial in *The Boston Medical and Surgical Journal* (predecessor of *The New England Journal of Medicine*) summarized the profession's prevailing opinion:

> We suspect few physicians have escaped the suggestion in a hopeless case of protracted suffering to stand aside passively and give over any further attempt to prolong a life which has become a torment to its owner. . . . Shall not a man under such circumstances give up the fight, take off the spur of the stimulant and let exhausted nature sink to rest? . . . may there not come a time when it is a duty in the interest of the survivors to stop a fight which is only prolonging a useless and hopeless struggle?[7]

At that writing, "the spur of the stimulant" was almost the sole means of attempting to push breathing and heartbeat a bit further. Within the next half century, the effective means of sustaining life multiplied. Two unprecedented problems then faced the practitioner: first, how was clinical death to be defined and determined and, second, when should means of life support be withdrawn? These two questions were linked by the

most effective of the life-sustaining technologies, the respirator, a machine which confounded even the definition of death.

The Definition and Determination of Death

Homer describes the death of the hero, Sarpedon, "Even as Sarpedon spoke, the end of
death enfolded him, closing his eyes and nostrils. Patroclus set his foot upon the chest
and drew forth from his midriff both the spear and the soul of Sarpedon."[8] These signs
of death, and their intimation that the familiar yet mysterious element called life or soul
is gone, have long seemed tragically obvious: a moving, speaking person becomes mo-
tionless and silent; eyes close, breathing ceases, and "the soul" is gone. At this point,
the family begins to mourn, or the victor, like Patroclus, exults. Religious rituals are
performed and the body is prepared for disposition. If a physician has been in atten-
dance during the dying, he or she withdraws. Unless invited back to study the remains,
the physician's duties end at death. Although the physiology of death itself was, and
still is, mysterious, the last breath is a compelling sign. Myth, religion, common sense,
and common law have enshrined that moment as the end of life. In many languages,
"breath" and "spirit" share the same word, and in many cultures and religions, the last
breath marks the departure of the spirit of the person, or of nature, or of God from the
body it had animated. Jewish law from the most ancient times has respected that sign:
Maimonides wrote, "If, upon examination, no sign of breathing can be detected at the
nose . . . he is already dead."[9]

Civil and criminal law has always been interested in the time of death, since what
causes death, and when it occurs, can have momentous legal consequences. Law has
directed doctors, as their final duty toward the patients, to declare death according to
their best knowledge. That best knowledge was the simple observation of the signs that
every person could recognize. Since the sixteenth century, medical science slowly began to appreciate the relation between respiration and circulation of the blood; whatever the cause, failure of the lungs to deliver oxygen to the blood leads rapidly to unconsciousness and death. *Black's Law Dictionary* defines death as "the cessation of life
. . . defined by physicians as a total stoppage of the circulation of the blood and a cessation of the animal and vital functions consequent thereon, such as respiration, pulsa-
tion, etc."[10]

Efforts to support failing respiration are reported as far back as Vesalius who, in his
classic *De Humani Corporis Fabrica* (1543), describes use of a bellows to inflate the
lungs of an animal. Dr. John Daziel, an eighteenth-century Scots physician, invented a
body-enveloping tank with a bellows to create negative pressures in synchrony with inspiration. The British and American Life Saving Services of the nineteenth century
trained their men to perform various resuscitative techniques on persons drowned. Surgeons working with the new and dangerous anesthetics struggled to revive patients who
suffered cardiac arrest on the operating table. These efforts were usually futile. How-

ever, the epidemics of poliomyelitis, which racked the United States and Europe during the 1930s and 1940s, made the development of effective respiratory support a priority. In the bulbar form of that disease, lung muscles are paralyzed. Parents and physicians watched children "become more and more dyspneic . . . silent, wasting no breath for speech, wide-eyed, frightened, conscious almost to the last breath."[11]

In 1929, Philip Drinker and Charles McKhann invented a tank respirator to support breathing of polio patients whose lung muscles were paralyzed. The patient was enveloped in a metal tank and an electric pump drew air in and out, creating a negative–positive vacuum cycle that pushed the chest up and down.[12] These devices, known officially as Drinker Tanks and unofficially as iron lungs, saved many patients during the critical phase of their paralysis. At the same time, their use raised a perplexing question. In 1941, Dr. James Wilson wrote, "The question concerns the ultimate value of the respirator in the treatment of poliomyelitis, and it arises because of the painful experience that physicians have had with patients who have survived after long and expensive dependence on a respirator but who are so extensively paralyzed that one can wonder as to the value of their lives to themselves or to others. . . . one moves quickly to questions of philosophy and ethics which are not necessary to discuss here." Dr. Wilson's philosophical and ethical questions were not widely discussed, although many a physician, family and patient must have agonized over them.[13]

A polio epidemic raged through Denmark in 1952. In an attempt to provide a more effective means of assisting patients, Dr. Bjorn Ibsen, chief anesthesiologist of the Beegdam Hospital, brought the techniques of operating room anesthesia to the bedside. He inserted a tube into a patient's windpipe and applied positive pressure by squeezing a hand-held bag. Seventy-five patients were kept alive by 250 medical students who sat by the bedside pumping the bag. A mechanical substitute for medical students was quickly invented and the modern ventilator was born. The mechanical air pump spread rapidly through the hospitals of the world. Patients brought to the hospital with stroke, myocardial infarction, or diabetic coma, with their breathing severely impaired, could be tided over by this miraculous machine until they could breathe again.

As physicians worked with the respirator, they realized that some patients failed ever again to breathe on their own and some patients slipped into deep unconsciousness, kept alive only by the pumping respirator. What was the right course: should they allow these patients to die? should they judge them already dead? Leaders in the field of anesthesiology took the opportunity to submit these moral questions to one of the world's moral authorities, Pope Pius XII. At a gathering of medical scientists in Rome on November 24, 1957, the Pope responded to three questions posed by Dr. Bruno Haid, chief anesthesiologist at the University of Innsbruck Hospital. First, is one obliged to use modern artificial respiration equipment in all cases, even those which in the doctor's judgment are completely hopeless? Second, does one have the right to remove the respiration apparatus when, after several days, the state of deep unconsciousness does not improve if, when it is removed, blood circulation will stop within a few minutes? third, must a patient in deep unconsciousness through paralysis of the respiratory centers, whose life—that is, circulation—is maintained through artificial respiration, and who does not improve after several days, be considered . . . dead?

The Pope opened his response with a little treatise on the contemporary state of the art of "reanimation," then "willingly" answered the questions.[14] He stated that, in principle, persons are obliged to use "only ordinary means—that is means that do not involve any grave burden for oneself or another" to preserve life. Thus, when respiratory support is an extraordinary means, it can be withdrawn. This depends, however, upon the patient's permission or on the family's permission based upon the presumed wish of the patient. He reformulated the third question as, "has death already occurred after grave trauma of the brain, which has caused deep unconsciousness and central breathing paralysis, the fatal consequences of which have been retarded by artificial respiration? Or does death occur only with complete arrest of circulation?" The answer, he said, does not lie within the competence of the Church and cannot be deduced from any religious or moral principle. It is an open question. The Pope then invited physicians to invent a clear and precise definition of death. Yet the Pope also said, "human life continues as long as its vital functions—as distinguished from simple life of organs—manifests itself." This added a complexity to the medical question of fact and invited the doctors to approach the questions of philosophy and ethics that Dr. Wilson had shied away from years before. Dr. Julius Korein, a pioneer in the neurology of death and coma, has written that the Pope's answer to Dr. Haid was "the initiation of the major events in the evolution of criteria . . . that will allow the physician to diagnose brain death."[15]

As the Pope was speaking to the anesthesiologists, medical research was being done that might help close the open question. In the late 1950s, French neurologists were studying groups of patients who were in profound coma, so profound that the researchers coined the phrase, *coma depassé* or "ultra-coma." They correlated absence of electrical activity of the brain with irreversible dysfunction of that organ. *Coma depassé* was a sort of "death of the brain," diagnosable by technical means, with a reliable prognosis that consciousness would never return. This clinical work suggested that a new way of determining death could be added to, or could substitute for, the cardiorespiratory signs that had been traditionally used.[16]

This medical information interested anesthesiologists who had been liberated from the operating suite and were now managing the new intensive care units. They had patients who had suffered severe head injuries and who were in *coma depassé*. *Coma depassé* was even of greater interest to another group with a new therapy, the transplanters. Their problem was how to retrieve from cadavers organs for transplant that still had the physiological properties that would enable them to function within their new host. Is a person in deep coma a cadaver from whom organs can be removed? Is *coma depassé* the same as death?

The 1966 Ciba Foundation Conference on Transplantation devoted considerable attention to the unanswered questions about the determination of the death of organ donors. Dr. G. P. J. Alexandre of the University of Louvain Hospital told the conferees that some European transplant surgeons had begun to remove organs from persons in *coma depassé*. He said "irreversible damage to the central nervous system is an indication of physiological death that permits us to take an organ from a body that is already a cadaver." He proposed four criteria: "bilateral dilatation of pupils, absence of reflexes, absence of spontaneous respiration, falling blood pressure and flat electroencephalogram." The conferees expressed great interest. Dr. Joseph Murray remarked, "These criteria are excellent. This is the kind of formulation that we will need before we can approach the legal profession."[17] The legal profession was not quite ready to be approached. Jurisprudent David Daube warned that "a re-definition (of death) with an avowed purpose might well create doubts in the mind of the layman; he might fear that there is room here for a transition from a definition to euthanasia." Some of Murray's transplant colleagues were also hesitant. Dr. Thomas E. Starzl stated, "I doubt that any of the members of our transplantation team could accept a person as being dead as long as there was a heart beat." A skeptical British transplanter, Roy Y. Calne, commented, "I am sure the public would at present reject Dr. Alexandre's criteria of death."[18]

The medical literature manifested uncertainty; persons who were the sources of organs were described as "dead" or "immanently dead" or "irreversibly dying." Problematic legal cases had already arisen. In England, for example, organs were taken from a Mr. Potter who, to the transplanter, was "virtually dead," and to the coroner, was still alive.[19] In the U.S., Clarence Nicks was beaten "to death" by an assailant but, after being placed on a respirator, his heart continued to beat until it was transplanted into John Stuckwish. The prosecutor worried that an indictment against Mr. Nicks's assailant would be clouded by the surgeon's action. The defendant's attorney said, "It will be our contention that Nicks wasn't dead."[20] At least two transplanters, Dr. Norman Shumway and Dr. John Hume, were in legal jeopardy for removing hearts.

Harvard Definition of Brain Death

A bold stroke to dispel the uncertainty appeared: *Journal of the American Medical Association* for August 5, 1968 published "A definition of irreversible coma: report of the ad hoc committee at Harvard medical school to examine the definition of brain death."[21] The report began, "Our primary purpose is to define irreversible coma as a new criterion for death." This is an astonishing sentence: death, which appears as the divinely appointed end of life only 49 verses into the *Book of Genesis* (Genesis 2: 17), is to be newly defined! The ad hoc committee was the creation of Dr. Henry Beecher who, with the concurrence of Dean Robert Ebert, called it together early in 1968. In addition to eight physicians, including transplant surgeons John Merrill and Joseph Murray, three non-medical faculty were invited to join: William Curran, Professor of Health Law in the School of Public Health, Everett Mendelsohn, a professor of the history of science, and Ralph Potter, a professor of social ethics in the School of Divinity. Potter recalls relatively little dispute over the development of a policy. Dr. Beecher and Professor Curran were the drafters, with the aid of Neurosurgeon William Sweet. The committee worked swiftly and approved the draft with relatively minor changes.

"A definition of irreversible coma" recognizes both the intensive-care and the transplantation problems. Paul Ramsey later imputed base utilitarian motives to Dr. Beecher's eagerness to redefine death, citing Beecher, "If these new criteria of brain death are accepted, tissues and organs now consigned to the grave can be utilized to restore those who, although critically ill, can be saved." However, Professor Curran recalls that Dr. Beecher was sincerely concerned about the intensive-care problem, although the organ-salvage problem was clearly in the minds of a committee on which two transplanters sat.[22] The report reflects these priorities in its opening remarks; the revision of the criteria for defining death was needed because "(1) improvements in resuscitative and supportive measures have led to increased efforts to save those who are desperately injured. Sometimes these efforts have led to partial success so that the result is an individual whose heart continues to beat but whose brain is irreversibly damaged. . . . (2) obsolete criteria for definition of death can lead to controversy in obtaining organs for transplantation."

The report is a pastiche, stitching together some medical information, a legal opinion, and a theological statement. It opens with a list of the physical and neurological characteristics of "irreversible coma": unresponsiveness, no movements or breathing, no reflexes, and, "of great confirmatory value, a flat electroencephalogram." These were essentially the criteria mentioned by Dr. Alexandre at the Ciba Conference. The criteria are followed by a legal commentary, written by Professor Curran, that describes the current state of law, which considers "the definition of death to be a settled, scientific, biological fact," properly described by the commonly accepted cardiorespiratory signs. Several cases are mentioned to demonstrate this fact. The report takes the position that legislative action would rarely be necessary to adopt new criteria, since "the law treats this question as one of fact to be determined by physicians." The committee then "suggests that responsible medical opinion is ready to accept new criteria for pronouncing death to have occurred in an individual sustaining irreversible coma as a result of permanent brain damage." Treating physicians, who should consult and who should avoid conflict of interest, should make the decision. The report sutures this medical–legal text to the solemn words of Pope Pius XII. Dr. Beecher was himself present when the Pope spoke those words (a photo of the event shows him standing next to the Pope).[23] Dr. Murray had heard an Italian transplant surgeon, Dr. Raffaello Cortesini, quote that same speech at the Ciba conference. The Harvard report reduces the Pope's allocution to two affirmations: first, it is "not within the competence of the Church" to determine the moment of death; second, "extraordinary means are not obligatory in hopeless cases." Thus, editorializes the report, "It is the church's view that a time comes when resuscitation efforts should stop and death be unopposed." The theologian on the committee, Ralph Potter, admitted years later that he could not recall having made any theological contribution. "After all, wasn't the Pope enough?" he mused.[24] Finally, another medical piece is patched on, emphasizing that the "brain death syndrome" of which the report speaks, is intended to cover "coincident paralysis of brainstem and basal ganglionic mechanisms."

The ad hoc committee asserted that "responsible medical opinion" was ready for its new criterion of death. No evidence of that readiness is provided. Indeed, an editorial in the *Journal of the American Medical Association,* appearing in the same year as the Harvard report, commented, "It seems ironic that the end point of existence, which ought to be as clear and sharp as in a chemical titration, should so defy the power of words to describe it and the power of men to say with certainty, 'it is here.'"[25] The Harvard ad hoc committee issued a needed and welcome clarification in the midst of these doubts and reaction was rapid. In 1970, Kansas enacted legislation that recognized the "new criterion," allowing "absence of spontaneous brain function" to serve alongside "absence of spontaneous respiration and circulation" as a definition of death.[26] Many states followed suit with widely differing statutory language. It was possible to be dead one way in one state and dead in another way in the neighboring state. The confusion that the Harvard ad hoc committee had hoped to dispel returned.

The Harvard report, despite its fame, is odd in many ways. Its science is done without a single reference to any neurological research (indeed, it has only one citation— the Pope's speech!). It mixes two distinguishable situations, "irreversible coma" and the abolition of function at "brain-stem levels." Its very title confuses "irreversible coma" with "brain death." It is never clear whether "stopping life support to allow death" or whether "stopping respiratory support on a dead body" is the issue. Finally, although the title proclaims it and the text constantly states it, the report does not "define" death.

Nevertheless, the report became authoritative soon after its publication. It canonized the concept of brain death, gave physicians guidance in diagnosing this condition, and gave transplanters access to fresh organs. Courts could avoid the embarrassing situation of indicting transplant surgeons as murderers. States could more easily justify statutes that recognized these "new criteria" (for the legal situation was not as simple as the report had suggested). After the Kansas legislation, twenty-six states had passed laws by the end of the decade. Several model statutes were proposed by the American Bar Association (1975), the American Medical Association (1979), and by lawyer Alexander Capron and physician Leon Kass.[27] Two other statements on brain criteria for death appeared in the same year, with almost the same criteria—one from the French Ministry of Health and the other from the Council for International Organizations of Medical Sciences.[28]

Despite this progress in understanding and in legislation, uncertainty remained about brain death. The scientific basis of the Harvard report and its formulations did not satisfy some observant readers.[29] The difference between permanent unconsciousness, usually caused by cerebral damage, and to which the term "brain death" was often applied, and the state of total organic disintegration perplexed physicians and the public. The statutes framed during the 1970s contained poorly drafted language. Some laws seemed to abolish the old criteria, while others seemed to require elaborate medical verification of every death. The most crucial problem was a properly philosophical one: what are the human functions that define human life and how are their presence and absence recognized?

The first persons to address this problem were two scientists: Professor Robert Morison and Dr. Leon Kass, who debated the definition of death during a Hastings-sponsored symposium at the 1970 meeting of the American Association for the Advancement of Science. Professor Morison proposed that death was not an event but a process commencing at the beginning of life and progressing through its entirety. He argued that "redefining" death, while reasonable as an effort to solve practical problems such as transplantation, was inadvisable because it fixed death to a particular set of physiological phenomenon. The process of death required a more comprehensive evaluation of the entire organism and its functions. "As the complexity and richness of the interactions of an individual human wax and wane," maintained Morison, "his 'value' can be seen to change in relation to other values." In his carefully argued riposte, Kass posited that death was an event, which should be defined by specific physiological criteria; above all, the ethics of discontinuing life support must fix on the value of the dying person to himself, not, as he had heard Morison say, on his value to others. This philosophical argument by scientists was a luminous moment in the initial days of bioethics.[30]

Hans Jonas was the first philosopher to speak on this topic. In his essay "Reflections on human experimentation," he commented on the recently published Harvard report with some disquiet. While he agreed with the Harvard report's first rationale for the redefinition of death, namely, allowing permanently unconscious patients to die, he strongly disagreed with the second rationale, that is, the designation of a permanently unconscious person as dead for the purpose of removing organs for transplant.[31] Jonas's objection "drew fire from within the medical profession" and he subsequently "engaged in private exchanges . . . with medical friends . . . conducted in the most amicable spirit of shared concern . . . which sharpened [his] theoretical case." Those private exchanges were with my own medical friends, Drs. Otto Guttentag, Samuel Kountz, and Harrison Sadler of the University of California, San Francisco, School of Medicine, all members of the committee on brain death that Dr. Engleburt Dunphy had invited me to join in 1969. Dr. Guttentag, a friend of Jonas, asked him to expatiate on his earlier opinion for the benefit of the UCSF committee. When I first met this group, they already had in their hands Professor Jonas's paper, which was later published as "Against the stream."[32]

Jonas positioned himself against the torrent of efforts to redefine death that made the organism of human beings, once lacking all higher functions, a mine of organs and, in the long run, a thing of which any socially beneficial use could be made. "We must remember," he said, "that what the Harvard group offered was not a definition of irreversible coma as a rationale for breaking off sustaining action, but a definition of death by the criterion of irreversible coma as a rationale for transposing the patient's body to the class of dead things, regardless of whether sustaining action is kept up or broken off

. . . [this was] motivated not by the exclusive interests of the patient but with extraneous interests in mind . . . [and thus] they serve the ruling pragmatism of our time which will let no ancient fear and trembling interfere with the relentless expanding of the realm of sheer thinghood and unrestricted utility."[33] Jonas saw the second rationale for redefinition as evidence of the utilitarian attitude that he had also condemned in experimentation.

Paul Ramsey agreed with Jonas in an erudite chapter, "On updating procedures for stating that a man has died." He praised efforts to update criteria for determining death that were meant to dissipate ambiguities about death, imminent death, and virtual death. But updating criteria to increase the supply of organs available for transplantation was to be repudiated. "The canons of highest loyalty to the primary patient can best be assured," he wrote, "if neither the procedures for stating death nor a decision that death has occurred are distorted by any reference to someone else's need for organs."[34]

Robert Veatch was a vocal critic of the Harvard criteria: "That report stated in its first sentence that 'Our primary purpose is to define irreversible coma as a new criterion of death.' It said this in spite of the fact that nowhere following that sentence was there even a hint of an argument . . . that irreversible coma was synonymous with the death of the person as a whole." The report, Veatch correctly recognized, was a statement of technical criteria to predict the irreversibility of prolonged coma. But, he wondered, should persons in irreversible coma be treated as if they were dead. A serious reflection on the definition of death was still needed. He stipulated that an entity was considered dead "when there is a complete change in the status of that entity characterized by the irreversible loss of those characteristics that are essentially significant to it." Veatch suggested four different concepts of death that might make more specific this general stipulation: irreversible loss of the soul, irreversible stopping of "vital" body fluids, irreversible loss of bodily integration, and irreversible loss of consciousness or capacity for special interaction. Each of these concepts of death has been widely believed; each represents a different view of what constitutes the "characteristics that are essentially significant"; and each concept has its own problems of empirical verification.[35] The Harvard report fails to address any of these issues.

During the decade after the Harvard criteria appeared, philosophers found a properly philosophical task of offering analyses of personhood and of personal identity that might support one or another of the practical formulations for the determination of death. Theologians also claimed a right to speak, for theology has reflected upon the meaning of death, if not its definition, from time immemorial.[36] The Harvard report, then, was less a conclusion than a beginning.

The President's Commission: Defining Death

Sufficient doubt, confusion, and concern persisted during the decade after the Harvard report that those who framed the mandate for the President's Commission directed the commissioners to study "the ethical and legal implications of the matter of defining death, including the advisability of developing a uniform definition of death."[37] This was the Commission's first mandate, which was discussed at the initial meeting, January 14, 1980. Immediately, the commissioners realized that the question of a uniform statute for the definition of death was closely related to the more general problem of discontinuing life support. They decided to pursue this second question in a separate report.

At the Commission's second meeting, staff philosopher Dan Wikler surveyed the conceptual issues involved in defining death, distinguishing between arguments based on the loss of essential characteristics (such as rationality), arguments based on a concept of personal identity, and arguments that rested on certain valuations of life. Robert Veatch explained the policy issues associated with social decisions to treat a person as dead. He reminded the commissioners of the distinct meanings of death that he had described in his previous writings. He warned against the use of the term "brain death," which could refer either to cessation of brain functions or to the death of a person based upon that cessation. Both Wikler and Veatch stressed the importance of deciding whether the definition of death should turn on loss of "higher" human functions or on a more total organic disintegration. At its July meeting, a series of round table discussions helped the Commission understand the scientific aspects of the question and the religious issues that it raised.[38] The first draft of a report was presented for discussion at the September meeting; a second draft met general approbation at the November meeting. The Commission endorsed the final report, *Defining Death,* on July 9, 1981.[39]

In *Defining Death,* the Commission evaluated whether the best legal policy was to leave the definition of death to medical judgment, leave it to court decisions, or to recommend statutory legislation. It concluded that legal jurisdictions should enact the following Uniform Determination of Death Act:

> An individual who has sustained either (1) irreversible cessation of circulatory and respiratory functions, or (2) irreversible cessation of all functions of the entire brain, including the brain stem, is dead. A determination of death must be made in accordance with accepted medical standards.[40]

This formulation expressed the Commission's conclusion that death was a unitary phenomenon that can be demonstrated either on the traditional grounds of irreversible cessation of heart and lung function, or on the basis of irreversible loss of all functions of the entire brain. We had listened to some philosophers arguing that a "higher brain" definition was theoretically more convincing. At the same time, we were acutely conscious that such a definition would be revolutionary: it would classify as "dead" a multitude of breathing persons whose organic functions were intact, either precipitating their disposal or opening their bodies to the utilitarian purposes that had troubled Hans Jonas. The unitary definition was admittedly conservative: it recognized that "brain death" and "cardiopulmonary death" were physiologically the same phenomenon, but recognizable by different clinical signs. Thus, the Commission's definition did not move far from current clinical practice, legal understanding, and public attitudes. At the same time, it allowed physicians to remove mechanical life support from "breathing" cadavers and to designate certain individuals who were dead, but still organically viable, as organ donors. The several organizations that had proposed model statutes quickly agreed to the Commission's formulation, and within the next several years, almost every state had enacted the uniform definition into a statute or endorsed it in case law.[41]

Defining Death brought conceptual clarity to a confused issue and helped to make good law. But it also contributed to the evolution of bioethics as a discipline and as a form of discourse. The report resulted from a careful inspection of the state of the dispute, as found in the literature and in the discussions of many scholars and scientists. The commissioners had the opportunity to hear alternative viewpoints. They weighed the cogency of certain theoretical philosophical opinions against the practical problems those arguments raised. They formulated conclusions that they judged had adequate conceptual and logical support and that could also be useful for policy formulation and legal determination. This form of doing ethics, which moved between the logic of moral philosophy and the exigencies of practical policy, had now become a characteristic of bioethics as discipline and as public discourse.

Neonatal Intensive Care

The killing of infants at birth has a long, dark history. In many cultures, babies too weak to survive, or marked with some defect, or unwanted by their parents have been exposed to the elements, drowned, or smothered.[42] When physicians became involved in birthing, they sometimes became accomplices in ending new life. This was usually done surreptitiously.[43] Yet most physicians struggled to save newborn life with the meager means at their disposal. A pioneer in the care of the newborn, the late Dr. Clement Smith of Harvard, described his experience as a young pediatrician in the 1930s: "If a two pound baby of 30 weeks gestation could not survive when drained of mucus and placed in a warm environment of extra oxygen, no procedure then known to us seemed very likely to increase his chances. If he died, we presumed he was, in simple terms, unable to live."[44]

Incubators that controlled heat and humidity for premature babies were invented by a French physician in the 1880s; the first clinic for premature infants was opened at La Maternité in Paris in 1893. Dr. Julius Hess opened the first American clinic at Chicago's Michael Reese Hospital in 1922. The technology to deal with lung immaturity, the major lethal problem of these tiny babies, did not become available until the 1950s. In that decade, advances in the understanding of lung physiology, techniques of ventilatory support, and methods to monitor blood gases were developed. The term "neonatology" first appeared in Alexander Schaffer's 1960 text *Diseases of the Newborn*.[45]

During the next twenty years, neonatology grew apace. In 1963, this new specialty served a famous patient, Patrick Bouvier Kennedy, son of President and Mrs. John F. Kennedy. Born on August 7, he was five and one half weeks premature and weighed slightly less than five pounds. After transfer from the Cape Cod hospital where he was born to Childrens' Medical Center in Boston, he died of "ideopathic respiratory distress syndrome" after only 38 hours. By 1982, 600 neonatal intensive care units, with 7,500 beds, had come into existence, a growth stimulated by state legislation throughout the country that mandated private insurance payment for neonatal intensive care.[46] One thousand board certified neonatologists, a subspecialty of pediatrics established in 1975, presided over these units. The patients, some 230,000 babies, or seven percent of all live births, were primarily of low birth weight (2,500 grams or less), born between a month and a few weeks before their due date. The primary affliction of these tiny patients is "ideopathic respiratory distress syndrome," due to the immaturity of their lungs, but along with this problem, they suffer many other cardiac, neurological, and gastrointestinal problems. These infants are at high risk of death in the first days of life; the smallest are certain to die within hours of birth. However, during the decade 1970–1980, the death rate in the first month of life was almost cut in two; half of the infants born at 1,000 grams (2.2 pounds) survived, compared with only 10 percent in 1960.

Yet the survivors were not guaranteed a healthy life. Many suffered chronic lung disease and, even more distressing, neurological insults that often led to mental retardation. In the early years of neonatal intensive care, the terrible suspicion arose that the treatment itself—administration of oxygen—was causing retrolental fibroplasia, damage to the eyes that results in blindness.[47] Thus, the ambiguity that plagues modern medical treatment was a constant threat in the intensive care nursery: treatment could save a life, but at the same time, leave that life terribly damaged. The tiny tragedies of the nursery were about to be projected on a large screen.

On Saturday, October 16, 1971, a large audience gathered at the Kennedy Center for the Performing Arts to attend The Joseph P. Kennedy Jr. Foundation International Symposium on Human Rights, Retardation and Research, "Choices on our Conscience." The symposium opened with a shocking 30-minute movie. Filmed a few weeks before by Werner Schuman, who had made the Bobby Kennedy presentation film for the 1968 Democratic convention, and financed largely by the John Simon Guggenheim Foundation, the short movie was designed as a lightning rod for debate around the topic of the symposium—the rights of the retarded, a subject close to the hearts of the Kennedy family, who cherished their retarded sister, Rosemary. The film told the story of two young parents who refused to permit a simple operation that would save the life of their newborn baby. The baby was, in the language of the day, a "mongol," stricken with the genetic disorder Down's syndrome, which always promises a future of mild to severe mental retardation. This baby had a frequently associated defect, a blockage between esophagus and stomach that prevented the passage of food. Surgeons can easily correct this defect, but the child's developmental future is uncorrectable.

The film was a composite of three cases that had occurred in the pediatric depart-

ment of the Johns Hopkins Medical School. The chairman of the department was Dr.
Robert E. Cooke, who had two children with developmental disabilities. He had become a close friend of the Kennedy family, which had established a research institute
on mental retardation at Johns Hopkins. Eunice Kennedy Shriver asked Dr. Cooke to
suggest a case that could serve as a vivid opener for the symposium. Cooke called the
chief pediatric resident, Dr. Norman Fost, and the intern who had been involved in the
most recent case, Dr. William Bartholome. Dr. Bartholome suggested that a film might
be more provocative than an oral presentation, and Mrs. Shriver enthusiastically
agreed.

   Schuman decided to use as actors Dr. Bartholome, the surgeon Dr. Alex Haller, and
several nurses who had been involved in the most recent case. These amateurs performed with compelling credibility. Young Dr. Bartholome was distressed by the events
of the case. Years later, he described himself as "an angry young man, a product of the
60s, who had chosen to be a saver of children." As an undergraduate at the Jesuit college in Kansas City, he wrote his senior thesis on the Catholic teaching about the ethics
of ectopic pregnancy. When, during the early months of his first residency year, he
found himself caring for a baby whose parents had refused life-saving surgery, he "experienced a sense of moral outrage . . . it was simply wrong, unjust, intolerable."[48]
As the little drama was being written and filmed, Bill Bartholeme formed a reasoned
opinion that children with Down's syndrome were full members of the human community, with the same claim on medical care as any other person. No one in the film expressed a moral opinion about the events, but Dr. Bartholome's "moral outrage" was
evident in his face and body language. The film ended with a discussion in which Dr.
Cooke, psychologist Sydney Callahan, health law professor William J. Curran, sociologist Renée Fox, and ethicist John C. Fletcher participated. As the final scene faded, a
grieving nurse carried the baby into a back corner of the nursery to die and Fletcher's
hushed voice was heard, "Wow!"

   After the movie, Roger Mudd of CBS News moderated a panel consisting of Professors Paul A. Freund of Harvard Law School and James M. Gustafson of Yale Divinity
School, social critic Michael Harrington, social psychologist Dr. Sydney Callahan, and
Senator Walter Mondale, who discussed the legal, ethical, social, psychological, and
public policy aspects of the case. The speakers were obviously moved by the film. In
the afternoon, groups of prominent persons, from Nobelists Joshua Lederberg and
James Watson to novelist William Styron, discussed various aspects of the general
topic. After the conference, the speakers gathered for dinner at the Shrivers' home,
Timberlawn, where they drew up a "call to action," urging the world community to
consider more seriously the problems raised by scientific advances: "Present legal
structures must be examined to ascertain whether, under the conditions established by
the new technologies, some persons, especially the powerless and helpless, such as infants, the sick, the retarded, the elderly, have rights that stand in need of defense."

   Although *The New York Times* summarized the tenor of the Timberlawn statement, it
was published in an obscure journal some months after the conference and never came

into public view.⁴⁹ The proceedings of "Choices on our Conscience" were never published and only Gustafson's comments and Paul Freund's remarks saw the light of day.⁵⁰ The short film, however, became a landmark in the history of bioethics. As Bartholeme said, "It was for bioethics like a crystal in a supersaturated solution—it attracted attention, gave bioethics something concrete to teach and talk about."⁵¹

The film on the Johns Hopkins baby thrust neonatal intensive care into the ambit of the early bioethics and stimulated some of the earliest serious bioethical analysis. Gustafson's commentary on the film, which was delivered at the symposium and published in *Perspectives in Biology and Medicine,* is a careful dissection of the ethical problem and a notable contribution to the early bioethics literature. An article by two pediatricians, Drs. Raymond S. Duff and A. G. M. Campbell, moved the problem from the prismatic case of a single child into the statistical world of the intensive care nursery. Drs. Duff and Campbell reported that out of 299 consecutive deaths in their nursery at the Yale-New Haven Hospital, 43 (14%) resulted from deliberate decisions to withdraw or withhold life-saving treatment.⁵² This article revealed to the world what neonatologists understood only too well: many premature babies who need the technology of the intensive care nursery fail the therapeutic rigors of that technology and are allowed to die by being deliberately removed from the ventilators. The article caused a furor. Many letters of protest were written to the *New England Journal.*⁵³ Yale's President Brewster later told me that he had never received so many outraged letters about an event on his campus (this was several years before the racial protests that caused President Brewster even more pain).

Father Richard McCormick reflected on the Duff and Campbell article in "To save or let die,"⁵⁴ in which he revisited the familiar Catholic distinction between ordinary and extraordinary care. The term "extraordinary" was large enough to justify the omission of life-sustaining treatments on the basis of expected diminished quality of life, defined in terms of the potential for human relationship. John Fletcher's "Abortion, euthanasia and care of the defective newborn" and H. Tristram Engelhardt's "Ethical issues in aiding the death of young children" soon appeared—the former defending passive, but not active, euthanasia for the seriously compromised newborn; the latter contending that maintenance of life for such children should be seen as inflicting the "injury of continued existence."⁵⁵

Lawyer John Robertson carefully analyzed the legal issues raised by pediatric euthanasia and in collaboration with pediatrician Norman Fost, co-authored a sobering article, "Passive euthanasia of defective infants: legal considerations," in which they reminded doctors and parents about potential criminal liability for withholding care. They admitted that "parents and health professionals with experience in the complex and heart-wrenching decisions . . . might justifiably react to this legal analysis with shock and rage." They understood why Duff and Campbell had called "for the law to be changed" and suggested that either criteria be drawn up to designate precisely those classes of infants who can be allowed to die or, preferably, a due process for decision-making be formulated.⁵⁶

The Johns Hopkins film was also a landmark in my own career as a bioethicist. In the fall of 1972, when I was a new arrival on the UCSF Medical School campus, I received a telephone call from Dr. William H. Tooley, Chief of Neonatology. He said that he had seen a film at a pediatrics meeting that he wished to show to his second-year medical students in the course on reproductive medicine, and he asked whether I would discuss the film with the students. Professor David Louisell, of the University of California Law School, whom I knew, had already accepted his invitation to discuss the film. This was my first entry into the classroom as a bioethicist. The film stunned the class; Louisell, Tooley, and I did our best to explain the ethical and legal issues, but our concepts were still as immature as the babies whose fate we discussed.

Dr. Tooley suggested to me that the time might be right for a conference on decision making in the nursery. We gathered twenty persons from medicine, law, theology, philosophy, and social science at the Westerbeck ranch in the Valley of the Moon, Sonoma, California, in May 1974. Papers were presented, but the heart of the conference consisted of the discussion of difficult cases. The participants were polled on four questions. Unanimous affirmative answers were given to two questions: would it ever be right not to resuscitate an infant at birth? and would it ever be right to withdraw life support from a clearly diagnosed, poor prognosis infant? To the question, would it ever be right to intervene directly to kill a self-sustaining infant, seventeen participants answered yes, two answered no, and one was uncertain. To the final question, would it ever be right to displace a poor prognosis infant in order to provide intensive care to a better prognosis infant? eighteen participants answered yes and two responded no. Participants were allowed to qualify their answers. One person who had answered yes to the active euthanasia question remarked, "If the parents administered the syringe of potassium chloride prepared by the judge, and all the lawyers, priests, economists, psychologists and journalists within a 50 mile radius were witnesses and no physicians, nurses or medical or nursing students were allowed to be present."[57]

The Valley of the Moon conference did not escape the vigilance of Paul Ramsey. He devoted one of his Bampton lectures to a scathing critique. The conclusions of the conference, expressed in an essay written by myself and my colleague in the UCSF medical ethics program, Dr. Michael Garland, had affirmed the moral legitimacy of foregoing life support, the primacy of parental decisions in doing so, and, in exceptional cases, the ethical propriety of hastening an infant's death. Ramsey vigorously repudiated the final conclusion and criticized the reasoning we used to support the other two conclusions. His most salient objection bore on "the circularity between the ethical principles assumed and the resultant policy." He judged that our attempt to state a "moral policy" for neonatal intensive care was, in effect, sadly confused: we failed to establish any primacy or priority for ethical principles, and we buried what principles we affirmed under a broad agreement about how difficult medical cases should be practically managed. Ramsey expressed his scorn for the reasoning and conclusions of the conference by commenting on the name of its site, the Valley of the Moon. He wrote, "The symbolism . . . should not be lost: a valley on a dead satellite of our mother earth."[58] Professor Ramsey's critique was harsh and I learned from it. Still, our "moral policy," with the exception of our slender endorsement of exceptional active euthanasia, seems to have been appreciated by those who worked in the trying settings of neonatal intensive care.

The Valley of the Moon conference exemplified a way of doing ethics that was becoming increasingly common in the emerging world of bioethics: a varied group of educated and experienced persons debate the difficult cases, their responses are tested against basic moral intuitions, and general conclusions, with designated exceptions, are drawn. This process, far from Ramsey's rough wrestling with concepts and principles and logic, I had called, to Ramsey's "immoderate glee," a sort of "infraethics." Despite the defect of circularity that Ramsey indicted, this manner of doing ethics seemed to meet the need of many concerned persons for a morally articulate understanding of plaguing problems. It became a common style of bioethical deliberation.[59]

Baby Doe

Between 1971 and 1981, the Johns Hopkins film was shown before students of medicine and nursing, law, and philosophy. After every showing, the rights and wrongs of what was done were debated. Most debaters acknowledged the complexity of the issues raised by the case. However, the complexity of these questions did not discourage politicians from attempting to solve them by legislation. Such an attempt gave rise to one of bioethics' most peculiar events: the Baby Doe story.

A baby very much like the Johns Hopkins baby was born in Bloomington, Indiana in early April 1982. The parents, learning that their baby was affected with Down's syndrome and had an esophageal atresia, declined permission for surgery to correct the atresia. One of the attending physicians disagreed with the parents and the hospital sought a court order for the surgery. The Indiana courts upheld the parents' decision; the United States Supreme Court declined review. Reporters covering the Supreme Court learned of the case and, several days after Baby Doe's death on April 15, *The New York Times* and *The Washington Post* both ran editorials deploring the parents' decision.[60] It is said that President Reagan saw the story on television news and immediately ordered his Secretary of Health and Human Services, Richard Schweiker, to prevent such outrageous behavior in the future. "The President," said Secretary Schweiker, "has instructed me to make absolutely clear to health providers in this nation that federal law does not allow medical discrimination against handicapped infants."[61]

In response to President Reagan's request, Secretary Schweiker issued an Interim Final Rule in March 1983, requiring that intensive care nurseries and maternity wards display notices stating "discriminatory failure to feed and care for handicapped infants in this facility is prohibited by Federal law."[62] The notices posted the number of a toll-free Handicapped Infant Hotline through which suspected violations could be reported to a DHHS "Baby Doe Squad" for investigation. The American Academy of Pediatrics immediately challenged the Interim Final Rule. Judge George Gesell of the U.S. District Court of the District of Columbia held that the rule had been improperly issued.[63] The DHHS reissued it in accord with proper procedures. The reissued rule diminished the size of the warning sign but remained substantially the same. The Academy of Pediatrics challenged it again on substantive grounds, charging that Section 504 of the Rehabilitation Act of 1974, which Secretary Schwieker had invoked as the basis for his regulation, was not applicable to the care of newborns. The Supreme Court agreed. Justice John Paul Stevens wrote, "The Federal Government has no power to overrule parental decisions . . . the Administration had presented no evidence that would justify Federal intervention in an area traditionally controlled by the state."[64]

While the departmental regulations were under judicial scrutiny, congressional anti-abortion advocates sought a judge-proof way to attain their end. They attached a Baby Doe Amendment to the Child Abuse Prevention and Treatment Amendments of 1984, a bill which authorized federal funding to states for Child Protection Services. The legislative language was crafted in an extraordinary collaboration between the sponsoring congressmen and representatives of interested organizations, the Academy of Pediatrics, the American Medical Association, and the Association of Handicapped Persons. Public Law 98-457 passed both houses and was signed into law by President Reagan on October 9, 1984. On the third anniversary of Baby Doe's death, April 15, 1985, the Department of Health and Human Services issued regulations and interpretive guidelines to implement the new federal law. The regulations required that all medically indicated treatments be provided to infants unless "such treatment would merely prolong dying, not be effective in ameliorating or correcting all of the infant's life-threatening conditions, or otherwise be futile in terms of the survival of the infant."[65] Warning signs and hotlines disappeared from the rules. States were required to carry out surveillance of neonatal intensive care units for violations of the rules or lose federal funding for their Child Protective Services. Some states, such as California, preferred to give up their funding rather than implement the regulations. Other states implemented them with varying degrees of vigilance. Regardless of their legal enforcement, the Baby Doe rules appeared to prompt overtreatment rather than prevent undertreatment.[66]

The Baby Doe regulations fused the ethical issues associated with care of the small premature infant with the notably different issues raised by infants with congenital anomalies.[67] The "premies" whose lungs would not mature or who, if their lungs did mature, were left with tragic defects, posed the most common ethical problem in the intensive care nursery. Congenital anomalies are a less common problem: only a fraction of the babies who enter neonatal intensive care are born with congenital anomalies (about 4% of the 3.3 million annual births), such as spina bifida, a neural tube defect that leads to severe physical problems and is often accompanied with mental retardation, and with chromosomal anomalies, the most frequent of which is Down's syndrome (one out of 700 live births). The Johns Hopkins baby, Baby Doe, and several other babies whose cases went to court during the 1970s, were such infants.[68]

A debate over appropriate treatment of infants born with spina bifida began in the early 1970s. The spinal cord protruding out of the open spine is prey to infections that are often lethal. Surgery can close the lesion and protect it from infection, but surgery cannot repair the original neurological damage. Children who survive suffer major physical and sometimes mental defects. Dr. John Lorber, a British neurologist, proposed criteria for determining which infants should be candidates for palliative surgery. Lorber's criteria referred to the location of the lesion on the spine and the presence of hydrocephalus. Infants with high spinal lesions and hydrocephalus had a poor prognosis, therefore they should not be operated on and should be allowed to die of subsequent infection of the exposed cord.[69]

Dr. Lorber's criteria, which seemed reasonable guidance for perplexed surgeons and families, quickly became the subject of debate. Robert Veatch saw them as a prime example of the "technical criteria fallacy." He wrote:

> The decision [to treat or not treat] must also include evaluation of the meaning of existence with varying impairments. Great variation exists about these essentially evaluative elements among parents, physicians, and policy makers. It must be an open question whether these variations in evaluation are among the relevant factors to consider in making a treatment decision. When Lorber uses the phrase, 'contraindications to active therapy,' he is medicalizing what are really value choices.[70]

One participant in the debate took a radical stance. Pediatric neurologist John Freeman suggested that some of the unoperated babies might not die as expected. Thus, because their death had been intended, it would be logical to administer active euthanasia to achieve the goal envisioned by Lorber's exclusion from surgery.[71]

The complex problems surrounding clinical decision for these infants were aired at a 1975 conference organized by pediatric surgeon Chester Swinyard and sponsored by the Foundation for Child Development. Dr. Lorber was present to defend his criteria. A number of the early bioethicists participated and, despite an almost universal criticism of Dr. Lorber's approach, considerable differences of opinion remained at the end of the three days. In a poignant moment, one of the few laypersons attending the conference, the mother of a young man with spina bifida, said, "I am very sorry that there are not more spina bifida parents here, and even more important, young spina bifida adults to express their feelings. . . . Perhaps some of you should go into the homes and look at children with spina bifida playing an effective role in family life."[72] Perhaps no other issue in the early bioethics so clearly illustrated the difficulty of factoring quality of life into a life-or-death decision.

The President's Commission devoted one chapter of *Deciding to Forego Life-Sustaining Treatment* to seriously ill newborns. The Commission had at hand the large literature that had accumulated around this problem. It held a hearing at which neonatologists presented their views and ethicists analyzed the options. The Commission affirmed the legitimacy of parental authority to make decisions in the best interests of their infant and then attempted to specify "best interests" in a way relevant to the circumstances. The chapter endorses the ethical propriety of foregoing clearly futile therapy and proposes a "very restrictive standard" to govern the foregoing of treatments that might sustain life but with attendant defects. For those cases, "such permanent handicaps justify a decision not to provide life-sustaining treatment only when they are so severe that continued existence would not be a net benefit to the infant. . . . The surrogate is obliged to try to evaluate benefits and burdens from the infant's own perspective."[73] The Commission recommended that hospitals formulate criteria for decision making and establish review mechanisms. The commissioners took the occasion to criticize the Baby Doe regulations that would create an "adversarial atmosphere" and add "further uncertainty to an already complex situation."[74]

The Johns Hopkins film, which told the story of private agony in the neonatal intensive care unit, and the Baby Doe episode, which projected that private agony onto the large screen of public policy, had placed the ethics of neonatal intensive care on the agenda of bioethics. The ethical questions raised in neonatology are rather different from the general questions raised by the care of the dying. These dying babies are usually premature newborns whose death sometimes comes even before the date of their expected birth. They are, as was Shakespeare's McDuff, "untimely ripp'd" from their mother's wombs.[75] Their death takes place within the tangle of tubes and machines that represent one of medicine's most advanced technologies, and the hope of preventing death depends on sophisticated scientific management of pulmonary physiology in the months before birth and the hours afterward. The hope seems so great and the loss so devastating to parents that the decision to give up is particularly agonizing. The possibility of success is often so close that the zeal of neonatal physicians is sometimes excessive. Bioethics and neonatology had much to learn from each other.

Cardiopulmonary Resuscitation

The heart stops beating; the person dies: this was an unbreakable link for centuries. Was it possible to revive a heart that had stopped beating and save a person from death? In 1898, French surgeons reported that when a patient's heart stopped after an appendectomy, they briefly revived it by rhythmic compression.[76] Their technique, manual compression of the surgically exposed heart, was occasionally used in the desperate circumstances of surgery and sometimes in emergency situations. More effective cardiopulmonary resuscitation had to await the development of cardiotonic drugs such as adrenaline and procaine, and electrical techniques for defibrillation during the early 1940s.[77] External cardiac massage was proven effective in 1960.[78] Hospitals began to organize groups of doctors, nurses, and technicians, sometimes called "code teams," that responded quickly with drugs, electrocardioversion, and chest massage to a sudden cardiac arrest on the wards. The American Heart Association and The National Academy of Sciences established standards for cardiopulmonary resuscitation in 1974, which stated, "Cardiopulmonary resuscitation is not indicated in certain situations such as in cases of terminal irreversible illness where death is not unexpected."[79]

This rather obvious admonition was more difficult to observe in practice than to state in policy. Code teams responded rapidly in emergency situations, often ignorant of the patient's general medical condition. Patients who were expected soon to die from cancer were resuscitated. There was a growing realization that this dramatic life-saving intervention was being used too often and with more harmful than helpful results.[80] A few hospitals found it useful to give more specific guidelines about resuscitation. The peculiar concept of an "order not to resuscitate" (DNR) appeared, the only order in medicine *not* to do something. In 1976, two of America's leading hospitals, the Massachusetts General Hospital and the Beth Israel Hospital of Boston, published their guidelines in the same issue of *The New England Journal*.[81]

Hospitals around the country followed their lead, writing policies that described the situations in which resuscitation was inappropriate and requiring physicians to record their reasons for such decisions in the patient's record. This new policy was in stark contrast to previous practice in which legal counsel often suggested that any such orders should be written in pencil and erased after they were implemented. Even as guidelines appeared, episodes of non-resuscitation shocked the public. As late as 1979, the Los Angeles Board of Supervisors was astonished to learn that a patient in a county facility had been allowed to die because of a deliberate order by the physicians. The Board outlawed such orders. Only after a joint committee of the county bar association and the medical society, with the guidance of lawyer-ethicist Leslie Rothenberg, elaborated a policy, was the DNR order made legal in Los Angeles County.[82]

In the early 1980s, the DNR order was no longer unfamiliar to medical and nursing personnel. The law was learning of it as well. A Massachusetts appellate case, *In Re Dinnerstein,*[83] declared legal an order not to resuscitate a 67-year-old woman in "vegetative state" since resuscitation would effect nothing more than "a mere suspension of the act of dying." The ethical rationale for the new policies and their legal and medical acceptance was "futility"—that is, the clinical judgment that a patient's underlying illness was so advanced that either a resuscitation would not be effective, or if it was effective, it would need to be repeated within a short time. Studies began to appear that verified the futility of resuscitation for certain classes of patients, such as those with metastatic cancer or in septic shock.[84] Although many DNR policies required obtaining the patient's permission or at least informing the patient of the medical decision, most policies assumed that the decision was the doctor's business. The problem of withholding cardiopulmonary resuscitation seemed to have been resolved. However, as the decade progressed, ambiguities arose. The meaning of futility was questioned; the specificity of such terms as imminent death and terminal condition was unclear; and the relative importance of quality of life over medical futility was problematic. Above all, the importance of consent by the patient or family remained ill defined.

The President's Commission devoted a chapter in *Deciding to Forego Life-Sustaining Treatment* to cardiopulmonary resuscitation. In accord with its general approach, the Commission heightened the importance of the consent of patient and family. The report contained an algorithm showing the relationship between the physician's assessment of benefit and the patient's preference. Its most controversial cell read, "Physician assessment: CPR would not benefit patient: Patient favors CPR=Try CPR; review decision."[85] The controversy over whether a patient has a moral right to demand a treatment that physicians judge to be futile would erupt in the 1990s.[86] However, the ethical analysis of the arguments over resuscitation shed considerable light on a perplexing practice.

Adult Intensive Care

We have seen Dr. Bruno Haid consulting the Pope about the moral dilemmas that he encountered in his novel intensive care unit. Despite the Pope's lucid and liberal response, the dilemmas that troubled Dr. Haid continued to perplex the doctors and nurses who staffed intensive care units and the patients and families who needed their technology. Twenty years later, the graduation photo of a young woman that appeared incessantly in the news media became the haunting image of those perplexities. Karen Ann Quinlan's biological, organic life was being sustained, even when it appeared that she would never recover, in the words of the New Jersey Supreme Court, "to a conscious and sapient state."

On April 15, 1975, 21-year-old Karen Ann Quinlan was brought comotose to the emergency department of Newton Memorial Hospital in Newton, New Jersey. Her coma apparently resulted from ingestion of barbiturates, Valium, and alcohol. She had been celebrating a friend's birthday at a bar, where she consumed several gin and tonics, became woozy, and was taken home and put to bed by friends. Fifteen minutes later, her roommate discovered that she was not breathing and called the police. A policeman resuscitated her and took her to the hospital, where she was put on a respirator to assist her breathing. Nine days later, Quinlan, who had not recovered consciousness, was transferred to St. Claire's Hospital in Denville. During the course of the next five months, her neurological condition deteriorated. In September 1975, Karen Ann was described in these grim terms:

> Her eyes are open and move in a circular manner as she breathes; her eyes blink approximately three or four times per minute; her forehead evidences very noticeable perspiration; her mouth is open while the respirator expands to ingest oxygen, and while her mouth is open, her tongue appears to be moving in a rather random manner; her mouth closes as the oxygen is ingested into her body through the tracheotomy and she appears to be slightly convulsing or gasping as the oxygen enters her windpipe; her hands are visible in an emaciated form, facing in a praying position away from her body. Her present weight would seem to be in the vicinity of 70 pounds. Her legs appear to be tucked toward her body rather than in the normal extended position.[87]

This description was written by Daniel Coburn, a lawyer who had been appointed Karen's legal guardian by Judge Robert Muir, Jr. Mr. and Mrs. Joseph Quinlan had decided, after much prayerful agony and consultation, to request the doctors to remove Karen's breathing tube and allow her to die. After consulting the hospital's lawyer and ascertaining that discontinuing life support might lead to criminal charges, her physician, Dr. Robert Morse, declined to discontinue Karen's respirator, "based on his conception of medical standards, practice and ethics." Mr. Quinlan sought legal help from Paul Armstrong, a Legal Aid lawyer (on behalf of his indigent daughter). Armstrong petitioned the court for an injunction requiring the hospital to desist from medical treatment of Karen Ann Quinlan. The court then appointed the guardian *ad litem*.

This portentous case wound its way through the courts, ultimately reaching the New Jersey Supreme Court. On March 31, 1976, the justices rendered an eloquent opinion which concluded that, under the protection of an implicit privacy right granted by the Constitution, Karen Ann, "if miraculously lucid for an interval . . . and perceptive of her irreversible condition, could effectively decide upon discontinuance of the life-support apparatus even if it meant the prospect of natural death" and that Karen's parents were appropriate surrogates to exercise that right for her. The state has no compelling interest in forcing Karen "to endure the unendurable, only to vegetate a few measurable months with no realistic possibility of returning to any semblance of cognitive or sapient life."[88] There would be no civil or criminal liability should life support be discontinued. Mr. Quinlan again ordered the discontinuance of the respirator; physicians began to wean her from the machine and removed her totally from it on May 20. Unexpectedly, she began to breathe spontaneously. On June 9, she was moved from St. Claire's Hospital to Morris View Nursing Home where she lived in a persistent vegetative state for ten years, dying on June 11, 1985, at the age of 31.

The Quinlans sought moral advice from a traditional source, their parish priest and their bishop, both of whom supported their appeal on grounds of the Catholic doctrine of "extraordinary means." They also sought counsel from a novel source, a bioethicist. The Quinlan's lawyer, Paul Armstrong, called Robert Veatch, Staff Director of the Death and Dying Group at The Hastings Center, who met three times with the Quinlans and Armstrong. Veatch reflected on the significance of the Quinlan case:

> It took the life-support debate to the front pages and to the lead story of the evening news. It made clear that the physician who happened to inherit a patient in an emergency room did not automatically have custody of that patient and could not automatically insist that life-support continue against the wishes of patient or surrogate. It brought surrogate decision making to the stage front and center. It identified privacy as a decisive legal and moral category. It introduced in a muddled way the concept of an ethics committee for the first time into the public discussion of life-support.[89]

Karen Ann Quinlan had not died in vain. Because of the sad ending of her short life, the American public learned the tragic side of the miracle of intensive care. American law began to move toward views that could accommodate the undesirable consequences of technological medicine. American doctors began to attend more seriously to the ethical dimensions of clinical decisions to forego life-sustaining treatment. American bioethics inherited the task of delineating the principles and values that should shape those ethical dimensions.

Tragic as Karen Ann Quinlan's case was, it provided a relatively easy ethical problem in that she was a person who would never again recover health or consciousness. Another dilemma is even more common in the intensive care unit. The critically ill patient who is not in a persistent vegetative state but who, no longer able to communicate, develops increasingly complex medical problems. As one organ system after another falters and new mechanical and pharmaceutical interventions are applied without success, the hoped-for recovery fades. The technological imperative begins to rule clinical decisions: if a technology exists, it must be applied. Patients, as a matter of course, are moved to higher and higher levels of care, finally becoming enmeshed in a tangle of tubes that extinguish their identity and needs as persons. Family members become distressed; physicians become puzzled. Is further care futile? Will another intervention or another day make a difference? Even if life can be saved, will it be a life worth living? These questions are commonplace in critical-care medicine. The intensity of intensive care, despite its marvelous success for some patients, began to burden many patients, their families, and their physicians. And so, the question that titles this chapter, "who should live? who should die?" had to be asked as soon as life-sustaining technologies came into the hands of physicians.

Still, during the 1960s, these agonizing questions were not broadly debated. The few articles that did appear in professional journals repeated with little elaboration the same distinctions about ordinary and extraordinary means and acts of commission and omission that the Pope had propounded to the anesthesiologists.[90] In 1970, sociologist Diana Crane found that 28 percent of the physicians whom she interviewed would not turn off a respirator of a patient who met the criteria for brain death; 50 percent of the doctors who would turn off the respirator would require the families' consent. Many of the physicians whom she interviewed considered that discontinuing respiratory support, even under these conditions, was a criminally liable act of commission. Her study revealed a strong inclination to treat patients very aggressively, even when their prognosis and quality of life were very poor. "It is imperative," concluded Crane, "to resolve some of the differences which now separate the perspective of the physician on these matters from that of the layman and the lawyer."[91] Imperative though it was, only after the Quinlan case did the medical and legal discussion ignite. Soon after the New Jersey Supreme Court had rendered its decision in that case, an editorial appeared in the *New England Journal of Medicine* entitled "Terminating life-support: out of the closet."[92]

Although death in the intensive care unit was not much discussed during the 1960s and early 1970s, a parallel discussion about appropriate ways of dying under the conditions of modern medicine contributed indirectly to the awareness of this problem. Two women physicians led that discussion. In England, Dr. Cicely Saunders recognized that a "good death" was often impeded rather than facilitated by medicine. Before entering medical school, she had worked in St. Luke's House for the Dying Poor, one of the many "hospitals for the dying" that were operated, usually by nuns, in England (and also in the United States). Later, as a physician, Dr. Saunders felt that the compassionate care provided in these institutions could be combined with scientific palliation of pain. Such an arrangement might provide an alternative to difficult death in a high-technology hospital. In 1967, she opened St. Christopher's Hospice in a London suburb where the terminally ill would be treated in a scientific, humane, and in Dr. Saunders' view, Christian way. She became a familiar lecturer in the United States. When she visited Yale University in the mid-1960s, she discovered a like-minded group, headed by Dean of Nursing, Florence Weld and Director of Religious Ministries, Ed Dobihal. The convergence of ideas and sympathies led to the first modern American hospice which opened in New Haven in 1971. During my "internship" with Dr. McKegney at Yale-New Haven Hospital, I meet Reverend Dobihal and learned from him about the emerging hospice movement.[93]

In 1969, Psychiatrist Elisabeth Kübler-Ross published *On Death and Dying*.[94] This book reported the experiences of some 500 patients facing death and developed the thesis that acceptance of death came in defined stages. Persons who learn that they are suffering from a fatal disease first experience denial and isolation, then become angry over their fate, then bargain with life to gain more time, then become depressed, and finally emerge into a calm acceptance of their impending death. Although Kübler-Ross says little about dying under the conditions of intensive care, many of her readers inferred from her thesis that medical technology impeded the patient's passage through these stages. Although not itself a treatise on ethics, Kübler-Ross's book contributed to the discussion of the appropriate care of the dying, summed up under the rubric, "death with dignity."[95]

Allowing To Die

My first encounter with the problem "who shall live? who shall die?" occurred during my Yale internship. Dr. Pat McKegney asked the question, not about the dilemmas of the intensive care unit, but about another of the early life-sustaining technologies, the dialysis machine. He was studying the phenomenon then called "dialysis suicide": patients would choose to discontinue the dialysis treatments that kept them alive. I recall my attempt to illuminate my mentor by explaining the Catholic doctrine of ordinary and extraordinary means. That teaching, as I understood it, solved the moral problem: persons could morally stop a form of life-sustaining treatment that was extraordinary. I was satisfied that this classic Catholic distinction was clear and convincing. Dr. McKegney, as I remember, was not so sure.[96]

Paul Ramsey used the same Catholic doctrine as the center of his analysis of the ethics of caring for the dying in *The Patient as Person*. The chapter "On (Only) Caring for the Dying" begins with the questions "shall a patient suffering from terminal disease be given life-sustaining treatment . . . be placed on a respirator, and is there reason for ever turning off the respirator if such treatment was hopefully begun? Is there any moral difference between not starting the respirator, compared to turning it off once started?"[97] Ramsey then expounds on what, to my knowledge, is the first extensive analysis of these questions as they apply to modern critical-care medicine. Ramsey and other ethicists guided ethics of care for the dying in the direction set by availability of critical-care technologies: under what conditions should these technologies be applied and under what conditions should they be removed? The preceding thirty years of medical development had made that the consuming question.

Ramsey asserts that "The medical ethics developed in western Christianity set its face resolutely against direct killing of terminal patients which it judged to be murder, whatever warrants may be alleged in favor of the practice."[98] At the same time, a long tradition among physicians and moralists alike has permitted persons to die as the result of omission of life-saving efforts. Although powerful life-saving and life-sustaining technologies did not exist until almost the time Ramsey wrote, Roman Catholic theologians had long considered the moral question, "may a person morally omit the means to preserve his life?" The answer had always been that, although persons had a moral obligation to preserve life under the divine imperative of the Fifth Commandment, "thou shalt not kill," that obligation extended only to ordinary and not to extraordinary means. Ramsey examines this traditional doctrine, as explained by a contemporary Catholic theologian, Father Gerald Kelly, for its adequacy as an answer to the moral problem.[99] Ramsey shows that for the traditional moralists, the distinction between "ordinary" and "extraordinary" refers not only to the nature of the medical intervention but also to the "morally relevant, nonmedical features of a particular patient's care: his 'domestic economy,' his familial obligations, the neighborhood that has become a part of his human existence, the person and the common good and whether a man's fiduciary relations with God and with his fellow man have been settled."[100]

Ramsey, following Kelly, first affirms that any medically usual, or "ordinary" treatment becomes "extraordinary" at the point that it has no remedial value—that is, when it has no "reasonable hope of success," for "there is no obligation to do what is useless." In Ramsey's dramatic phrase, when a "man is seized by his own unique dying," he and his physicians have no obligation to oppose death. However, even when death is not imminent, persons may refuse life-saving interventions as extraordinary—that is, when they no longer serve "a patient's estimate of the higher importance of the worth and relations for which his life was lived."[101] Having demonstrated that there are situations in which the duty of fidelity no longer requires life-sustaining medical interventions but only requires loving care for the dying, Ramsey admits one situation in which a direct taking of life might be permitted, namely, when the patient has passed beyond the ability to experience fidelity. When the patient is "irretrievably inaccessible to human care," death may be hastened.[102] Otherwise, he argues vehemently against Joseph Fletcher's endorsement of direct, active euthanasia, as "a serious misunderstanding of the ethics of only attending the dying," and a serious departure from the fidelity we owe them.[103]

The arguments outlined in "On (Only) Caring for the Dying" came to medical ethics at an appropriate time. The clinical problem was whether to apply the new life-saving technologies and, once applied, when to discontinue their use. Ramsey, drawing on a long tradition, offered persuasive arguments that a physician's duty encompassed not only saving life but also allowing to die in the context of only caring. Over the next few years and in the hands of many ethicists, this argument became a central doctrine of the new medical ethics. Ramsey later retreated from one important element in his argument. Eight years after the publication of *The Patient as Person,* he published his Bampton Lectures, delivered at Columbia University in 1975, as *Ethics at the Edges of Life. Medical and Legal Intersections.* In the six chapters gathered under the title, "The Last of Life," the Ramsey of the Beecher Lectures, like St. Augustine of old, issued uncustomary retractions of former positions. Of his interpretation of the Catholic ordinary/extraordinary distinction, he claimed that "historically, this was a mistake," and, even more abjectly, he admitted that he had to "make certain retractions in my past ethical analysis."[104] The mistake, historically and ethically, was to allow into his analysis room for the future quality of the patient's life.

Turning much more polemical than he had been in *Patient as Person,* Ramsey attacked a bevy of ethicists who had made room for such considerations; McCormick, Veatch, Reich, and I were among his targets. He affirmed only the first of the conditions for elective care, namely, the utility of the treatment as a remedy for the patient's condition. This he called "a medical indications policy," considering that it reflected only the objective medical condition of the patient and not the subjective, capricious, and often selfish evaluations of quality of future life that are often to the detriment of the most vulnerable and voiceless. He also repudiated the notion that had become widespread in the ethics literature, namely, that patients had a moral right to refuse life-sustaining care, in the sense that the patient's choice was the ultimate norm for foregoing life support. This notion, he claimed, "enthroned an arbitrary freedom. . . . there are medically indicated treatments . . . that a competent conscious patient has no moral right to refuse, just as no one has a moral right deliberately to ruin his health."[105] Even though Ramsey had sculpted the original shape of the ethics of life support, his later work took a conservative path that few ethicists were willing to follow. Yet, even in his most conservative moments, they appreciated his warnings that certain paths were dangerous to follow.[106]

Deciding to Forego Life-Sustaining Treatment: The President's Commission

Between Ramsey's discussion and the President's Commission report, *Deciding to Forego Life-Sustaining Treatment,* came a decade of debate. The *Quinlan* decision was the stimulant and fulcrum of that debate, and a torrent of articles ensued.[107] When the President's Commission turned to the problem of the ethical and legal implications of life-sustaining treatment it benefited from an ample literature produced by philosophers and theologians. The literature devoted to the ethics of experimentation with human subjects made up, as it were, the original library of bioethics; the outpouring of writing on the ethics of life support was the next major addition to the collection.

The Commission devoted two years to the preparation of *Deciding to Forego Life-Sustaining Treatment*. After many public meetings and much testimony from physicians, scholars, patients and families, a picture of how medicine manages the seriously ill and dying patient emerged. The introduction to the report summarized that picture: First, it showed how the "biomedical developments of the past several decades . . . have made death more a matter of deliberate decision. . . . Matters once the province of fate have now become a matter of human choice." Second, it maintained that "medical technology often renders patients less able to communicate or direct the course of treatment. . . . Consequently, in recent years there has been a continuing clarification of the rights, duties and liabilities of all concerned."[108]

The commissioners affirmed their central commitment: decisions about health care ultimately rest with competent patients. The report then goes on to explain how that central commitment can be realized in the complex and agonizing situations of serious and terminal illness. Various chapters discuss the most problematic situations: when patients lack decisionmaking capacity, when they suffer from permanent loss of consciousness, when hospital resuscitation is indicated, and when the patient is an imperiled newborn. The report's major conclusions affirm that "(1) the voluntary choice of a competent and informed patient should determine whether or not life-sustaining therapy will be undertaken; and, (2) health-care professionals serve patients best by maintaining a presumption in favor of sustaining life, while recognizing that competent patients are entitled to choose to forego any treatments, including those that sustain life."[109] These fundamental positions are supplemented by many other suggestions about the role of surrogate decisionmakers, institutional policy, and legal reforms. Hospital ethics committees are endorsed as forums for discussion of difficult decisions in particular cases, and the legal devices of the living will and the durable power of attorney are recommended as means for anticipating these difficult decisions.

Central to the entire report is the chapter "Elements of Good Decision Making." The story of how that chapter was written was told in Chapter 4. Its conclusion reads, "the Commission has found that a decision to forego treatment is ethically acceptable when it has been made by suitably qualified decisionmakers who have found the risk of death to be justified in light of all the circumstances."[110] No form of treatment, such as nutrition and hydration or resuscitation or antibiotics, can be considered universally warranted and obligatory. This conclusion is sometimes described as the principle of proportionality, in which an assessment of the proportion of benefits to burdens, as evaluated by patients, physicians, and families, dictates the ethical conclusion.[111] In the principle of proportionality, the long discussions by Ramsey, McCormick, and many others during the 1970s converge to a common conclusion that contradicted the prevailing medical ethic that aggressive application of critical-care interventions was always obligatory; there are clearly times and circumstances when life-saving and life-sustaining means need not be applied. This conclusion, much to the surprise of many people, was not a modern artifact. As medical historian Darrel Amundsen has demonstrated, the obligation to prolong life was a medical duty "without classical roots."[112]

The Commission's espousal of the principle of proportionality was dramatically illustrated by a case that became a paradigm in bioethics; it is known as "Dax's Case." On July 23, 1973, Donald "Dax" Cowart and his father were engulfed by an inferno caused by a propane explosion. They were rushed to the burn unit at Dallas's Parkland Hospital. The senior Cowart died en route. Dax's life was saved and he was entered into an extensive rehabilitation program. Almost from the beginning of his treatment, he insisted that he did not want to live. Before the accident, he had been a handsome, vigorous young man and had recently returned home from service as an Air Force pilot in Vietnam. In the hospital, he was vividly aware that he would never be the same person again. He was totally disabled and dependent on others for help in the activities of daily life. Despite his insistence that he be allowed to die, the medical team, encouraged by Dax's mother and dubious about their legal liability, pressed on. During his hospitalization at the University of Texas Medical Branch, Galveston, where he had been transferred for rehabilitation, he consented to being videotaped.

The video showed a horribly disfigured patient undergoing terribly painful treatments, then talking quite rationally and eloquently with Dr. Robert White, a psychiatrist, about his wish to die. That video, "Please Let Me Die," although intended only for in-house educational use, quickly "became a classic among professionals concerned with the treatment and care of the hopelessly ill and hopelessly deformed. It was shown at professional meetings around the world and was regularly used for classroom instruction at medical, law and divinity schools."[113] A second video, "Dax's Case" appeared in 1985, in which the professionals who had been involved in the case express their views about what they had done. It also showed Dax in his subsequent life, scarred and crippled but married and successful in business. Even then, he insisted that he should have been allowed to die.

I first saw "Please Let Me Die" at a meeting sponsored by the organization Concern for Dying, in San Francisco in 1977. I obtained a copy and used it regularly in the ethics course at UCSF School of Medicine. By the end of the 1970s, students could be told that the law had become clearer about honoring a patient's wish to discontinue life-saving therapy. They could be given a medical article from a leading burn center that endorsed the right of the badly burned patient to decline treatment.[114] By 1983, the lucid arguments of *Deciding to Forego Life-Sustaining Treatment* could be expounded. Still, the principle of the patient's right to refuse treatment, so clear in statement, becomes agonizingly complicated when physicians, nurses, and medical students contemplate "Dax's Case." The video "Please Let Me Die" joined the Johns Hopkins film, "Who Shall Live," as standard educational tools in bioethics courses across the country.

Euthanasia or Assisted Suicide

The question whether a suffering human being might deliberately end that suffering by ending their life has long touched the human conscience. The Stoic philosopher Seneca recalls a friend suffering from "a disease not incurable, but protracted and troublesome," who anguished over the question of suicide until someone said to him, "you must not worry as if you were making a great decision. There is nothing so very great about living—all your slaves and animals do it—what is, however, a great thing is to die in a manner honorable, enlightened, courageous." Whereupon the sick man made a peaceful end to his life.[115] The suicide of the sick was not unusual in the pre-Christian West. Even if the phrase of the Hippocratic Oath, "I will neither give a deadly drug to anybody even if asked, nor make a suggestion to that effect," does refer to assisting persons who choose to end their sufferings (it may refer to collusion in murder), ancient physicians seem not to have been hindered. Ludwig Edelstein wrote, "throughout antiquity many people preferred voluntary death to endless agony. . . . many physicians actually gave their patients the poisons for which they asked." He believed that the phrase was honored only by those physicians who adhered to Pythagoreanism. Apart from occasional references to assisting death, as when the Roman physician Scribonius Largus condemns physicians who take life, the medical literature of antiquity ignores the subject.[116]

By the fourth century of the Christian era, Christian teaching about the divine authority over life and death branded suicide a mortal sin. After some vacillation among the early church fathers, who sometimes saw martyrdom as a form of laudable suicide, St. Augustine thundered a powerful and exceptionless condemnation.[117] St. Thomas Aquinas agreed: "Suicide is the most serious of sins because one cannot repent of it."[118] Only rarely did Christian thinkers dare suggest otherwise, yet a Catholic saint, Thomas More, and an Anglican Dean, John Donne, contemplated the moral goodness of suicide of the suffering.[119] A skeptical philosopher, David Hume, demolished the rational arguments against suicide.[120] Still, a strong moral reprobation over many centuries pushed suicide of the sick and dying out of mind.

During the nineteenth century, as noted at the beginning of this chapter, the term "euthanasia" appeared in the medical literature to describe the physician's duties to ease the death throes. Some physicians advised restraint in the use of heroic medicine for the dying and emphasized the palliation of suffering. But the earliest overt suggestions that physicians should hasten the death of the dying come not from the medical profession but from laypersons. In the 1870s, two English essayists, Samuel Williams and Lionel Tollemache, wrote articles advocating this practice. Williams wrote, "in all cases of hopeless and painful illness it should be the recognized duty of the medical attendant, whenever so desired by the patient . . . to destroy consciousness at once and put the sufferer at once to a quick and painless death."[121]

The proposals of those English authors attracted some attention from the public in their own country but little response from the medical profession. In the United States, the topic was occasionally broached, but with ambiguity rather than advocacy. An 1884 editorial in *The Boston Medical and Surgical Journal* compromised, favoring "a passive rather than an active attempt at euthanasia . . . to surrender to superior forces is not the same thing as to lead the attack of the enemy upon one's own friends."[122] Very rarely, an article would forthrightly urge that physicians be given the legal authority to end the lives of patients who requested a peaceful end to a hopeless and agonizing sickness.[123] Although these rash suggestions met strong public and professional opposition, occasional efforts to introduce such legislation were made. Just after the turn of the century, euthanasia bills were introduced in the Iowa, Ohio and New York legislatures.[124]

Nothing came of these efforts, but a small band of convinced partisans continued to promote the cause. The Voluntary Euthanasia Legislation Society, founded in the 1930s in Great Britain, was influential in bringing to the House of Lords a private member's bill to legalize voluntary euthanasia in 1936. The bill was defeated after a fascinating debate in the world's oldest debating society. Viscount Dawson of Penn, physician to His Majesty George V, eloquently argued that any such decision should be a matter between a doctor and his patient; legislation would inexcusably intrude upon the intimacy of that relationship. Many years later, it was revealed that he had hastened the death of the terminally ill monarch.[125] The Euthanasia Society of America, which was founded in 1937, also moved quickly to promote, in a polite but persistent way, the passage of euthanasia legislation. Under its influence, a renewed drive to enact legalization was launched. Its first effort was a bill introduced in the Nebraska Legislature on February 2, 1937, which allowed "competent adults who were suffering from incurable and fatal disease or were helpless and suffering from the infirmities of old age" to apply to the state "referee in euthanasia . . . [for] a permit for euthanasia." Guardians and next of kin could apply for mentally incompetent adults and children.[126] Other states considered such legislation, including Connecticut in 1959, Idaho in 1969, and Oregon and Montana in 1973. None of these attempts succeeded.

The horrors of the Holocaust cast a dark cloud over even the most restrained advocacy of euthanasia. Although few persons were aware that German medicine had reached a broad tolerance for "mercy killing" of the incurably ill before the Nazi ascendancy, it was commonly known that once in power, the Nazi regime had included that practice among its genocidal policies.[127] Yet, just a year before the revelations of those events, an American physician advocating euthanasia wrote:

> To end a life that is useless, helpless and hopeless seems merciful. The end should be welcome. The act is then kind rather than ruthless and the result could not but benefit the living. . . . The useless, helpless and hopeless are of many kinds. . . . The opinion of many would include in this classification idiots and the insane, imbeciles and morons, psychopaths, both mild and severe, criminals and delinquents, monsters and defectives, incurables and the worn-out senile. . . . Not only are they a great burden upon society but, supported and protected, they are fast increasing their dead weight by reproducing their kind."[128]

This commendation of mercy killing ignores all distinctions between active and passive or voluntary and involuntary, is totally indiscriminate about the conditions that might justify mercy killing, and justifies the practice by reference to the benefits to society rather than to the patients. Words such as these, written even by benevolent persons (I knew the author, who was an emeritus professor at UCSF), were ominously close to the Nazi condemnation of "useless eaters." The horrors of the Holocaust and the muddle-headedness of some advocates did not commend the cause of euthanasia to the public or to the profession.

Some brave souls persisted in their cause. Joseph Fletcher, an early member of the Euthanasia Society, devoted a chapter in *Morals and Medicine* to clarifying the issues. He argued that the values of personhood and autonomy should prevail over mere prolongation of life. He criticized the traditional moral condemnation of suicide and differentiated the motives and ends of euthanasia from those of murder. He criticized the relevance of the claim that God alone decrees the time when death should come. He also dismissed common arguments against euthanasia: physicians can make mistakes about prognosis, patients can make impulsive decisions. He made an impassioned plea for voluntary euthanasia in terminal illness as an act of creative rationality and courage, and in passing, and without extended defense, he also approved of "involuntary euthanasia for monstrosities at birth and mental defectives, a partly personalistic and partly eugenic position."[129] Fletcher commended a law that the Euthanasia Society was about to introduce in the New York Assembly which allowed a competent adult with an incurable, painful, and fatal disease to petition a court for euthanasia, whereupon the court would appoint a commission to investigate the case and, upon a report that the case met the conditions of the law, grant permission to a physician or to any other person to perform euthanasia.[130] This modern proposal is an exact copy of the suggestion offered in 1516 by Sir Thomas More for the citizens of Utopia. Unimpressed by that intellectual lineage and by the support of 1,776 New York physicians and the distinguished citizens of the Euthanasia Society, the New York bill, like every other bill that had been submitted, never became law.

Scholarly discussion, however, had been stimulated. Philosopher Marvin Kohl solicited essays for and against euthanasia from a group of reputable scholars for his volume, *Beneficent Euthanasia*. John Behncke and Sissela Bok published a collection of essays, *Dilemmas of Euthanasia*. Daniel Maguire broke Catholic theological ranks to publish *Death by Choice*.[131] In all these discussions, the scholarly opinion moved perceptibly toward a conception of voluntary euthanasia that repudiated mercy killing of the unconsenting and endorsed the right of competent persons in pain and nearing death to be aided in ending their lives. Still, the debate over active euthanasia was confined to small circles. The question of the conditions for ethically foregoing life support, as we saw in the previous section, absorbed most of the scholarly attention. Even the Euthanasia Society changed its name to Concern for Dying to disassociate itself from the mercy-killing position and to promote living wills and rational decision making about life support. The bible of death-and-dying ethics, *Deciding To Forego Life-Sustaining Treatment*, mentions voluntary euthanasia only incidentally. In one passage, the report notes that courts have held that refusal of life support differs from suicide.[132] In another place, the Commission concludes its discussion of the distinction between acting and omitting with an endorsement of the standing legal prohibition against active causation of death: "The Commission finds this limitation on individual self-determination to be an acceptable cost of securing the general protection of human life afforded by the prohibition of direct killing."[133] The commissioners saw no need to say anything more on the subject.

The Commission endorsed what many commentators then called "passive, voluntary euthanasia," or the foregoing of life support at the request of a competent patient or an appropriate surrogate. The medical profession acquiesced. The American Medical Association approved the following statement in 1988: "For humane reasons, with informed consent, a physician may do what is medically necessary to alleviate severe pain, or cease or omit treatment to permit a terminally ill patient whose death is imminent to die. However, he should not intentionally cause death."[134]

The more ambiguous moral problem of active euthanasia was pushed to the background—but not for long. Some philosophers and even some physicians wondered how a decision to omit life-sustaining treatment was not "intentionally causing death." Some authors questioned the logical and psychological validity of the distinction between active and passive, omission and commission.[135] *Deciding To Forego Life-Sustaining Treatment* even signaled agreement with those criticisms.[136] Other authors warned that an acceptance of passive euthanasia would set society inevitably on the route to active euthanasia.[137] A broad public debate over euthanasia erupted in the late 1980s. In a one-page essay, "It's Over, Debbie," appearing in *The Journal of the American Medical Association*, an anonymous physician-author told a story (true or fictional, no one knew) about helping a dying woman to die more quickly. That brief essay stirred up a storm of dispute among physicians and was, in the view of many observers, the spur to a more open discussion of euthanasia within the profession.[138] A new society, called Hemlock, appeared and its leader published a book, *Final Exit*, that not only argued for legal euthanasia but provided directions for those who chose such an exit.[139] One nation, The Netherlands, embarked on an experiment with legally tolerated euthanasia.[140]

By the early 1990s, the proponents of what was now called "assisted suicide" had generated enough strength to introduce initiatives in the states of Washington (1991), California (1992), and Oregon (1995) that would legally authorize physicians to hasten the deaths of requesting, competent, terminal patients. The Washington and California initiatives narrowly failed, but the citizens of Oregon accepted (also narrowly) their initiative, the Death with Dignity Act, and granted that "an adult may make a written request for medication for the purpose of ending his or her life in a humane and dignified manner."[141]

Death, Bioethics, and the Law

Law, of course, has always been interested in death. Forensic medicine, the use of medical testimony as evidence in criminal cases, has a history that goes back to antiquity. The protophysician of Pope Innocent X, Paolo Zacchia, wrote a monumental treatise, *Quaestiones medico-legales* (1621), which included detailed discussions of beatings, woundings, and poisonings. Dr. Percival's *Medical Ethics* devotes the longest of its four chapters to the "Professional Duties, in Certain Cases Which Require a Knowledge of the Law." A doctor should understand wills and testaments, and conditions for confinement of lunatics but, above all, a doctor should be able to testify about sudden death, suspected homicide, and infanticide. Dr. Percival instructed his readers, "When medicines administered to a sick patient, with an honest design, to produce the alleviation of his pain, or cure of his disease, occasion death, this is misadventure, in the view of the law, and the physician or surgeon, who directed them, is not liable to punishment criminally."[142]

From ancient times, everyone—doctors and patients alike—knew that medicine killed and injured. A standing joke called doctors "unpunishable murderers." The new medicine, particularly in the forms that sustained living processes, put a new twist on that old, sad joke. Now a patient's continued life could depend on persistent application of the supporting technology. To stop the technology was to cause death; causing death was homicide. The doctors who used the new respirators could become potential murderers. Even more dramatically, the surgeons who removed hearts for transplantation faced this threat, and in several cases, transplanters were on the verge of indictment. The old view still lingered with sufficient strength that this new problem appeared as a paradox: could modern doctors, acting in their professional capacity, cause death and still have the law view their actions as "misadventures?"

Judge-made law, rendered in many court cases, began to formulate a new medical jurisprudence closely associated with the new bioethics. A small library of cases about mercy killing, unauthorized experimentation, refusal of blood transfusions by Jehovah's Witnesses, and donation of organs had accumulated in American law before the 1960s. However, the case that thrust the questions of the new medicine into the legal and public limelight was *In the Matter of Karen Ann Quinlan, An Alleged Incompetent*. As attorney Daniel Coburn, court-appointed guardian for Karen Ann, remarked, it was "a case of first impression," that is, a case never before seen in American law.[143] The trial judge, Robert Muir, stated in a footnote to his decision, "The onus of the judicial decision of the judicial process for me, in this instance, is unparalleled."[144] He struggled to fit the facts of this unprecedented and unparalleled case into the framework of existing law. When Judge Muir's opinion was overturned by the New Jersey Supreme Court, the justices made a major contribution to the new bioethical jurisprudence. The Quinlan decision elevated the Constitution's "penumbral" right of privacy, as enunciated in the *Griswold v State of Connecticut* and *Roe v Wade* by the United States Supreme Court, to the center of the argument and granted, as Judge Muir would not, the right to exercise that right to Karen's parents and guardians. They had to exercise that right in accord with their daughter's "putative decision . . . to permit (her) non-cognitive, vegetative existence to terminate by natural forces."[145] The New Jersey Supreme Court's reasoning became precedent for the state of New Jersey and came into the ken of other courts that found themselves faced with similar cases.

Four months after *Quinlan* was decided, the Massachusetts Supreme Judicial Court heard arguments in the case *Superintendent of Belchertown State School v Joseph Saikewicz.* Mr. Saikewicz was a 67-year-old, profoundly retarded and institutionalized man who developed leukemia. Authorities of the institution where he lived petitioned the court to allow them to forego chemotherapy. The court opened its opinion as follows: "We recognize at the outset that this case presents novel issues of fundamental importance that should not be resolved by mechanical reliance on legal doctrine . . . [and seek] the collective guidance of those in health care, moral ethics, philosophy and other disciplines."[146] The justices reviewed the *Quinlan* decision and, stating substantial agreement with their New Jersey brethren, fashioned a doctrine of "substituted judgment" that "commended itself simply because of its straightforward respect for the integrity and autonomy of the individual." In formulating their concept, they cited bioethicist-lawyer John Robertson, who, citing John Rawls, had written, "maintaining the integrity of the person means that we act toward him, 'as we have reason to believe that he would choose for himself if he were capable of reason and deciding rationally.'"[147] In this philosophical excursus, the new bioethics begins to creep into the law. The court determined that Mr. Saikewicz, "having no capacity to understand his present situation or his prognosis . . . would have no comprehension of the reasons for the severe disruption of his formerly secure and stable environment occasioned by the (toxicity) of chemotherapy. He therefore would experience fear without the understanding from which other patients draw strength." They judged that Saikewicz, had he been able, would reasonably have refused chemotherapy and, hence, would have authorized the doctors to refrain from treatment.[148]

Another Massachusetts case, *In the Matter of Shirley Dinnerstein,* came one year later. In that case, an appellate court upheld the validity of a "no code order" for a 67-year-old woman suffering from advanced Alzheimer's disease.[149] In 1980, Massachusetts again permitted life-sustaining treatment (in this instance, dialysis) to be stopped for a senile man, and New York permitted a respirator to be removed from an elderly Catholic Brother in a persistent vegetative state.[150]

A 1986 California case shifted the "right to refuse care" away from its secondary application in surrogate judgment back to where it is more relevant and clear: when the choice is that of a competent adult. Elizabeth Bouvia, an almost totally paralyzed patient who had been hospitalized, requested that her tube feeding be discontinued so that she could starve to death. The hospital refused, citing a duty to continue necessary life-sustaining treatment, particularly "ordinary" treatment such as the provision of nutrition and hydration. After a long struggle and several court trials, Ms. Bouvia's right to refuse even that care was vindicated by a California appellate court.[151]

This series of legal cases from around the United States clearly endorsed the fundamental principle enunciated in *Quinlan*: persons have a constitutionally protected "privacy right" to refuse medical care, even if that care is life preserving. Other persons who are properly authorized may exercise that right for them in accord with their previously expressed preferences or in their best interests. While there are state interests that may impede the exercise of this right, those interests will prevail only in the most unusual circumstances. The jurisprudence that commenced with *Quinlan* culminated with the first case to reach the Supreme Court of the United States, *In the Matter of Nancy Cruzan*. Decided in 1990, this case, which was quite similar to that of Karen Ann Quinlan, upheld the right of the state of Missouri to require strict standards of evidence regarding the patient's preferences but, at the same time, affirmed the fundamental principle of a patient's right (called in this case, "a liberty interest") to forego life-sustaining treatment.

As the series of cases were adjudicated, some of the confusion that had attended early cases was resolved. Bioethical reflection, running parallel to the judicial cases, helped to dispel the confusion. In *Quinlan,* the plaintiffs had included the claim that Karen Ann was "brain dead." The Harvard report had been available for several years, and expert witnesses had testified that Karen Ann did not meet the report's criteria for death; she was in a persistent vegetative state. The court was thus able to reject that pleading. The court did not so easily escape other confusions. Its dramatic words, "We have no doubt, in these unhappy circumstances, that if Karen were herself miraculously lucid for an interval . . . and perceptive of her irreversible condition, she could effectively decide upon discontinuance of the life-support apparatus, even if it meant the prospect of natural death,"[152] represented a subjective value judgment by a panel of reasonable, healthy people. It might be a judgment in which most other reasonable, healthy persons would concur, but should it serve as the basis for a surrogate's judgment to allow another person to die?

The same problem plagued the "substituted judgment" that the Massachusetts justices rendered for Joseph Saikewicz. In both cases, the judgments involved assessments of quality of life which, as the Massachusetts court said, is "vague and perhaps ill chosen."[153] So, the standards for substituted judgment required further scrutiny. The New Jersey court provided that scrutiny almost ten years after it had decided *Quinlan*. *In the Matter of Claire Conroy* presented the court with a case in which the plaintiff, Mr. Thomas Whittemore, legal guardian of his aunt, Miss Claire Conroy, sought permission to have feeding tubes removed from his 84-year-old ward who was afflicted with serious and irreversible physical and mental impairments. The justices could now consult *Deciding to Forego Life-Sustaining Treatment*. They could read a number of appellate level cases and a number of essays written by philosophers, theologians, physicians, and lawyers working in the field of bioethics.[154] Citing much of this ample reflection on the problem that faced them, the justices reaffirmed the right of privacy authorizing the patient to refuse care, and crafted an elaborate schema for the exercise of that right by a surrogate in the best interests of the patient. The justices hoped that their schema would render the surrogate judgment more objective and bring it closer to the patient's putative wishes than any prior formulation.

In 1983, a California appellate court cited the section of *Deciding to Forego* in which the concept of proportionate treatment was explained. The court refused to indict two physicians who had discontinued life support of a patient in persistent vegetative state: "Proportionate treatment is that which, in the view of the patient, has at least a reasonable chance of providing benefits to the patient, which benefits outweigh the burdens attendant to the treatment . . . a treatment course which is only minimally painful or intrusive may nonetheless be considered disproportionate to the potential benefits if the prognosis is virtually hopeless for any significant improvement in condition." The court's attention was drawn to the Commission's text by an expert witness, Jesuit bioethicist Father John Paris, who had been a consultant to the Commission.[155]

While each case had its own singular features, and each opinion reflected a unique reading of the law by different courts, common features began to emerge. It became clear that physicians had no duty to continue life-sustaining treatment to forestall death "forever." There were circumstances in which physicians, with appropriate instructions from the patient or surrogates, could refrain from providing life-sustaining treatment without fear of liability. Patients had a right to refuse life-sustaining care; that right remained even after they had lost the ability to communicate their wishes. Appropriate surrogates could exercise that right for them, basing their decisions either on their knowledge of the patient's wishes or on their assessment of the patient's best interests.

Legislation accompanied the stream of court cases. In the same year as the Quinlan case, the California legislature passed landmark legislation that contributed greatly to the jurisprudence of medical dying. Barry Keene, a member of the California Assembly (the lower house of the state legislature), introduced a "Natural Death Act," which authorized physicians to refrain from providing life-sustaining treatment to an incompetent person when presented with a signed document in which that person expressed a wish not to be treated. Keene intended to give legal status to the so-called living will that had been devised in the 1950s by Chicago lawyer Louis Kutner (Kutner's first signatories were the popular Catholic TV star Monsignor Fulton J. Sheen and film star Errol Flynn). A living will modeled on Kutner's text was promoted by the Euthanasia Council of New York and by many church groups.[156] In the opinion of most lawyers, the living will was nothing but a letter to one's physician, with essentially no legal effect. Keene's Natural Death Act Directive gave the living will some legal force. The law granted protection from legal liability to a physician who followed the patient's instructions (though it did not require the physician to follow the instructions). After much consultation and debate, and with continued redrafting to meet the objections raised by many persons, from the physicians of the California Medical Association to the Catholic bishops of California, the Natural Death Act passed and was signed into law.

I testified twice at the hearings of the California legislature on the Natural Death Act and talked with Mr. Keene about its provisions. I was strongly in favor of his efforts.

However, a hospital case in which I was involved as consultant suggested how difficult it could be to interpret the directive. With Dr. Stuart Eisendrath, a psychiatric consultant on the same case, I co-authored an article entitled "The living will: help or hindrance."[157] We pointed out the ambiguity of language and complexity of notions that sometimes confused rather than clarified the situation in which the decision to terminate treatment had to be made. The Natural Death Act was not without its critics on other grounds. The Catholic Bishops feared that it was the first step toward euthanasia (although its language explicitly forbade mercy killing). Some ethicists worried that physicians would become even more reluctant to forego life support if they did not have a directive in hand.[158] Still, the California law was emulated in state after state. In the six years after the passage of Keene's bill, fifteen states passed identical or similar legislation. *Deciding to Forego Life-Sustaining Treatment* endorsed the use of the Natural Death Act and also recommended that an old legal device, the durable power of attorney, be extended from its usual limited place in property law to end-of-life decisions.[159]

Conclusion

"Who shall live? who shall die?" is a favorite title for articles about bioethics: it almost deserves to be inscribed over the entrance to the discipline. Even though life and death is not the sole theme of bioethics, from the earliest glimmering of interest in the questions raised by the new biology and new medicine, these questions have commanded attention. Bioethicists have meditated on these questions, and they have clarified the relevant concepts and logic of argument. They have also recommended practical strategies about care of the dying. Not too many years ago, death had been banished from polite discussion in American society. Today, death and dying are openly discussed; they are a matter of education, policy, and law. Many persons have learned a vocabulary and a grammar of principles and values with which to discuss the painful questions. Many patients have been given the freedom to choose their course of treatment. The extent to which the technology of modern medicine is more discriminatingly applied is unclear, but as one who has watched these developments over twenty-five years, I am convinced that many physicians have become more thoughtful about applying their powerful technologies, and many patients have become more aware of their risks as well as their benefits.[160] Bioethics has offered helpful, even if not definitive, answers to the plaintive and perennial question, "who shall live? who shall die?"

Notes for Chapter 8

1. William Shakespeare, *King Henry IV Part II*, act 3, scene 2, line 41.
2. "[Medicine] does away with the suffering of the sick, lessens the violence of their diseases,

and refuses to treat those who are overmastered by their diseases, realizing that in such cases medicine is powerless." Hippocrates, *Art*, III In W. H. S. Jones (trans.), *Hippocrates with an English Translation*, (Cambridge, Mass.: Harvard University Press, 1957), vol. 2, p. 193.

3. Chauncey Leake (ed.), *Percival's Medical Ethics* (Baltimore: Williams and Wilkins, 1927), II, iii, p. 91.

4. C. F. H. Marx, "Medical euthanasia," *Journal of the History of Medicine and Allied Sciences* 7 (1972): 404–416. See William Munk, *Euthanasia or Medical Treatment in Aid of an Easy Death* (London: Longmans, Green and Co., 1887). Dr. Munk praises the use of opium to relieve pain but warns that if administered when respiration is compromised, "it is hazardous and may cause death." p. 81.

5. James Patterson, *The Dread Disease: Cancer and Modern American Culture* (Cambridge, Mass.: Harvard University Press, 1987).

6. "Euphoria vs. euthanasia," *Journal of the American Medical Association* 32 (1899): 674; "Euthanasia," *Journal of the American Medical Association* 41 (1903): 1094; *British Medical Journal* 1 (1906): 1094; "Euthanasia: degenerated sympathy," *Boston Medical and Surgical Journal* 154 (1906): 330–331; Abraham Jacobi, "Euthanasia," *Medical Review of Reviews* 18 (1912): 362–363; "May the physician ever end life?" *British Medical Journal* 1 (1897): 934; William Osler, "Our attitude toward incurable disease," *Boston Medical and Surgical Journal* 141 (1899): 531; "The problem of euthanasia," *Journal of the American Medical Association* 60 (1913): 1897; William Munk, "Review of euthanasia: a medical treatment in aid of an early death," *British Medical Journal* 1 (1888): 473; Louis J. Rosenberg and N. E. Aronstam, "Euthanasia: a medico-legal study," *Journal of the American Medical Association* 36 (1901): 108–110; Sir Robert A. Wilson, "Medico-literary causerie: euthanasia," *Practitioner* 56 (1896): 631–635; Charles B. Williams, "Euthanasia," *Medical and Surgical Report* 70 (1894): 909–911.

7. "Permissive euthanasia," *Boston Medical and Surgical Journal* 20 (1884), quoted in Stanley Joel Reiser, "The dilemma of euthanasia in modern medical history: the English and American experience," in Reiser, Arthur J. Dyck, and William J. Curran (eds.), *Ethics in Medicine: Historical Perspectives and Contemporary Concerns* (Cambridge, Mass.: The MIT Press, 1977), p. 490.

8. Homer, *Iliad*, XVI, 502.

9. Maimonides, *Mishneh Torah*, Hilchot Shabbat 2:19; see Fred Rosen, *Modern Medicine and Jewish Ethics* (New York: Yeshiva University Press, 1986), chapter 18, and J. D. Bleich, "Establishing criteria of death," in *Contemporary Halakhic Problems* (New York: Ktav, 1977), pp. 372–393.

10. *Black's Law Dictionary,* 4th ed. (St. Paul, Minn.: West Publishing Co., 1968), p. 488.

11. Cited in Stanley Joel Reiser, "The intensive care unit: the unfolding ambiguities of survival therapy," *International Journal of Technology Assessment* 8 (1992): 382–394; Vesalius, *De Humani Corporis Fabrica*, 5; 23; David K. Brooks, *Resuscitation* (Baltimore: Wilkins and Wilkins, 1967); Tony Gould, *A Summer Plague: Polio and Its Survivors* (New Haven: Yale University Press, 1995).

12. Philip Drinker and Charles F. McKhann, "The use of a new apparatus for the prolonged administration of artificial respiration," *Journal of the American Medical Association* 92 (1929): 1658–1660; J. H. Maxwell, "The iron lung: halfway technology or necessary step," *Milbank Quarterly* 64 (1986): 3–29.

13. J. L. Wilson, "The use of the respirator," *Journal of the American Medical Association* 117 (1941): 278–279. I have tried in vain to find ethical commentary on this problem during the 1940s and 1950s.

14. Pope Pius XII, *Acta Apostolicae Sedis* 49 (1957): 1027–1033 *The Pope Speaks* 4 (1958): 393–398. The Pope's answer invoked the distinction long familiar to Roman Catholic moralists

between ordinary and extraordinary care. See Chapter 2 and later in this chapter for the meaning of this distinction. Although one source (*The Pope Speaks*) describes the gathering as "an International Congress of Anesthesiologists," the more authoritative *Acta* states that the Pope addressed "a meeting of distinguished physicians and medical educators invited to Rome by the Gregor Mendel Institute of Genetics." Several senior anesthesiologists have told me that they cannot recall any International Congress in 1957.

15. Julius Korein, "Problem of brain death: development and history," in Korein (ed.), *Brain Death: Interrelated Medical and Social Issues (Special Issue), Annals of the New York Academy of Sciences* 315 (1978): 19–38, quote on p. 19. The words of the papal discourse were quoted at the Ciba Conference on Transplantation in 1966, in the Harvard Report on Definition of Death in 1969, in the judicial opinion on the Quinlan case, and in innumerable articles on the care of the dying.

16. Pierre Mollaret and M. Goulon, "Le coma dépassé," *Revue Neurologique* 101 (1959): 3–15.

17. Ciba Foundation Symposium, *Ethics in Medical Progress*, G. Wolstenholme and M. O'Connor eds. (London: J. & A. Churchill Ltd., 1966), p. 69.

18. Ciba, *Ethics in Medical Progress*, pp. 69, 155, 157, 190.

19. "Moment of Death," *British Medical Journal* 2 (1963): 394.

20. From Paul Ramsey, *The Patient as Person*, (New Haven: Yale University Press, 1970), p. 72; "Texas heart transplants raise legal questions," *New York Times*, May 13, 1968: 18; "Two indicted in death of heart donor," *New York Times*, January 28, 1969: A3. I recall the Shumway and Hume cases but cannot find their verification.

21. Report of the Ad Hoc Committee at Harvard Medical School to Examine the Definition of Brain Death, "A definition of irreversible coma," Journal of the American Medical Association 205 (1968): 337–340. See Vincent J. Kopp, "Henry Knowles Beecher and the redefinition of death," *Bulletin of Anesthesia History* 1997; 15: 6–8.

22. Interview with William Curran, 16 March 1996. See Henry Beecher, "Scarce resources and medical advancement: ethical aspects of experimentation with human subjects," *Daedalus* 98, no. 2 (1969): 275–313, 294; see also Ramsey, *The Patient as Person*, p. 107, where Ramsey compares Beecher's diverse opinions rather crudely: "We must appeal from the late Beecher drunk to the early Beecher sober."

23. Pope Pius XII, *Discoursi ai Medici*, F. Angelini ed. (Rome: Orizzante, 1959), p. 607.

24. Personal communication to Albert Jonsen, April 12, 1996.

25. "What and when is death? An editorial," *Journal of the American Medical Association* 204 (1968): 539–540.

26. Kansas Stat. Ann. 77-202 (Supp. 1971), quoted in the President's Commission for the Study of Ethical Problems in Medicine and Biomedical and Behavioral Research, *Defining Death: A Report on the Medical, Legal, and Ethical Issues in the Determination of Death* (Washington, D.C.: Government Printing Office, 1981), p. 62.

27. Alexander M. Capron and Leon R. Kass, "A statutory definition of the standards for determining human death: an appraisal and proposal," *University of Pennsylvania Law Review* 121 (1972): 87–118. This paper, while original, was gestated in the discussion of the Hastings Center Death and Dying Research Group.

28. French Ministry of Health, *Circulaire Jeanneny*, April 24, 1968; "Heart transplantation," *Council for International Organizations of Medical Sciences* (CIOMS), Geneva, June 13–14, 1968. Dr. David Rutstein of Harvard Medical School was the rapporteur for the latter. See also Henry Beecher, "After the 'Definition of Irreversible Coma,'" *New England Journal of Medicine* 281 (1969): 1070.

29. Frank J. Veith, Jack M. Fein, Moses D. Tendler, et al., "Brain death I: a status report of medical and ethical considerations," *Journal of the American Medical Association* 238 (1977): 1651–1655; "Brain death II: A status report of legal considerations," *Journal of the American Medical Association* 238 (1977): 1744–1748; Peter McL. Black, "Brain death," parts one and two, *New England Journal of Medicine* 299 (1978): 338–344; 393–401.

30. Robert Morison, "Death: process or event?" and Leon Kass, "Death as an event: a commentary on Robert Morison," *Science* (1971): 173: 694–702. At the same symposium, Beecher spoke on the criteria for brain death and Veatch criticized him for confusing technical and ethical matters.

31. Hans Jonas, "Reflections on human experimentation," *Daedalus* 98 (1969): 243–245.

32. Hans Jonas, "Against the stream," in *Philosophical Essays: From Ancient Creed to Technological Man* (Englewood Cliffs: Prentice Hall, 1974), pp. 132–140.

33. Jonas, "Against the stream," pp. 138, 140.

34. Paul Ramsey, "On updating procedures for stating that a man has died," in *The Patient as Person*, p. 112.

35. Robert M. Veatch, "The definition of death: ethical, philosophical and policy confusion," in Julius Korein (ed.), *Brain Death* (New York: The New York Academy of Sciences, 1978), pp. 307–318. Veatch describes these concepts somewhat differently in other writings; see, for example, Veatch, *Death, Dying and the Biological Revolution: Our Last Quest for Responsibility* (New Haven: Yale University Press, 1976), chapter 1.

36. H. Tristram Engelhardt, Jr., "Defining death: a philosophical problem for medicine and law," *Annual Review of Respiratory Disease* 112 (1975): 587; Robert M. Veatch, "The whole brain oriented concept of death: an out-moded philosophical formulation," *Journal of Thanatology* 3 (1975): 13–30; Michael B. Green and Dan Wikler, "Brain death and personal identity," *Philosophy and Public Affairs* 9 (1980): 105; J. L. Bernat, C. M. Culver, B. Gert, "On the definition and criterion of death," *Annals of Internal Medicine* 94 (1991): 389–394; Bernard Gert, "Personal identity and the body," *Dialogue* 10 (1971): 458–478; Stanley Hauerwas, "Religious concepts of brain death and associated problems," in Korein, *Brain Death*, pp. 329–336; Fred Rosner, "Definition of death: in *Modern Medicine and Jewish Ethics* (New York: Yeshiva University Press, 1986) p. 241–254. William May, "Attitudes toward the newly dead," *Hastings Center Report* 1, no. 1 (1973): 3–15.

37. "The Public Health and Welfare," 42 USC 1802 (1978).

38. Transcripts, papers, and drafts of the May and July meetings are in President's Commission Archive Boxes 25 and 37, National Reference Center for Bioethics Literature, Georgetown University, Washington, D.C.

39. President's Commission on Ethical Problems in Medicine and Biomedical and Behavioral Research, *Defining Death: A Report on the Medical, Legal, and Ethical Issues in the Definition of Death* (Washington, D.C.: U.S. Government Printing Office, 1981).

40. President's Commission, *Defining Death*, p. 2.

41. Although the Commission's definition closely followed the suggestions made by its director, Alex Capron, and his co-author, Leon Kass, it simplified Capron and Kass's complex definition and added the crucial words "including the brain stem," which made clear that the definition embraced the total organic disintegration that follows the destruction of the brain's respiratory centers rather than only the permanent loss of consciousness. See Capron and Kass, "A statutory definition of the standards for determining human death."

42. Darrel W. Amundsen, "Medicine and the birth of defective children: approaches of the ancient world," in Richard M. McMillan, H. Tristram Engelhardt, Jr., and Stuart F. Spicker (eds.), *Euthanasia and the Newborn: Conflicts Regarding Saving Lives* (Dordrecht/Boston: D. Reidel

Publishing Company, 1987), pp. 3–22; Maria W. Piers, *Infanticide* (New York: Norton, 1978); Cindy Bouillon-Jensen, "Infanticide," in Warren T. Reich (ed.), *Encyclopedia of Bioethics* (2nd ed.) (New York: Simon and Schuster Macmillan, 1995), pp. 1200–1205.

43. In 1910, however, Dr. Harry Haiselden, a Chicago surgeon, publicly declared that he ended the lives of defective children; a dramatic silent film, with Haiselden in the starring role, justified this practice by a eugenic ethic. See Martin S. Pernick, *The Black Stork: Eugenics and the Death of "Defective" Babies in American Medicine and Motion Pictures* (New York: Oxford University Press, 1996).

44. Clement A. Smith, "Neonatal medicine and quality of life: an historical perspective," in Albert R. Jonsen and Michael J. Garland (eds.), *Ethics of Newborn Intensive Care* (Berkeley: Institute for Governmental Studies, 1976), p. 33.

45. Alexander Schaffer, *Diseases of the Newborn* (Philadelphia: Saunders, 1960).

46. P. Budetti and P. McManus, "Assessing the effectiveness of neonatal intensive care," *Medical Care* 20 (1982): 1027; President's Commission on Ethical Problems in Medicine and Biomedical and Behavioral Research, *Deciding to Forego Life-Sustaining Treatment: A Report on the Ethical and Legal Issues in Treatment Decisions* (Washington, D.C.: U.S. Government Printing Office, 1982), chapter 6.

47. William Silverman, "The lesson of retrolental fibroplasia," *Scientific American* 236 (1977): 100–107.

48. Interview with William Bartholome, January 15, 1995.

49. *International Documentation of the Contemporary Church*, 11 Dec. 1971, p. 56; Harold Schmeck, "Parley discusses life and death ethics," *New York Times* Oct 17, 1971, A33.

50. Paul A. Freund, "Mongoloids and 'mercy killing'" in Reiser et al., *Ethics in Medicine*, pp. 536–538; James M. Gustafson, "Mongolism, parental desires and the right to life," *Perspectives in Biology and Medicine* 16, no. 4 (1973): 529–557; Albert R. Jonsen, "Can an ethicist be a consultant," in Virginia Abernethy (ed.), *Frontiers in Medical Ethics: Applications in a Clinical Setting* (Cambridge, Mass.: Ballenger Publishing Company, 1980), 157–172.

51. Interview with William Bartholome, January 15, 1995.

52. Raymond S. Duff and A. G. M. Campbell, "Moral and ethical dilemmas in the special-care nursery," *New England Journal of Medicine* 289 (1973): 890–984.

53. Letters to the Editor, *New England Journal of Medicine* 290 (1974): 518–520.

54. Richard A. McCormick, "To save or let die," *Journal of the American Medical Association* 229 (1974): 172–176.

55. John C. Fletcher, "Abortion, euthanasia and care of the defective newborn," *New England Journal of Medicine* 292 (1975): 75–79; H. Tristram Engelhardt, Jr., "Ethical issues in aiding the death of young children," in Martin Kohl (ed.), *Beneficent Euthanasia* (Buffalo, N.Y.: Prometheus Books, 1975), pp. 180–192.

56. John Robertson and Norman Fost, "Passive euthanasia of defective newborn infants," *Journal of Pediatrics* 88 (1976): 883–889; John Robertson, "Involuntary euthanasia of defective newborns: a legal analysis," *Stanford Law Review* 27 (1975): 213–269.

57. Jonsen and Garland, *Ethics of Newborn Intensive Care*, p. 190; Albert Jonsen, William Tooley, Roderick Phibbs, and Michael Garland, "Critical issues in newborn intensive care: a conference report and policy proposal," *Pediatrics* 55 (1975): 756–768; Barbara Culliton, "Intensive care for newborns: are there times to pull the plug?" *Science* 188 (1975): 133–134.

58. Paul Ramsey, "An ingathering of other reasons for neonatal infanticide," in *Ethics at the Edges of Life: Medical and Legal Intersections* (New Haven: Yale University Press, 1978), pp. 228–267, 250.

59. "Infraethics" was my early effort to explain what I later designated as "casuistry"; the term appears in Albert R. Jonsen and Lewis Butler, "Public ethics and policy," *Hastings Center*

Report 5, no. 4 (1975): 17–31 and is ridiculed by Ramsey in *Ethics at the Edges of Life*, p. 242.

60. "The Bloomington baby," *Washington Post*, April 18, 1982: B6; "Private death," *New York Times*, April 27, 1982: A22.

61. George J. Annas "The Baby Doe regulations: governmental intervention in neonatal rescue medicine," *American Journal of Public Health* 74 (1984): 618–620. It is difficult to verify President Reagan's role in this story. The Schweiker quote in the Annas article is referenced to Norman Fost, "Putting hospitals on notice" *Hastings Center Report* 12, no. 4 (1982): 5–8, but Fost's article does not mention the President or Secretary Schweiker.

62. *Federal Register* 48 (1983), 9630–9632.

63. *In re Infant Doe*, No GU8204-00 (Cir. Monroe Conty, Ind, Apr. 12, 1982), *State ex rel infant Doe v Baker* (Ind Sup Ct. May 27, 1982) cert. Den. 464 US 961 (1983). A parallel New York case, with rather different facts, called Baby Jane Doe, was contested during the same period. See *Baby Jane Doe: Weber v Stonybrook Hospital*, 476 NYS 2d (1983); *U.S. v University Hospital* 729 F.2d 144, 156 (2d Cir. 1984).

64. *Bowen v American Hospital Association* 476 U.S. 610, 106 S. Ct. 2101 (1986).

65. *Federal Register* 50 (April 15, 1985), 14888.

66. L. M. Kopelman, T. G. Irons, and A. E. Kopelman, "Neonatologists judge the 'Baby Doe' regulations," *New England Journal of Medicine* 318 (1988): 677–683; Fost, "Putting hospitals on notice," pp. 5–8; Nancy M. P. King, "Federal and state regulation of neonatal decision-making," in McMillan et al., *Euthanasia and the Newborn*, Thomas H. Murray, "The final, anticlimactic rule on Baby Doe," *Hastings Center Report* 15, no. 3 (1985): 5–9; Nancy K. Rhoden and John D. Arras, "Withholding treatment from Baby Doe: from discrimination to child abuse," *Milbank Memorial Fund Quarterly* 63 (1985): 18–51.

67. Albert R. Jonsen, "Ethics, law and the treatment of seriously ill newborns," in A. Edward Doudera and J. Douglas Peters (eds.), *Legal and Ethical Aspects of Treating Critically and Terminally Ill Patients* (Ann Arbor, Mich.: AUPHA Press, 1982), pp. 236–241.

68. *Maine Medical Center v Houle*, 74–145, Cumberland Co., Maine, Feb 14, 1974, *In Matter of Kerrin Ann McNulty* #1960 Essex Co., Mass., Feb. 15, 1978. During the thalidomide tragedy in 1963, a Belgian mother, Corinne Van de Put, killed her infant, born with no arms, a disfigured face and imperforate anus. She was tried for murder and acquitted on the grounds that she did not have the motive requisite for murder. The story was followed avidly in the United States. See *New York Times*, November 11, 1962: A35; November 16, 1962; A1, A7.

69. John Lorber, "Results of treatment of mylomeningocele," *Developmental Medicine and Child Neurology* 13 (1971): 279; "Results of selective treatment of spina bifida cystica," *British Medical Journal* 4 (1973): 201.

70. Robert M. Veatch, "The technical criteria fallacy," *Hastings Center Report* 7, no. 4 (1977): 15–16; T. Ackerman, "Meningomyelocele and parental commitment: A policy proposal regarding selection for treatment," *Man and Medicine* 5 (1980): 201; Stuart F. Spicker and J. R. Raye, "The bearing of prognosis on the ethics of medicine: congenital anomalies, the social context and the law," in Stuart F. Spicker, Joseph M. Healey, Jr., and H. Tristram Engelhardt, Jr. (eds.), *The Law-Medicine Relation: A Philosophical Exploration* (Dordrecht/Boston: D. Reidel Publishing Company, 1981), pp. 189–216; R. B. Zachary, "Commentary: on the death of a baby," *Journal of Medical Ethics* 7 (1981): 5; Chester A. Swinyard, *Decision Making and the Defective Newborn. Proceedings of a Conference on Spina Bifida and Ethics* (Springfield, Ill.: Charles Thomas, 1978).

71. John Freeman, "The shortsighted treatment of myelomeningocele: a long term case report," *Pediatrics* 53 (1974): 511; R. Reid, "Spina bifida: the fate of the untreated," *Hastings Center Report* 7, no. 4 (1977): 16.

72. Swinyard, *Decision Making and the Defective Newborn*, p. 608. The bioethicists present

were Joseph Fletcher and John Fletcher, Norman Fost, Paul Ramsey, Warren Reich, Robert Veatch, John Robertson, Rabbi David Bleich, and myself.

73. President's Commission, *Deciding to Forego Life-Sustaining Treatment*, pp. 218–219, 225–226.

74. President's Commission, *Deciding to Forego Life-Sustaining Treatment* chapter 6, pp. 197–229; Raymond S. Duff and A. G. M. Campbell, "Moral and ethical dilemmas in the special-care nursery," *New England Journal of Medicine* 289 (1973): 890–894; Anthony Shaw, "Dilemmas of 'informed consent' in children," *New England Journal of Medicine* 289 (1973): 885–890; Jeff Lyon, *Playing God in the Nursery* (New York: Norton, 1985); Earl E. Shelp and R. Weir, *Selective Nontreatment of Handicapped Newborns* (New York: Oxford University Press, 1984); Robert Stinson and Peggy Stinson, *The Long Dying of Baby Andrew* (Boston: Little, Brown, 1983).

75. *Macbeth*, Act V, scene viii, l. 16.

76. T. Tuffier and L. Hallion, "De la compression rhythmie du coeur dan la syncope cardiaque par embolie," *Bulletin de la Société de Chirurgie de Paris* 24 (1898): 937.

77. H. D. Adams and L. V. Hand, "Twenty minute cardiac arrest with complete recovery," *Journal of the American Medical Association* 118 (1942): 133; C. S. Beck, "Resuscitation for cardiac standstill and ventricular fibrillation occurring during operation," *American Journal of Surgery* 54 (1941): 273; C. S. Beck, W. H. Pritchard, and H. S. Feil, "Ventricular fibrillation of long duration abolished by electric shock," *Journal of the American Medical Association* 135 (1947): 985–986.

78. W. B. Kouwenhoven, J. R. Jude, and G. G. Knickerbocker, "Closed chest cardiac massage," *Journal of the American Medical Association* 173 (1960): 1064; see also Lael Wertenbaker, *To Mend the Heart* (New York: Viking Press, 1980); Mickey S. Eisenberg, *Life in the Balance: Emergency Medicine and the Quest to Reverse Sudden Death* (New York: Oxford University Press, 1997).

79. "Standards for cardiopulmonary resuscitation (CPR) and emergency cardiac care (ECC)," *Journal of the American Medical Association* 227 (7) (1974): Suppl. 841–860.

80. J. Castagna, H. Shubin, and M. H. Weil, "Cardiac arrest in the critically ill patient," *Heart and Lung* 2 (1973): 847.

81. M. Rabkin, G. Gillerman, and N. R. Rice, "Orders not to resuscitate," *New England Journal of Medicine* 295 (1976): 364; "Optimum care for hopelessly ill patients: a report of the Critical Care Committee of the Massachusetts General Hospital," *New England Journal of Medicine* 295 (1976): 362.

82. President's Commission, *Deciding to Forego Life-Sustaining Treatment*, pp. 237, 510–511.

83. *In Re Dinnerstein*, 1978 Mass App 380 NE2d, at 138.

84. W. A. Tweed, "Evaluation of hospital-based cardiac resuscitation," *California Medical Association Journal* 301 (1980): 122–126; M. DeBard, "Cardiopulmonary resuscitation: analysis of six years experience and review of the literature," *Annals of Emergency Medicine* 10 (1981): 408–412; Susan Bedell, Thomas Delbanco, E. Francis Cook, and Franklin Epstein, "Survival after cardiopulmonary resuscitation in the hospital," *New England Journal of Medicine* 309 (1983): 569–576; Stuart J. Youngner, "Do not resuscitate orders: no longer secret, but still a problem," *Hastings Center Report* 17, no. 1 (1987): 24–33.

85. President's Commission, *Deciding to Forego Life-Sustaining Treatment*, p. 244.

86. Lawrence J. Schneiderman and Nancy S. Jecker, *Wrong Medicine: Doctors, Patients, and Futile Treatment* (Baltimore: Johns Hopkins University Press, 1995).

87. "Affidavit of Guardian ad Litem, Daniel Coburn," *In the Matter of Karen Quinlan. The*

Complete Legal Briefs, Court Proceedings and Decision, Volume I (Arlington, Va.: University Publications of America, 1975), pp. 19–20.

88. *In re Quinlan* 70 NJ, 335 A2d, at 663.

89. Robert Veatch, "Foregoing life support," (paper read at the Birth of Bioethics Conference, Seattle, Wa., Sept. 23–24, 1992), transcript pp. 185–187.

90. Vincent Collins, "Limits of moral responsibility in prolonging life: a guide to decisions," *Journal of the American Medical Association* 206 (1968): 389–392; George Fletcher, "Legal aspects of the decision not to prolong life," *Journal of the American Medical Association* 203 (1968): 66.

91. Diana Crane, "Physicians' attitudes toward the treatment of critically ill patients," *The Radcliffe Quarterly* 62 (March, 1976): 18–21, 21; Diana Crane, *The Sanctity of Social Life: Physicians' Treatment of Critically Ill Patients* (New York: Russel Sage Foundation, 1975); see also Franklin H. Epstein, "The role of the physician in the prolongation of life," Eugene A. Stead, Jr., "Death as you wish it," and Robert S. Morison, "Alternatives to striving too officiously," in Franz J. Ingelfinger, Richard V. Ebert, Maxwell Finland, and Arnold S. Relman (eds.), *Controversy in Internal Medicine*, Vol. II (Philadelphia: W. B. Saunders, 1974), pp. 103–109, 110–112, 113–121.

92. Charles Fried, "Terminating life-support: out of the closet," *New England Journal of Medicine* 295 (1976): 390–391.

93. Cathy Siebold, *The Hospice Movement: Easing Death's Pain* (New York: Maxwell Macmillan International, 1992); Sandol Stoddard, *The Hospice Movement: A Better Way of Caring for the Dying* (New York: Stein and Day, 1978); Dame Cicely Saunders and Mary Baines, *Living with Dying: The Management of Terminal Disease* (New York: Oxford University Press, 1983).

94. Elisabeth Kübler-Ross, *On Death and Dying* (New York: Macmillan, 1969).

95. Paul Ramsey, "The indignity of 'death with dignity,' " *Hastings Center Studies* 2, no. 2 (1974): 47–62.

96. Gerald Kelly, *Preserving Life, Medico-Moral Problems* (St. Louis: Catholic Hospital Association, 1958); F. Patrick McKegney and P. Lange, "The decision to no longer live on chronic hemodialysis," *American Journal of Psychiatry* 128 (1971): 264–273; H. S. Abram, "The psychiatrist, the treatment of chronic renal failure and the prolongation of life," *American Journal of Psychiatry* 126 (1969): 157–167.

97. Paul Ramsey, *The Patient as Person*, p. 114.

98. Ramsey, *The Patient as Person*, p. 119.

99. Gerald Kelly, "The duty of using artificial means of preserving life," *Theological Studies*, 11 (1950): 203–22; "The duty to preserve life," *Theological Studies* 12 (1951): 550–556.

100. Ramsey, *The Patient as Person*, p. 122.

101. Ramsey, *The Patient as Person*, p. 137.

102. Ramsey, *The Patient as Person*, p. 161.

103. Ramsey, *The Patient as Person*, p. 148.

104. Ramsey, *Ethics at the Edges of Life,* pp. 159, 189. St. Augustine, one of Western culture's most dogmatic thinkers, issued *Retractiones* at the end of his life, in which he admitted to his few doctrinal errors.

105. Ramsey, *Ethics at the Edges of Life*, pp. 156–157.

106. See James F. Childress, *Who Should Decide?: Paternalism in Health Care* (New York: Oxford University Press, 1982), pp. 164ff; Ronald Carson, "Paul Ramsey, principled protestant casuist," in *Medical Humanities Review* 2 (1988): 24–35.

107. James Rachels, "Active and passive euthanasia," *New England Journal of Medicine* 292

(1975): 78–80; *The End of Life: Euthanasia and Morality* (New York: Oxford University Press, 1986); John Ladd, *Ethical Issues Relating to Death and Dying* (New York: Oxford University Press, 1979) (based on a conference at Brown University, 1974); P. J. Fitzgerald, "Acting and refraining," in Samuel Gorovitz, Andrew Jameton, Ruth Macklin, et al., (eds.), *Moral Problems in Medicine* (Englewood Cliffs: Prentice-Hall, 1976), pp. 284–289; Bonnie Steinbock (ed.), *Killing and Letting Die* (Englewood Cliffs: Prentice-Hall, 1980); Jonathan Glover, *Causing Death and Saving Lives* (New York: Penguin Books, 1977). Subsequent to the Commission's study, The Hastings Center Working Group on Death and Dying produced a comprehensive statement, *Guidelines on the Termination of Life-Sustaining Treatment and Care of the Dying* (Bloomington, Ind.: University of Indiana Press, 1987).

108. President's Commission, *Deciding to Forego Life-Sustaining Treatment*, pp. 1–2.

109. President's Commission, *Deciding to Forego Life-Sustaining Treatment*, p. 3.

110. President's Commission, *Deciding to Forego Life-Sustaining Treatment*, p. 89.

111. The words "proportionate" and "disproportionate" are not in the text of the report, but they do appear in a footnote on the same page as the above-quoted conclusion, in a citation from the Vatican's *Declaration on Euthanasia* (June 26, 1980), which is reprinted in an appendix to the report. While there are subtle differences of meaning between the Vatican's concept of proportionate care and the Commission's conclusion, there is a common theme: a treatment is not morally obligatory when, in the patient's view, it produces greater burdens than benefits. See President's Commission, *Deciding to Forego Life-Sustaining Treatment*, p. 88.

112. Darrel W. Amundsen, "The physician's obligation to prolong life: a medical duty without classical roots," *Hastings Center Report* 8, no. 4 (1978): 23–30.

113. L. D. Kliever, *Dax's Case: Essays in Medical Ethics and Human Meaning* (Dallas: Southern Methodist University Press, 1989), p. xv.

114. S. Imbus and B. Zawacki, "Autonomy for burn patients when survival is unprecedented," *New England Journal of Medicine* 300 (1977): 301–311.

115. Seneca, *Letters From a Stoic*, letter lxxvii, 77 (Harmondsworth: Penguin, 1969), p. 126.

116. J. S. Hamilton, "Scribonius Largus on the medical profession," 60 (1986): 209–216. See also Ludwig Edelstein, "The Hippocratic Oath: text, translation and interpretation," in Owsei Temkin and C. Lilian Temkin (eds.), *Ancient Medicine: Selected Papers of Ludwig Edelstein* (Baltimore: The Johns Hopkins Press, 1983), p. 12; Danielle Gourevitch, "Suicide among the sick in classical antiquity," *Bulletin of the History of Medicine* 43 (1969): 501–518; Paul Carrick, *Medical Ethics in Antiquity* (Dordrecht: D. Reidel Publishing Company, 1985), chapter 7; John M. Cooper, "Greek philosophers on euthanasia and suicide," in Baruch A. Brody (ed.), *Suicide and Euthanasia: Historical and Contemporary Themes* (Dordrecht/Boston: Kluwer Academic Publishers, 1989), pp. 9–38.

117. St. Augustine, *City of God* I, 16; See Darrel Amundsen, "Suicide and early christian values," in Brody (ed.), *Suicide and Euthanasia*, pp. 77–154.

118. St. Thomas Aquinas, *Summa Theologiae*, II–II, q. 64, a. 5.

119. St. Thomas More, *Utopia*, in *The Complete Works of St. Thomas More*, Edward Surtz and J. H. Hexter eds. (New Haven: Yale University Press, 1963), IV, p. 186; John Donne, *Biathanatos*, Margaret Battin and Michael Rudick eds. (New York: Garland Publishing, 1982).

120. David Hume, "On Suicide," in *Essays Moral, Political and Literary* (London: Oxford, 1963), pp. 586–596.

121. Samuel Williams, "Euthanasia," *Popular Science Monthly* (May 1873): 91; Lionel Tollemache, "The new cure for incurables," *Fortnightly Review* (Feb. 1873): 218–230.

122. "Permissive euthanasia," *Boston Medical and Surgical Journal* 110 (1884): 19–20.

123. Charles B. Williams, "Euthanasia, 1894," *Medical and Surgical Report*, 70 (1894): 909–911; see also Stanley Joel Reiser, "The dilemma of euthanasia in modern medical history:

The English and American experience," in John A. Behnke and Sissela Bok (eds.), *The Dilemmas of Euthanasia* (New York: Anchor Press, 1975), pp. 27–49, and reprinted in Reiser et al., *Ethics in Medicine*, pp. 488–494; W. Bruce Fye, "Active euthanasia. An historical survey of its conceptual origins and introduction to medical thought," *Bulletin of the History of Medicine* 52 (1979): 492–501; Brody, *Suicide and Euthanasia.*

124. Stanley J. Reiser, "The dilemma of euthanasia in modern medical history: The English and American Experience," in Reiser et al., *Ethics in Medicine*, p. 490. Apparently, the first legislative attempt was in the Ohio legislature in 1906. A complete dossier of proposed legislation is provided in David Forster, "Slippery Slope Arguments against Physician-Assisted Suicide: The Challenge to the Legislative Drafter," Master's thesis, University of Washington, 1996.

125. Reprinted in Reiser et al., *Ethics in Medicine,* pp. 498–500. Text is reprinted in O. Ruth Russell, *Freedom to Die: Moral and Legal Aspects of Euthanasia* (New York: Human Science Press, 1977), pp. 291–294. As the king lay comotose and clearly dying, the Privy Council (of which Dawson was a member) expressed concern that should he survive the night, the news of his death would appear in the evening tabloids rather than in the newspaper of record, *The Times of London*; Lord Dawson obligingly prepared a morphine injection and His Majesty expired just after midnight. "Life of King George V ended prematurely." *Times of London*, Nov. 27, 1986, p. 1; "The King's Peace?" *Times of London*, Nov. 28, 1986, p. 17.

126. Legislature of Nebraska, Bill No 135 (1937), reprinted in Forster, "Slippery Slope Arguments," pp. 122–128.

127. Leo Alexander, "Medicine under dictatorship," *New England Journal of Medicine* 241 (1949): 39–47; Robert N. Proctor, *Racial Hygiene: Medicine Under the Nazis* (Cambridge: Harvard University Press, 1988).

128. Frank Hinman, "Euthanasia," *Journal of Neurological and Mental Diseases* 99 (1944): 640.

129. Joseph Fletcher, *Morals and Medicine* (Princeton: Princeton University Press, 1954), p. 207.

130. Fletcher, *Morals and Medicine*, chapter 6, in particular, pp. 187–189.

131. Marvin Kohl (ed.), *Beneficent Euthanasia* (New York: Prometheus Books, 1975); Daniel C. Maguire, *Death by Choice* (New York: Doubleday, 1973); John A. Behnke and Sissela Bok (eds.), *The Dilemmas of Euthanasia* (Garden City, N.Y.: Anchor Press, 1975).

132. President's Commission, *Deciding to Forego Life-Sustaining Treatment*, pp. 37–38.

133. President's Commission, *Deciding to Forego Life-Sustaining Treatment*, p. 73.

134. *Code of Medical Ethics Annotated Current Opinions of the Council on Ethical and Judicial Affairs of the American Medical Association* (Chicago: American Medical Association, 1992), section 12, p. 46, currently Opinion 2.20, "Withholding and withdrawing life-prolonging medical treatment" (1996–1997 edition of the *Code of Medical Ethics*).

135. James Rachels, "Active and passive euthanasia," *New England Journal of Medicine* 292 (1975): 78–80.

136. President's Commission, *Deciding to Forego Life-Sustaining Treatment,* pp. 60–88.

137. Yale Kamisar, "Some non-religious views against proposed 'mercy killing,'" *Minnesota Law Review* 42 (1968): 969–1042.

138. "It's over Debbie," *Journal of the American Medical Association* 259 (1988): 272; Willard Gaylin, Leon R. Kass, Edmond D. Pellegrino, and Mark Siegler, "Doctors should not kill," Kenneth Vaux, "Debbie's death: mercy killing and the good death," and George Lundberg, "'It's over Debbie' and the euthanasia debate," *Journal of the American Medical Association* (1988): 259: 2139–2143.

139. Derek Humphry, *Final Exit: The Practicalities of Self-Deliverance and Assisted Suicide for the Dying* (Secaucus, N.J.: The Hemlock Society, 1991).

140. See Carlos F. Gomez, *Regulating Death: Euthanasia and the Case of the Netherlands* (New York: The Free Press, 1991); Richard Fenigsen, "Physician-assisted death in The Netherlands: impact on long-term care," *Issues in Law and Medicine* 11 (1995): 283–297; M. A. M. de Wachter, "Active euthanasia in The Netherlands," *Journal of the American Medical Association* 262 (1989): 3316–3319; Henk Rigter, Els Borst-Eilers, and H. J. J. Leenen, "Euthanasia across the North Sea," *British Medical Journal* 297 (1988): 1593–1595. See also the special issue of *Issues in Law and Medicine, Euthanasia and the Netherlands* (1988) 3: 361–452. The Netherlands has not revoked its law against euthanasia, but physicians are allowed to practice it, in accord with strict guidelines, without threat of liability.

141. *Oregon Death With Dignity Act*, Section 2, 127. 805. Although the subsequent legal actions regarding assisted suicide take place in the years beyond this history, it is worth nothing that on June 26, 1997, the U.S. Supreme Court decided two cases, *Washington et al. v Glucksberg et al.* and *Vacco, Attorney General of New York, et al. v Quill et al.*, in which the justices determined that, while there was no constitutionally protected right or liberty for assisted suicide, the problem deserved continued debate; states may legislate permissively, and palliative care should be fostered. While the arguments are framed in legal terms, the decisions are almost a compendium of the bioethical arguments of the last decade.

142. Leake, *Percival's Medical Ethics*, chapter IV, 7, p. 130.

143. *In re Quinlan*, Affidavit of Guardian ad Litem, Daniel Coburn, *In the Matter of Karen Quinlan. The Complete Legal Briefs, Court Proceedings and Decision* (Arlington, Va.: University Publications of America, 1975), vol. I, pp. 19–20.

144. *In the Matter of Karen Quinlan*, Vol. I, p. 555, fn 5.

145. *In the Matter of Karen Quinlan*, Vol. II, p. 306.

146. *Superintendent of Belchertown State School v Saikewicz*, Mass Supreme Court, 1977. 373 Mass. 728, 736 (p. 7).

147. John Robertson, "Organ donations by incompetents and the substituted judgment doctrine," *Columbia Law Review* 76 (1976): 48; John Rawls, *Theory of Justice*, p. 209.

148. *Superintendent of Belchertown State School v Saikewicz*, Mass Supr. Ct. 373 Mass. 728, 750–755 (1977), pp. 15, 16, 17.

149. *In re Shirley Dinnerstein*, 6 Mass App. 466, 380 N.E.2d 134 (1978).

150. *In re Spring*, 380 Mass. 629, 405 N.E.2d 115 (1980); *In re Eichner*, 73 A.D.2d 431, 426 N.Y.S.2d 517 (1980). Other cases followed: Barber (California, 1983), Bartling (California, 1984), Conroy (New Jersey, 1985), Jobes (New Jersey, 1987), and Brophy (Massachusetts, 1986).

151. *Bouvia v Superior Court*, 179 Cal. App. 3d 1127, 225 Cal. Rptr. 297 (1986).

152. *In re Quinlan*, 355 A.2d 647, p. 663.

153. *Superintendent of Belchertown State School v Saikewicz*, Mass Supr. Ct. 373 Mass. 728, 754 (1977), p. 17.

154. *In the Matter of Claire Conroy*, Supreme Court of New Jersey 98 N.J. 321; 486 A. 2d 1209; 48 A.L.R. 4th 1, 1985; Sidney H. Wanzer, S. James Adelstein, Ronald E. Cranford, et al., "The physician's responsibility toward hopelessly ill patients," *New England Journal of Medicine* 310 (1984): 955–959; Arthur Dyck, "Ethical aspects of care for the dying incompetent," *Journal of the American Geriatric Society* 32 (1984): 661; K. Danner Clouser, "Allowing or causing: another look," *Annals of Internal Medicine* 87 (1977): 622; Joanne Lynn and James F. Childress, "Must patients always be given food and water?" *Hastings Center Report* 13, no. 5 (1983): 17–21; Bernard Lo and Loren L. Dorenbrand, "Guiding the hand that feeds: caring for the demented elderly," *New England Journal of Medicine* 311 (1984): 401.

155. *Barber v Superior Court* 147 Cal App 3d 1006, 195 Cal Rptr, at 1232; President's Commission, *Deciding to Forego Life-Sustaining Treatment*, pp. 88–89. The court pulled from a foot-

note the Commission's citation of the Vatican statement recommending that the words "proportionate" and "disproportionate" replace "ordinary" and "extraordinary."

156. Robert F. Weir, *Abating Treatment: Ethical and Legal Limits to the Prolonging of Life* (New York: Oxford University Press, 1989), p. 181.

157. Albert R. Jonsen and Stuart Eisendrath, "The living will: help or hindrance," *Journal of the American Medical Association* 249 (1983): 2054–2058.

158. Karen Lebacqz, "On 'natural death,'" *Hastings Center Report* 7, no. 2 (1977): 14; Michael J. Garland, "Politics, legislation and natural death: the right to die in California," *Hastings Center Report* 6, no. 5 (1976): 5–6.

159. President's Commission, *Deciding to Forego Life-Sustaining Treatment*, chapter 4.

160. A disconcerting report has recently appeared that casts doubt on how deeply the lessons of bioethics have penetrated medical practice; see The SUPPORT Principle Investigators, "A controlled trial to improve care for seriously ill hospitalized patients," *Journal of the American Medical Association* 274 (1995): 1592–1598.

9

O Brave New World: The Ethics of Human Reproduction

Socrates' friends once asked him to describe family life in his ideal republic and "how citizens will bring children into the world and rear them when they have arrived." Socrates replied, "The answers to these questions are far from easy. . . . I approach the subject with great reluctance."[1] He overcame his reluctance enough to declaim about how to choose the fittest parents and even proposed that wives and offspring be held in common. His novel suggestions astonished Socrates' friends. During the second half of the twentieth century, novel ways of procreating children astonished the world. The settled ethics about how people beget children and rear them has been disturbed by the scientific ability to conceive children without sexual intercourse, by joining sperm and ovum outside the body and inserting the resulting zygote into a womb. These novel ways of procreation raised questions that, as Socrates admitted, are far from easy to answer. The questions are even difficult to comprehend without understanding the old ethics about reproduction that placed the generation of children within the legal and moral setting of monogamous marriage, discouraged the deliberate inhibition of conception, and prohibited abortion. This chapter begins, then, by tracing many almost forgotten paths of the old ethics of reproduction and goes on to review the questions and answers about the ethics of the new reproductive technologies.

The begetting of children has been a matter of morality and religion in most cultures and over many centuries. The various unions of men and women that are expected to generate children have been regulated by custom, law, and ritual. The birth of infants has been surrounded by taboos and rites. The sexual behavior physiologically associated with reproduction has fallen under a multitude of strictures. None of this is surprising: sex and reproduction mesh with a myriad of other vital social practices and institutions. Historian James Brundage writes, "Sexual beliefs and practices exert power, not only over individual conduct, but also over the ways in which institutions themselves grow and develop. Marriage, adultery, fornication, prostitution, rape, sodomy and celibacy—all have significant bearings upon property interests, household structure and notions about morality."[2] Out of the long history of how Western society has viewed this sphere of morality, we can pick out the general lineaments, seeing only the ideas, insulated from the intense emotions that have surrounded these matters in private and social life.

The origins of marriage as a cultural device to structure sexual behavior around reproduction are lost in the mists of the past. Monogamous marriage appears in the most ancient records of the Near Eastern cultures and in Greek and Roman antiquity. The Code of Hammurabi and the Laws of Solon enforce monogamous unions. All philosophical sects of the Hellenic and Hellenistic worlds offer reflections on sexuality, marriage, and procreation. Even when a wide variety of sexual practices was tolerated, monogamous marriage appears as a central social institution. The Mosaic law, which initially permitted polygyny, rigidly regulated sexual behavior. Important above all was the imperative for every Jewish male to marry and beget children, and rabbinic law carefully designed the family structure that enabled Yahweh's command to Adam and then to Noah, "be fruitful and multiply," to be fulfilled (Gen. 1:28; 9:1; 9:7). The Gospels that relate the story and words of Jesus say relatively little about sexuality and marriage. Among Jesus' few comments, one becomes central to the Christian view of marriage, "Have you not read that he made them male and female . . . so a man shall leave father and mother and they shall be one flesh. . . . what therefore God hath joined together, let not man put asunder" (Matt. 19:4–6).

The writings of Paul, one of Jesus' first followers, are filled with literal and symbolic references to marriage. Citing these same words of Jesus, Paul comments, "Husbands, love your wives, even as Christ loved the church and gave himself for it" (Eph. 5:26). Despite this solemn injunction, Paul evinces a negative attitude toward sexuality. All sexual activity outside marriage was condemned and sex within marriage grudgingly approved. "Flee fornication . . . he that committeth fornication sins against his own body. . . . It is good for a man not to touch a woman. Nevertheless, to avoid fornication, let every man have his own wife and every woman her own husband" (I Cor. 6: 18; 7:2). These Pauline notions fueled a disdain and even repugnance for sexuality in many influential figures of early Christianity.[3]

Catholic thought about sex and marriage was profoundly affected by the church's vigorous repudiation during the fourth and fifth centuries of a rival religious doctrine, Manichaeism. Mani, an Iranian prophet, elaborated Iranian folk religion, which divided creation into a Kingdom of Light ruled by the Living Spirit and a Kingdom of Darkness dominated by the Prince of Darkness. The Prince of Darkness created human beings and the material world. Matter, including the human body, was evil. Manichaean scripture proclaimed, "Evil become[s] the framer of bodies, deriving from bodies the generative forces to fashion them."[4] The act of human procreation multiplied evil in the world. Human salvation was won by cleansing oneself of the material world, which involved repudiation of procreation.

The church's champion against Manichaeism was an African of deep learning and powerful eloquence, Augustine, Bishop of Hippo. As a youth, Augustine had been attracted to Manichaean beliefs. He also led a luxurious and debauched life. When converted to the Catholic faith at the age of thirty, he repented his former ways, attributing his slowness in seeing the truth to the power of lust, and turned ardent opponent of Manichaean doctrine. His personal experiences combined with Pauline prudery to form a theological ethics of sexuality that dominated Catholic thinking for centuries. On the one hand, he refuted the Manichean teaching that procreation was collusion in evil: procreation, Augustine asserted, was good within a holy marriage. The very purpose of marriage was "offspring, mutual fidelity and holiness (*proles, fides, sacramentum*)."[5] On the other hand, his repugnance at his own youthful lust made him see all sexuality as tainted with sin. Sexual behavior was redeemed only when intended to procreate children. Within marriage, sexual activity had to be strictly held to that purpose; outside marriage, it was wholly sinful. His distaste for sex was transmuted into a theological doctrine when, in arguing against another heretic, Pelagius, he associated sexual desire with Adam's Original Sin that would damn the entire human race, had it not been for its redemption by Jesus Christ.[6] Augustine's teachings reinforced the ambiguity surrounding marriage and sexuality that had been intimated in the writings of Paul the Apostle. The growing church incorporated that ambiguity.

The church's theology of marriage settled into clear doctrine during the early Middle Ages. It developed further as the church encountered many customs among the evangelized peoples of Northern Europe that it aimed to extinguish, particularly concubinage and dissolvable marriage. Out of these battles emerged a doctrine of marriage as a sacrament sealed by the church between a single man and woman, indissoluble during life and dedicated to the procreation and education of children. Sexual intercourse within marriage for the purpose of procreation was morally good; sexual behaviors that were not procreative were sinful. All sexual activity outside marriage was seriously sinful, including masturbation, homosexuality, and fornication. Abortion and contraception were prohibited. Imposition of celibacy on the clergy set up an ideal that in comparison made marriage, despite its sacral nature, deficient. Church law, borrowing from the Roman law of marriage, made marriage a legal institution with many rules, over which the church claimed primary jurisdiction. A theology of marriage taught the laity their duties and required that they confess their failures to their priests. This view of marriage, sexuality, and reproduction dominated the Western world. Even after the Roman church lost its universal authority after the Reformation, the reformed churches espoused essentially the same theology and influenced the legal regulation of marriage by the state. This view of marriage and sexuality, in its moral and legal dimensions, prevailed, even in an attenuated form, when the new reproductive technologies appeared in the twentieth century.

Abortion

Abortion is sparsely mentioned in the literature of the ancient world. After Socrates described how the union of men and women should generate the most suitable children, he advised that there be strict laws to assure that, "any embryo (conceived outside the legally prescribed unions) must be prevented from seeing the light and, if any are born, parents must understand that such offspring cannot be maintained and arrange accordingly."[7] Aristotle also proposed laws about marriage that would guarantee "that the frames of the children who are reared may be as good as possible." He not only counseled on the best age for procreation ("Women who marry early are apt to be wanton; and in men the bodily frame is stunted if they marry while the seed is still growing.") but also advised in case of failure: "Let there be a law that no deformed child shall live . . . and if couples have children in excess, let abortion be procured before life and sense have begun."[8] The concluding phrase reflects Aristotle's belief that living things were "ensouled," that is, physical matter was given form and purpose at various stages of development. Although his teaching is difficult to interpret, he seems to claim that a human becomes human, that is, is informed with a rational soul, sometime during the second trimester of pregnancy. The first signs of fetal movement in the womb, or "quickening," was later taken as evidence of that event.[9] This Aristotelian embryology, and the ethics that went with it, profoundly influenced thinking about abortion for centuries.

The Hippocratic Oath contains the phrase, "I will not give to a woman an abortifacient pessary." The phrase is not entirely clear in meaning or intent. It may be an expression of the Pythagorean belief that requires all humans to respect and preserve life in all its forms.[10] Only physicians belonging to this cult would have honored that prohibition of the Oath. The phrase refers only to one technique for abortion, although many techniques were known to ancient medicine, and probably many more were familiar to women and those who would assist them to end a pregnancy. The ancient texts of gynecology that describe these techniques rarely comment on the morality of the practice. One rare comment appears in the gynecological treatise by the second-century A.D. physician, Soranus, who notes two schools of thought about a physician's cooperation in abortion. Some physicians "banish abortives, citing the testimony of Hippocrates . . . and also because it is the specific task of medicine to guard and preserve what has been engendered by nature." Others will prescribe an abortifacient but only for a proper medical reason, such as a deformed *os uteri;* they would not prescribe "to destroy the embryo conceived in adultery or to preserve youthful beauty." Soranus does not choose between these views, but he does recommend contraception over abortion because it is safer.[11] Roman physician Scribonius Largus invoked the Oath to condemn a physician's collaboration in abortion.[12] Ancient literature, then, shows the inkling of an ethics about physicians' cooperation in abortion, but it appears that, in general, abortion was common, unsanctioned morally, and aided by physicians.

One text in the Hebrew Bible, Exodus 21:22–23, mentions abortion in the context of a miscarriage caused by someone pushing a pregnant woman. The text is concerned with the payment of appropriate compensation for the loss of the fetus. Rabbinical commentators all agree that a fetus does not attain the status of *nephesh,* a living human, until it breathes the air of the world; a fetus is part of the mother's body until birth. Thus, the deliberate death or destruction of fetal life is not the killing of a human being. One talmudic text says forthrightly, "it is permissible to kill an unborn fetus."[13]

Despite these teachings, the predominant talmudic and rabbinical opinions repudiate abortion in all cases except to save the mother's life. Many reasons are given—abortion is analogous to forbidden expulsion of semen in coitus interruptus, abortion is a prohibited wounding of the self, abortion destroys a potential life—but the principal reason arises from the fact that the major Mishnaic text on abortion, *Oholot,* deals with it in the context of a defense of maternal life, and almost all subsequent commentary, from the great Maimonides onward, interprets abortion solely within that light.[14] Rabbi Immanuel Jakobovits writes, "The Jewish attitude to the destruction of foetal and nascent human life is complex and but sparsely defined in our chief sources. . . . While, according to the consensus of rabbinical opinion, (foetal) life is not protected by any definite legal provisions, the artificial termination of a pregnancy is strongly condemned on moral grounds, unless it can be justified for medical or, possibly, other grave reasons."[15]

The Christian scriptures do not mention abortion. One early Christian writing, *Didache,* contains the stark injunction, "You shall not kill the fetus by abortion or destroy the infant already born." Those who do so are "destroyers of the work of God."[16] Many subsequent writers include abortion among their catalogues of serious sins: it is akin to murder. Yet, despite all this testimony, no argument is adduced to explain why abortion is akin to murder or even to clarify what is meant by abortion. Theological and canonical texts do not clearly distinguish between abortion, contraception, sterilization, and infanticide.[17] The twelfth-century canonist Gratian, who collated the principal texts of ancient church law, mentions the doctrine, derived from Aristotle and preserved through the Middle Ages, of the difference between the "formed" and the "unformed" fetus. Only the killing of a formed fetus counts as homicide.[18] This distinction was adopted in a definitive collection of church law issued by Pope Gregory IX. The medieval theologians and most later theological and canonical writers accepted this view; abortion is to be condemned as equivalent to homicide and subject to ecclesiastical penalty only if the fetus is "formed" or "animated" or "vivified." Destruction of a fetus before animation was considered a sin against the primary good of marriage, procreation, but not as a homicide, and did not incur ecclesiastical penalties.[19]

The question most urgent for medical ethics, namely, the legitimacy of abortion to save the mother's life, was not discussed by Catholic theologians or canonists until the fourteenth century. The founder of moral theology, Archbishop Antoninus of Florence, concluded that a physician may and should procure an abortion when the continued pregnancy threatens maternal life but only if he is morally certain that the fetus is "unformed." In such cases, the mother has a prior right (*jus potius*) to life. If the fetus is "formed," the physician must refrain from abortion even should the mother die. The physician who destroys a formed fetus kills it physically and spiritually, since it will die without baptism. He is not morally responsible for the death of the mother since it is the disease that causes her death.[20] Antoninus's opinion carried great weight among subsequent theologians and canonists.

Authors after Antoninus introduced another significant distinction. Many of them permit the killing even of a formed fetus if its death is caused by a medicine or treatment necessary for the mother's medical care. A physician who recommends bleeding or baths or gives drugs to assuage fever, knowing that an abortion might result, may do so; he must never give a drug only to procure the abortion. In the former case, abortion is an accidental, unintended effect; in the latter, it is the direct and intended effect.

The settled doctrine began to unravel in the seventeenth century. In the early years of that century, Thomas De Feynes, a professor of medicine at Louvain, challenged the Aristotelian teaching about delayed animation of the fetus, claiming that ensoulment must come immediately or very soon after conception. In 1621, Dr. Paolo Zacchia, who bore the grand title General Protophysician of the Whole Roman Ecclesiastical State, also repudiated the Aristotelian doctrine. At the same time, he admitted that, for practical purposes, the distinction between animated and unanimated fetuses could guide the decisions of doctors and confessors.[21] By the early nineteenth century, scientific opinion had shifted entirely from Aristotle to De Feynes. With the distinction between formed and unformed fetus eliminated, the major argument justifying abortion of an unanimated fetus fell. Pope Pius IX finally erased the distinction from church law in 1869, and the ecclesiastical penalties for abortion fell on anyone who procured an abortion of a human fetus at any stage of its development.[22]

The problem of the threatened mother remained. Theologians during the nineteenth century generally continued to allow "indirect" abortion to save the life of the mother; induction of premature delivery would be, in their view, an indirect killing of the fetus. Some even tolerated craniotomy, which clearly was a direct physical attack on the fetus, but they justified it as an "indirect" killing in the moral sense: it was analogous, these authors argued, to self-defense in which a person may kill another who is attacking him, an unintended side-effect of protecting one's self. The fetus whose existence in the womb endangered its mother could be considered an "unjust aggressor" on the mother's life. A furious debate ensued among the theologians. An official response from the Vatican on May 31, 1884, appeared to settle the debate: "It may not be safely taught that a craniotomy is permissible when otherwise both mother and fetus will perish, but with the operation, although the child will perish, the mother's life will be saved."[23] Despite this official statement, Catholic theologians continued speculative argument about the problem. The final word came in 1930, when Pope Pius XI solemnly condemned all abortions for medical, eugenic, or social reasons. The Pope explicitly repudiated the "unjust aggressor" theory, saying indignantly, "who can call an innocent child an unjust aggressor?"[24]

Catholic physicians of that era were taught that any direct attack on fetal life by a procedure such as craniotomy or embriotomy or by giving an abortifacient drug was a mortal sin and incurred the ecclesiastical penalty of excommunication. They were also taught that they could perform certain procedures, such as hysterectomy of a gravid but cancerous uterus or excision of a fallopian tube containing an ectopic fetus. These procedures were directly intended to save the mother's life and only "indirectly" or unintentionally caused the death of the fetus.[25] This application of moral theology's principle of double effect offered the physician a narrow way out of some difficult cases but, for the most part, Catholic physicians and mothers were held to a rigid, often tragic, morality. Although abortion was commonly recommended in the medical texts of the early twentieth century for pregnant women with heart disease or renal disease, Catholic doctors were forbidden that therapeutic option, to the peril of the Catholic mother.

Protestant theology said little about abortion during the period that the Catholic moralists were elaborating their casuistry on the topic. The major figures of the Reformation had followed the patristic and medieval condemnation of those who destroy life in the womb. When abortion was mentioned by preachers, it was usually to condemn those women who aborted to hide adultery or to abandon the unwanted burden of sexual indulgence. The Protestant churches in America, however, found another reason to condemn abortion. American religion was intensely family centered. Children were seen as God's greatest blessing; women derived their worth from being devoted wives and mothers. Abortion negated these cherished beliefs and weakened the moral fiber of American life. At the same time, pastors who preached against abortion may have been tolerant of the personal crises that compelled some women to seek it.[26] A public attitude of disapproval, mitigated by a tolerance for problem cases, was the general stance of the principal Protestant denominations (the later fundamentalist sects emphasized the disapproval to the detriment of the tolerance). Protestant doctors seem to have taken a position almost as strict as their Catholic counterparts, one that was more liberal only in admitting direct abortion to save maternal life. Only rarely could a woman seeking an abortion approach her physician: she was forced into "the back ally," where disreputable and dangerous medical and laypersons were waiting to help.

This situation was aggravated by the law. The English common law view that abortion be considered criminal only after quickening prevailed in the United States. In 1821, Connecticut passed the first statute prescribing life imprisonment for anyone "who shall willfully and maliciously administer . . . any deadly poison . . . with an intention to cause or procure the miscarriage of any women then being quick with child."[27] Within the next twenty years, fourteen other states passed similar statutes; several states, such as New York, added the phrase, "unless the same shall have been necessary to preserve the life of such woman, or shall have been advised by two physicians to be necessary for that purpose."[28] These statutes were part of a general move to revise American civil and criminal law; they did not arise from any broad public concern about abortion and essentially made little difference in the legal view that had prevailed in Anglo-American jurisdictions for centuries.

During the 1840s, abortion came into view as a social problem. It appears that the incidence of abortion had risen dramatically. These procedures were in large part sought by upper-class, white, Protestant women who desired to limit their childbearing. Abortions were very frequently performed by abortionists, called "wise women" or "lady doctresses," and by other "irregular practitioners." Newspapers carried advertisements for abortifacients or consultation for "private female diseases." Sensational cases, such as that of abortionist Madame Restell, who ran a large commercial abortion enterprise from New York, made the papers. In 1857, Dr. Horatio R. Storer, a Boston obstetrician, initiated a campaign to organize regular physicians against abortion and in favor of stricter law. Within two years he had generated enough support that the AMA, meeting in Louisville, resolved "publicly to enter an earnest and solemn protest against the unwarranted destruction of human life" and, recognizing the traditional duties of "its grand and noble calling, to urge the several legislative assemblies of the Union to revise abortion laws."[29] The revision most desired was the extension of criminality to the destruction of fetal life from conception, not just from "quickening" (medical opinion considered quickening irrelevant) and the clear indictment of any procurer of abortion who acted without sound medical judgment that the abortion was necessary to save the mother's life. James C. Mohr, historian of these events, concludes, "The vigorous efforts of America's regular physicians would prove in the long run to be the single most important factor in altering the legal policies toward abortion in this country."[30]

This was the situation in the 1950s, when efforts surfaced to liberalize the state abortion laws. Under the aegis of Planned Parenthood, the case for reform was built. The major argument was based on the large number of women who died or became sterile as the result of illegal abortions (although great debates raged about exact numbers). Ironically, the doctors' campaign for restrictive abortion law had also urged this argument: abortion performed by non-physicians, they claimed, led to death and sterility. Now, half a century after the doctors had won their cause, death and sterility continued. Women who could not meet the strict criteria for therapeutic abortion still sought out abortionists.

Medical abortions were surrounded by barriers. While I was doing my "ethical internship" at Yale-New Haven Hospital, Dean Fritz Redlich invited me to attend the committee that approved abortion requests. Connecticut law required medical affirmation that abortion was necessary for the health of the mother. The committee was composed mostly of physicians, and my friend, Dr. McKegney, as the psychiatrist member, was often the determining voice, since most abortion requests urged "mental health" as justification. On one occasion, he expressed his dismay at the role he had been given: "These are not," he said heatedly, "matters of mental health for a psychiatrist—they are emotional, social and economic problems for these women. Don't look to me for wisdom!"

Several major conferences on reform of abortion law were held, one by the National Committee on Maternal Health in 1944, another by Planned Parenthood in 1955. By the mid-1950s, sufficient concern had been generated to prompt the American Law Institute to draft a model statute for abortion.[31] Published in final form in 1962, it permitted abortion if a licensed physician believed "there is substantial risk that continuance of the pregnancy would gravely impair the physical or mental health of the mother, or that the child would be born with grave physical or mental defect, or that the pregnancy resulted from rape, incest, or other felonious intercourse."[32] In the same year, media coverage of the case of Sheri Finkbein alerted the public to the problem of restrictive law. Mrs. Finkbein had taken thalidomide during her pregnancy. Fearing that her fetus might be deformed, she sought an abortion, but was refused permission by the medical authorities. After much travail, she went to Sweden where a deformed fetus was aborted.[33]

Medical opinion was shifting toward a less restrictive view of abortion. In 1871, during its campaign for stricter laws, the AMA resolved that "it is unprofessional for any physician to induce abortion or premature labor without the concurrent opinion of at least one respectable consulting physician and then always with a view to the safety of the child—if that be possible." One hundred years later, after acrimonious debate, the AMA amended its stance, allowing abortion "that is performed according to good medical practice and under circumstances that do not violate the laws of the community in which he practices. . . . good medical practice requires due consideration for the patient's welfare and not mere acquiescence to the patient's demand."[34] The physicians most intimately involved in abortion, the obstetricians, adopted a policy on therapeutic abortion in 1968: consent of patient and husband (if the patient is married) was required and a consultative opinion from two physicians had to affirm that the procedure was medically indicated—that is, continuance of the pregnancy would endanger the woman's health (as viewed within her "total environment, actual or reasonably foreseeable") or the pregnancy would result in the birth of a child with grave physical deformities or mental retardation. Only two years later, the Executive Board of the College of Obstetricians and Gynecologists issued a briefer statement of policy: "It is recognized that abortion may be performed at a patient's request, or upon a physician's recommendation."[35]

During the summer of 1964, after my first year of graduate studies, I was plunged quite unexpectedly into the politics of the abortion debate. I was teaching an ethics course in the Summer School at the University of San Francisco. While walking across the campus one foggy morning, I was hailed by another visiting professor, Father Joseph Fuchs, a distinguished German theologian from the Gregorian University in Rome. Father Fuchs asked if I knew the name Sargent Shriver. When I told him that Mr. Shriver was the brother-in-law of the late President Kennedy, he said that Mr. Shriver had invited him to the Kennedy compound at Hyannisport for a meeting of a few Catholic theologians to discuss the political aspects of abortion. Mr. Shriver had explained that Senator Edward Kennedy was standing for re-election in Massachusetts, and Robert Kennedy was running in New York. The Kennedys hoped to formulate a political stance on abortion that would be compatible both with Catholic teaching and with the political climate of the country. Father Fuchs had responded that he knew nothing about the American political climate, but he agreed to attend the meeting if he could bring along a young American theologian. Mr. Shriver agreed. Father Fuchs then asked me to accompany him. For the next two days, I briefed the courtly German Jesuit on American law and attitudes toward abortion. We flew to Boston and we were driven at breakneck speed to Hyannisport by fellow Jesuit Robert F. Drinan, then Dean of Boston College Law School and later a Democratic congressman. The small group met on the ocean terrace of Robert Kennedy's home. Both Kennedy brothers were briefly present, while Shriver, Dr. André E. Hellegers, Father Richard A. McCormick, Father Charles E. Curran, professor of moral theology at Catholic University, Father Fuchs, Father Drinan, and I, the novice among them, struggled with the problem posed to us.

Father McCormick was particularly articulate. I recall his careful exposition of the thesis of our fellow Jesuit scholar, the late John Courtney Murray, that distinguished between the moral aspects of an issue and the feasibility of enacting legislation about that issue.[36] McCormick applied this thesis to the contemporary abortion debate in America prior to the *Roe v Wade* decision. He concluded—and to the best of my memory, the other theologians present concurred—that the translation of a rigorously restrictive ethics of abortion into law was unlikely to be enforceable or to achieve its positive goals without significant attendant social evils. These theologians, in close agreement on the immorality of abortion as taught by their church, favored a public policy that followed the lines of the American Law Institute's proposed model statute on abortion that had been drafted in 1962, and at the time of the Hyannisport conclave had been enacted in about a dozen states. Some years later, Father McCormick wrote:

> When I try to fit the Christian evaluation of fetal life into the contemporary American scene and to develop a feasible protective law, I believe it is realistic (feasible) to say that many people would agree that abortion is legally acceptable if the alternative is tragedy, but unacceptable if the alternative is mere inconvenience. Furthermore, I believe that Americans are capable of distinguishing the two in policy. . . . Such a policy would prohibit abortion unless the life of the mother is at stake; there is a serious threat to her physical health and to the length of her life; the pregnancy is due to rape or incest; fetal deformity is of such magnitude that life-supporting efforts would not be considered obligatory after birth. . . . This list is for all practical purposes and with a few changes the American Law Institute's proposals. . . . I (do not) judge them to be exceptions that are morally right. I do so only because at the present time many people believe that continuing the pregnancy in such circumstances is heroic and should not be mandated by law . . . also because among the evils associated with any law, these seem to represent the lesser evil. I am confident that such a policy will completely satisfy no one.[37]

Father McCormick was correct: his mediating proposal pleased no one completely. By the time he wrote these words in 1979, the debate had already hardened into "pro-life" and "pro-choice," each side espousing absolutist positions. He knew that the bishops of his own church had condemned the *Roe v Wade* decision as "erroneous, unjust, and immoral" and were calling for highly restrictive legislation.[38] But at the end of the 1960s, many thought that some middle ground of public policy could be staked out, accommodating those who firmly held to the immorality of abortion and those who advanced a more flexible position.

In September 1967, Harvard Divinity School and the Joseph P. Kennedy Jr. Foundation sponsored an international conference on abortion that drew a distinguished audience. The Solicitor General of the United States, Erwin Griswold, and two Supreme Court justices, Potter Stewart and Abe Fortas, attended. A powerful team of Catholic and Protestant theologians participated, together with prominent scientists. Although a few liberals espoused the cause of abortion reform, most presenters defended the ethical basis, as well as the political and legal prudence, of restrictive law. The tone of the conference was illustrated in the popular book that issued from it, *The Terrible Choice: The Abortion Dilemma,* in which Lennart Nilsson's famous photographs of a fetus *in utero* occupied a prominent place.[39] Despite the generally conservative tone of the gathering, the participants recognized the need for a public policy that would be acceptable in a democratic nation. Rev. Robert Drinan stated in public the position he had stated at the private Kennedy conclave in Hyannisport: "One way to avoid the necessity of making these choices [posed by the American Law Institute model law on abortion] would be for the law to withdraw its protection from all fetuses during the first 26 weeks."[40]

For many who favored abortion law reform, the morality was simple: illegal abortion killed women (the defense of abortion on demand as a woman's right appears only tentatively in the late 1960s).[41] Many who argued against reform espoused as simple a view: abortion was morally wrong, therefore it should be illegal. Some commentators realized, however, how intricate the ethical problem was. Paul Ramsey's first excursions into medical questions were prompted by the perplexities of abortion: his "Points in deciding about abortion," presented at the Harvard/Kennedy Conference, outlined the intricacy of the debate over abortion law reform. He proposed that five issues needed clarification if there was to be "greater sanity in the debate over abortion laws": the proper place of religious views in public policy, the distinction between sin and crime, the moral status of the fetus and embryo, the difference between feticide and infanticide, and the implications of various views of abortion on fetal and neonatal medicine.[42]

Ramsey produced five major essays and devoted two of his 1975 Bampton lectures to the topic.[43] He built his argument on the theological premise that the sanctity of human life, with its implication of inviolability, is "an overflow from God's dealings with man and not primarily an anticipation of anything he will ever be by himself alone. . . . the value of a human life is ultimately grounded in the value God is placing on it."[44] In view of this sanctity, the arguments over the "beginning of life" are relatively unimportant; God spreads his protection over humankind, "before I formed thee in the womb, I knew thee . . . I sanctified thee" (Jeremiah 1:5). Nascent human life, at all its stages, is most vulnerable and most in need of protection. However, after these theological claims, Ramsey had to say, "Nothing in the foregoing solves any problems."[45] Beyond the theological claims about the sanctity of life and the equality of all human lives, whether in the womb or in the world, the "direction and ingredients of actual moral decisions in the matter of abortion" had to be scrutinized.

The problem arises when one life is pitted against another, when the saving of the fetus imperils the mother or vice versa. Ramsey employed the doctrine of double effect, as do the Catholic theologians, to analyze these situations, finding that indirect taking of fetal life may be permitted to save maternal life. He went beyond the Catholic analysis to permit direct killing when both fetus and mother are in peril. In such cases, the incapacitation of the fetus as danger to the mother, not its killing, is intended. Ramsey recommended that "the Protestant Christian should wrestle with his Catholic brother over the verdict each delivers upon this proposed action."[46] And "wrestle" he did. Over the next decade, Catholic theologians McCormick and Curran and Catholic philosopher Germain Grisez challenged Ramsey on this point.[47]

Another of the first figures of bioethics, Dan Callahan, entered the field through the rapids of the abortion debate. When he began to write *Abortion: Law, Choice and Morality,* he had expected to write a defense of the traditional moral prohibition of abortion. As he pondered the facts, issues, and arguments, he found himself working from a critique of two positions, which he called "one-value solutions"—the Roman Catholic position that abortion is always wrong, and the women's rights position that abortion is a matter of personal choice only—toward a "very large and ambiguous middle ground" that he hoped would provide space for a public consensus on public policy and law. The middle ground was "a bias . . . a broad stance . . . in favor of protecting human life. . . . it is good, so far as humanly and morally possible, to favor and promote the preservation of human life." This position, resting on general considerations about "the sanctity of life," is carefully developed. The arguments surrounding the moment of the beginning of human life and its moral relevance are reviewed, and those of the "developmental school," favoring a staged emergence of the fetus into moral standing, are approved as most convincing. Surveying the desirability of restrictive law, moderate law, or no law, he chose a balanced jurisprudence that would give women optimal freedom, manifest society's serious concerns about abortion, and express society's respect for unborn life. In the end, "abortion decisions should be left to the women themselves," but public policy should be designed to promote the protection of unborn life by many means: liberal availability of contraception, social alternatives to abortion, counseling, and education.[48]

Not surprisingly, Callahan's middle ground met harsh criticism. Paul Ramsey was particularly critical. Callahan, he said, had structured his argument on the incorrect premise that there can be inequality when life is in conflict with life.[49] Richard McCormick did not criticize the principle but the conclusions. Callahan, he wrote, was "still trying to have it both ways," arguing for a bias in favor of human life and at the same time admitting that abortion was a moral solution for many problems. McCormick judged that Callahan's "honest and sensitive" analysis ended not with a balance of rights but the effective elimination of one right altogether.[50] An earnest search for a quiet harbor of compromise on abortion had run on the rocks of moral contention.

Public policy, however, was moving toward the liberal legal solution that Callahan had sought. By 1970, a dozen states had revised their abortion statute to reflect the American Law Institute's model statute. The tide of reform had barely begun when the Supreme Court of the United States struck down even those revised codes. On January 22, 1973, the Court announced its decision in two related cases, *Roe v Wade* and *Doe v Bolton*. The first case was brought by a Texas woman against Dallas County. She charged that the state's criminal abortion statute, which excepted from criminality only a life-saving procedure, prevented her from obtaining a desired abortion. The second case challenged the revised abortion statutes of Georgia. In *Roe v Wade,* the Supreme Court held that state law could not restrict the right of a woman, in accord with her doctor, to obtain an abortion during the first trimester of pregnancy, that states could make laws regulating the safety of abortion procedures relative to maternal health during the second trimester, and that during the third trimester, when the fetus was "viable," law could prohibit abortion except when necessary to preserve the life and health of the woman. The Court justified these holdings by asserting that the Constitution contains a "penumbral" right to privacy, implied by several explicit provisions of the Bill of Rights. The Court also affirmed that a fetus is not a person as interpreted under the 14th Amendment and, thus, does not have the rights guaranteed by the Constitution. The justices ruminated, "We need not resolve the difficult question of when life begins. When those trained in the respective disciplines of medicine, philosophy and theology are unable to arrive at any consensus, the judiciary, at this point, in the development of man's knowledge, is not in a position to speculate as to the answer." Nevertheless, the Court allowed that the medical determination of viability, "the capability of meaningful life outside the womb," could be a "compelling point" at which a state might legitimately protect fetal life.[51]

The Court's decision radically reformed American law but at the time, it appeared consistent with Americans' more liberal attitude toward abortion. This appearance proved deceptive. As state after state revised their old statutes to conform with the Supreme Court, multitudes of citizens began to express their dissent, led at first by Catholics, who were soon joined by fundamentalist Protestants. By the mid-1970s, abortion had become a major political issue, and the abstract arguments of philosophers and theologians were caught up in the whirlwind of public debate.

Most philosophers had paid little attention to the abortion question, considering it either a theological or a legal issue (Callahan's interest was a philosophical idiosyncrasy). However, as its intricacies began to unfold in the public debate, philosophical interest was piqued. Judith Thomson, Gerald Dworkin, and Baruch Brody, the philosophy faculty at the Massachusetts Institute of Technology, devised a course entitled "Contemporary Moral Issues" in order to attract scientifically minded students to philosophy. The professors decided to include a few classes on abortion, even though all agreed that there was nothing really interesting to say about it, since every woman should be able to have an abortion if she wished. As the philosophers and their students argued, they realized the conceptual complexity of the problem. The course produced two pieces of literature that argued for contrary positions. Brody's *Abortion and the Sanctity of Human Life* was almost unique among the philosophical discussions (apart from the Catholic philosophers) in supporting a conservative position.[52] He argued that, since it is impossible to determine whether or not the fetus is a person, the law should incline toward the protection of life. Abortion should be permitted only in the most extreme circumstances of saving maternal life; the fetus must be imminently dying, for then "he whose life is taken loses nothing of significance." Brody's philosophical analysis echoed the rabbinical arguments of his Jewish heritage.

That course also produced what may be the article best known to American students enrolled in an introductory ethics course, Judith Thomson's "A defense of abortion," which appeared as *Philosophy and Public Affairs*' first "bioethics" article.[53] The essay opens with a bizarre case: you awaken and find that a famous, dying violinist is hooked to your body and only by remaining hooked can he continue to live. Is it morally right to unhook him? Thomson then drew an analogy with the fetus, hooked up to a woman's body for life support: just as you could unhook the violinist intruding on your body, so a woman could disconnect the fetus. Baruch Brody recalls his arguments with Judith Thomson over that analysis: "I claimed that she missed the crucial distinction between letting someone die and killing them . . . I asked students whether they would be happy to separate themselves from the violinist if they had to cut him to pieces?" The discussion of this bizarre case, commented Brody, is similar to much of the abortion debate: it forced one to come up with a yes or no without allowing any discussion of in-between positions, of the circumstances that might make an abortion right in some and wrong in others. He reflected, "The literature about abortion that comes from the analytic school, is a literature of the highest intellectual quality, with rich argumentation, analytically very clear, vigorous . . . and yet it has had, as far as I can see, no influence anywhere outside the classroom."[54]

Brody's opinion did not deter other philosophers from entering the debate. Most favored Thomson's opinion over Brody's, arguing that the doubt justifies giving priority to the woman's choice. They accepted and elaborated Thomson's thesis, which, despite its bizarre example, elevated the autonomy of women to the central—indeed, sole—moral principle. One philosopher, Michael Tooley, felt that Thomson had not gone far enough. He not only justified abortion but also infanticide, on the principle that an organism can be said to have rights "only if it possesses a concept of self as a continuing subject of experiences and other mental states, and believes that it is itself such a continuing entity."[55] In Tooley's view, embryos, fetuses, and newborn babies had equally negligible moral status. This conclusion, so counterintuitive, was not widely welcomed. Other philosophers delved into complex questions about the beginning of personhood, the definition of personal identity, and the relevance of viability as a marker for protection of fetal life. A few philosophers, following Callahan's lead, attempted to formulate a middle way between the two horns of the dilemma, the fetus's right to life and the woman's right over her body.[56]

Abortion, ancient moral question that it is, faded from the agenda of bioethics. Although a burning public issue around the time of bioethics' birth, the public policy questions seemed to have been settled by the Supreme Court's decision, which drew the morally contentious practice under the protection of the Constitution. The complex philosophical arguments seemed to disappear under the glare of the principle of autonomy and of women's rights. Among the theologians, the divide seemed unbreachable: some of them maintained the ancient doctrine of the inviolable sanctity of unborn life, others had less faith in that ancient doctrine, given doubts about the personhood of the fetus and growing appreciation of the moral autonomy of persons. So, early in the life of bioethics, the law had spoken, the philosophers had exhausted their arguments, and the theologians found argument fruitless in closing doctrinal gaps. As we shall see later this chapter, the emotionally charged and ethically complex problem was carefully skirted in the public policy discussions of issues that touched abortion, such as research with the human fetus and in vitro fertilization.

One abortion question did arise during these years of general silence among bioethicists. Amniocentesis and ultrasound revealed the sex of a fetus in the womb. Some ethicists raised the question of "selective abortion," that is, aborting a fetus because it was of an unwanted gender, and one ethicist, Karen Lebacqz, criticized selective abortion on the grounds that it violated equality.[57] John Fletcher justified sex selection abortion because he thought it inconsistent to reject this one reason for abortion when the law had sanctioned a woman's unconditional right to abortion in the first and second trimester of pregnancy. Fletcher later reconsidered his position, holding that sex selection was unethical because the harms to society of devaluing females and unbalancing the sex ratio outweigh the benefits to individuals, and because the practice violates the principle of fairness between male and female fetuses.[58]

Contraception

Presumably, attempts to prevent conception have been made by humans since they realized the causal connection between intercourse and pregnancy. Ancient medical literature reports many contraceptive measures, mostly drawn from a great store of folk beliefs. Some of these methods may have been effective (although families were probably more effectively limited by abortion and exposure of infants) since concern over underpopulation occasionally led to official sanctions. King Philip V of Macedonia, for example, forbade contraception, abortion, or infanticide, prompted more by his worry that a depopulated land could not be a military power than by moral scruples.[59]

While moral concern about contraception rarely appears in Greek or Roman culture, it does surface in the Jewish and Christian writers of antiquity. The duty imposed upon every Jewish man to generate children renders deliberate contraceptive intercourse problematic. In general, rabbinical sources disapprove of contraception except to protect the physical or mental health of the wife.[60] Christian teaching blessed the moral use of sex only within a monogamous and procreative marriage. Contraception and abortion (not always clearly distinguished) both fell under condemnation. Contraception not only frustrated one of the essential ends of marriage, the generation of children, but signaled that a married couple had been seduced by the pleasure that was akin to sin. Official Catholic teachings that condemn contraception appear in the Middle Ages when the Church fought against another unorthodoxy, Catharism, which flourished in southern France (known also as Albigensianisn). Catharism was similar to Manichaeism, condemning as evil physical life and prohibiting as sinful sexual relationships that resulted in procreation. A new text was added to church law, aimed at the Cathars: "If conditions are set against the substance of marriage, for example, if one says to the other, 'I contract with you if you avoid offspring,' . . . the matrimonial contract lacks effect."[61] Catholic teaching remained consistent down to the thundering condemnation of contraception by Pope Pius XI in *Casti Connubii* as a "base stain" on marriage and a perversion of the natural order.[62] Family planning was permitted only by abstinence or "periodic continence," and only for grave reasons.

Christian churches of every persuasion shared similar views on the sanctity of monogamous marriage and on the duty of bearing and educating children, although Protestant teaching was more tacit about contraception. A discreet silence from the pulpit on the subject and a greater tolerance for personal conscience does not signify that most Protestant moralists of the past would approve a marriage marked by consistent contraceptive practices.[63] American Protestant denominations had never shown enthusiasm for birth control. In the late nineteenth century, the hotly debated "Women's Question" about the role of women in society usually found the churches on the conservative side and, insofar as birth control was discussed, it was seen as a means of freeing woman from their duties as mothers and wives and, hence, as degrading to their feminine nature. One author summarizes the Protestant attitude: "The American churches, the official guardians of respectability, only cautiously and belatedly gave birth control their official attention. . . . Insofar as American Protestants listened to their churches in such matters, for a long time they could find there no comfort of conscience about contraception."[64] In 1931, the Committee on Marriage and the Home of the Federal Council of Churches issued *Moral Aspects of Birth Control,*[65] in which a cautious approval of birth control was stated. The report, while quietly acknowledged as a belated approval of a practice already readily accepted by most parishioners, met adamant opposition. The Southern Presbyterian Church and the Northern Baptist Convention disavowed the report's conclusions. Opposition was strong enough to block the acceptance of the report by the entire council.

One influential religious body took a distinctly liberal direction. The bishops of the worldwide Anglican communion, meeting at Lambeth Palace in 1930, stated that all forms of contraception were morally legitimate; yet they cautioned, "Where there is a clearly felt moral obligation to limit or avoid parenthood, the method must be decided on Christian principles. The primary and obvious method is complete abstinence from intercourse . . . but where there is a morally sound reason for avoiding complete abstinence, the conference agrees that other methods may be used, provided that this is done in the light of the same Christian principles."[66] The bishops urged "perplexed couples" to seek competent medical and spiritual advice. T.S. Eliot, a devout Anglican, was moved to remark that "the honest minority which seeks 'competent advice' . . . will have to appeal to a clergy just as perplexed as itself."[67] The Lambeth statement prompted a more scathing criticism from Pope Pius XI whose encyclical *Casti Connubii* followed only a few months later with pointed reference to the Anglican relaxation of moral rigor. Still, the Lambeth statement reflected ideas that had been maturing within the mainstream Protestant churches, and its teaching was heard by American ministers.

Although religious discussion of contraception was muted, there was sufficient popular repugnance to support enactment of restrictive law in the United States and Great Britain. The common law had never spoken about contraception, but populist moral reformers during the nineteenth century haled the law's attention. Among these moral reformers, the most zealous was Anthony Comstock, a pious grocery clerk who, in 1873, successfully lobbied Congress to pass, almost without debate, a law "for the suppression of trade in and circulation of articles for immoral use." Comstock was appointed special agent of the United States Postal Service to oversee the implementation of the law, and held that post for forty years. Under his vigilant eye, any literature that hinted at sexuality could be seized and confiscated and its senders prosecuted. He saw obscenity everywhere, and even scientific attempts to explain and promote birth control fell beneath his baleful glare. Comstock's Society for the Suppression of Vice encouraged state legislatures to pass laws penalizing the sale and possession of materials branded as obscene by broad definition, including contraceptive information and devices. States restricted the availability of contraceptives to those prescribed by physicians for the cure of disease and outlawed birth control clinics.

By the turn of the century, twenty-two states had "little Comstock laws." Comstock died in 1915, but traces of the legislation he inspired lingered at the federal and state levels until the 1960s. A historian writes, "Though Comstock's activities represent the extremes of bigotry he was, in a sense, merely reflecting the predominant attitude of his time."[68] The public supported this censoriousness. Preachers were pleased by it (Comstock was often cited in sermons as an exemplary Christian). Physicians, either sympathetic to the censoriousness or cowed by legal threats, often refused to advise contraception. While information about condoms, pessaries, and cervical caps was sometimes available to the wealthy and middle class, poorer and less educated women were uninformed about their contraceptive options.

After World War I, American attitudes toward marriage, sex, and family began to shift in a liberal direction. Public discussion of sex became less reticent; indeed, many believed that it had become excessive. Freudian thought invaded the scholarly world and filtered through the popular mind. Divorce began to fray the bonds of the traditional family. Into this changing environment marched the militant Margaret Sanger, social radical and advocate for woman's liberation and for birth control. She lectured and organized incessantly to promote these causes. In 1915, her husband, who shared her views, was personally arrested by Anthony Comstock, and Mrs. Sanger was indicted but not prosecuted under the Comstock law. In the next year, she opened her first birth control clinic in New York City. She was arrested often, once at the behest of New York's Patrick Cardinal Hayes, after which she said, "[This is] now the battle of a republic against the machinations of the hierarchy of the Roman Catholic Church."[69] Gradually her message hit its mark. A broader public began to sympathize with her crusade to abolish restrictive law, and many physicians began to see birth control as a matter of their patients' health.

In 1952, Mrs. Sanger was introduced by her friend, philanthropist Katherine Dexter McCormick, to biologist Gregory "Goody" Pincus. Pincus had done pioneering work in reproductive endocrinology and genetics during his early career at Harvard and, after 1944, he continued his work at the Worcester Foundation for Experimental Biology. He was particularly interested in hormonal control of mammalian reproduction. The intrepid Mrs. Sanger recruited him in a search for an oral contraceptive, and Mrs. Mc-Cormick provided generous financial support.

The collaboration was rapidly productive. Biological research into the hormonal factors of conception was performed with great creativity by Goody Pincus and his colleagues. Searle Company translated their research into pharmaceutical chemistry, producing "the Pill," a combination of two synthetic steroids, progesterone and estrogen, which was given the commercial name "Enovid." Initial clinical studies were planned and implemented by Dr. John Rock, chairman of Obstetrics/Gynecology at Harvard, during 1954–1955 and, in April 1956, large-scale clinical trials were inaugurated in Rio Piedras, a poor, crowded suburb of San Juan, Puerto Rico. The women of Rio Piedras were described as "a population ripe for a fertility study."[70] Although the "patient failure" rate was high because of noncompliance with the regimen, the coordinator of the trial, Dr. Edris Rice-Wray, reported in January 1957 that Enovid was "100% effective against pregnancy in 10 mmg doses taken over twenty days for nine months by 221 women."[71] Dizziness, headaches, and nausea were noted as side effects. Trials were expanded to other locales in Puerto Rico and to Haiti. Searle obtained FDA approval to market Enovid for threatened miscarriage and menstrual disorders in the same year. Three years later, the evidence of its contraceptive effects justified approval for that indication, and in May 1960, Enovid was approved as an oral contraceptive. Within three years of this approval, over two million American women were on the Pill. Author, congresswoman, and diplomat Clare Booth Luce said of this reproductive revolution, "Modern woman is at last free as a man is free, to dispose of her own body, to earn a living, to pursue the improvement of her mind, to try a successful career."[72]

The Pill posed, in new forms, a very old ethical question: was it an unethical contravention of nature and God's law to prevent conception? That question was not, as some today believe, an exclusive concern of the Roman Catholic church: it had bothered Christian America through the nineteenth century. The advent of the Pill raised the question again. For Catholics, it asked whether chemical contraception was morally equivalent to physical contraception. This form of contraception (together with the intrauterine ring) injected confusion into the previously clear teaching on the immorality of contraception. This scientific development urged a re-examination of the history of that teaching and the nature of the arguments used to support it.[73] For the general public, which had widely accepted contraception as morally unproblematic, the question was whether the ready availability of an effective, easy contraceptive would revolutionize the social and sexual life of Americans.

In 1965, the U.S. Supreme Court, in *Griswold v Connecticut*, struck down Connecticut's 1879 remnant of the Comstock era, a statute criminalizing "use of any drug, medical article or instrument for the purpose of preventing conception."[74] Justice Potter Stewart called this "an uncommonly silly law," but noted that the Court could not strike down laws for silliness. Instead, the Justices created constitutional history by ruling that a law forbidding the use of contraceptives could not be enforced without invading "a right of privacy older than the Bill of Rights—marriage is a coming together for better or worse, intimate to the degree of being sacred." Even then, a right of privacy, old as it might be, must be found in the Constitution of the United States. The founding document contains no direct reference to such a right, so the Justices discovered that right as "penumbra emanating from those (specific) guarantees that help give them life and substance . . . various guarantees create zones of privacy."[75] The Court elevated the doctrine of "the penumbral right to privacy" that had been explicated in an 1890 *Harvard Law Review* article by a future Supreme Court Justice, Louis Brandeis, into a central doctrine of jurisprudence in family law.[76] It was to appear again in the abortion decisions of 1972, and in subsequent cases concerning the refusal of life-sustaining medical care. The Griswold decision removed the last legal barrier to effective promotion of contraception.

In itself, the Pill aroused little controversy. Its consequences for the liberalization of sexual life caught the ethical eye of some moralists, but it was generally considered a boon. Women readily sought it and doctors willingly prescribed it. Catholics, however, were not liberated by the Pill. One of its co-inventors, Dr. John Rock, who was a Catholic, felt that his invention might avoid the general church prohibition of artificial methods of contraception, since the hormonal effect on the reproductive cycle seemed to him "natural." Joseph Fletcher, in the preface to a revised 1960 edition of his *Morals and Medicine,* optimistically wrote of the steroidal contraceptives: "Since the same medicines can also be used to regulate or stabilize the menstrual cycle, Roman Catholic priests will be able to justify this form of birth control as an 'indirect effect' . . . of menstrual therapy."[77] Episcopalian Fletcher underestimated the tenacity of his Catholic brethren: it was not to be so easy.

A few Catholic authors dared venture further than Fletcher had suggested. They felt that the new contraceptives in themselves were less important than a thorough revision of Catholic teaching about the morality of human sexuality and of marriage. These writers claimed the teachings were based upon a narrow vision of the human person and upon a "physicalist view" that inferred moral rules from the physical configuration of the human organism; they sought a more "personalist" ethics and a fuller view of married sexuality. Father Charles Curran, Professor of Moral Theology at the Catholic University of America, wrote, "The discussion should not be confined to the organs in question and their relationship to the organism but rather the good of the whole man and his relationship to his family, community and the larger society must be taken into account."[78] A flurry of debate ensued. Liberal Catholics had their hopes raised when Pope Paul VI announced, on June 23, 1964, that he was establishing a commission to study disputed questions about marriage and birth control; among the 58 members was Dr. André Hellegers. The hopes for revision of the traditional teaching were disappointed two years later when the Pope rejected the commission's liberalizing report. In 1968, a major papal encyclical entitled *Humanae Vitae* affirmed the traditional teaching in the most solemn tones.[79]

The papal decision aroused a debate over the nature of ecclesiastic authority. That debate was an intramural Catholic affair. However, it did have an indirect effect on bioethics. The contraception debate had drawn Dan Callahan, who had taken a lead among Catholic laity in urging a revision of the teaching, closer to bioethical issues.[80] It drove others away from their original home in Catholic moral theology into the new field of bioethics. Two nontenured professors of moral theology at the Catholic University of America, Warren Reich and George Kanoti, signed a respectful dissent to the *Humanae Vitae* and were invited to leave the university. Reich moved to the Kennedy Institute at Georgetown University, and Kanoti moved to John Carroll University in Cleveland and then to the Cleveland Clinic as its first bioethicist in residence.[81] I had just joined the faculty of the Department of Theology at the University of San Francisco when the encyclical appeared. I had followed the doctrinal dispute avidly and sided with the liberals. I was dismayed to see that position rejected by the Pope, even after a thorough and thoughtful re-examination by his appointed advisors. It began to dawn on me that as a newly minted moral theologian, I would not be comfortable or conscientious teaching the traditional doctrine on abortion and contraception. The intramural debate over contraception, then, inadvertently promoted the growth of bioethics by increasing the ranks of the new bioethicists.

Apart from the problem posed to Catholic married couples and to Catholic doctors who might consider contraception or sterilization appropriate for a particular patient (and also to non-Catholic doctors working in Catholic hospitals, where the *Ethical Principles of the Catholic Hospital Association* forbade sterilization procedures), contraception was not generally a contentious matter. However, an issue in which contraception was intricately involved attracted much attention in the 1960s.

The "population explosion" was on the agenda of the emerging bioethics. At Dartmouth's 1960 Great Issues of Conscience in Medicine Conference, the Honorable Mahomedali Chagla, Indian Ambassador to the United States, recounted the figures of astonishing population growth in his own country and in other underdeveloped nations, with the attendant increase in poverty, and then declared, "Government and official institutions fight shy of doing research in the problem of human fertility. Why? . . . The real solution of this problem in India is a cheap oral contraceptive . . . [yet] it is very often not respectable here to speak of birth control or family planning."[82] Even as he spoke, clinical studies on Enovid were being conducted. He was correct, however, in lamenting the reluctance of governments to face questions of human fertility. The questions raised by Ambassador Chagla on a political and international level, as well as by the pioneers in birth control for individual women and families, had met with reticence, resistance, and restrictions.

Toward the end of the 1960s, the troubling questions raised by Ambassador Chagla burst into a crisis. Three scholars—Paul Ehrlich of Stanford University, along with Garrett Hardin and Kingsley Davis of the University of California—published analyses of the "population explosion," proposing that the dynamics of population growth were pushing the inhabited world toward a complex of crises: famine, pollution, resource depletion, and environmental degradation. These authors argued that attempts to deal with this problem by voluntary means of family planning were wholly inadequate.[83] Garrett Hardin wrote, "No technical solution can rescue us from the misery of overpopulation. Freedom to breed will bring ruin to all . . . the only way we can preserve and nurture other more precious freedoms is by relinquishing the freedom to breed." Freedom to breed, Hardin said, should be curtailed by government policies that limit family size, restrict the right to marry, tax children, and require contraception, sterilization, and abortion. Benighted religious doctrines, he continued, are complicit in the crime.[84]

Such provocative proposals bred instant opposition. Scholars challenged the demographic science behind the analyses; churchmen condemned the moral premises; politicians shied away from compulsory measures. A Protestant theologian, Arthur Dyck, who held the Saltenstall Professorship of Population Ethics at Harvard University, saw the camps dividing into the "Crisis Environmentalists," who maintain that population growth and environmental depletion will continue without explicit government coercion, the "Family Planners," who proposed education and voluntary birth control, and "the Developmental Distributivists," who argued that improved socioeconomic conditions ameliorate population strains. Dyck elucidated the moral values underlying these positions and argued, referencing Rawls's theory of justice, that it is unfair to burden the poor by coerced or even voluntary family planning unless their lot is otherwise relieved. A notion of justice must underlie population policy.[85] Several pioneers of bioethics were deeply involved in the population question: Dyck, along with Ralph Potter of Harvard Divinity School, held appointments in Harvard's Center for Population Studies; André Hellegers came to Georgetown University as director of The Center for Population Research.

By the mid-1970s, however, population ethics had moved to the bottom of the bioethical agenda. The reasons for this shift are obscure, but Professor Potter believes that the question was originally raised by effective publicists who "exploded" it out of proportion and that it soon became clear that the real problems would be in the hands of politicians rather than philosophers.[86] International organizations began to mount policies and nations began to undertake programs. Only the linkage between abortion and population control in some nations, such as China, remained contentious.

Bioethics opened with classical moral concerns about reproduction, abortion, and contraception, to which the contemporary concern over the population explosion was added. The ethics of contraception soon disappeared from the agenda. The ethics of abortion quickly became the politics of abortion and philosophical discussions of its complexity were buried beneath adamancy and rancor. The ethics of population control remained on the agenda for a decade. All these traditional ethical questions bear on the prevention of reproduction. Totally new questions now appeared.

Reproductive Technologies

While humans sometimes desire to prevent birth, they more often desire to make children and failure to succeed causes deep distress. Medical attempts to assist reproduction have an ancient history. Classical texts, such as Soranus' *Gynecology,* are filled with prescriptions to assure that coitus will produce offspring.[87] Most of these attempts, based on drugs, diet, and physical manipulation, were futile. They were also morally inoffensive within a generally pronatalist religious culture (except insofar as they smacked of magic, which the church repudiated). The scientific work of Goody Pincus and many others in reproductive endocrinology did not simply produce an effective contraceptive; it contributed to the growing ability to understand and control the entire reproductive process and advanced the search for a remedy for infertility.

As science explored the physiology of human reproduction in the nineteenth century, these attempts to remedy infertility became more focused and effective. Mechanically assisted insemination was first reported at the end of the eighteenth century: an Italian priest-scientist, Lazaro Spallanzani, achieved success with toads, and British surgeon John Hunter effected a successful pregnancy of a linen draper's wife using her husband's sperm.[88] In the 1860s, American gynecologist J. Marion Sims attempted artificial insemination sixty-six times for six women with their husband's sperm, producing one pregnancy. In the 1880s, William Panacost and John Dickenson of Jefferson Medical College in Philadelphia used donor sperm from "the handsomest medical student in the class" to impregnate a woman whose husband was infertile. This event was surrounded by the greatest secrecy and was only reported in 1909. Once revealed, it aroused more admiration than criticism (though it was assailed by some clergy as "medical adultery"). The young man whose conception had been facilitated was able to find his father, now a prosperous practitioner, to their mutual delight.[89] During the 1930s and 1940s, two gynecologists, Sophia Kleegman in the United States and Margaret Jackson in England, did much to explain the procedure to the profession and the public. Stored frozen sperm was first used in 1953, and the 1970s saw a fourfold increase in demand for donor insemination.

The legal status of children born of artificial insemination was uncertain. In the United Kingdom, a committee of the Department of Health recommended as late as 1960 that the status of illegitimacy be retained for such children. A New York appellate court ruled similarly in 1963; but, in 1968, the California Supreme Court granted legitimacy to a child conceived by AID, the clever acronym for Artificial Insemination by Donor. Oklahoma enacted a statute deeming such children legitimate in 1967.[90]

The Catholic Church, despite its pronatalist doctrines, took a firm stance against any procedure that was seen to violate the natural process of intercourse leading to conception. An official statement from the Vatican in 1897 had condemned "artificial fecondation," and Pope Pius XII, speaking to the Fourth International Convention of Catholic Physicians in 1949, made clear that the prohibition included spousal as well as donor insemination.[91]

Even as the practice became medically more common, many religious groups, Christian and Jewish, remained hesitant, particularly about donor insemination. In 1972, the Ciba Foundation sponsored a Symposium on Legal and Other Aspects of Artificial Insemination by Donor (AID) and Embryo Transfer. This symposium was suggested to the foundation by Lord Kilbrandon who said, "The subject matter of this conference first occurred to me during a conference run by the Institute of Society, Ethics and the Life Sciences at the Fogarty Center in 1971."[92] All the speakers at the Ciba symposium agreed that artificial insemination was medically simple, desired by infertile couples, and frequently effective. Rev. G. R. Dunstan, Professor of Moral and Social Theology at King's College, London, who would become a respected voice in British medical ethics, provided an ethical review, noting the general skepticism of religious groups. "No Christian Church in the United Kingdom," he said, "has explicitly favored the practice and the judgment of Jewish Orthodoxy is hostile."[93] He deplored the deception and secrecy fostered by the legal status of illegitimacy. He analyzed the implications of the practice for the married couple and for the child, and discussed the responsibilities of the donor and the question of payment for semen, which he strongly repudiated. On the whole, Dunstan gave qualified moral approval to a practice that was becoming common and accepted.

The title of the Ciba symposium included the words, "embryo transfer." The symposium had taken a large step beyond the relatively simple topic of AID by inviting Professor R. G. Edwards, a Cambridge physiologist, and Mr. Patrick Steptoe, an obstetrician in private practice in Oldham, outside Manchester, England. These two had been collaborating for several years on perfecting the conditions for retrieval of oocytes, fertilization of the retrieved oocytes under laboratory conditions (in vitro) and implantation of the fertilized embryo in the womb. In 1965, Edwards succeeded in fertilizing a human ovum with his own sperm in a petri dish and, for the first time, human life was created outside a woman's body. Subsequent attempts to effect pregnancy by "embryo transfer" into a womb for gestation were unsuccessful. Their paper at the Ciba symposium claimed that embryo transfer might "soon be possible," explained the procedure and the results of animal experiments. Their concluding remarks defended the ethics of their experiments: "We believe that our studies conform with the Hippocratic Oath in that they are for the benefit of patients and not for their hurt or any wrong—indeed we believe they hold out the prospect of widespread benefit."[94]

Harvard law professor Charles Fried reflected during the conference on the "unease" many persons felt over the new reproductive technology. He advised that the unease arose from the threat to personal identity that came from the possibility of genetic manipulation and advised that reproductive assistance be limited to those who take responsibility to care for the child resulting from their genetic material.[95] Fried's critique was gentle, but Dr. Edwards had been the target of a much harsher judgment, delivered by Paul Ramsey at the 1967 Kennedy symposium, Choices on Our Conscience. Edwards recalled the moment:

> I had to endure a denunciation of our work as if from some nineteenth-century pulpit. . . . Our work was, he thundered, "unethical medical experimentation on possible future human beings and therefore it is subject to absolute moral prohibition." I was as much surprised as made wrathful by this impertinent scorching attack. He abused everything I stood for.[96]

Ramsey's principal objection to in vitro fertilization and embryo transfer was that it was experimentation without the consent of the subject experimented upon. The potential for damage to the embryo was not insignificant, but Ramsey's rhetoric carried him beyond his logic. In Dr. Edwards' astonished words, "[How] disturbing, but perhaps to be expected from an extremist, is the hope half-offered by one theologian that the first child born through these methods will be abnormal and will be publicly displayed. The wrath of the pulpit is obviously to be heaped on the heads of sinners!"[97] Dr. Edwards had met bioethics in its most monitory mood. Eleven years later, the experiments of Edwards and Steptoe came to fruition in a healthy, perfectly formed baby girl.

On July 25, 1978, Mrs. Leslie Brown delivered by Cesarean section a healthy girl baby who was named Louise Joy. John and Leslie Brown, an English working-class couple, had reason to call their baby "Joy." After nine years of trying to become pregnant, Mrs. Brown was told that her fallopian tubes had been damaged by an earlier ectopic pregnancy and that she would not be able to conceive. They were referred to Mr. Steptoe, who consulted with Professor Edwards. Ova were retrieved from Mrs. Brown by laparoscopy, fertilized with Mr. Brown's sperm in vitro, and reimplanted in Mrs. Brown. Mrs. Brown was the first patient to carry her implanted embryo to term. The American and British media heard rumors of the event, descended on Oldham hospital, and on the morning after Louise's birth the newspapers proclaimed the birth of the world's first, "test tube baby."

Professor Edwards and Mr. Steptoe, with the cooperation of Mr. and Mrs. Brown, had accomplished a long-sought dream, a technical remedy for female infertility. That technical remedy could bring the joy of a child to couples whose infertility was due to physical constrictures of the fallopian tubes. As the scientist and obstetrician offered that remedy, they stirred an ethical maelstrom. The ethics of reproduction, accustomed to features of human life that seemed fixed and natural, encountered a strange and seemingly unnatural possibility: the conception of a child without sexual coitus. Their technique remedied the personal tragedy of infertility but it also placed within reach the human conceptus, opening possibilities for manipulating, designing, and cloning human beings. Not only could the question be asked whether making babies in a petri dish rather than within a mother was ethical, but also whether fashioning humans according to design should ever be a human option.

Edwards and Steptoe had anticipated these questions. They said at the Ciba symposium: "Some of the comments that are made about the wider implications of embryo transfer appear to be irrelevant or misleading. Debates on the imminence of genetic engineering are highly imaginative. The spectre of cloning is often raised, although no adult offspring have yet been produced after nuclear transfer in any species. Excessive concern over the "camel's nose . . . that cloning must follow from embryo transfer, seems unworthy of serious consideration. . . ."[98]

A few scholars, however, did consider cloning, remote though it might be, worthy of consideration. Ramsey engaged in combat with Nobel prizewinner, Joshua Lederberg on this issue. Lederberg ruminated about the possibilities of human cloning in a 1966 essay, "Experimental genetics and human evolution."[99] Although the tone of this essay is ironic and Lederberg himself warns that its readers should not "mistake comment for advocacy," his discussion of "vegetative reproduction," or cloning, is provocative: "if a superior individual—and, presumably, then, genotype—is identified, why not copy it directly, rather than suffer all the risks, including those of sex determination, involved in the disruptions of recombination?" Many scientists believed that cloning, the making of exact genetic copies of an individual, was about to become a common laboratory technique of the new molecular genetics. Lederberg says, "The internal properties of the clone open up new possibilities, for example, the free exchange of organ transplants with no concerns for graft rejection" and neurological similarities that could conceivably enhance communication between clones working together on complex tasks, "say a pair of astronauts . . . or a surgical team."[100]

Even though Lederberg qualified this suggestion with cautions, it provoked Ramsey to a strong response. His article "Should we clone a man" is brilliant Ramseian prose, showing him as both ethical polemicist and profound moral thinker. Nobelist Lederberg, even if he intended only ironic commentary, is given no quarter. Not only his claims, but even his qualifications are attacked by logic, counterargument, and ridicule. When Lederberg hesitates over the risks involved in the first attempt to clone a human, Ramsey seizes on that hesitation to make his major point: "The formidable moral objection [is] . . . what to do with the mishaps? . . . In case a monstrosity—a subhuman or parahuman individual results, shall the experiment simply be stopped and this artfully created human life be killed?" Lederberg, he argued, does not take this "grave moral question" seriously.[101] After a punctilious dissection of Lederberg's argument, Ramsey again invoked, in the only explicit theological passages in this essay, the Christian understanding of the covenant link between personal union and procreation in marriage. Many of the eugenic proposals, he averred, simply ignore or misunderstand the Christian and human understanding of parenthood.

The essay concludes with a disquisition on "the total life view at work in the grand design of mixing clonal with sexual reproduction in the control of man's own evolution." This world view, expressed not only by scientists but also "symptomatic of modern thought forms in general," is one that some would call *hybris* or "playing God." Modern *hybris* is a paradoxical combination of boundless determinism with boundless freedom which eliminates "all reason for man to respect and honor any feature of the creation."[102] Ramsey concludes with the demurrer that nothing he has said should be held against the moral use of genetic information in medicine which must pursue the prevention and cure of genetic disorders. He recommends genetic counseling and testing, even mandatory premarital genetic testing, to protect the innocent and unborn. Gene "surgery," should it ever become possible, "would raise no moral questions at all . . . that are not already present in the practice of medicine . . . [that is], a reasonable and well-examined expectation of doing more good than harm."[103] In all this, we must never lose sight of the real patients—the man, the woman and the child; these real patients should not be replaced by "non-patients, the species, or our control of human evolution."[104]

While the prospects for human cloning were scientifically remote, the theoretical possibility of reproducing copies of human individuals and designing them with particular talents intrigued many scientists and caught the public imagination. Remote science was made to seem imminent.[105] Regardless of the scientific remoteness of human cloning, the ethical debate touched on a perennial human concern, the nature and value of human identity and the limits of its manipulation. The cloning debate between Ramsey and Lederberg was one of the opening rounds of bioethical discourse. When human cloning again leapt into the headlines in the 1990s, the debate echoed Ramsey's thoughts of almost thirty years before.[106]

Many scholars less vehement than Paul Ramsey were reflecting on the ethical ramifications of the new science and practice of reproduction. Within a few years of Baby Louise's birth, a veritable nursery of other babies had come into being, some by the same process as Baby Louise, others by more elaborate manipulations. Reproductive endocrinology was surging ahead and the dreams (and nightmares) of the past were turning real. Questions about ownership of fertilized embryos, rightful claims of parenthood among the multiple contributors to a child's being, and preimplantation research and diagnosis pressed on public policy and the law. Each of those questions provided ample material for the reflections of bioethicists.

One of the first to speak was Joseph Fletcher, whose 1974 *Ethics of Genetic Control* is a paean of praise for the new techniques of reproduction which would allow rational humans to "end reproductive roulette." After reviewing the various advances in reproductive science, he wrote, "These answers are based upon a humane concern for the well-being of people, according to actual needs in actual situations . . . sometimes abortion would be right, sometimes wrong; sometimes egg transfers would be a good thing, sometimes not. The same holds true with test-tube conceptions, sterilizations, artificial gestations, preselection of sex, cloning, insemination and enovulation from storage banks. . . . This is the 'clinical' approach typical of biomedical ethics."[107] This was the biomedical ethics typical of Dr. Fletcher but not of many others who watched the same developments.

The firmest repudiation of the panoply of reproductive technologies came from bio-chemist/physician, Leon Kass. Employed as Executive Secretary of the Committee on Life Sciences and Social Policy, National Research Council, he began to indulge his philosophical inclinations, long submerged beneath his scientific training, in papers dealing with the new developments in genetics and reproduction. "Making babies: the new biology and the 'old' morality" first appeared in 1972, six years before Baby Louise was born. Kass revised the essay after her birth to reflect the fact that the first baby was born, not deformed, but quite normal.[108] Still, Kass asked whether we have the wisdom to manufacture babies and to deal with the broad implications that will flow from "divorcing the generation of human life from human sexuality and ultimately from the confines of the human body?"[109] He reviewed the implications: problems raised by the disposal of spare embryos, by surrogate gestational mothers, by the com-modification of gametes and embryos, by the desire to design "perfect" children and by the depreciation of defective ones, by ambiguity over personal identity and, finally, by the dehumanization of sexuality, marriage, and procreation. He expatiates on each of these problems with insight and sensitivity and answers his own question about whether we have the wisdom to make babies in these new ways with a resounding no. Each problem raises so many questions to which we have not the inkling of an answer that, "when we lack the sufficient wisdom . . . wisdom consists in not doing. Re-straint, caution, abstention and delay are what this second best (and maybe only) wis-dom dictates with respect to baby manufacture." If this wisdom not to do is unheeded (and by the time Kass revised his essay, the cat—or the baby—was out of the bag), then we must establish procedures to monitor and regulate what is done and establish "effective international control so that one nation's folly does not lead the world into degradation."[110]

The science of reproductive endocrinology and its concomitant technologies rushed ahead. In vitro fertilization (IVF) quickly became a relatively simple laboratory proce-dure, although efficiently produced pregnancies remained elusive. In short order, oocytes were not only fertilized with ease, but the resultant embryos could be frozen and stored for later implantation or for other uses.[111] These rapid developments stimu-lated rapid response from the public and from policymakers. Australia, home of a thriv-ing reproductive science, was the first to prepare policy. In 1982, the State of Victoria established a Committee to Consider the Social, Ethical and Legal Issues Arising from In vitro Fertilization, chaired by Law Reform Commissioner Louis Waller. The com-mittee produced several reports, the most significant of which dealt with the disposition of frozen embryos. (A Melbourne team had produced the first baby from a frozen em-bryo in March, 1984).[112] The Waller Committee agreed that "respect" was owed the human embryo but, like almost every other group that has faced these issues, they pro-vided neither a clear definition of respect nor much guidance about what it entails in practice. The report suggested that couples be given three options about disposition of embryos: donation to another couple, research use, or destruction. If destruction was chosen, its performance would be the moral equivalent of "withdrawing life support" for the embryo: removing the ampoule from the freezer and allowing it to thaw.[113] Research was permitted on embryos prior to fourteen days of development.[114] Although there was considerable disagreement among the committee on many particular points, the Victoria Legislature accepted the report as the basis for the Infertility Act of 1984, the world's first legislation on IVF.

When faced with a real question of destroying actual embryos, the same Parliament backtracked. An American couple named Rios went to the Melbourne Fertility Clinic and, after several failed attempts to initiate a pregnancy, left two frozen embryos in storage for another try. Two years later, they were killed in a plane crash. The Waller Committee recommended destruction of the orphan embryos, but the Parliament, in face of a public outcry, amended the Infertility Act to require that these embryos be donated to another couple.[115] Other Australian states and federal bodies also produced their own reports on reproductive technology; these reports were in substantial agreement on the policy issues and equally without extensive philosophical grounding for those policy issues.[116]

Great Britain had the opportunity to provide the philosophical grounding that Australia failed to lay. In June 1982, one of England's leading philosophers, Mary Warnock, was appointed chair of a Royal Commission "to examine the social, ethical and legal implications of recent, and potential developments in the field of human assisted reproduction." After wide consultation with scientific, professional, and religious bodies and individuals, the Warnock Report appeared in June, 1984. It recommended that commercial surrogacy be made illegal and it permitted research on spare, and on deliberately created embryos, up to the fifteenth day of development.

Given the reputation of the chairperson as a moral philosopher, it could have been expected that the report's conclusions would rest on solid philosophical reasoning. Although the report is lucidly written, with careful attention to conceptual issues, there is little effort to formulate theoretical arguments. Ethically intriguing topics, such as surrogacy and frozen embryos, are brushed lightly with philosophy but resolved by pragmatic considerations.[117]

I was living at Oxford during the Royal Commission's early deliberations. As a former member of the National and Presidential Commissions, I paid Professor Warnock a call. In the drawing room of Hertford College, she and I, together with her husband, Geoffrey Warnock, an equally respected moral philosopher who was then Master of Hertford and vice-chancellor of Oxford University, discussed the American experience with commissions, and with fetal research in particular. Mary Warnock spoke of the problem of reaching agreement among persons of quite different beliefs. During that conversation, at least, we did not touch on the particular role of moral philosophy. In her preface to the published report, the now Dame Warnock remarks on that problem, emphasizing that both deontological and utilitarian views were unsatisfying to the committee, who "were bound to have recourse to moral sentiments, to try . . . to sort out what our feelings were and to justify them." In her conclusion, she states forthrightly a relativist position: "It cannot be too strongly emphasized that in questions of morality, though there may be better or worse judgments, there is no such thing as a correct judgment."[118] Some of Dame Warnock's philosophical colleagues were disappointed by the insipid philosophical tone of the report. R. M. Hare felt that, instead of doing "a lot of hard philosophical work," to elucidate the defensible reasons for the conclusions, the commissioners merely tried to find some conclusions which most of them could sign. He sighed, "I have a lingering doubt as to whether, if Mary's philosophical views had been more as I think they should be, she might not have produced a more effective report."[119]

The next chance to elaborate public policy about in vitro fertilization fell to the United States. Leon Kass concluded his 1972 "Making babies" with the advice that in vitro fertilization and embryo transfer not be done. He commented, "Fortunately, there are no compelling reasons to proceed. . . . Though it saddens the life of many couples, infertility is hardly one of our major health problems."[120] Ironically, it was precisely the sadness of infertile couples that impressed the first and only American governmental project to evaluate the new reproductive technologies. Dr. Pierre Soupart of Vanderbilt University submitted to the National Institutes of Health a proposal to do laboratory research on embryos fertilized in vitro. Dr. Soupart's study was approved for scientific merit and then forwarded, as law required, to the Ethics Advisory Board (EAB) of the Department of Health, Education, and Welfare. The Board decided to take up the entire question of in vitro fertilization as a research procedure and in September 1978 (two months after Baby Louise Brown was born) initiated a study that was completed in May 1979. The Board imitated the National Commission by inviting scholars of all stripes to submit studies of the scientific, medical, psychological, ethical, and legal aspects of in vitro fertilization. It also held hearings around the United States. In the course of those hearings, many infertile couples testified about the pain and emptiness of their lives and their desire for a remedy for their infertility. The members of the Board were deeply moved and the perception that infertility was not an urgent problem was modified.

The EAB Report, *HEW Support of Research Involving In Vitro Fertilization and Embryo Transfer,* was carefully crafted. It began by expressing the Board's agreement with the opinion of the National Commission that "the human embryo is entitled to profound respect, but this respect does not necessarily encompass the full legal and moral rights attributed to persons."[121] It stated the Board's conclusion that research on in vitro fertilization is acceptable under defined conditions: the research should be designed to demonstrate safety and efficacy of the procedure; embryos will be sustained in vitro only for fourteen days; human gametes should be obtained after appropriate informed consent and, if embryo transfer is to be effected, it will be done only "with gametes obtained from lawfully married couples."[122] The EAB also encouraged the drafting of a model law to clarify the legal status of children born as the result of in vitro fertilization and embryo transfer. At the insistence of EAB member Father Richard Mc-

Cormick, the report answered Secretary Califano's question about whether in vitro fertilization could be considered "ethically acceptable" with the less definitive remark that it could be considered "acceptable public policy."[123]

This carefully researched and thoroughly debated report had a sad fate. It was deposited on Secretary Califano's desk on May 4, 1979. The EAB ceased to exist a year and six months later. During that time, silence surrounded the fate of the report. The Secretary did not acknowledge its receipt nor was notice published in the *Federal Register*. After the EAB lapsed, *Research Involving In Vitro Fertilization* disappeared from view and has not been heard from since. Most probably, the controversial topic frightened the politicians away. Dr. Soupart died before he knew the fate of his proposal. An opportunity to get in front of a major ethical issue was lost; the technology and clinical practice moved on without federal support for research and, thus, without oversight over its practices.

The techniques of in vitro fertilization and embryo transfer were developed to assist infertile couples like Mr. and Mrs. Brown. But, as Leon Kass feared, "once introduced for the purpose of treating intramarital infertility, in vitro fertilization can now be used for any purpose. There is no reason why the embryo need be implanted in the same woman from whom the egg was obtained."[124] Fertilized eggs could be used for research; they could be bartered and sold. Although the ethics commissions and boards around the world had dealt extensively with research use of embryos, these other possibilities of IVF were not so carefully examined. The EAB and the Warnock Report recommended that IVF be confined to married couples. Yet the technology made other procreative arrangements possible. The most obvious of those possibilities was that a woman, other than the woman whose egg had been fertilized, might serve as a gestator for the growing fetus. This practice, for which the term "surrogate mother" was coined, had already been employed for the much less technical process of artificial insemination. The New Jersey Commission on Legal and Ethical Problems in the Delivery of Health Care estimated that between 1976 and 1989, some 33 brokers had made arrangements that led to the birth of 1,200 children and that another 1,000 babies were born to parties who had made their own arrangements. The brokers' fees averaged $30,000. It is not known how many of these surrogacy arrangements involved the new technology of in vitro fertilization.

A few bioethicists noticed this phenomenon. In 1983, Professor John Robertson of the University of Texas School of Law, wrote "Surrogate mothers: the case for and against."[125] Robertson argued that surrogacy is analogous to adoption and can benefit all parties involved. However, he recognized problems: surrogate mothers might find it excruciating to give up the baby they had borne; they might even claim the baby as their own. The child might be harmed by uncertainty about the identity of its parents. Monetary exchange, generally forbidden by adoption laws, raised the question of "child selling" and the danger of perceiving a child as an article of commerce (the phrase "commodification of children" was coined to express this problem). Robertson saw no need to prohibit surrogacy but suggested that we have much to learn about how it should be done.

The quiet practice of surrogate gestation became noisy with the case of Baby M. In 1985, William and Elizabeth Stern agreed to pay Mary Beth Whitehead $10,000 to bear a baby conceived by artificial insemination from Mr. Stern. The Infertility Center of New York facilitated the arrangements for a fee of $7,500. After the baby, named in legalese, "Baby M," was delivered, Ms. Whitehead refused to surrender the child, claiming that she was its natural mother. The Sterns sued to enforce the contract; the Superior Court of Bergen County, New Jersey, upheld the contract and the Supreme Court of New Jersey, on February 3, 1988, upheld that decision. The case was followed avidly in the media, and the language of "surrogate," "gestational mother," "birth mother," entered the public vocabulary.

The Baby M case did not involve in vitro fertilization (such a case, in which "genetic" mother argued against "gestational" mother, had already appeared in an unappealed Michigan case of 1986) but it pushed all forms of surrogate motherhood—the old form by insemination and the new form by IVF and embryo transfer—into public attention. The new technology of assisted reproduction befuddled the identity of parents and the heritage of children even more than had artificial insemination: it was estimated that, with the help of the new science, as many as eight men and women could collaborate to make a baby. A number of surrogacy cases were brought to the courts. Many states adopted laws, most of which made the practice of commercial surrogacy illegal. The New Jersey Commission on Legal and Ethical Problems in the Delivery of Health Care initiated a study of surrogacy soon after the Baby M case was decided.[126]

The scientists and physicians involved in assisted reproduction recognized the problems that their work was creating. In 1984, the American Fertility Society appointed one of their most distinguished members, Dr. Howard Jones, to chair a committee to develop an ethical stance on the new reproductive technologies and to make recommendations about a wide range of issues. The committee included bioethicists Richard McCormick, John Robertson, and LeRoy Walters. A substantial report was published as a supplement to *Fertility and Sterility*, the scientific journal of the American Fertility Society.[127] While most techniques of assisted reproduction won the committee's approval, gestational surrogacy was viewed with skepticism. Father McCormick dissented from the committee's endorsement of the use of sperm, ova, or womb of a party outside a marriage covenant. Among the reasons for his dissent, he criticized, "the stud-farm mentality . . . with its subtle but unmistakable move toward eugenics."[128]

As the period that defines our history comes to an end, the serious bioethical discussion of reproductive technologies was just beginning. All participants in that discussion can appreciate the truth of Socrates' remark, "The answers to these questions are far from easy; many more doubts arise about this than about any of our previous conclusions."[129] The questions may be even more difficult than they were for Socrates, for they are posed against a two-thousand-year tradition of sexual and reproductive morality within monogamous and procreative marriage. That paradigm, deeply impressed upon Western culture, makes the new questions seem either outrageous or challeng-

ingly problematic. The long-standing condemnation of abortion, with its attendant casuistry, has left a legacy of concern about the moral standing of the fetus that compli-
cates discussions about the "manipulation" of embryos that are now, as never before,
available to be created, split, frozen, transferred, discarded, and experimented upon.
The long-standing condemnation of contraception tightly linked coitus to conception
and circumscribed coitus within the bonds of marriage; the unlinking of conception
from coitus and from marriage continues to trouble the modern conscience, relaxed as
it is about sexual morality. The long traditions still sound loudly in some places: in
1987, the Vatican Congregation for the Doctrine of the Faith issued a resounding condemnation of all reproductive technology.[130] In other places, the long tradition is more
muted, but it still can be heard in restrictive views and legislation. Commissions in several countries, such as West Germany, France and Italy, recommended restrictive law.
An international convention, sponsored by the Council of Europe, through its Steering
Committee on Bioethics, established a common framework for the protection of human
rights in genetics, reproductive technology, and other bioethical issues.[131] However,
even though these moral memories linger, the bioethical debates over the reproductive
technologies have yielded some answers that have been widely accepted as reasonable.
English philosopher Jonathan Glover prefaced his report to the European Commission
on the new reproductive technologies with the reflection, "The deep divisions over present developments are partly about whether they are in themselves acceptable. But
partly they reflect concern that we may be sleepwalking, step by step, into a world
which few of us would now choose."[132] One of the values of bioethical discourse is to
keep the walkers awake as they trek into the futures to which the reproductive and genetic sciences point.

The ethical debates that surround reproductive technology frequently cite Aldous
Huxley's 1932 novel, *Brave New World*. In that frightening vision of the future, all babies are produced in state hatcheries where government scientists preconditioned and
decanted "socialized human beings, as Alphas or Epsilons, as future sewer workers or
world controllers." Huxley lifted the title of his book from the last act of Shakespeare's
The Tempest. That wondrous play is filled with strange creatures, some beautiful like
Ariel, others horrible like Caliban, all engineered by Prospero's magic art, and they
dance and howl at his behest. But these sprites and monsters are not the creatures that
evoke the phrase "brave new world." Miranda, Prospero's daughter, who was raised
among the strange creatures of her father's magic, utters that phrase when she sees her
first humans other than her father and her fiancée, Ferdinand. She greets the retinue of
noble gentlemen cast by storm upon her island with the exclamation, "O, wonder! how
many goodly creatures there are here! How beauteous mankind is! O brave new world
that has such people in it."[133] She is astonished—not at the bizarre creatures she has
lived with all her life—but at quite normal, ordinarily proportioned and modestly talented humans. The difficulty of unraveling the ethics of reproductive technology may
be due to our impoverished ability to recognize and appreciate what is normal about
being human.

Notes for Chapter 9

1. Plato, *The Republic*, V, 449–450.

2. James A. Brundage, *Law, Sex and Christian Society in Medieval Europe* (Chicago: University of Chicago, 1987), p. 1.

3. Louis Epstein, *Sex Laws and Customs in Judaism* (New York: Ktav Publishing House, 1967); Eric Fuchs, *Sexual Desire and Love: Origins and History of the Christian Ethic of Sexuality and Marriage*, trans. Marsha Daigle (New York: Seabury Press, 1983).

4. *The Fundamental Epistle of Mani*, quoted in John T. Noonan, Jr., *Contraception: A History of Its Treatment by the Catholic Theologians and Canonists* (Cambridge, Mass: Harvard University Press, 1965), p. 111.

5. Augustine, *The Good of Marriage*, 29:32, in *The Fathers of the Church*, vol. 27, *Treatises on Marriage and Other Subjects*, trans. Charles T. Wilcox, ed. Roy J. Deferrari (New York: Fathers of the Church, Inc., 1955), pp. 9–51. See Peter Brown, *Augustine of Hippo* (Berkeley and Los Angeles: University of California Press, 1967).

6. Augustine, *Marriage and Concupiscence*, in *Works of Aurelius Augustinus*, ed. Marcus Dods, (Edinburgh: T. & T. Clark, 1874), vol. xii, pp. 137–202.

7. Plato, *The Republic* V, 461e.

8. Aristotle, *Politics* VII, 16, 1335b.

9. Aristotle, *History of Animals*, VII, 3, 583b; *De Anima* 414a–415b.

10. Ludwig Edelstein, "The Hippocratic Oath: text, translation and interpretation," in Owsei Temkin and C. Lilian Temkin (eds.), *Ancient Medicine: Selected Papers of Ludwig Edelstein* (Baltimore: Johns Hopkins University Press, 1967), pp. 18–20.

11. Soranus of Ephesus, *Gynecology*, trans. Owsei Temkin (Baltimore: Johns Hopkins University Press, 1956), I, xix, p. 63.

12. Scribonius Largus, *On Remedies*, trans. J. S. Hamilton, *Bulletin of the History of Medicine* 60 (1962): 209–216; see Paul Carrick, *Medical Ethics in Antiquity* (Dordrecht/Boston: D. Reidel Publishing Company, 1985).

13. Tosafot, *Niddah* 44b, cited in Fred Rosner, *Modern Medicine and Jewish Ethics* (Hoboken, N.J.: Ktav Publishing House, 1986), p. 144. Rosner comments, "Some rabbinic authorities accept these words verbatim, while others are of the opinion that Tosafot is not to be interpreted literally, yet others believe that Tosafot is in error."

14. Mishnah, *Oholot*, 7:6; Maimonides. Hil. Ratz'ah 9, cited in Immanuel Jakobovits, *Jewish Medical Ethics: A Comparative and Historical Study of the Jewish Religious Attitude to Medicine and Its Practice* (New York: Bloch Publishing Company, 1959), p. 184.

15. Jakobovits, *Jewish Medical Ethics*, p. 190.

16. *The Didache*, trans. James A. Kleist (Westminster, Md.: Newman Press, 1948), 2.2, 5.2.

17. The text that would become a principal source of church law about abortion is maddeningly unclear. A brief paragraph in a tenth-century canon law text, called after its first words *Si aliquis*, reads, "If anyone to satisfy his lust or in deliberate hatred does something to a man or woman so that no children be born of him or her, or gives them to drink so that he cannot generate or she conceive, let it be held as homicide." *Penitential of Regino of Prum*, cited in Noonan, *Contraception*, p. 168. This text does not contain the word "abortion" and appears to refer more to sterilization and contraception, even involuntary at that, yet it stood in church law until the revision of canon law in 1917. Another important text of church law (*Aliquando*), excerpted from St. Augustine reads, "Sometimes this cruel lust comes to this, that they (husband and wife) obtain poisons of sterility and, if these do not work, extinguish and destroy the fetus in some way in the womb, preferring that their offspring die before it lives, or if it was already alive in the womb to

kill it before it was born." *Marriage and Concupiscence*, I, 15–17, cited in Noonan, *Contraception*, p. 136.

18. Gratian, *Decretum* 2.32.2.7; Gregory IX *Decretales*, 5.12.20, *Corpus Juris Canonici* ed. Emil Friedberg (Leipzig, 1879–1881).

19. John R. Connery, *Abortion. The Development of the Roman Catholic Perspective* (Chicago: Loyola University Press, 1977); John T. Noonan, "An almost absolute value in history," in Noonan (ed.), *The Morality of Abortion: Legal and Historical Perspectives* (Cambridge, Mass.: Harvard University Press, 1970), pp. 1–59.

20. Antoninus, *Summa Theologiae Moralis* II, 7.2.2.

21. Paolo Zacchia, *Quaestiones medico-legales* (Lyons, 1701). In 1679, Pope Innocent XI condemned the opinion that permitted abortion before animation, not so much to salvage the old doctrine but because he disapproved of the reason given by the censured theologians, namely, to save a pregnant girl (*puella*) from being killed or defamed by an enraged father or cuckolded husband. See Heinrich Denzinger and Adolfus Schonmetzer, *Enchiridion Symbolorum Definitionum et Declarationum de Rebus Fidei et Morum*, 33rd ed. (Rome: Herder, 1965), #2134.

22. See U. Diamond, "Abortion, animation, and biological hominization," *Theological Studies* 36 (1975): 305–324. Civil jurisdictions abolished the Aristotelian distinction during the same period. It was removed from English statutes on abortion in 1837, and American jurisdictions dropped it gradually during the first half of the 19th century. In both cases, progressive scientific opinion influenced the law.

23. Denzinger and Schonmetzer, *Enchiridion Symbolorum*, #3258.

24. Denzinger and Schonmetzer, *Enchiridion Symbolorum*, #3719–3721; Noonan, "An almost absolute value in history," p. 40.

25. Austin O'Malley, *The Ethics of Medical Homicide and Mutilation* (New York: Devin-Adair, 1919); T. Lincoln Bouscaren, *The Ethics of Ectopic Pregnancy* (Chicago: Loyola University Press, 1933).

26. James B. Nelson, "Abortion: Protestant perspectives," in Warren T. Reich (ed.), *Encyclopedia of Bioethics* (New York: The Free Press, 1978) Vol. 1, pp. 13–17, and Beverly Wildung Harrison, "Abortion: Protestant perspectives," in Warren T. Reich (ed.), *Encyclopedia of Bioethics, Revised Edition* (New York: Simon and Schuster Macmillan, 1995), Vol. I, pp. 34–38.

27. Public Statute Laws of the State of Connecticut, Crimes and Punishment, 1821, section 14; James C. Mohr, *Abortion in America: The Origins and Evolution of National Policy 1800–1900* (New York: Oxford University Press, 1978), p. 21.

28. Revised Statutes of New York, 1828–1835, I, Title VI, Ch. I, Part IV, section 21; Mohr, *Abortion in America*, p. 27.

29. Report on Criminal Abortion, *Transactions of the American Medical Association*, XII (1859): 75–78; Mohr, *Abortion in America*, p. 157.

30. Mohr, *Abortion in America* p. 157.

31. Mary Steichen Calderone (ed.), *Abortion in the United States* (New York: Hoeber-Harper, 1958); Frederick J. Taussig, *Abortion, Spontaneous and Induced: Medical and Social Aspects* (St. Louis: The C. V. Mosby Company, 1936); Harold Rosen, *Therapeutic Abortion: Medical, Psychiatric, Anthropological, and Religious Considerations* (New York: Julian Press, 1954); Proceedings of a Conference of the National Committee on Maternal Health, *The Abortion Problem* (Baltimore: Wilkins and Wilkins, 1944); see also Mohr, *Abortion in America*; Daniel Callahan, *Abortion: Law, Choice, and Morality* (New York: Macmillan, 1970), pp. 131–136.

32. American Law Institute, *Model Penal Code: Proposed Official Draft* (Philadelphia: ALI, 1962), sec. 230.3.

33. Bill Becker, "Abortion to bar defective birth is facing legal snag in Arizona," *New York*

Times, July 25, 1962, A22; "Mrs. Finkbine undergoes abortion in Sweden," *New York Times*, August 19, 1962: A69.

34. *Transactions of the American Medical Association* 33 (1871): 258; Proceedings of AMA House of Delegates, June 1970, 220.

35. American College of Obstetricians and Gynecologists, *Standards for Obstetric-Gynecological Hospital Services* (Washington, D.C.: ACOG, 1969), p. 53; *Statement of Policy: Abortion* (Washington, D.C.: ACOG, August, 1970).

36. John Courtney Murray, *We Hold These Truths: Catholic Reflections on the American Proposition* (New York: Sheed and Ward, 1960).

37. Richard A. McCormick, "Public policy on abortion," *Hospital Progress* 60 (1979): 26–30; *How Brave a New World: Dilemmas in Bioethics* (Garden City: Doubleday, 1981), p. 200.

38. National Conference of Catholic Bishops Administrative Committee, "Pastoral message," *Hospital Progress* 54 (1973): 83ff.; also included in McCormick, *How Brave a New World*, p. 117.

39. Robert E. Cooke, André E. Hellegers, Robert Hoyt, and Herbert Richardson (eds.), *The Terrible Choice: The Abortion Dilemma* (New York: Bantam, 1968). *The Morality of Abortion* also issued from that conference.

40. Cooke et al., *The Terrible Choice*, p. 57.

41. Lawrence Lader, *Abortion* (Indianapolis: Bobbs-Merrill, 1966); The National Association for Repeal of Abortion Laws, 1969.

42. Paul Ramsey, "Reference points in deciding about abortion," in Noonan, *The Morality of Abortion*, p. 60.

43. Paul Ramsey, "The morality of abortion," in Daniel H. Labby (ed.), *Life or Death: Ethics and Options* (Seattle: University of Washington Press, 1968), pp. 60–93; "Reference points in deciding about abortion," in Noonan, *The Morality of Abortion*, pp. 60–100; "Feticide/Infanticide on request," *Religion in Life* 39 (1970): 170–186; "The ethics of a cottage industry in an age of community and research medicine," *New England Journal of Medicine* 284 (1971): 700–706; "Abortion: A review article," *The Thomist* 37 (1973): pp. 174–226; "The Supreme Court's bicentennial abortion decision: Can the 1973 abortion decisions be justly hedged?" and "Abortion after the law: conscience and its problems," in *Ethics at the Edges of Life. Medical and Legal Intersections* (New Haven: Yale University Press, 1978), pp. 3–42, 43–93.

44. Ramsey, "The morality of abortion," p. 71.

45. Ramsey, "The morality of abortion," p. 78.

46. Ramsey, "The morality of abortion," p. 81.

47. Richard A. McCormick, "Past church teaching on abortion," *Proceedings of Catholic Theological Society of America* 23 (1968): 137–140; Charles E. Curran, *Politics, Medicine and Christian Ethics: A Dialogue with Paul Ramsey* (Philadelphia: Fortress Press, 1973), pp. 111–131; Germain G. Grisez, *Abortion: the Myths, the Realities, and the Arguments* (New York: Corpus Books, 1970).

48. Callahan, *Abortion: Law, Choice, and Morality* pp. 19, 495; see also Callahan, "Abortion: thinking and experiencing," *Christianity and Crisis* 32 (1973): 295–298.

49. Paul Ramsey, "Abortion: a review article," *The Thomist* 37 (1973): 174–226.

50. Richard A. McCormick, "The abortion dossier," in *How Brave a New World*, p. 160; originally in *Theological Studies* 34 (1974): 312–359.

51. *Roe v Wade,* Supreme Ct US 410 US 113; 93 S. Ct 705 (1973). See Larry Gostin (ed.), *Justice Harry A. Blackmun: The Supreme Court and the Limits of Medical Privacy* (special issue), *American Journal of Law and Medicine* 13, nos. 2 and 3 (1987): 153–525.

52. Baruch A. Brody, *Abortion and the Sanctity of Life* (Cambridge, Mass.: MIT Press, 1975);

"Abortion and the sanctity of human life," *American Philosophical Quarterly* 10 (1973): 133–140; "Abortion and the law," *Journal of Philosophy* 357 (1971): 357–369. Representative of the Catholic philosophical argumentation is Germain Gabriel Grisez and John Finnis, "The rights and wrongs of abortion," *Philosophy and Public Affairs* 2 (1973): 117–45.

53. Judith Jarvis Thomson, "A defense of abortion," *Philosophy and Public Affairs* 1 (1971): 47–67.

54. Baruch Brody, "From abortion to reproductive technology: abortion," (paper read at the Birth of Bioethics Conference, Seattle, Wa., Sept. 23–24, 1992), transcript, pp. 221–33. A recent contribution from the analytic tradition that fits Brody's description is Frances Myrna Kamm, *Creation and Abortion: A Study in Moral and Legal Philosophy* (New York: Oxford University Press, 1992).

55. Michael Tooley, "Abortion and infanticide," *Philosophy and Public Affairs* 2 (1972): 37–65; *Abortion and Infanticide* (Oxford: Clarendon Press, 1983).

56. H. T. Engelhardt, Jr., "The ontology of abortion," *Ethics* 84 (1974): 217–234; Mary Anne Warren, "On the moral and legal status of abortion," *Monist* 57 (1973): 43–61; L. W. Sumner, *Abortion and Moral Theory* (Princeton: Princeton University Press, 1981); R. M. Hare, "Abortion and the golden rule," *Philosophy and Public Affairs* 4 (1975): 201–222; see also Marshall Cohen, Thomas Nagel, and Thomas Scanlon (eds.), *Rights and Wrongs of Abortion* (Princeton: Princeton University Press, 1974), essays originally published in the journal *Philosophy and Public Affairs;* Joel Feinberg (ed.), *The Problem of Abortion*, 1st ed. (Belmont, Calif.: Wadsworth Publishing Company, 1973) (contains Noonan, Donceel, Devine, Sumner, Warren, Tooley, Benn); William Bondeson, H. Tristram Engelhardt, Jr., Stuart Spicker, and Daniel Winship (eds.), *Abortion and the Status of the Fetus* (Dordrecht/Boston: D. Reidel Publishing Company, 1983), especially LeRoy Walters, "The fetus in ethical and public policy discussions from 1973 to the present," pp. 15–30.

57. Karen Lebacqz, "Prenatal diagnosis and selective abortion," *Linacre Quarterly* 40 (1973): 109–27.

58. John Fletcher, "Ethics and amniocentesis for fetal sex identification," *New England Journal of Medicine* 301 (1979): 550–553; "Amniocentesis for sex identification," *New England Journal of Medicine* 302 (1980): 525; "Is sex selection ethical?" *Progress in Clinical and Biological Research* 128 (1983): 333–348.

59. Carrick, *Medical Ethics in Antiquity*, pp. 104–107; Norman E. Himes, *Medical History of Contraception* (Baltimore: The Williams and Wilkins Company, 1936); Soranus, *Gynecology*, pp. 62–66.

60. Rosner, *Modern Medicine and Jewish Ethics*, chapter 8; David M. Feldman, *Birth Control in Jewish Law* (New York: New York University Press, 1968).

61. *Decretals of Gregory IX*, 4.5.7 "*Si conditiones*"; Denzinger and Schonmetzer, *Enchiridion Symbolorum*, #827; Noonan, *Contraception*, chapter VI, p. 178.

62. Denzinger and Schonmetzer, *Enchiridion Symbolorum*, #3715–3718.

63. As late as the 1950s, Protestant theologian Karl Barth issued a stern warning: "Sexual intercourse as the physical completion of life-partnership in marriage can always be . . . an offer of divine goodness. . . . Hence every act of intercourse which is technically obstructed or interrupted, or undertaken with no desire for children, or even refrained from on this ground, is a refusal of this divine offer, a renunciation of the widening and enriching of married fellowship." Barth does not conclude that contraceptive intercourse is forbidden but calls for "grave reasons if the gravity of this renunciation . . . is to be dispelled." Karl Barth, *Church Dogmatics*, trans. A. T. Mackay, T. H. L. Parker, et al. (Edinburgh: T. & T. Clark, 1961), III 4, pp. 269–270.

64. David M. Kennedy, *Birth Control in America: The Career of Margaret Sanger* (New Haven: Yale University Press, 1970), p. 141.

65. Committee on Marriage and the Home of the Federal Council of Churches, *Moral Aspects of Birth Control* (New York, 1934).

66. Lambeth Conference of 1930, Resolution 15, quoted in William Redmond Curtis, *The Lambeth Conferences: The Solution for Pan-Anglican Organization* (New York: Columbia University Press, 1942), p. 332.

67. T. S. Eliot, *Thoughts After Lambeth* (London: Faber and Faber, 1931), p. 17.

68. Clive Wood and Beryl Suitters, *The Fight for Acceptance: A History of Contraception* (Aylesbury: Medical and Technical Publishing Company, 1970), p. 151.

69. Quoted in David Halberstam, *The Fifties* (New York: Villard Books, 1993), p. 286.

70. Paul Vaughn, *The Pill on Trial* (London: Weiderfeld and Nicholson, 1970), p. 39.

71. Vaughn, *The Pill on Trial*, p. 47.

72. Quoted in Halberstam, *The Fifties*, p. 605.

73. John T. Noonan, Jr., *Contraception: A History of Its Treatment by Catholic Theologians and Canonists* (Cambridge: Harvard University Press, 1965).

74. General Statutes of Connecticut, rev. 1958, section 53-32.

75. *Griswold v Connecticut* 381 US 479, 85 S. Ct. 1678.

76. Louis Brandeis and Charles Warren, "The right to privacy," *Harvard Law Review* 4 (1890): 193.

77. Joseph F. Fletcher, *Morals and Medicine*, 2nd ed. (Boston: Beacon Press, 1960), p. xv.

78. Charles Curran, *New Perspectives in Moral Theology* (University of Notre Dame Press, 1976), pp. 205–206; see also Curran, *Contraception: Authority and Dissent* (New York: Herder and Herder, 1969); Louis K. Dupré, *Contraception and Catholics: A New Appraisal* (Baltimore: Helicon, 1964).

79. Pope Paul VI, *Humanae Vitae*. It is often said that the Pope favored the minority opinion, but the commission's report had no minority opinion; rather, several conservatives, led by American Jesuit John Ford and encouraged by arch-conservative Cardinal Ottaviani, devised an alternative position that was presented to the Pope. See Robert Blair Kaiser, *The Politics of Sex and Religion, A Case History in the Development of Doctrine, 1962–1984* (Kansas City: Leven Press, 1985).

80. Daniel Callahan (ed.), *The Catholic Case for Contraception* (New York: Macmillan, 1969).

81. Sandro Spinsanti, *La Bioetica: Biografie per una Disciplina* (Rome: FrancoAngeli, 1995), pp. 127, 227.

82. Proceedings, *The Great Issues of Conscience in Modern Medicine*, Dartmouth College, September 8–10, 1960, published in Dartmouth Alumni Magazine 53, no. 2 (Nov. 1960), p. 20.

83. Paul Ehrlich, *The Population Bomb* (New York: Ballantine Books, 1968); Garret Hardin and Kingsley Davis, "Population policy: will current programs succeed," *Science* 158 (1969): 730–739.

84. Garrett Hardin, "The tragedy of the commons," *Science* 162 (1968): 1243–1248, quote on p. 1248.

85. Arthur Dyck, "Assessing the population debate," *The Monist* 61 (Jan. 1977); Ralph Potter, *The Simple Structure of the Population Debate: The Logic of the Ecology Movement* (Hastings-on-Hudson: Institute of Society, Ethics and the Life Sciences, 1971).

86. Ralph Potter, interview, March 5, 1996.

87. Soranus, *Gynecology*, I, ch. xix, pp. 62–68.

88. John Kobler, *The Reluctant Surgeon: A Biography of John Hunter* (Garden City, N.Y.: Doubleday and Company, 1960), p. 283. John Hunter's account of this case was published posthumously in 1799.

89. A. D. Hard, "Artificial impregnation," *Medical World* 27 (1909): 136.

90. Department of Health and Human Services, *Report to the Departmental Committee on Human Artificial Insemination (The Feversham Committee)* (London: His Majesty's Stationery Office, 1960); *People v Sorensen*, 66 Cal Rptr. 7, 437 p. 2d 495 (1968); see also A. H. Rosenberg, "Legal aspects of artificial insemination," *New England Journal of Medicine* 278 (1968): 552–554.

91. Holy Office, March 17, 1897, Denzinger and Schonmetzer, *Enchiridion Symbolorum*, #3323; Allocution, Sept. 29, 1949, *Acta Apostolicae Sedis* 41 (1949): 5591ff; see Charles J. Mc-Fadden, *Medical Ethics*, 2nd ed. (Philadelphia: F. A. Davis, 1949).

92. Ciba Foundation, *Law and Ethics of AID and Embryo Transfer* (Amsterdam/New York: Elsevier, 1973).

93. Rev. G. R. Dunstan, "Moral and social issues," in Ciba Foundation, *Law and Ethics of AID and Embryo Transfer*, p. 51.

94. R. G. Edwards and Patrick Steptoe, "Biological aspects of embryo transfer," in Ciba Foundation, *Law and Ethics of AID and Embryo Transfer*, p. 12.

95. Charles Fried, "Ethical issues," in Ciba Foundation, *Law and Ethics of AID and Embryo Transfer*, pp. 41–45.

96. Robert Edwards and Patrick Steptoe, *A Matter of Life: The Story of a Medical Break-through* (London: Morrow, 1980), p. 113; Ramsey, "Shall we 'reproduce'? I. The medical ethics of *in vitro* fertilization," *Journal of the American Medical Association* 220 (1972): 1346–1350; "Shall we 'reproduce'? II. Rejoinders and future forecast," *Journal of the American Medical Association* 220 (1972): 1480–1485.

97. R. G. Edwards, "Fertilization of human eggs *in vitro*: Morals, ethics and the law," *Quarterly Review of Biology* 49 (1974): 3–26, 23, responding to Ramsey, "Shall we 'reproduce'? II"

98. R. G. Edwards and Patrick Steptoe, "Biological aspects of embryo transfer," in Ciba Foundation, *Law and Ethics of AID and Embryo Transfer*, pp. 17–18.

99. Joshua Lederberg, "Experimental genetics and human evolution," *American Naturalist* 100 (1966): 519–531 and *Bulletin of the Atomic Scientist* 22 (1966): 4–11.

100. Lederberg, "Experimental genetics and human evolution," *Bulletin of the Atomic Scientist*, pp. 9–10.

101. Ramsey, *Fabricated Man: The Ethics of Genetic Control* (New Haven: Yale University Press, 1970), p. 78.

102. Ramsey, *Fabricated Man*, p. 94.

103. Ramsey, *Fabricated Man*, pp. 99–100.

104. Ramsey, *Fabricated Man*, p. 100.

105. A few years after the Ramsey–Lederberg exchange, a popular book by David Rorvik, *In His Image: The Cloning of a Man* (Philadelphia: J. B. Lippincott Company, 1978) convinced many people that a human clone had already been created, and a popular film, *The Boys From Brazil*, based on a book of the same name by Ira Levin (New York: Random House, 1976), made the public shudder at the prospect of a clan of cloned Adolf Hitlers. And, of course, constant references were made to Aldous Huxley, *Brave New World* (New York: Harper and Brothers, 1946).

106. Allan Verhey, "Cloning: revisiting an old debate," *Kennedy Institute of Ethics Journal* 4 (1994): 227–234; Michael Specter and Gina Kolata, "After decades and many missteps, cloning success," *The New York Times*, March 3, 1997, A1, A8–10; Ian Wilmut, A. E. Schnicke, J. McWhir, et al., "Viable offspring derived from fetal and adult mammalian cells," *Nature* 385 (1997): 810–813.

107. Joseph Fletcher, *Ethics of Genetic Control: Ending Reproductive Roulette* (Garden City: Anchor Press, 1974), p. 147.

108. Leon Kass, "Making babies: the new biology and the 'old' morality," *The Public Interest* 26 (Winter, 1972) 26: 18–56; the revised version appears in Kass, *Toward a More Natural Sci-

ence: Biology and Human Affairs (New York: The Free Press, 1985), pp. 43–79.

109. Kass, *Toward a More Natural Science*, p. 47.

110. Kass, *Toward a More Natural Science*, p. 78; see also Kass's "New beginnings in life," in Michael P. Hamilton (ed.), *The New Genetics and the Future of Man* (Grand Rapids: William P. Eerdmans Publishing Company, 1972), pp. 15–63.

111. LeRoy Walters, "Human *in vitro* fertilization: a review of the ethical issues," *Hastings Center Report* 9, no. 4 (1979): 23–43.

112. Committee to Consider the Social, Ethical and Legal Issues Arising from *In vitro* Fertilization, *Report on the Disposition of Embryos Produced By In vitro Fertilization* (Melbourne: Victoria Government Printer, 1984).

113. Ibid., 29, para 2.12.

114. Ibid., 46, para 3.29.

115. "Australians reject bid to destroy 2 embryos," *New York Times*, October 24, 1984, A18.

116. Pascal Kasimba and Peter Singer, "Australian commissions and committees on issues in bioethics," *Journal of Medicine and Philosophy* 14 (1989): 403–424.

117. Department of Health and Human Services, *Report of the Committee of Enquiry into Human Fertilisation and Embryology* (London: Her Majesty's Stationery Office, 1984) secs. 8,10.

118. Mary Warnock, *A Question of Life* (Oxford: Blackwell, 1985), pp. x, 96.

119. R. M. Hare, "*In vitro* fertilization and the Warnock Report," in Ruth F. Chadwick (ed.), *Ethics, Reproduction and Genetic Control* (London: Croom Helm, 1987), pp. 71–90. In this paper, which was first presented at a 1985 meeting of the Hastings Center at Oxford, Hare compares the Warnock Report with the Report of the Committee on Obscenity and Film Censorship, chaired by philosopher Bernard Williams: "It must be admitted that, perhaps because it was so enlightened, the Williams Commission did not get nearly such a good press as the Warnock Commission, and its recommendations were not taken up. But it may have in the end a more lasting influence because . . . the reasons are all here and will eventually be absorbed." See also Alastair V. Campbell, "Committees and commissions in the United Kingdom," *Journal of Medicine and Philosophy* 14 (1989): 385–401; G. R. Dunstan, "Warnock reviewed," *Crucible* (Oct.–Nov., 1985): 152–153; M. Lockwood, "The Warnock Report: a philosophical appraisal," in Lockwood (ed.), *Moral Dilemmas in Modern Medicine* (New York: Oxford University Press, 1985), pp. 155–186.

120. Kass, *Toward a More Natural Science*, p. 79; see Margaret Marsh and Wanda Ronner, *The Empty Cradle: Infertility in America from Colonial Times to the Present* (Baltimore: Johns Hopkins, 1996). It was Father McCormick who told me how moving the testimony of infertile couples was.

121. Ethics Advisory Board, DHEW, *Report and Conclusions: HEW Support of Research Involving Human In vitro Fertilization and Embryo Transfer*, May 1979 Conclusions 1 & 2, p. 101.

122. Ethics Advisory Board, DHEW, *Report and Conclusions: HEW Support of Research Involving Human In vitro Fertilization and Embryo Transfer*, May 1979 Conclusions 1 and 2, pp. 104–107.

123. Ethics Advisory Board, *Report and Conclusions*, Conclusion 5, p. 113.

124. Kass, *Toward a More Natural Science*, p. 59.

125. John A. Robertson, "Surrogate mothers: the case for and against," *Hastings Center Report* 13, no. 5 (1983): 28–34; Herbert T. Krimmel, "The case against surrogate parenting" *Hastings Center Report* 13, no. 5 (1983): 35–39; George Annas, "The baby broker boom," *Hastings Center Report* 16, no. 3 (1986): 30–32. A symposium called "Surrogate Motherhood: An Ethical Perspective" was held at Wayne State University on November 20, 1982, and another one was held at Santa Clara University, called "Manufactured Motherhood," on April 22, 1988; see *Logos* 9 (1988).

126. New Jersey Commission on Legal and Ethical Problems in the Delivery of Health Care, *After Baby M: The Legal, Ethical and Social Dimensions of Surrogacy* (Trenton, 1992). The New York State Task Force on Life and the Law issued *Surrogate Parenting: Analysis and Recommendations for Public Policy* (New York, 1988). Both state bodies recommended that their jurisdiction discourage surrogate parenting.

127. "Ethical Considerations of the New Reproductive Technologies," *Fertility and Sterility* 46 (Suppl. 1) (1986). In 1991, The American Fertility Society and the American College of Obstetricians and Gynecologists initiated the National Advisory Board for Ethics and Reproduction (NABER). This group, which soon became independent of its initiators, continues to provide ethical advice on new issues that arise in reproductive medicine. I was its first chairman, serving from 1991 to 1995; bioethicist Cynthia Cohen was its first director. See, for example, a recent work commissioned by NABER. Cynthia B. Cohen (ed.), *New Ways of Making Babies: The Case of Egg Donation* (Bloomington: Indiana University Press, 1996).

128. *Ethical Considerations*. Appendix A, 82S. See also Richard T. Hull, *Ethical Issues in Reproductive Technologies* (Belmont: Wadsworth Publishing Company, 1990); Bonnie Steinbock, *Life Before Birth: The Moral and Legal Status of Embryos and Fetuses* (New York: Oxford University Press, 1992); Jonathan Glover, *Ethics of New Reproductive Technologies: The Glover Report to the European Commission* (DeKalb, Ill.: Northern Illinois University, 1989); Kenneth Alpern (ed.), *The Ethics of Reproductive Technology* (New York: Oxford University Press, 1992); Carson Strong, *Ethics in Reproductive and Perinatal Medicine: A New Framework* (New Haven: Yale University Press, 1997).

129. Plato, *Republic* V, 450.

130. Congregation for the Doctrine of the Faith, *Instruction on Respect for Human Life in its Origins and on the Dignity of Procreation* (Boston: St. Paul Press, 1987).

131. Council of Europe, *Explanatory Report to the Convention for the Protection of Human Rights and Dignity of the Human Being with Regard to the Application of Biology and Medicine* (Strasbourg: Directorate of Legal Affairs, 1997).

132. Glover, *Ethics of New Reproductive Technologies*, p. 20.

133. William Shakespeare, *The Tempest* V, i. ll 181–183.

III

DISCIPLINE, DISCOURSE, AND ETHOS

10

Bioethics As a Discipline

Bioethicists sometimes worry whether bioethics should be called a discipline. This concern is a mark of the academic mind, wondering whether one's peculiar interest has a place in the panoply of subjects that have standing within the university. Many bioethicists were trained in the classical disciplines, such as philosophy, theology, or law, that have long held such standing and they know that their new interest lies outside the familiar territory of those disciplines. Yet, in the modern university, the clear lines of many classical disciplines have diffused into mosaics: even the most definitive ones, such as mathematics and physics, are complex collections of subdisciplines with quite diverse theories, methods, and even definitions of the field. So, is bioethics a discipline if it contains, as it does, pieces of philosophy, law, medicine, anthropology, and theology? Or can a stronger claim be made that bioethics has emerged as a discipline in its own right?

Bioethics As Discipline

The word "bioethics" was canonized in the Library of Congress catalogue on an entry that cited an article by Dan Callahan, "Bioethics as a Discipline." In that essay, written for the first issue of the *Hastings Center Studies*, Callahan remarked, "Bioethics is not yet a full discipline . . . [lacking] general acceptance, disciplinary standards, criteria of excellence and clear pedagogical and evaluative norms." This very lack offered bioethics an unprecedented opportunity to define itself. It could move toward "definition of issues, methodological strategies and procedures for decision-making." In defining issues, bioethics would need "the rigor of the unfettered imagination," the ability to envision alternatives, to get into people's ethical agonies. In developing methodologi-

325

cal strategies, bioethics must use the traditional modes of philosophical analysis—logic, consistency, careful use of terms, seeking rational justifications—supplemented by sensitivity to feelings and emotions as well as to the political and social influences on behavior. Finally, the discipline must provide procedures "to reach reasonably specific, clear decisions . . . in the circumstances of medicine and science." Callahan concluded: "The discipline of bioethics should be so designed, and its practitioners so trained, that it will directly—at whatever cost to disciplinary elegance—serve those physicians and biologists whose positions demand that they make the practical decisions." This sort of discipline, according to Callahan, requires a knowledge of the sociology of the profession and of health care, scientific training, historical knowledge of regnant value theories, facility with methods of ethical analysis common in the philosophical and theological communities, and their limitations when applied to cases—an "impossible list of demands," admitted Callahan, but approachable by "a continuing, tension-ridden dialectic . . . kept alive by a continued exposure to specific cases in all their human dimensions."[1]

Early bioethicists became aware of that impossible list of demands. As soon as they began to discuss the issues with concerned persons, they realized that every question led them into unfamiliar territory. Philosophers found that the levels of abstraction demanded by their discipline flew high above the problems posed by the practitioners of medicine and science. Theologians sensed that the doctrinal commitments from which their discipline flowed were not acceptable to all conversants. Sociologists realized that the descriptive capacities of their discipline did not close normative gaps. Lawyers learned that the law's minatory face frightened off many to whom they spoke in good faith. Scientists and physicians, often encased in the epistemological positivism and ethical skepticism pervasive at that time, could not easily transcend their highly subjective view of values. It was difficult to imagine a new discipline emerging from any of these traditional disciplines; it was equally difficult to conceive of how they could talk to each other with interdisciplinary congeniality.

The early bioethicists, however, were not deterred. Although they all came from disciplinary bases and could not easily abandon disciplinary habits, they tried to shed the more chauvinistic ones. The theologians restrained their reference to scriptural or doctrinal sources and sought to translate the lessons that those sources taught into ecumenical formats. They tempered their use of theological language, although some of that language, such as "sanctity of life," drifted into secular discourse. The philosophers became less arcane, trying to step down from the rarefied air of deontological and teleological theory into the world of moral discourse more familiar to non-philosophers. The lawyers ventured from the sure paths of procedural justice into unsettled law where little precedent ruled. The physicians and scientists opened their minds to the "soft" data they had previously ignored. These first tentative steps out of familiar disciplinary worlds led the early bioethicists on the paths that Callahan had indicated: a search for theory, an articulation of principles, and the formulation of methods for making decisions.

The Search for Theory

One of the common features of a discipline is the presence of a central theory (and sometimes alternative theories). Theories are sets of propositions that explain how data are identified, fitted together, and evaluated. Philosophers of science work hard at clarifying the notion of scientific theory, and the relationships between hypotheses, observation, prediction and data that such theories purportedly explain.[2] Moral philosophers have been much more casual about theory. In one sense, they use the word simply to report that, through history, writers have described the moral life in different ways and perceptive observers can abstract from those descriptions certain salient features. In this sense, Cambridge don C. D. Broad discovered *Five Types of Ethical Theory* in the works of Kant, Hume, Spinoza, Butler, and Sidgwick.[3]

Some philosophers go further. Richard Brandt, in his book *Ethical Theory*, wrote, "Ethical theory has been interested in finding a set of valid ethical principles, which is complete in the sense that all true ethical statements can be deduced from it . . . and which is also as economical as possible, in distinct concepts and principles."[4] George Kerner introduced his *Revolution in Ethical Theory* with the following definition: "By ethical theory we must mean, essentially, the logical analysis of ordinary moral languages—in other words, an investigation into the nature of the terms and modes of reasoning which are actually employed in discussing and settling moral issues in practice."[5] John Rawls's *A Theory of Justice* defines theory as a "guiding framework" of definitions and analyses of concepts, "designed to focus our moral sensibilities and test our considered judgments in matters of justice."[6] So, sometimes, the phrase "ethical theory" will appear as a title for the various conceptions of freedom, virtue, duty, and the good life proposed by any moral philosopher; sometimes, it is used in a more limited sense as a title for the prominent approaches to normative ethics, such as utilitarianism (sometimes called consequentialism or teleology) and deontology (sometimes called formalism); and, again, it may sometimes describe various metaethical analyses of moral discourse, such as naturalism, intuitionism, and noncognitivism.[7]

Although this vagueness clouded the notion of ethical theory, Callahan suggested that the traditional methods of philosophy would continue to be central to bioethics. His suggestion implies that the bioethicist would know the ins and outs of the normative and the metaethical theories. The first proper professor of bioethics, Danner Clouser, felt obliged to explain what medical ethics was and what it wasn't and in so doing, expounded a thesis close to Callahan's. Bioethics, he asserted, was nothing more than standard ethical theory applied to the problems of medicine. "Medical ethics is no big deal," he wrote, " . . . [it] is simply ethics applied to a particular area of our lives . . . and has no special principles or methods or rules. It is the 'old ethics' trying to find its way around in a new, very puzzling circumstance." Clouser, in consort with his friend, Dartmouth philosopher Bernard Gert, viewed morality as the agreement of rational persons to observe those rules which forbid harming oneself and others: all rational persons would wish to avoid death, pain, loss of freedom, opportunity, and pleasure, and "therefore, the rules most likely to be advocated by all rational people are those which proscribe behavior harmful to others." Although the new biomedicine does raise unusual questions about what constitutes good and harm, none of these questions goes beyond the basic rules of traditional ethics. "Bioethics," Clouser wrote, "would seem to be the response of traditional ethics to particular stresses and urgencies that have emerged by virtue of new discoveries and technology. Ethics is pressed, not to find new principles or foundations, but to squeeze out all the relevant implications from the ones it already has."[8]

The ethicist helps in this search by "structuring the issues," or specifying conflicting ethical principles and isolating concepts that need clarification. This structuring reveals "where various arguments and actions lead, what facts would be relevant, what concepts are crucial, and what moral principles are at issue and probably in conflict." Clouser leaves the impression that ethical theory, that is, the deontological/teleological theories of normative ethics and the naturalist/non-naturalist theories of metaethics, provides the tools to structure the issues. Good reasoning constructs the structure and "everyone is needed and each must listen to the other."[9] Ethicists are not reformers, Clouser advised, nor do they provide solutions.

In 1973, André Hellegers and I presented a joint lecture at a Conference on Health Care and Changing Values sponsored by the Institute of Medicine. Our lecture was titled "Conceptual foundations for an ethics of medical care." Our foundations were not novel; we proposed that the new medical ethics needed a "comprehensive theory of human morality," and that this comprehensive theory should include three theories that explore the three principal questions of morality: a theory of virtue, a theory of duty and a theory of justice. "A theory of virtue," we wrote, "concerns those dispositions and qualities that define uprightness of life for those who . . . engage in care. The theory of duties concerns criteria that enable the practitioner to recognize what he or she must do and not do for those who seek his help. The theory of justice concerns the establishment of fair and equitable institutions for the provision of care." We assumed that these three theories—familiar to classical moral theology and philosophy—would form a "comprehensive theory of human morality"; we did not seek a higher theory that would unify them or provide critical judgment upon them.[10]

Paul Ramsey criticized our lecture. He admitted that our "threefold canopy of general ethics," was well and good, but that it failed to "address the problem of a lexical ordering, or some other value ranking, among the three. . . . Within the amplitude . . . of general ethics, our authors fail to address clearly and rigorously the issue: which of these moral claims has priority (e.g., in case of conflict)? Therefore, the shape of medical ethics and the weights to be assigned to its constitutive norms are left undetermined."[11] Ramsey had hit home: the problem of value ranking was central to the construction of theory and we had failed to address it. Within the next few years several books ventured where we had not.

Beauchamp and Childress produced the first edition of *Principles of Biomedical Ethics* in 1979. The first chapter, "Morality and Ethical Theory," contained a diagram that became widely known among students of bioethics; it showed four "hierarchical levels or tiers which we call levels of moral justification." At the bottom level, judgments about what ought to be done in particular situations are justified by reference to moral rules; moral rules are justified by reference to principles, and principles are grounded in ethical theories. "Theories," they wrote, "are bodies of principles and rules, more or less systematically related," in view of which judgments, rules, and principles can be justified. In this sense, moral theories "seek to formulate and defend a system of moral principles and rules that determine which actions are right and which are wrong." Theory must be consistent and coherent, complete and comprehensive, simple in having no more principles than necessary and complex enough to account for the full range of moral experience. Beauchamp and Childress then explain the two normative theories that recent moral philosophers had espoused, utilitarianism and deontology.[12]

Beauchamp and Childress followed Callahan and Clouser in suggesting that the work of bioethics should be done by situating new problems within the familiar theoretical forms of normative ethics. Reasoning about these new problems would move between the facts that raised the questions and the moral theories that justified the answers. None of these sophisticated philosophers supposed that the movement of the mind between these levels was facile. Despite the simplicity of the diagram in *Principles*, no straight line ran between question and answer and, for Callahan particularly, the movement was as much one of "unfettered imagination" as it was of logic.

Several pioneer bioethicists felt that the new bioethics deserved a more unique theoretical foundation than the routine invocation of the standard theories of moral philosophy. Robert Veatch took up the challenge to produce a general theory for the field. His 1981 volume, *A Theory of Medical Ethics*, contended that many particular questions had been recently debated and that many different "unsystematic, unreflective ethical stances or traditions" had contributed to the arguments.[13] Veatch intended to articulate foundations for a general medical ethic that were rooted in philosophical thought. He analyzed the major sources that had contributed to the current understanding of medical ethics: the Hippocratic tradition, the Judeo-Christian ethos, and liberal political thought. Each of these sources, he argued, was unique and often led to contradictory conclusions about professional duties. The most revered of these sources, the Hippocratic tradition, is fatally flawed, since it rests on the discretion of the physician alone to determine what is beneficial to patients, determines right action by consequences alone, ignores deontological duties, and limits the relevant consequences to those affecting the patient alone to the neglect of social benefits and justice. Veatch insisted that the Hippocratic tradition had little influence on the later Judeo-Christian medical ethics, and should have none on the modern bioethics.[14]

Veatch found his own source for a more consistent, more universal ethic in the contract theory that had wound its way through Anglo-American moral philosophy from Hobbes, Hume, and Locke down to Richard Brandt and his own teacher, John Rawls, and which we have seen Norman Daniels adapt to the circumstances of allocation of scarce resources. Veatch elaborated this theory with a "triple contract" for medical ethics. The first contract is the general social contract in which enlightened, self-interested parties, taking the moral point of view in which each person's welfare counts equally, agree to the fundamental principles under which they choose to live together. Within that social contract, the professions and society-at-large devise a contract that establishes their mutual responsibilities. Finally, a third contract determines the terms that govern the relationship between professionals and the laity. Although these contracts are hypothetical, they create the ideals that actual persons relating to each other may approximate.

Veatch then analyzed the standard principles of medical ethics—beneficence, autonomy and justice (adding the principles of contract-keeping, honesty, and avoiding killing)—in light of the hypothetical contracts. This analysis shows, he contended, that nonconsequentialist principles such as respect for autonomy, promise-keeping, avoiding killing, and justice have priority over the consequentialist principles of beneficence and nonmaleficence. The book concludes with a covenant for medical ethics in which a hypothetical moral community of responsible people state, in order of priority, the principles that constitute their dealings with each other: the moral necessity of keeping promises, treating each other as autonomous members of the moral community, dealing honestly with each other, avoiding the taking of morally protected life, striving for equality, and, finally, the moral necessity of producing good for one another insofar as this is compatible with the other basic principles.[15]

In 1986, H. Tristram Engelhardt produced his *Foundations of Bioethics*. Convinced that the traditional sources of moral authority in society had fragmented beyond repair, Engelhardt proposed that ethics be conceived as "an enterprise in controversy resolution" which consists in seeking, by free agreement to commonly accepted procedures, to resolve controversies without recourse to force. Engelhardt attempted to show how this enterprise would generate the foundational principles of respect for autonomy and beneficence. Respect for freedom is "the necessary condition for the possibility of resolving moral disputes without force and for sustaining a minimum ethical language of praise and blame. . . . It provides the empty process for generating moral authority in a secular pluralistic society through mutual agreement." Beneficence affirms that morality consists in a common community of welfare and sympathies. As a principle, beneficence is as empty as autonomy and is given content by the efforts to fashion "a web or nexus of commitments and understandings, both explicit and implicit, which sustain a fabric of moral understandings . . . usually open to revision."[16] These two "content poor" principles provide the boundaries of morality, which are filled in by continual efforts to resolve disputes peaceably. This effort constitutes a "secular ethic" of minimal conditions that can reach across many communities in a pluralist society. In addition to this secular ethic, persons may participate in the richer moral life of cultural and religious communities which share a vision of the good not appreciated by outsiders.

Both Veatch and Engelhardt recognized the problem of "conflict of principles and values." Both resolved that problem by positing a lexical ordering that placed deonto-logical principles above consequentialist ones; giving to the deontological principle of autonomy higher priority than beneficence in the resolution of a moral problem. Such a lexical ordering turned the Hippocratic tradition, based in medical beneficence, on its head.

Edmund Pellegrino and David Thomasma desired to preserve that tradition for the new medical ethics. They collaborated on a general theory of medical ethics set firmly on medical beneficence, elaborated in two books, *A Philosophical Basis of Medical Practice: Toward a Philosophy and Ethic of the Healing Professions*, and *For the Patient's Good: The Restoration of Beneficence in Health Care*.[17] Pellegrino, a physician and medical administrator, holds no degree in philosophy or history, but he demon-strates a deep familiarity with those subjects. From his undergraduate days at St. John's University, he has been a dedicated Aristotelian and neo-Thomist, and it was natural that he form a scholarly friendship with Dominican-trained David Thomasma, who studied philosophy of medicine with him as an Institute of Human Values in Medicine Fellow in 1975.

Their admiration for Aristotle led them to seek in the empirical and experienced fea-tures of the healing relationship between patient and physician an ontology of medicine as a practice. The nature of illness, the vulnerability of the patients, and the profession of the physician converge into a practice governed by three axioms: do not harm, re-spect the vulnerability of the patient, treat each patient as a representative of the human race. The principle of beneficence is reinterpreted as beneficence-in-trust, that is, beneficence is not merely the physician's paternalistic determination of the patient's good; it is the physician's duty to incorporate, by dialogue with the patient, the patient's values into a conception of the patient's welfare. The principle of autonomy, so exalted in modern medical ethics, is reduced to a place within the broader beneficence dictated by the dedication of the physician faced by the vulnerability of the patient. Each of these key ideas is worked out in detail, with the goal of grounding the medical morality in a philosophy of medicine.

Veatch, Engelhardt, Pellegrino, and Thomasma were explorers in the search for a general theory for bioethics. Each brought useful insights to the search. Their theories made a philosophical and historical case for the origin, binding force, and priority of normative principles and values. Still, none of these valiant attempts won the entire al-legiance of bioethicists. Veatch's triple contract was too hypothetical, Engelhardt's "logic of pluralism" too morally thin, Pellegrino and Thomasma's beneficence-in-trust too ontological to win the critical approval of the majority of their colleagues.[18] No sin-gle theoretical base for bioethics has been enthusiastically endorsed by the bioethics community.

The absence of enthusiasm may be explained by another reason quite remote from the philosophical merits of these attempts. Bioethics took a practical tack early in its evolution. Bioethicists became engaged in actual disputes and in the perplexing deci-sions forced upon practitioners and patients. They often found that theory, as they had learned it in their original disciplines, was too remote from these concerns, and seldom shed much light on the dark paths of decision. Even if theory was helpful, commitment to one theory to the exclusion of another did not seem necessary: one could be a deontologist for one problem and a utilitarian for another without contradiction. Finally, theoretical disquisitions from philosophically inclined ethicists lulled the attention of many participants in the bioethical discussions. By the mid-1980s, interest in creating a general bioethical theory seemed to wane. However, the short silence was only prologue to a renewed debate over theory that arose in the 1990s. That debate pitted "principlism" against "casuistry" and promoted approaches to ethical reasoning not previously stored in the mental warehouses of ethicists.[19]

Principles

Unlike theory, which is a term of relatively recent vintage in moral philosophy, the language of principles appears throughout the ethical literature of the Western tradition. That language, however, carries many different meanings. Some authors, such as Aristotle, Aquinas, and Kant, have used the word "principle" (or reasonable translations of it) to refer to the broadest foundations for moral reasoning.[20] Other writers, particularly the seventeenth- and eighteenth-century English moral philosophers, apply the term to the "sources" of morality in human nature, such as "sentiment," "reason," "sympathy," "conscience."[21] In more recent moral philosophy, authors speak of principles as norms that guide action (the term "action-guides" became a popular synonym for principle); principles are distinguished from rules as the general from the particular.[22] In the 1960s, American and British moral philosophers were concerned about how "moral" or "ethical" principles differed from other principles, such as legal, artistic, technical, and prudential principles.[23] This discussion, which was carried out within the atmosphere of metaethics, narrowed the content of morality down to principles, with scant attention to other topics of classical moral philosophy, such as ultimate goods, values, virtues and vices, motives and intentions.

The relationship between ethical principles and moral theories takes diverse forms. Utilitarian theory is identical with its single, dominant principle: that action is right which maximizes the greatest good for the greatest number. Various deontological theories, such as those of British philosopher W. D. Ross and American philosopher Bernard Gert, are collections of many common-sense moral principles held together by a general view of the nature and purpose of morality.[24] Surprisingly, close inspection of moral theory suggests that both dominant forms of moral theory appear to be compatible with the same sort of moral principles. In the first edition of their *Principles of Biomedical Ethics*, Tom Beauchamp confessed a preference for rule utilitarianism; James Childress admitted an inclination to rule deontology. After examining the strengths and weaknesses of both theories, they concluded, "We find that many forms of rule utilitarianism and rule deontology lead to identical rules and actions. It is possible from both utilitarian and deontological standpoints to defend the same rules . . . and to assign them roughly the same weight."[25] Finally, moral principles can be affirmed without commitment to any theory, as the contemporary casuists suggest.[26] Despite all these complexities of moral philosophy, people espouse principles and invoke them constantly in their moral reflections, deliberations, and decisions. Principles are the common coin of moral discourse.

It is not surprising, then, that the legislation which set the mandate for the National Commission for the Protection of Human Subjects of Biomedical and Behavioral Research instructed the commissioners "to conduct a comprehensive investigation and study to identify the basic ethical principles which should underlie the conduct of biomedical and behavioral research involving human subjects." This is a surprising sentence in the text of a federal law. Legislation rarely ventures into the area of ethics and, when it does, its concern is more about policy than principles. The call for a "comprehensive investigation" sent the commissioners into strange territory, far from the inquiries that legislatures make into government policies or activities. And "identifying basic ethical principles" poses a challenge quite different from identifying a violation of law or an opportunity for tax revenue. The Commission initiated the comprehensive study by asking philosophers Kurt Baier and Alasdair MacIntyre and theologian James Childress to clarify what it meant to "identify" an ethical principle. Each scholar surveyed the current ethical literature and revealed how complex (indeed, according to MacIntyre, intractable) were the questions raised by the mandate.[27]

After reading these impressive essays, the commissioners might have concluded that identifying basic ethical principles was too daunting a task and made its apologies to the Congress. But federal commissions are not allowed such discretion. Despite the theoretical complexity, the Commission plunged ahead, asking several other scholars—philosophers Tom Beauchamp and Tristram Engelhardt and theologian LeRoy Walters—to identify some principles, a process that eventually produced the three basic ethical principles of *The Belmont Report*: respect for persons, beneficence, and justice.[28]

The "comprehensive investigation," together with the preoccupation of contemporary moral philosophers with principles and rules as the sole elements of morality, endowed the emerging bioethics with a conceptual shape. Almost from its birth, bioethics was an ethics of principles, formulated as "action-guides" and little else. Again, as with theory, this orientation suited its function, for bioethics was generated out of an interest in solving problems, not merely thinking about them. This confined scope gave the early bioethics the appearance of a set of rules and procedures and truncated its growth in certain directions, particularly in the realms of moral character and virtue. It is notable that Beauchamp and Childress entitled the book that would become magisterial in the field *Principles of Biomedical Ethics*, with its main chapters devoted to the principles of autonomy, non-maleficence, beneficence, and justice. While the authors acknowledged other realms of the moral life by adding a concluding chapter, "Ideals, Virtues and Integrity," they set the agenda for the next decade.

Early in bioethics' life, a principle variously called " respect for persons" or "respect for autonomy" began to dominate the moral principles. The ideas behind that principle have run a long and complex course through the history of Western philosophy; for centuries, those ideas played an important, but modest, role as the conditions for free will and, in more recent times, particularly since the Renaissance, a more dramatic role as a proclamation of human liberty from divine dominance or social tyranny.[29] Despite the rich store of ideas that those traditional discussions offered, modern moral philosophy had relatively little interest in the concept of autonomy as such. The phrases "respect for autonomy" or "respect for persons" do not even appear in the indices of the moral philosophy textbooks by such luminaries as William Frankena and Richard Brandt, nor are they found as entries in the *Encyclopedia of Philosophy* or even in the 1978 *Encyclopedia of Bioethics*![30] Philosophers Robert Downie and Elizabeth Telfer noted the pervasiveness of the general idea of "the individual as of supreme worth" and its importance in major philosophers such as Kant and Mill, but remarked on the absence of a sustained examination of that idea.[31] As bioethics began, then, the notion that was to become its hallmark, respect for autonomy, was rare in the ambient philosophical air.

The first defining moment for bioethics, the debate over human experimentation, pushed forward a problem that needed a principle. Should the social good to which the results of biomedical experimentation contributed overrule the freedom, wishes, and choices of individuals? As we saw in Chapter 5, Hans Jonas had answered that question negatively. He insisted that the research subject not only give voluntary consent, as the Nuremberg Code required, but also embrace as his own the ends of the research by "full, autonomous identification . . . [with the purposes and ends] of research. . . . An authentic identification with the cause."[32] When the time came to formulate the "ethical principles that should govern research" in *The Belmont Report*, "respect for autonomy" seemed to sum up the trend of the literature about research ethics. The Commission defined respect for autonomy as giving "weight to autonomous persons' considered opinions and choices while refraining from obstructing their actions unless they are clearly detrimental to others."[33]

Tristram Engelhardt had prepared the way for that formulation. In his essay for the National Commission, he wrote, "The literature [on the ethics of research] focuses on three cardinal ethical issues. The first concerns respect for persons as a logical condition for morality. Such respect for persons is not a value among other values. It is rather the basis for our sense of moral responsibility, and is considered apart from any interest we might have in respecting other persons (e.g., that such respect is useful or that giving such respect will tend to protect us)." He states in a footnote, "I am proposing a view of freedom and morality that draws heavily upon Immanuel Kant, that freedom is a presupposition for both claims to knowledge and morality."[34]

Kant, who spoke of "respect for the moral law" and "the autonomy of the will," rather than respect for persons clearly placed these notions at the deepest roots of his conception of morality. His five formulations of the categorical imperative repeat those notions in various ways. The third formulation, in particular, has caught the fancy of modern ethicists, "act so that you treat humanity, whether in your own person or in that of another, always as an end and never as a means only."[35] Not only did the notion of respect for persons fit the problem of experimentation with human subjects; it also seemed an appropriate principle for bioethics, indeed, for all ethics. Veatch endorsed it as such, pointing out that Rawls sees autonomy as basic to the contractarian theory; Engelhardt, in his *Foundations of Bioethics*, saw autonomy as a basic presupposition for his secular ethics.[36]

By the time Beauchamp and Childress issued *Principles of Biomedical Ethics*, the principle of autonomy had become firmly fixed among the principles of bioethics. They defined "autonomy" as "a form of personal liberty of action where the individual determines his or her own course of action in accordance with a plan chosen by himself or herself." Respect for autonomy is defined as "to recognize with due appreciation their own considered value judgments and outlooks even when it is believed that their judgments are mistaken." When they formulate the principle of autonomy, they fuse the Kantian concept of respect for persons with John Stuart Mill's quite different notion of liberty; that is, persons' choice of actions should not be obstructed unless those actions infringe upon the liberty of others. The principle of respect for autonomy, then, dictates that "persons should be free to perform whatever action he wishes—even if it involves serious risk for the agent and even if others consider it to be foolish."[37]

Folding together the distinct views of Kant and Mill blurred the edges both of the Kantian and the Millsian notions. Although Beauchamp and Childress refined their treatment of the principle of autonomy in each successive edition, giving it more careful definition and application, in the wider bioethical discourse the more careful definitions were often lost. Although autonomy had been launched as one of a quartet of principles, along with beneficence, nonmaleficence, and justice, it seemed to dominate the rest and even swamp them. Autonomy floated through bioethical discourse in a cloud of confusion for some years. The confusion, however, did not detract from its attraction.

That attraction came, of course, from its similarity to personal liberty, a firm fixture of the American ethos, as we shall see in Chapter 12. But there were other reasons. In a pluralistic society, where broad agreement on the content of morality seemed to be fading, a principle of autonomy, as the sole or primary moral principle, solved many a conundrum: one merely respects the wishes and choices of every person without passing judgment on further moral grounds. This shallowest meaning of respect for autonomy, unfortunately, seemed the most readily grasped. Also, the principle of autonomy meshed nicely with the emphasis on rights abroad in the land. Rights are claims of autonomous persons either to be left alone or to be entitled to something. In this guise, the principle of autonomy showed up as a defense for refusals of care and as a justification for claims to care. In addition, the accumulating body of law about bioethical questions drew heavily on the jurisprudential principle of self-determination and on the Constitution's penumbral right of privacy. The ethical principle of autonomy, particularly in its

Millsian form as protection of the individual from intrusion of others, seemed to correspond nicely with that jurisprudence. But, perhaps, the principle of autonomy won most attention as a counter to professional authority and to paternalism.

The professional standing of physicians in the United States altered dramatically during the twentieth century. At the beginning of the century, doctors generally belonged to the socioeconomic middle class, living in conditions similar to their patients and enjoying considerable social respect, despite their meager medical armamentarium. By mid-century, physicians had moved into the upper-middle and the upper class; were increasingly isolated, socially and professionally, from their patients; had a growing technical armamentarium; and were slowly losing the aura that had surrounded them. Sociologists—such as Talcott Parsons and Eliot Freidson—described physicians' work in terms of power and "professional dominance."[38] Ivan Illich warned of the "medical nemesis," and Thomas Szasz described "the myth of mental illness," in which physicians were indicted as the cause of disease rather than its healers.[39] A special section in the October 1960 *Harpers*, "The crisis in American medicine," explored the reasons for what the editors saw as widespread dissatisfaction among Americans about doctors and health care. One author opened his essay, "The physician has found himself in a chillier climate of national opinion in recent years. He has undergone what often seems to him like systematic and studied deprecation." Among the reasons for this change of climate, the author noted, was that "we [physicians] are, perhaps, more and more alienated from the common run of people. . . . We have drifted into an upper-class status identification that prevents us from recognizing the wishes and needs of the great mass of our patients."[40] Doctors had become, in the phrase that historian David Rothman chose as the title of his history of bioethics, "strangers at the bedside."[41]

It became common to assert that physicians were paternalistic, or inclined to make decisions about the welfare of their patients that patients were entitled to make for themselves. A Hippocratic maxim advised that patients did best when "under orders." "Paternalism," coined during a debate over enforcement of morals that had excited the world of jurisprudence in the 1960s, was readily transferred to the medical world.[42] At the 1972 Hastings Conference on Teaching Medical Ethics, Willard Gaylin linked most issues in medical ethics to "the larger problem of the redefinition of the physicians' role." He spoke of "the power of the medical model . . . [that] stems from the existential fear of death. . . . The preserver of life has often been exempted from normal limits of behavior. . . . The universal terror of illness operating under the imprimatur of the medical establishment will make coercion in the traditional sense unnecessary. . . . By redefining morality and values in medical terms we are expanding the mechanism for controlling human behavior."[43]

Robert Veatch, in his first major contribution to the literature of bioethics, criticized the assumption of moral authority by persons with technical competence as the "generalization of expertise," the covert introduction of personal values into their diagnostic judgments and treatment recommendations, subverting the values of the patient.[44] In this climate, the assertion of the principle of patient autonomy appeared as a direct challenge to professional paternalism. Although a kernel of genuine ethical value was hidden within the paternalism discussion, namely, under what circumstances can the liberty of one person be overridden for his or her own good, the paternalism–autonomy dichotomy became a constant theme during the first decade of bioethics.[45]

The principle of autonomy or respect for autonomy that gained such prominence in bioethics is, in my view, an amalgam. It is annealed from three quite different sources: a theological doctrine about the sacredness of the individual, a philosophical stress on the creativity of the individual, and the centrality of the individual in the American ethos. The latter two ingredients will be discussed in Chapter 12, where we discuss the American ethos; the theological origins of autonomy deserve notice here. The theological doctrine is the Christian message about the salvation of individuals. Christianity, from its beginnings, has stressed the salvation of the individual through a theologically complex interplay of God's grace and personal responsibility. Salvation does not come from social status or tribal identity. St. Paul declared, "There is neither Jew nor Gentile, slave or free, male or female: for you are all one in Jesus Christ. . . . Let each one test his own work, and then his reason to boast will be in himself and not in his neighbor" (Gal. 3:28; 6:4). This Christian doctrine sharpened the Judaic belief that each human life is sacred as God's unique creation: "Before I formed thee in the belly I knew thee; and before thou camest forth from the womb I sanctified thee. . . ."(Jer. 1.5).

Paul Ramsey eloquently preached this central doctrine; in the opening pages of *Patient as Person*, he proclaimed: "Just as man is a sacredness in the social and political order, so he is a sacredness in the natural, biological order. . . . The sanctity of human life prevents ultimate trespass upon him even for the sake of treating his bodily life, or for the sake of others who are also only a sacredness in their bodily lives." Earlier he had written, "One grasps the religious outlook upon sanctity of human life only if he sees that this life is asserted to be surrounded by a sanctity that need not be in a man; that the most dignity a man ever possesses is a dignity that is alien to him. . . . A man's dignity is an overflow from God's dealings with him, and not primarily an anticipation of anything he will ever be by himself. Thus, every human being is a unique, unrepeatable opportunity to praise God."[46] This theological belief is hardly "autonomy," for the unique human being remains folded into the embrace of the laws of God; it would take Renaissance and Enlightenment thought to reach Kant's autonomy, in which rational beings are "self-legislators" and, further, even creators of their own moral values. Ramsey repudiated the unfettered and contentless freedom that autonomy had come to signify, yet his invocation of the theological tradition provided one essential element of autonomy: the center of ethics is the person, irreducible and inviolable.

Ramsey preached his doctrine of the religious sanctity of the individual at the Reed College symposium, "The Sanctity of Life." At the same event, sociologist Edward Shils reflected on the meaning of sanctity of life "in the decline of Christian belief." Shils' lecture reveals the shift from sanctity to autonomy. He finds that, even as the world of faith fades, human life is "self-evidently sacred. Its sacredness is the most primordial of experiences" and that in one of its forms, it guides us in dealing with "the individual human being, as an individuality located in a discrete organism, possessing consciousness of itself as an agent and patient both in the past and present, having the capacity for psychic 'self-locomotion.' "[47]

Dan Callahan later took the Reed Conference lectures as the basis of an extended essay, "The sanctity of life."[48] Callahan established a philosophical framework, based on Henry Aiken's "four levels of ethical discourse," within which he analyzed the meaning and function of this "basic western principle." Callahan reviewed both the Christian theological view and Shils's natural view of the sanctity of life, proposed that a non-theological formulation was possible, and suggested how such a formulation might serve as a moral principle and the basis for a variety of moral rules "ranging from the preservation of the species to the inviolability of human bodies." He concludes, "The principle of 'the sanctity of life' even if given a religious grounding, is best protected by the recognition that it is human beings who must form, implement, and set the conditions of those rules designed to protect and foster that sanctity."[49] From Ramsey through Shils to Callahan, sanctity of life is secularized into the moral principle of autonomy.

In this secularization of the Christian principle of the sanctity of the individual, it is possible to see a central element of the ethical principle of respect for autonomy. The individual person, as a perceiving, willing, choosing, suffering entity, is placed at the center of value; his or her liberty to form a life is to be tolerated, fostered, and protected. This secular remnant of sanctity of life discards the sovereignty of divine authority that, in the traditional doctrine, existed in such tension with human freedom. The freedom of each individual stands alone, no longer faced by a transcendent legislator. The traditional doctrine had also seen human freedom as formed within, and limited by, the authority of communities. The secular remnant loses touch with those communities and each person's freedom faces the freedom of every other person. The autonomy of the person becomes not only the center of value, but the sole value. Among the early contributors to bioethics, theologian Stanley Hauerwas was an articulate dissenter from this view. He observes, "only within a degree of moral consensus derived from past judgments can those engaged in a practice have confidence in one another . . . This challenges the presupposition of American liberalism which assumes that freedom consists in having individuals freed from all commitments other than those that they have freely contracted. . . . There must also be a hierarchy of goods, for medical, as well as other forms of authority, to function well."[50] This dissent remained unheeded during the formative years of bioethics but slowly forced itself on the attention of the maturing discipline. The exaggeration of autonomy became obvious to many bioethicists, who began to define the concept more carefully and to situate it more safely within "a hierarchy of goods" and principles.[51] Even with their principles in better balance, the bioethicists were unsure how their theories and principles should fit together in the analysis of moral problems in medicine. One other crucial element of a discipline was still lacking—a methodology.

Methodology

A discipline requires a method that allows its practitioners to order their materials in recognizable ways, to evaluate the relevance of various bits of that material, and to analyze the relationships between those bits. Above all, a method guides the thinker in constructing approaches to the problem, whether it be an experiment in biochemistry, a mathematical puzzle, or a philosophical quandary. "Method," wrote philosopher-theologian Bernard Lonergan, "is a normative pattern of recurrent and related operations yielding cumulative and progressive results."[52] Method, in this sense, is most clearly manifested in mathematics and the physical sciences. In an attempt to emulate the productivity and clarity of those sciences, theologians, and philosophers, as well as historians and social scientists from the eighteenth century onward, endeavored to articulate methods that fit the matter of their disciplines.

The early bioethicists, who were trained in those disciplines, were familiar with the search for method and with the canons that their parent disciplines had set in place to guide investigation.[53] Yet, in the middle of the twentieth century, it would be an exaggeration to claim that any agreed methods held sway over philosophical or theological ethics. Modern moral philosophy can mark its beginnings with a book called *Methods of Ethics*, in which Henry Sidgwick endeavored to demonstrate the superiority of utilitarian reasoning for the construction of a system of ethics, yet moral philosophers continued to disagree with Sidgwick and with every other colleague who dared propose a method for ethics.[54] Among theologians, Roman Catholic moralists worked with a long-accepted method of natural law reasoning and casuistry, yet these methods had been variously interpreted over the centuries and were, at the beginning bioethics, being seriously challenged.[55] Protestant ethicists veered between fundamentalists whose method was a pious reading of the Scriptures to situationists who seek the divine command in the shifting context of human life.[56] Despite this confusing variety, most ethicists acknowledged the desirability of devising a method that could "yield cumulative and progressive results."

Bioethics began, as we have seen, at conferences where the issues were aired by concerned persons whose methods were not those of philosophical or theological ethics. As these people began to invite theologians and philosophers to their conferences, the outlines of method began to appear in the lectures presented by those guests. The lecture and the essay are the forte of the philosopher and the theologian. Complex and obscure ideas are formatted and drawn toward simplicity and clarity by definition, division, distinction, and example. Problems are set into historical contexts and referenced to the data appropriate to the issue. The essay, with its beginning, middle, and end, began to draw into order the randomness of conversations and became the method of the early bioethics.

James Gustafson's 1970 "Basic ethical issues in the biomedical fields" exemplified orderly exposition, and at the same time, it offered a distinctive method for analysis of ethical issues. Professor Gustafson listed the many questions being asked and then stated, "in the hope of clarifying this situation . . . I shall distinguish nine pertinent issues and state some conflicting propositions directed to each. I shall develop these issues and propositions in such a way that some of the reasons for contrasting judgments become clear. In some instances, the reasonable position appears to be a dialectical one between two *prima facie* opposing propositions. A fully developed constructive or systematic position cannot be elaborated here, but the direction which I believe a more complete development ought to take does become clear."[57] Gustafson's methodology—articulating contrasting responses to moral questions and attempting to draw from them a common ground for agreement—represented a style of doing ethics that many ethicists (often not conscious of Gustafson's articulation) employed. Some bioethicists, having been Gustafson's students, consciously used it.

Such an analytic method requires not only logical acuity; it needs sources of data. The data of ethics are opinions shored up by arguments. In 1974, theologian Kenneth Vaux produced *Biomedical Ethics: Morality for the New Medicine*. In that short book, he presented as the sources of ethical insight the traditions of the past, the concrete situation of the present, and the possibilities of the future. Ethics, he claimed, works by retrospection, introspection, and perspective. "Responsible decision-making and planning," he wrote, "should be aware of these three vectors impinging on any particular decision-making context." He then applied these "vectors" to the questions in genetics, reproductive science and organ transplantation.[58] Vaux's thoughts on these subjects were provocative, but it remained unclear how the vectors, only vaguely sketched, actually generated his conclusions. At the same time, Vaux was doing what many other bioethicists were doing: seeking lines of ethical guidance in moral and religious traditions, in the facts of present life, medicine, and technology, and in a future of possible benefits and detriments.

Methods are devised for different purposes: there are methods for scholarly inquiry and methods for teaching the results of that inquiry. Although these methodologies will overlap, it is teaching that often presses random inquiry into methodological study. As bioethics began to be taught in a formal way, the urgency for method grew. As we shall see in the next chapter, courses in bioethics spread through health sciences education and college undergraduate curricula. Courses create the need for texts, and texts must be methodically organized. The earliest texts, however, were anthologies that gathered essays and lectures, scientific articles and newstories, with no demonstrable method.[59] In 1976, two more methodologically mature texts appeared. *Moral Problems in Medicine*, produced by Samuel Gorovitz and his colleagues at Case-Western Reserve University, retained the anthology form, but they juxtaposed selections from philosophical ethics with articles on biomedical problems. In the section on truth-telling, for example, four pages from Immanuel Kant and two pages from Nicolai Hartmann join Donald Oken's empirical study, "What to tell cancer patients: a study of medical attitudes." Students and professors were invited to draw together the theoretical and the practical.[60]

Howard Brody's *Ethical Decisions in Medicine* took a further methodological step: the student and professor are given a specific ethical decision-making technique, a sort of rough consequentialism. The decision-maker is given cases arranged systematically to identify the consequences of various courses of action and is invited to compare these consequences with his or her values and to compare personal values with critically assessed values. The critical assessment is made by reference to "a bioethical injunction consistent with the survival imperative: wherever possible, seek to solve a problem by hierarchical growth rather than hierarchical regression. In this way, adaptability for future crises will be best preserved." Future growth comes by advancing the uniqueness of individuals and the ability to participate in complex social interactions.[61] In the next few years, a plethora of textbooks appeared, giving increasing attention to the problem of methodology.[62]

An additional methodological challenge appeared. Cases lured bioethicists toward the clinical, as they became teachers of medical students and consultants on hospital wards. The method for teaching ethical decision-making had to be tailored to the clinic as well as to the classroom. Medical students are taught how to do a physical "workup" on patients; David Thomasma suggested a technique for an "ethical workup."[63] He proposed a six-step process of moral reasoning that would help the student identify the underlying ethical norms in any case, and to criticize one's own assumptions about the case. During a 1979 conference at Vanderbilt University School of Medicine, I asked whether an "an ethicist could be a consultant," and answered that an ethicist could consult by becoming familiar with the antique mode of moral reasoning called "casuistry." Catholic moral theologians, from the fourteenth century onward, sought to unravel moral perplexities by interpreting moral rules in light of the various circumstances of particular cases. I had become familiar with this method during my Jesuit career and believed that it might serve the needs of ethicists working with medical cases. Stephen Toulmin and I had already begun our rehabilitation of historical casuistry to serve the needs of modern bioethics.[64]

In an article that achieved wide notice, "How medicine saved the life of ethics," Stephen Toulmin asserted that the interest in medical ethics had drawn philosophers away from the subjectivist and relativist views fostered by metaethics and toward analysis of real cases, real human tasks and duties. This enlivened the abstractions with which moralists had been concerned and drew attention to practical judgment, an area in which, as Aristotle claimed, "the theoretical rigor of geometrical analysis is unattainable (but where) we should strive above all to be reasonable rather than insisting on a kind of exactness that the 'nature of the case' does not allow."[65] This reasonableness was exercised in the analysis of concrete cases and required a new "casuistry." Toulmin concluded,

> By reintroducing into ethical debate the vexed topics raised by particular cases, they have obliged philosophers to address once again the Aristotelian problems of practical reasoning, which had been on the sidelines for too long. In this sense, we may indeed say that, during the last 20 years, medicine has 'saved the life' of ethics, and that it has given

back to ethics a seriousness and human relevance which it had seemed—at least, in the
writings of the interwar years, to have lost for good.[66]

In an attempt to introduce casuistry to bioethics, I joined my casuistical competence
with Mark Siegler's clinical acumen and William Winslade's familiarity with case law
to produce *Clinical Ethics*, a text that drew ethical reasoning closer to clinical decision
making.[67]

The concerns about methodology continued to grow. In 1986, philosopher Larry Mc-
Cullough remarked on "a shift that is under way in our literature . . . the shift to inquiry into the basic methodological concerns in the field of bioethics." McCullough reviewed the major contributions to bioethics, such as the books by Beauchamp and
Childress and by Robert Veatch, and found them examples of what Arthur Caplan had
called "the engineering model of medical ethics." The analogy presumes that, in ethics
as in engineering, there are definite bodies of elaborated theory that could be simply
"applied" to the case at hand. Another quite different approach bases medical ethics on
the study of the responsibilities of physicians as professionals and on the virtues that
professionals must display. McCullough analyzed the values and shortcomings of these
approaches and concluded that not only are the familiar models of philosophical and
professional theory relevant to bioethics, but to many other methods as well, such as
Marxism, feminist, ethnic, even deconstructive approaches to ethics. He notes that government bodies are being commissioned to do "federal ethics" about medicine and
wonders what methods and theories these bodies will adopt.[68]

In the following decade, methodological discussions became even more intense.
New methodologies, such as the ones mentioned by McCullough (with the exception of
Marxism!), claimed a prominent place. "Federal ethics" became a significant source of
opinion in bioethics as public moral discourse took place not only on federal premises
but also in state agencies, professional societies, institutional committees, and public
forums. The form and influence of this public discourse will be reviewed in the next
chapter.

Bioethics, Law, and Other Disciplines

From its beginnings, bioethics has been a *mélange* of disciplines. While philosophers
and theologians shaped theories and methods, many other scholars contributed to the
content. The discipline that has mixed most prominently with bioethics has been law.
Many bioethical matters have been translated into law: the National Commission recommended federal regulations to govern research with human subjects; state legislatures have enacted statutes about the definition of death and advance directives. Above
all, courts have adjudicated decisions to forego life-sustaining treatment. A bioethical
jurisprudence has been fostered by a few scholarly lawyers who found the field fascinating.[69] A rather moribund American Society of Law and Medicine was revived by an

influx of interest in bioethics. It began to hold conferences on bioethical and legal questions in the mid-1970s and slowly emerged as a principal sponsor of the new jurisprudence. It produced two journals: one of them started as *Medicolegal News*, which transmuted first into *Law, Medicine and Health Care* and then into *Law, Medicine and Ethics*; the other journal, the *American Journal of Law and Medicine,* began to publish lengthy scholarly articles on the intersection between law and ethics. In 1992, the society changed its name to the Society for Law, Medicine and Ethics.[70]

Bioethics and the new jurisprudence of medicine have lived together for several decades. It is difficult to distinguish which discipline has influenced which. George Annas, a pioneer in law and bioethics, has no doubt about the answer:

> Bioethicists can be seduced by the law and by legal procedures. . . . American bioethics has been driven by the law. . . . The stress on autonomy and self determination comes from our Bill of Rights, our Declaration of Independence and the whole common law tradition. And law's primary contribution to bioethics is procedural. Lawyers are expert at procedure. The common law itself is based on deciding individual cases and using these cases as the basis for creating law. Bioethics has adopted this technique. In the United States, with its pluralism of beliefs and people, the law is what holds us together. There is no other ethos. Thus, the law—procedural, autonomy based and case focused—came into bioethics.[71]

Annas charges that bioethicists are seduced by law. Unquestionably, law and bioethics have had constant intercourse, but who seduced whom is not as clear as Professor Annas suggests. Certainly, the central concepts of American law, self-determination and rights, have loomed large in bioethics. But these concepts have a theological twin—the doctrine of the sanctity of the individual—which Paul Ramsey enunciated so powerfully from the earliest days of bioethical discourse. They also have a philosophical relative—the concept of respect for persons—which flows out of Renaissance philosophy through Kant and into American philosophical thought. All these ideas flourish in the American ethos. It is not easy to prove that it is only law that has imparted these emphases to bioethics.

Further, the law's notions of self-determination and the privacy that protects it are not quite the same as the philosopher's concept of autonomy. In American jurisprudence, the former notions delineate the limits of state power over individuals; in ethics, the latter concept, diffuse as it is, constitutes a moral principle of action. The law's use of cases differs from their use in bioethics: judges render decisions about the matter before them, tracing their decision through other cases with relevantly similar matter; bioethicists seek the relevant moral maxims in the circumstances of the cases delivered to them by practitioners. Procedure in law and procedure in bioethics are only remotely related. Legal procedure forces judges and lawyers along clearly marked paths as they carry a case through indictment, hearing, and verdict. In bioethics, philosophical speculation has been translated into guidelines and policies to which practitioners refer when making decisions.

It is true that bioethicists have often translated legal decisions too easily into bioethical arguments. They frequently fail to appreciate the case-bound nature of these decisions or to discern the differences between a jurisprudential concept of privacy and a philosophical concept of autonomy. At the same time, judges seem to have learned something about philosophy and theology from the bioethicists. Again and again, their opinions refer to the importance of seeing matters of life and death in a perspective wider and deeper than the law offers, and their best decisions, even when crafted within the limits of legal frameworks, often demonstrate that they have tried to do so. Yet Annas' analogy of seduction does have its point. Bioethics does look, at times, quite legalistic and often it is necessary for bioethicists to admonish each other that they are not doing law.[72]

Other disciplines have mixed with bioethics. The social sciences had a natural affinity: medical sociologists and anthropologists had already studied the education of physicians, medical decision-making, research with human subjects, and the care of dying patients.[73] They could describe the complex structures of medical work. They had already pioneered the teaching of behavioral sciences in medical schools. The studies of sociologist Renée Fox, for example, richly describe the textures and colors of the world which the bioethicists were just beginning to explore. Nevertheless, she could write, "the relation between bioethics and social science continues to be tentative, distant, and also susceptible to strain." Fox and her colleague, Judith Swazey, contrasted "medical morality" in China, embedded in Chinese cultural traditions and social structures, with American bioethics, which was isolated from the relationships, communities, and values of real life in sickness and health. The isolation produced an uneasy relationship between the social sciences and bioethics; bioethics, confined in its individualism and American chauvinism, rendered an "impoverished and skewed expression of our society's cultural tradition (which), in a highly intellectualized but essentially fundamentalistic way, thins out the fullness of that tradition and bends it away from some of the deepest sources of its meaning and vitality."[74]

This scathing critique may be motivated, in part, by Fox's resentment that this "impoverished" bioethics has shouldered aside the teaching of behavioral sciences to medical students, which she pioneered. Yet, she perceives a genuine gap in the theory and method of bioethics: there is no easy and consistent flow of empirical data into ethics. Methods for gathering that sort of data, for interpreting it and fitting it into normative analysis are seldom familiar to ethicists; the methods of ethicists are seldom known to behavioral scientists. In addition, the data of the behavioral sciences often reveal situations as more complex than ethicists perceive them to be, rendering a straightforward ethical analysis more difficult; sociologists and ethnographers often offer multiple, contrasting perspectives on what the layperson sees as a simple situation. The tensions between disciplines that should be collegial are manifest, yet the value of the behavioral sciences to ethics should compel collaboration. Dan Callahan's words spoken in 1980 have yet to be fully heeded: "Those in ethics must learn to work more closely with those in the law and the social sciences."[75]

Conclusion

We return to the question, "is bioethics a discipline?" In the simplest sense, it certainly is: a discipline is a body of material that can be taught, and bioethics is and has been a teachable and taught subject since the mid-1970s. In the strictest sense, it is not a discipline. A discipline is a coherent body of principles and methods appropriate to the analysis of some particular subject matter. Bioethics has no dominant methodology, no master theory. It has borrowed pieces from philosophy and theology. Its theological pieces are the secular remnant of the sanctity of the person, the urgency to examine human experience in light of some sort of transcendent values, and the concern to translate those values into practical life. It adopted several pieces of philosophy: the relatively recent division of ethical discourse into two normative theories, deontological and consequentialist, and the modern version of traditional contract theory. It also took another philosophical piece that is largely methodological, namely, the critical work of casting questions in logical form and inquiring about the premises behind them. In addition to these philosophical and theological pieces, fragments of law and the social sciences have been clumsily built onto the bioethical edifice.

Tristram Engelhardt, having tried to bring some order into this jumble, takes a dim view of the results. "Many theoretical reflections in bioethics have helped clarify the character of arguments, the force of claims, and the meaning of moral principles . . . the question is, though, whether bioethics has succeeded in securing a theoretical understanding of the various theoretical understandings of bioethics." He answered his question as follows:

> In bioethics, the journey from the religious orthodoxies of the Middle Ages, through the rationalist hopes of modernity, to the disappointments of post-modernity, spanned less than 30 years. One has during this brief period been brought to look for theoretical and rational guidance, and then one is shown how little guidance is in fact available. . . . This is not to say that there are not regnant fashions or views regarded as correct, according to some bioethical orthodox consensus. It is just that no particular contentful view can be secured as that which is rational and canonical. The challenge will be to live honestly in this impoverished condition.[76]

This is a somber assessment yet, in a sense, it confirms the nature of contemporary bioethics. The notion of a discipline as a body of principles and methods surrounding a dominant theory is attractive, but probably an archaism. Academic disciplines today are mosaics of theories, with principles and methods formulated in diverse ways. When practitioners argue about the state of theory within their discipline, they contribute to the vitality of the discipline itself. Those arguments stir up fresh views of the work, open new routes for exploration, and suggest the need for expanded empirical investigations. The debates over bioethics as a discipline are actually a sign that bioethics is maturing as a discipline.

As the period covered by this history draws to a close (and even a decade later), bioethics might be called a "demi-discipline." Only half of bioethics counts as an ordinary academic discipline: the half that has original and borrowed theory, principles, and methods. But only part of bioethics lies within the academy, where scholars worry about whether they have a discipline to teach and promote. The other half of bioethics is the public discourse: people of all sorts and professions talking and arguing about bioethical questions. That half of bioethics is the subject of the next chapter.

Notes for Chapter 10

1. Daniel Callahan, "Bioethics as a discipline," *Hastings Center Studies* 1 (1973): 66–73, quotes from pp. 68, 71, 72, 73. Warren Reich identified the catalogue entry at the Library of Congress, see Reich, "The word 'bioethics': its birth and the legacies of those who shaped its meaning," *Kennedy Institute of Ethics Journal* 4 (1994): 319–336.

2. See, for example, Karl Popper, *The Logic of Scientific Discovery* (London: Hutchinson, 1959); Stephen E. Toulmin, *Philosophy of Science: An Introduction* (London: Hutchinson, 1953).

3. C. D. Broad, *Five Types of Ethical Theory* (New York: Harcourt Brace, 1930).

4. Richard B. Brandt, *Ethical Theory: The Problems of Normative and Critical Ethics* (Englewood Cliffs, N.J.: Prentice-Hall, 1959), p. 5. In the same vein, Alan Donagan's *The Theory of Morality* (Chicago: University of Chicago Press, 1977) attempts to work out "a system of specific precepts . . . derived from a first principle the observance of which will have been shown to be a condition upon rational action" (p. 31).

5. George C. Kerner, *Revolution in Ethical Theory* (New York: Oxford University Press, 1966), p. 2.

6. John Rawls, *A Theory of Justice* (Cambridge, Mass.: Harvard University Press, 1967), pp. 46–53.

7. William Frankena, "Moral philosophy at mid-century," *Philosophy Review* (1951): 44–55; see also Henry Aiken's critique in "The multiple roles of the language of conduct," in *Reason and Conduct* (New York: Knopf, 1962), pp. 33–43.

8. K. Danner Clouser, "Bioethics," in Warren T. Reich (ed.), *Encyclopedia of Bioethics* (New York: The Free Press, 1978), pp. 124–125.

9. K. Danner Clouser, "Medical ethics: some uses, abuses, and limitations," *New England Journal of Medicine* 293 (1975): 384–387; "Some things medical ethics is not," *Journal of the American Medical Association* 223 (1973): 787–789; "Biomedical ethics: some reflections and exhortations," *The Monist* 60 (1977): 47–61.

10. Albert R. Jonsen and André Hellegers, "Conceptual foundations for an ethics of medical care," in Laurence R. Tancredi (ed.), *Ethics of Health Care* (Washington, D.C.: National Academy of Sciences, 1974), p. 19.

11. Paul Ramsey, "Commentary," in Tancredi, *Ethics of Health Care*, p. 23.

12. Tom L. Beauchamp and James F. Childress, *Principles of Biomedical Ethics*, 1st ed. (New York: Oxford University Press, 1979), chapter 1, p. 5. The fourth edition, extensively rewritten, appeared in 1994. The four-tier approach to ethics can be attributed to an important article by James Gustafson, who was Childress's mentor; Gustafson's formulation was itself attributed to an influential essay by philosopher Henry David Aiken. See James M. Gustafson, "Context versus principles: a misplaced debate in Christian ethics," *Harvard Theological Review* 58 (1965): 171–202; Henry D. Aiken, "Levels of moral discourse," in *Reason and Conduct*, pp. 65–87. I also was influenced by these essays, and I thank Robert Veatch for pointing out this geneology of ideas.

13. Robert M. Veatch, *A Theory of Medical Ethics* (New York: Basic Books, 1981).

14. The Hippocratic tradition, which is the body of Greek medical literature produced between the fifth and first centuries B.C.E. and its subsequent interpretation in classical times, is best explained in Ludwig Edelstein, *Ancient Medicine: Selected Papers of Ludwig Edelstein*, ed. Owsei Temkin and C. Lilian Temkin (Baltimore: Johns Hopkins Press, 1967) and Oswei Temkin, *Hippocrates in a World of Pagans and Christians* (Baltimore: Johns Hopkins University Press, 1991). The origins of the famous Hippocratic Oath is unknown but Edelstein considers it the work of physicians who were followers of the mystic philosopher Pythagoras. The phrases of the Oath match the tenets of that sect and do not reflect the wider ethical commitments of Greek physicians. See Ludwig Edelstein, "The Hippocratic Oath: text, translation and interpretation," in *Ancient Medicine*, pp. 3–64; also Vivian Nutton, "Beyond the Hippocratic Oath," in Andrew Wear, Johanna Geyer-Kordesch, and Roger French (eds.), *Doctors and Ethics: The Earlier Historical Setting of Professional Ethics*, Clio Medica 24 (Amsterdam/Atlanta: Rodopi, 1992).

15. Veatch, *A Theory of Medical Ethics*, p. 328.

16. H. Tristram Engelhardt, *The Foundations of Bioethics* (New York: Oxford University Press, 1986), pp. 39, 75. A much revised second edition of this important book appeared in 1995. This volume is one of the few American treatises on bioethics widely read in Europe (interview with Rev. Patrick Versperien, Directeur, Département de Bioethique, Centre Sevrès, Paris, April 16, 1996).

17. Edmund D. Pellegrino and David C. Thomasma, *A Philosophical Basis of Medical Practice: Toward a Philosophy and Ethic of the Healing Professions* (New York: Oxford University Press, 1981); *For the Patient's Good: The Restoration of Beneficence in Health Care* (New York: Oxford University Press, 1988).

18. For reviews of Veatch's book, see Howard Brody, "Review of *A Theory of Medical Ethics*," *Journal of the American Medical Association* 247 (1982): 2293; L. W. Sumner, "Does medical ethics have its own theory," *Hastings Center Report* 12 (1982): 38–39; John Kultgen, "Veatch's new foundation for medical ethics," *Journal of Medicine and Philosophy* 10 (1985): 369–386. Some reviews of Engelhardt's work are: David H. Smith, "Quest for certainty," *Medical Humanities Review* 1 (1987): 11–13; Erich H. Loewy, "Not by reason alone," *Journal of Medical Humanities and Bioethics* 8 (1987): 67–72; Soren Holm, "The peaceable pluralistic society and the question of persons," *Journal of Medicine and Philosophy* 13 (1988): 379–386. On Pellegrino's contribution, see H. T. Engelhardt, Jr. (issue editor), *Edmund D. Pellegrino's Philosophy of Medicine: an Overview and an Assessment*, (special issue) *Journal of Medicine and Philosophy* 15, no. 3 (1990): 237–341.

19. *Theories and Methods in Bioethics: Principlism and its Critics* (special issue), *Kennedy Institute of Ethics Journal* 5 (September 1995); Edwin DuBose, Ronald P. Hamel, and Laurence J. O'Connell (eds.), *A Matter of Principles?: Ferment of U.S. Bioethics* (Valley Forge, Pa: Trinity Press International, 1994); Raanon Gillon (ed.), "Part I: approaches to applied health care ethics," in *Principles of Health Care Ethics* (Chichester, U.K.: John Wiley and Sons, 1994), pp. 1–333; K. Danner Clouser and Loretta M. Kopelman (eds.), *Philosophical Critique of Bioethics* (special issue), *Journal of Medicine and Philosophy* 15, no. 2 (1990).

20. Aristotle refers to the *arche*, or the forces that move human action. If the *arche* are external, action is coerced; if the *arche* are internal, action is voluntary. "Man," says Aristotle in W. D. Ross's translation, "is a moving principle of action." Aquinas wrote of the *prima et communissima principia* of the natural law and identified them as self-preservation, preservation of the species by procreation and education of children, and preservation of social life. Kant states that the *Grundprinzip* of moral law is the categorical imperative whereby maxims of action can be willed to be universal. See Aristotle, *Nicomachean Ethics III*, 1112b; Thomas Aquinas,

Summa Theologiae I–II, Q. 94, a.2; Immanuel Kant, *Groundwork of the Metaphysic of Morals*, ed. and trans. H. J. Paton (New York: Harper and Row, 1994).

21. Bishop Butler wrote, "One of those principles of action [in man's nature], conscience or reflection, compared with all the rest . . . claims the absolute marks of authority over all the rest." Joseph Butler, "Preface," from *Sermons*, reprinted in L. A. Selby-Bigge (ed.), *British Moralists*, vol. 2 (New York: Dover Publications, 1965), p. 187.

22. Marcus G. Singer, "Moral rules and principles," in A. I. Melden (ed.), *Essays in Moral Philosophy* (Seattle: University of Washington Press, 1958), pp. 160–197.

23. William Frankena, "The principles of morality," in Curtis L. Carter (ed.), *Skepticism and Moral Principles: Modern Ethics in Review* (Evanston: New University Press, 1973), pp. 43–76.

24. W. D. Ross, *The Right and the Good* (Oxford: Clarendon Press, 1930); Bernard Gert, *The Moral Rules: A New Rational Foundation for Morality* (New York: Harper and Row, 1970).

25. Beauchamp and Childress, *Principles of Biomedical Ethics*, 1st ed., p. 40. A similar passage with a less confessional tone appears in the much more elaborate discussion of theory in the 4th edition (1994), p. 110.

26. Albert R. Jonsen and Stephen Toulmin, *The Abuse of Casuistry: A History of Moral Reasoning* (Berkeley and Los Angeles: University of California Press, 1988), especially chapter 15.

27. Kurt Baier, "Ethical principles and their validity"; Alasdair MacIntyre, "How to identify ethical principles"; James Childress, "The identification of ethical principles," in *The Belmont Report: Ethical Principles and Guidelines for the Protection of Human Subjects* (Washington, D.C.: U.S. Government Printing Office, 1979), Appendix I.

28. Tom L. Beauchamp, "Distributive justice and morally relevant differences"; H. Tristram Engelhardt, Jr., "Basic ethical principles in the conduct of biomedical and behavioral research involving human subjects"; LeRoy Walters, "Some ethical issues in research involving human subjects," in *The Belmont Reports*, Appendix I.

29. See Isaiah Berlin, *Two Concepts of Liberty* (Oxford: Oxford University Press, 1958). It must be noted that "respect for persons," "respect for autonomy," or "respect for personal autonomy" are not synonymous. Respect for persons seems a much wider concept than respect for autonomy. In contemporary bioethics, however, the phrases are carelessly interchanged.

30. William Frankena, *Ethics* 2nd ed. (Englewood Cliffs: Prentice-Hall, 1973); Brandt, *Ethical Theory*; see also John Rawls, "Rational and full autonomy," *Journal of Philosophy* 77 (1980): 524; Gerald Dworkin, *The Theory and Practice of Autonomy* (New York: Cambridge University Press, 1988).

31. Robert S. Downie and Elizabeth Telfer, *Respect for Persons* (London: Allen and Unwin, 1969), p. 9. This book, which I read just as the National Commission was beginning its work, put the phrase "respect for persons" in my moral vocabulary.

32. Hans Jonas, Philosophical reflections on experimenting with human subjects, *Daedalus* 98, no. 2 (1969): 236.

33. *The Belmont Report*, p. 4.

34. *The Belmont Report*, Appendix I, pp. 8–5, 8–40.

35. Immanuel Kant, *Groundwork of the Metaphysic of Morals*, ch. 2, p. 98.

36. Veatch, *A Theory of Medical Ethics,* pp. 193–195; Engelhardt, *Foundations of Bioethics*, pp. 43–46.

37. Beauchamp and Childress, *Principles of Biomedical Ethics*, 1st ed., quotes on pp. 56, 58, and 59, respectively.

38. Talcott Parsons, *The Social System* (Glencoe, Ill.: The Free Press, 1951); Eliot Freidson, *Professional Dominance: The Social Structure of Medical Care* (New York: Atherton Press, 1970).

39. Ivan Illich, *Medical Nemesis: The Expropriation of Health* (London: Calder and Boyars,

1975); Thomas Szasz, *The Myth of Mental Illness: Foundations of a Theory of Personal Conduct* (New York: Hoeber-Harper, 1961).

40. L. Beaton, "A doctor prescribes for his profession," *Harper's*, October 1960, 151–153, quote on p. 151.

41. David J. Rothman, *Strangers at the Bedside: A History of How Law and Bioethics Transformed Medical Decision Making* (New York: Basic Books, 1991).

42. Patrick Devlin, *The Enforcement of Morals* (London: Oxford University Press, 1965); H. L. A. Hart, *Law, Liberty and Morality* (Stanford: Stanford University Press, 1963). Hippocrates, *Precepts* ix.

43. Robert M. Veatch, Willard Gaylin, and Councilman Morgan (eds.), *Teaching Medical Ethics* (Hastings-on-Hudson: Institute of Society, Ethics and the Life Sciences, 1973), p. 8.

44. Robert M. Veatch, "Medical ethics: professional or universal?" *Harvard Theological Review* 65 (1972): 531–559.

45. Gerald Dworkin, "Paternalism," *The Monist* (1972): 64–89; Bernard Gert and Charles M. Culver, "Paternalistic behavior," *Philosophy and Public Affairs* 6 (1976): 45–57; Joel Feinberg, *Social Philosophy* (Englewood Cliffs, N.J.: Prentice-Hall, 1973).

46. Paul Ramsey, *The Patient as Person: Explorations in Medical Ethics* (New Haven: Yale University Press, 1970), p. xiii; "The morality of abortion," in Labby, *Life or Death*, pp. 71–72.

47. Edward Shils, "The sanctity of life," in Labby, *Life or Death*, pp. 19, 29.

48. Daniel Callahan, "The sanctity of life," in Donald R. Cutler (ed.), *Updating Life and Death: Essays in Ethics and Medicine* (Boston: Beacon Press, 1969), pp. 181–251.

49. Callahan, "The sanctity of life," pp. 208, 215.

50. Stanley Hauerwas, "Creating a discipline: community," (Seattle, Wa., Sept. 23–24, 1992), Birth of Bioethics Conference, pp. 415–431; see his *Peaceable Kingdom: A Primer in Christian Ethics* (Notre Dame: Notre Dame University Press, 1983).

51. Robert M. Veatch, "Autonomy's temporary triumph," *Hastings Center Report* 14, no. 5 (1984): 38–42; Daniel Callahan, "Autonomy: a moral good, not a moral obsession," *Hastings Center Report* 14, no. 5 (1984): 40–42; James F. Childress, "The place of autonomy in bioethics," *Hastings Center Report* 20, no. 1 (1990): 12–17; Dworkin, *The Theory and Practice of Autonomy*; David L. Jackson and Stuart Youngner, "Patient autonomy and 'death with dignity,'" *New England Journal of Medicine* 301 (1979): 404–408; Bruce L. Miller, "Autonomy and the refusal of lifesaving treatment," *Hastings Center Report* 11, no. 4 (1981): 22–28.

52. Bernard Lonergan, *Method in Theology* (New York: Herder and Herder, 1972), p. 4.

53. In 1974, a research group was formed at the Hastings Center to explore this very question under the title "Foundations of ethics and its relationship to science." The group published their work in four volumes, the last being the most germaine to the question of methods: H. Tristram Engelhardt, Jr. and Daniel Callahan (eds.), *Knowing and Valuing: The Search For Common Roots* (Hastings-on-Hudson: Institute of Society, Ethics and the Life Sciences, 1980).

54. Henry Sidgwick, *Methods of Ethics* (London: Longmans-Green, 1874).

55. John Maloney, *The Making of Moral Theology* (Oxford: Oxford University Press, 1987); Jonsen and Toulmin, *The Abuse of Casuistry*; Charles Curran, *Contemporary Problems in Moral Theology* (Notre Dame: Fides Press, 1970) and *Ongoing Revision: Studies in Moral Theology* (Notre Dame: Fides Press, 1975).

56. Carl F. H. Henry, *Christian Personal Ethics* (Grand Rapids: Wm. B. Eerdmans, 1957); Paul L. Lehmann, *Ethics in a Christian Context* (New York: Harper and Row, 1963). The best review of the problem of method in Catholic and Protestant ethics is James Gustafson, *Protestant and Roman Catholic Ethics: Prospects for Rapprochement* (Chicago: University of Chicago Press, 1978).

57. James Gustafson, "Basic ethical issues in the biomedical fields," *Soundings* 53 (1970):

151–180, reprinted in Gustafson, *Theology and Christian Ethics* (Philadelphia: Pilgrim Press, 1974), p. 247.

58. Kenneth L. Vaux, *Biomedical Ethics: Morality for the New Medicine* (New York: Harper and Row, 1974), p. 39.

59. One early course, created in 1966 by Robert Williams, Chairman of the Department of Medicine at the University of Washington School of Medicine, invited "prominent religious leaders, attorneys, psychologists, psychiatrists, geneticists, marriage counselors and other specialities, as well as criminals and sexual deviates" to discuss "how we live and how we expect our progeny to live." Dr. Williams collected many of these lectures—by Joseph Fletcher, Elisabeth Kübler-Ross, Arthur Dyck, and others—in a 1976 volume, *To Live and To Die: When, Why and How* (New York: Springer-Verlag, 1974). Other examples of the earlier anthology approach are E. Fuller Torrey (ed.), *Ethical Issues in Medicine. The Role of the Physician in Today's Society* (Boston: Little, Brown, 1968) and Richard W. Wertz (ed.), *Readings on Ethical and Social Issues in Biomedicine* (Englewood Cliffs: Prentice-Hall, 1973). In a review of a dozen of these early texts I wrote, "I can write a preface on ethical theory to my hypothetical book on the troubles of San Francisco (pollution, corrupt politics, homelessness, crime) or include a chapter from Hobbes or Nietzsche. This would not make it the ethics of San Francisco." Albert R. Jonsen, "Books on bioethics: a commentary," *Pharos* 41 (1978): 39–43, p. 41.

60. Samuel Gorovitz, Andrew Jameton, Ruth Macklin, et al. (eds.), *Moral Problems in Medicine* (Englewood Cliffs: Prentice-Hall, 1976).

61. Howard Brody, *Ethical Decisions in Medicine* (New York: Little-Brown, 1976), p. 291, #1003. Brody explicitly refers to Van Rensselaer Potter's *Bioethics* for his theory of value.

62. Robert M. Veatch and Roy Branson, *Ethics and Health Policy* (Cambridge: Ballinger Publishing Company, 1976); Dennis J. Horan and David Mall (eds.), *Death, Dying and Euthanasia* (Washington, D.C.: University Publications of America, 1977); James M. Humber and Robert F. Almeder, *Biomedical Ethics and the Law* (New York: Plenum Press, 1976); Thomas A. Shannon (ed.), *Bioethics* (Mahwah, N.J.: Paulist Press, 1976); Robert Hunt and John Arras (eds.), *Ethical Issues in Modern Medicine* (Palo Alto: Mayfield Publishing Company, 1977); Joel Reiser, Arthur J. Dyck, and William J. Curran (eds.), *Ethics in Medicine* (Cambridge, Mass.: MIT Press, 1977); Tom L. Beauchamp and LeRoy Walters (eds.), *Contemporary Issues in Bioethics* (Belmont: Wadsworth Publishing Company, 1978); Robert M. Veatch, *Case Studies in Medical Ethics* (Cambridge: Harvard University Press, 1977); Howard Brody, *Ethical Decisions in Medicine*.

63. David Thomasma, "Training in medical ethics: an ethical workup," *Forum on Medicine* 1 (12) (1978): 33–36. A more elaborate version of the "ethical workup" can be found in Pellegrino and Thomasma, *A Philosophical Basis of Medical Practice*, pp. 119–51.

64. Albert R. Jonsen, "Can an ethicist be a consultant?" in Virginia Abernethy (ed.), *Frontiers in Medical Ethics: Applications in a Medical Setting* (Cambridge, Mass.: Ballinger, 1980), pp. 157–171. Jonsen and Toulmin, *The Abuse of Casuistry*. Baruch Brody has also made significant contributions to casuistic analysis of moral problems; see his *Life and Death Decision Making* (New York: Oxford University Press, 1988).

65. See Aristotle, *Nicomachean Ethics*, I, iii, 1094b.

66. Stephen Toulmin, "How medicine saved the life of ethics," *Perspectives in Biology and Medicine* 25 (1982): 749–750.

67. Albert R. Jonsen, Mark Siegler, and William J. Winslade, *Clinical Ethics: A Practical Approach to Ethical Decisions in Clinical Medicine* (New York: Macmillan, 1982); Albert Jonsen, "Casuistry and clinical medicine," *Theoretical Medicine* 7 (1986): 65–84.

68. Laurence B. McCullough, "Methodological concerns in bioethics," *Journal of Medicine and Philosophy* 11 (1986): 17–37, quotes on pp. 33–34; Arthur L. Caplan, "Applying morality to advances in biomedicine: Can and should this be done?" in William B. Bondeson, H. Tristram

Engelhardt, Jr., Stuart F. Spicker, and Joseph M. White, Jr. (eds.), *New Knowledge in the Biomedical Sciences: Some Moral Implications of Its Acquisition, Possession, and Use* (Dordrecht: D. Reidel, 1982), pp. 155–168.

69. Jay Katz of Yale Law School is the dean of legal scholars in bioethics. George Annas, Alexander Morgan Capron, Angela Holder, John Robertson, Patricia King, William Winslade, and Joseph Healey have also made major contributions.

70. See, for example, Margery Shaw and E. Edward Doudera (eds.), *Defining Human Life: Medical, Legal and Ethical Implications* (Ann Arbor: AUPHA Press, 1983).

71. George Annas, "From selection to rationing: policy," Birth of Bioethics Conference, (Seattle, Wa.: Sept. 24–25, 1992), pp. 75–80.

72. John Ladd, "Legalism and medical ethics," in John W. Davis, C. Barry Hoffmaster, and Sarah Shorter (eds.), *Contemporary Issues in Biomedical Ethics* (New York: Humana Press, 1978), pp. 1–35; a shorter version was reprinted in *Journal of Medicine and Philosophy* 4 (1979): 70–80; see Stuart F. Spicker, Joseph M. Healey, Jr., and H. Tristram Engelhardt, Jr. (eds.), *The Law-Medicine Relation: A Philosophical Exploration* (Dordrecht/Boston: D. Reidel Publishing Company, 1981); Roger B. Dworkin, *Limits. The Role of the Law in Bioethical Decision Making* (Bloomington: Indiana University Press, 1996).

73. Among the many sociological studies relevant to bioethics are Bernard Barber, John J. Lally, Julia Loughlin Makarushka, and Daniel Sullivan, *Research on Human Subjects: Problems of Social Control in Medical Experimentation* (New York: Russell Sage Foundation, 1973); Charles Bosk, *Forgive and Remember: Managing Medical Failure* (Chicago: University of Chicago Press, 1979); Diana Crane, *The Sanctity of Social Life: Physicians' Treatment of Critically Ill Patients* (New York: Russell Sage Foundation, 1975); Renée Fox, *Experiment Perilous: Physicians and Patients Facing the Unknown* (Glencoe: The Free press, 1959); Renée Fox and Judith Swazey, *The Courage to Fail: A Social View of Organ Transplants and Dialysis* (Chicago: University of Chicago Press, 1978); Eliot Freidson, *The Profession of Medicine: A Study of the Sociology of Applied Knowledge* (New York: Harper and Row, 1970); Barney G. Glaser and Anselm L. Strauss, *Awareness of Dying* (Chicago: Aldine Press, 1965); Arthur Kleinman, *The Illness Narratives: Suffering, Healing and the Human Condition* (New York: Basic Books, 1988). I mentored two anthropologists in bioethics, Renée Anspach, "Life and Death Decisions in Neonatal Intensive Care: A Study in the Sociology of Knowledge" (Ph.D. dissertation, University of California, San Diego, 1982), published as *Deciding Who Lives: Fateful Choices in the Intensive Care Nursery* (Berkeley: University of California Press, 1983) and Barbara Koenig, "The Technological Imperative in Medical Practice: An Ethnographical Study of Therapeutic Plasma Exchange" (Ph.D. dissertation, University of California, San Diego, 1987).

74. Renée C. Fox, "The evolution of American bioethics: a sociological perspective," in George Weisz (ed.), *Social Sciences Perspective on Medical Ethics* (Philadelphia: University of Pennsylvania Press, 1990), pp. 201–220, p. 213. Renée Fox and Judith Swazey, "Medical morality is not bioethics—medical ethics in China and the United States," *Perspectives in Biology and Medicine* 27 (1984): 336–360, p. 358.

75. Daniel Callahan, "Shattuck lecture—contemporary biomedical ethics," *The New England Journal of Medicine* 302 (1980): 1228–1232.

76. H. Tristram Engelhardt, Jr., "Creating a discipline: theory," (paper read at the Birth of Bioethics Conference, Seattle, Wa., Sept. 23–24, 1992), transcript, pp. 404, 411, 415.

11

Bioethics As a Discourse

Bioethics does not belong to the bioethicists who worry about its disciplinary status. From its beginnings, bioethics has gotten people talking. It is public discourse carried on by many people in many settings. We opened the history of American bioethics with a walk through a decade of conferences in which savants exposed their problems of conscience about the new biology and medicine. We stopped in at the founding of two centers at which the conversations of those conferences were perennialized. We listened as government panels debated about how to convert those conversations into public policy and regulations. The early bioethicists called for wide public discussion about the ethical goals of medicine and science, and that discussion has taken place.

The native language of the savants was technical science; when they spoke about ethical and social problems, they often spoke haltingly (although with emotion and conviction). The vocabulary suited to moral and social issues did not come easily; their conference discourse was rhetorical rather than analytic, and the conference setting did not easily engage minds in the intense inquiry required to sharpen concepts and argument. The theologians came out of their churches and into the conferences, bringing a tradition of reflection on the moral life and a rich vocabulary. Academic philosophers, segregated from public philosophy by the arcane terminology of analytic philosophy, arrived at the conversation, eager to instill logic into arguments. Philosophers and theologians quickly realized that they needed not only to familiarize themselves with the world of science and medicine but also how to phrase arguments that the other conversants could understand and answer.

The summer conferences sponsored by the National Endowment for the Humanities provided places for closer philosophical inquiry, but at these gatherings, the philosophers often conversed without non-philosophical partners. The Hastings Center research groups provided better forums to foster genuine public discourse. Devoted to genetics, death and dying, behavioral modification, and population, these groups invited scientists, ethicists, and other scholars to argue out issues to the point of policy. The first two federal Commissions continued in this vein, with the added impetus of specific congressional mandates, and with the added help of scholarly staff and invited experts from all fields. The Commissions engaged the broader public: professionals, interested parties, and the general public were informed about the Commissions' agenda, and their comments were welcomed. The media reported the deliberations and new journals, such as the *Hastings Center Report* and the *Journal of Philosophy and Medicine*, published critical articles about the work and products of the Commissions.

Bioethics has been a discourse, a persistent and purposeful conversation open to diverse participants. The conversation has been persistent: it has taken up and followed certain problems over an extended time, seeking clearer definition for the terms of the conversation and more articulate and critical expression of the arguments for and against certain positions. The conversation has been purposeful: it has moved toward resolution of problems, both speculative and practical. These resolutions have often been tentative, partial, and in need of revision; at the same time, the conversants have been motivated to reach reasonable, helpful answers. The conversation has been open to a diversity of participants, for it was initiated by persons from different interests and backgrounds, all asking questions from their own perspective. Bioethics from its beginnings has been public discourse. This chapter examines how that discourse has contributed to the evolution of bioethics, first in private medical conversations, then in the classroom, in ethics committees and citizens' conclaves, and in the media.

Shared Decision-making

All this public conversation had an echo in some very private places—the closeted conversations between doctors and their patients about medical problems, and between researchers and the persons they invited to participate in their research. These most private conversations re-enact in small compass the public discourse about the ethical dimensions of those relationships. Physicians and patients, researchers and subjects speak to each other in the terms scripted by the educational and legal results of the wider bioethical debates.

Of course, doctors and patients have always conversed. Patients came to physicians complaining about a physical disorder and physicians explained how the disorder could be remedied. The decorum of medical ethics taught physicians to converse courteously and encouragingly. It also recommended reticence, even deception, when bad news had to be conveyed. Yet, despite centuries of medical conversation between physicians and patients, scholars cannot discern a consistent pattern about the ethics of medical communication. One author maintains that "disclosure and consent . . . have no historical roots in medical practice," while another finds that "truth-telling and consent-seeking have long been part of an indigenous medical tradition, based on medical theories that

taught that knowledge and autonomy had demonstrably beneficial effects on most patients' health."[1]

This ambiguity appears in the earliest evidence: Plato tells us that a free physician
treating free citizens would converse with them, attempt to understand their problems,
and "when he has brought the patient into his confidence, and then only, prescribe for
him." Physicians who treated slaves dispensed with the conversation and merely gave
orders, "like a tyrant."[2] The distinction between citizen and slave patients collapses in
other Hippocratic aphorisms: "If a patient be under orders, he will not stray; left to himself, he will give up the struggle and depart this life . . . so, [the physician must] take
the patient in hand."[3] Physicians are encouraged to assume authority, to give orders
firmly, and to urge obedience and to upbraid the delinquent. The physician's authority
directs the conversation with patients.

The physician's authority also sanctions what would otherwise be ethically suspect—the withholding and even distortion of truth. In Hippocratic times, the physician
was admonished, "Reveal nothing of the patient's future or present condition, for many,
on learning what is to come, have taken a turn for the worst."[4] The truth might kill.
Throughout medical history, physicians were encouraged to be reticent in talking about
impending death. Only a solemn decree of the church could drag medieval physicians
toward truthful disclosure: they were charged with the responsibility to see that a patient not die unshriven.[5] Despite that holy admonition, doctors remained reluctant to
warn of death. The prevailing opinion of medical moralists supported the "therapeutic
privilege," a physician may withhold the truth if he believe the patient will be harmed
by it. Dr. Percival argued against a moral philosopher's claim that physicians should always tell patients the truth, with the apothegm, "To a patient who makes inquiries
which, if faithfully answered, might prove fatal to him, it would be a gross and unfeel-
ing wrong to reveal the truth." Two American physicians fought vainly against the tide
by arguing that the truth should be told because, in fact, the truth is inevitably more
helpful than harmful.[6] For most of medical history, the complaint uttered by Dr.
Samuel Johnson, "Of all lying I have the greatest aborrence of this (medical lying), because I believe it has been frequently practiced on me," went unheeded by practitioners.[7] So, during several millennia of medical conversation, the content of that conversation and its candor remain obscure and only the generalities of the traditional decorum
guided its moral direction. The informational part of what we call today "informed consent" was, it appears, "up to the doctor."

The consent part of informed consent has an equally ambiguous history. Sick persons have usually put themselves willingly enough into the hands of a healer and, explicitly or implicitly, consented to their treatment. Patients could and often did walk
away or dismiss the physician. Yet, healers have often been summoned to the bedside
of a weak, and possibly unwilling, sufferer, and some physicians may have inveigled
their way into persons' lives, holding them as patients by fabricating illnesses or claiming healing skills they did not possess. Still, the liberty of persons not to be patients has
ancient origins: in medieval times, physicians were admonished never to come unbid-

den to the patient's bedside. The custom of requiring permission for a medical touching entered English common law in the fifteenth century; touching a patient without permission was trespass. A 1914 American case, *Schloendorff v Society of New York Hospitals*, gave classic expression to the common law principle: Justice Cardozo's words ring down the corridors of medical jurisprudence, "Every human being of adult years and sound mind has a right to determine what shall be done with his own body; and a surgeon who performs an operation without his patient's consent commits an assault, for which he is liable in damages."[8]

Justice Cardozo made no mention of a consent that was informed, and the relevance of information to consent (obvious as it might seem) was not given judicial blessing until 1957, when the California Supreme Court, in *Salgo v Leland Stanford Jr. University*, ruled that physicians "have the duty to disclose any facts which are necessary to form the basis of an intelligent consent by the patient to proposed treatment" and granted relief to Martin Salgo who, having undergone translumbar aortography without being told that paralysis was a risk, suffered that dreadful outcome.[9] Three years later, the Kansas Supreme Court, in *Natanson v Kline*, placed the new concept of informed consent into the legal framework of negligence rather than battery. Mrs. Natanson sued her radiologist for failing to inform her of the risk of serious burns from cobalt therapy.[10] In 1972, *Canterbury v Spence*, a Washington, D.C., case, provided the first expanded description of the new legal requirement of informed consent. Mr. Canterbury, after undergoing a laminectomy, fell from his hospital bed and suffered a serious paralysis. He sued his surgeon for failure to inform him of the risk of paralysis. The court ruled that the information was material to Mr. Canterbury's decision to undergo the surgery. The court declared:

> True consent to what happens to one's self is the informed exercise of a choice, and that entails an opportunity to evaluate knowledgeably the options available and the risks attendant upon each. The average patient has little or no understanding of the medical arts, and ordinarily has only his physician to whom he can look for enlightenment with which to reach an intelligent decision. From these almost axiomatic considerations springs the need, and in turn the requirement, of a reasonable divulgence by physicians to patients to make such a decision possible.[11]

During the 1960s, a new concept, informed consent, was being shaped within the legal doctrines of malpractice and negligence. The standards and the essential elements of informed consent were stated in legal fashion and incorporated into the statutory law of many states: physicians must inform their patients about the nature of their condition and its expected course, about the benefits and risks of any proposed treatment, and of alternative treatment or non-treatment. This new legal requirement was impressed upon physicians as a professional duty.

At the same time that this professional duty was being newly formulated in the law, the moral importance of informed consent was under critical examination in another discussion: the debate about the ethics of medical experimentation involving human subjects. As we saw in Chapter 5, the consent of volunteers to risky research had long been accepted as the ethical premise of research with human subjects. The Nuremberg Code declared consent "absolutely essential" and insisted that the consenting subject "have sufficient knowledge and comprehension of the elements of the subject matter involved as to enable him to make an understanding and enlightened decision."[12] Such a decision was even more obviously crucial for research than for treatment, since the research subject is offered an intervention aimed not at his or her own good, but rather at generating knowledge that might benefit future patients. Hans Jonas argued that the consent to research must be more than mere permission. It must be an act that truly engages a free and knowledgeable person in the project.[13] This is a high standard for consent. It goes much deeper than a mere "okay" to an obscure request; it even goes beyond a listing of risks and benefits, which might inform the subject well enough. It was not difficult to demonstrate that in most research situations, this deeper consent was rare.

John Fletcher's 1967 essay, "Human experimentation: ethics in the consent situation," discusses the results of an empirical study he conducted of the consent process, in which he interviewed researchers and their research subjects at the NIH Clinical Center in order to obtain an accurate picture of what happens as researchers attempt to provide information and gain consent from those whom they invited to be research subjects. As an ethicist rather than a sociologist, Fletcher was looking for the moral values expressed in the interaction between researchers and subjects: "I expected that these patients would give signs, gestures, and verbal expression to show how their experience in a risk-taking study reflected on their sense of having the status of a 'person.' . . . I assumed . . . that the real meaning of the rule (of informed consent) was to protect the status of personhood which is enshrined in the traditions of law, morality and religion surrounding the concept of consent."[14] Instead, Fletcher found a truncated, ritualistic process in which many pressures, from the side of both researcher and subject, constricted the sense of freedom. He suggested that the role of patient advocate be established to aid investigators and to support subjects in explaining and appreciating the full range of options to which the potential subjects' personhood and freedom entitled them.

In 1972, the same year that several American courts enshrined informed consent in medical practice, the scandal of the Tuskegee Syphilis Study revealed that American doctors, as well as Nazi war criminals, could ignore the Nuremberg Code's first principle of voluntary consent of research subjects. It was shockingly obvious that the subjects of the twenty-year study had not consented to being research subjects and had not been informed about why government doctors were taking their blood. Indeed, they had been deceived about what was being done to them. One member of the Tuskegee panel, Dr. Jay Katz, declared: "The most fundamental reason for condemning the Tuskegee Study . . . [is that the subjects] were never fairly consulted about the research project, its consequences for them and the alternatives available to them."[15]

Paul Ramsey placed John Fletcher's phrase, "ethics in the consent situation," at the head of his discussion of free and adequately informed consent as the chief canon of loyalty in the experimental relationship.[16] Consent, whether to experimentation or to therapy, is the external manifestation of the moral values of freedom and loyalty that renders the relationship between physicians and patients/subjects a moral one. Informed consent came to bioethics with impeccable credentials: it had the philosophical arguments of Jonas, the theological references of Ramsey, and the accumulating laws of the land.

The National Commission for the Protection of Human Subjects initiated its study of informed consent to experimentation by inviting several scholarly essays. Robert Veatch's contribution, "Three theories of informed consent: philosophical foundations and policy implications," set the pattern for a deeper exploration of the topic. Veatch examined three possible philosophical grounds for informed consent: first, the beneficent duty of physicians requires them to warn patients of possible harm associated with treatment; second, the utilitarian principle recommends consent as a means of maintaining the general trust between the scientific profession and society; third, the right to self-determination. He criticized the first two and strongly defended the third, arguing that an informed consent grounded in the right to self-determination implies a standard of disclosure based not on professional judgment but on the need of a reasonable person for information to make a decision.[17] The Commission accepted Veatch's analysis and located its discussion of informed consent in *The Belmont Report* under the general topic of "Respect for Persons."

The President's Commission for the Study of Ethical Problems in Medicine, asked by Congress to study informed consent for medical procedures, decided to broaden this topic from the narrow, legalistic scope implied by the phrase, "informed consent," toward one that examined "how to foster a relationship between patients and professionals characterized by mutual participation and respect and by shared decisionmaking." The Commission report, *Making Health Care Decisions*, described the qualities of such a relationship and criticized the virtual absence of these qualities in dealings between patients and physicians. It presented a philosophical argument based on the principle of autonomy—persons have an intrinsic right to direct their lives—and on the principle of beneficence—care is improved when the patient is a collaborator. The Commission recommended changes in practice and policy that would enhance the qualities of shared decision-making.[18]

Dr. Katz reviewed *Making Health Care Decisions* and judged its analysis and recommendations "a bold move to imprint on physician, patients, and society, the Commission's moral vision on how doctors and patients should make joint decisions." That vision was "noble," he said, but "formidable obstacles stood in the way of its implementation."[19] The obstacles were the absence of a tradition of shared decision-making, the lack of a coherent legal doctrine of informed consent, the pervasiveness of uncertainty, and the incapacity of physicians, due to their training and to deeper psychological reasons, to engage patients in shared decision-making. Katz judged that the Commission's linking of autonomy and beneficence as the ethical ground for shared decision-making had a fatal flaw: the dual justification allowed a physician's judgment about a patient's well-being to compromise their duty to engage the patient in dialogue. Dr. Katz expanded on these views in his eloquent book, *The Silent World of Doctor and Patient,* where he argued that physicians are educated away from frank communication with their patients.[20] A decade after Katz wrote the book, medical education and medical practice are still far from removing the obstacles that he noted. Nevertheless, it seems indisputable that physicians are now more aware that the patient is the final arbiter of treatment decisions, and informed consent is a part of their daily interaction, even if often meager and formalistic. Patients, too, are more aware of their right and need for more ample communication.

It may seem strange to locate this discussion of so private a business as informed consent in this chapter on public discourse. The reason for doing so is to show how the public discussion about the moral and legal obligation to obtain consent for therapeutic or investigational interventions shapes the private discourse that should take place between physicians and patients, researchers and subjects. Each conversation will be an improvisation, suited to situation and to the personalities, but the moral and legal requirement that there must be a conversation including certain elements has been dictated by the public discourse that took place in commissions and in courts.

Teaching Bioethics

The discourse about bioethics first entered the classroom via medical schools. Ethics had been a desultory part of medical education. A few lectures on the moral and legal duties of physicians were included in most medical curricula during the nineteenth century. The commencement address, usually by a distinguished physician, was often devoted to ethics. After the AMA Code was promulgated in 1847, some physicians urged that it should be systematically propounded in medical education. This was rarely done. One disgusted commentator wrote in 1861, "Some physicians are moral idiots in respect to the dignity and honor of the profession they follow. . . . It would take no serious interruption of the course of medical studies to have one lecture a week delivered on the subject of professional ethics."[21] Outside the Catholic medical schools, few courses in medical ethics were offered, and where such courses were taught, they were combined with medical jurisprudence.[22]

The Hastings Center organized a conference called "The Teaching of Medical Ethics" in New York, June 1–3, 1972, where Robert Veatch reported the results of a survey he had done in anticipation of the conference. One hundred two American medical schools were asked about ethics in their curriculum. Of those schools, 94 responded: 15 stated they had no ethics instruction, 56 reported that ethics was taught within other courses, such as social medicine, legal medicine, or psychiatry, and 33 schools reported that a specific ethics course was offered as an elective.[23] Six actual programs were described by the faculty that had designed them, beginning with

Veatch's presentation of the curriculum at the Columbia College of Physicians and Surgeons, which had been planned and implemented with the collaboration of The Hastings Center. The Columbia curriculum was ambitious: it included didactic lectures, case conferences in clinical rotations, dinner discussions, and elective courses, spread throughout the four years of the curriculum. Georgetown University School of Medicine had converted a century-old required course into a four-segment elective course described as "popular and provocative." Hershey Medical School's Department of Medical Humanities offered a menu of "selectives" in the humanities that were available to medical students, including several ethics courses. Harvard had inaugurated an Interfaculty Program in Medical Ethics, concentrating on graduate courses across disciplines and offering a course in Harvard College, although no medical school curriculum had been implemented. Dr. Otto Guttentag of UCSF described his course, "The Medical Attitude," as a highly theoretical introduction to medical philosophy; I attended this course along with a few medical students during my year as visiting professor. The patterns varied from the "popular and provocative" of Georgetown to the existential hermeneutics of Guttentag.

These patterns were to be tried, modified, discarded, and revived over the next two decades. The Columbia program, so ambitious in its conception, was soon reduced to a lecture course, without The Hastings Center's participation. Veatch later recalled that the course had engendered both enthusiasm and hostility among students and faculty and reflected, "Callahan, Gaylin and I got tired of 'retailing' medical ethics."[24] Still, many medical schools, particularly the newer and less prestigious ones, were willing to experiment with courses. These courses, while certainly of differing quality and thoroughness, brought new participants into the discourse. Many faculty, some of them with considerable standing in their schools, were willing to help with the teaching. Students heard the language of medical ethics and learned that there was such a thing, even if they may have left the courses having a somewhat vague notion about what medical ethics was.

Teachers of bioethics were trying to find the "teachable moment" in the long, complex medical education when students would be most likely to appreciate ethical discourse about medicine. It was commonly recognized that the first two years of medical education, when ethics lectures were usually offered, were too remote from the practice of medicine for ethics to be compelling. I attempted to solve this problem at UCSF by devising a course at the conclusion of the second two years, the clerkship rotation years, after the students would have experienced actual ethical problems in the clinics and wards and before they entered their residency as providers of care. Dr. J. Engleburt Dunphy pushed the concept through the faculty council, helped plan its content and format, and, unfortunately, became too ill to teach in its first presentation in 1979. This course, called "Responsibilities of Medical Practice," was innovative and, fortunately, popular with students.[25]

The number of medical school courses steadily increased. By 1974, 97 of 197 responding medical schools offered some kind of medical ethics instruction: 6 schools required an ethics course, 47 offered an elective, and in the rest, instruction was scattered through the curriculum. The number of schools "with major commitments to medical ethics teaching" had increased from 19 to 31 between 1972 and 1974.[26] By 1984, 84% of medical schools reported that they had required courses in medical humanities in the first two years, and 34% in the last two years.[27] Dr. Edmund Pellegrino editorialized, "The teaching of medical ethics . . . should help to prepare physicians for these new relationships [to patients and society]. It is an essential first step in returning critical intelligence to medicine and situating it more securely between the sciences and the humanities—where it has always belonged."[28]

In the beginning, courses were shaped by the professor's interests. Some stressed philosophical concepts and used the actual texts of the great philosophers. Other courses slighted philosophy and dwelt on the common topics of medical ethics, such as care of the dying, experimentation, and genetic screening, around which a body of literature was gathering. Still other courses combined philosophical ethics with novels, short stories, and films that illustrated the moral dimensions of medicine. During 1976, The Hastings Center sponsored a year-long study of bioethics teaching at all educational levels. Charles Culver, a psychiatrist at Dartmouth Medical School, and I wrote on medical school teaching. We recognized the current diversity of curriculum, but we particularly encouraged courses that seriously tried to impart skills of identifying, defining, arguing, and resolving practical problems. We preferred the seminar-discussion format over lectures to achieve these ends. We strongly supported teaching done by a team "of medically knowledgeable ethicists and ethically conversant physicians."[29]

In July, 1983, Dr. Culver convened a conference of medical school teachers of ethics to determine goals for ethics instruction. The report of that group began, "A medical school dean or curriculum committee surveying the current state of education in medical ethics might conclude that nothing has evolved that might serve as a national standard for adequate instruction." During the three-day meeting, the group concluded that a minimal basic curriculum should aim to instill in students seven abilities: to recognize the moral aspects of medical practice, to obtain valid consent for treatment, to know how to proceed with the incompetent patient, to manage a refusal of treatment, to decide when withholding of information is justified, to decide when a breach of confidentiality is justified, and to appreciate the moral aspects of care for the terminally ill. Several participants also advocated coverage of equitable distribution of health care and discussion of abortion.[30]

Although it is difficult to evaluate the efficacy of teaching ethics, several studies gratifyingly revealed that students seemed to know more about ethics after the course than before it.[31] Dr. Don Self of Texas A&M School of Medicine has contributed significantly to the evaluation of ethics teaching, basing his methods on James Rest's "Defining Issues Test," which is itself related to Lawrence Kohlberg's theory of moral development. Self concludes, "Contrary to apparent popular belief, it is not developmentally too late for growth in moral reasoning to occur in higher education students.

Indeed, several recent studies have shown significant increases in the moral reasoning skills of medical students as a result of taking a medical ethics course as part of their curriculum."[32]

It can be asked, of course, whether this success carries beyond medical school into medical practice. Dr. Pellegrino studied 3,000 practicing physicians who had graduated between 1974 and 1978. His study concluded, "Those who had courses in medical ethics perceived it to be of substantial benefit in confronting the actual ethical problems they encountered in daily practice." At the same time, the respondents ranked courses less effective than discussions with advisors, reading articles, and attending conferences; only 10% felt that formal instruction strongly influenced their moral behavior.[33]

It would seem that a teachable moment for ethics comes during the post-graduate training, or residency, which consists of three or more years of supervised care of patients, usually in a hospital setting. Newly graduated physicians are immersed in the reality of caring for very ill patients, dealing with families, engaging with consultants, and working under the organizational and economic constraints of institutions. The ethical problems that they may have discussed in a first-year classroom are now real. However, this teachable moment is less than ideal: the residents are exceedingly busy; there is much medicine to learn; time is fractured; curriculum is fragmented. These years are not under the authority of the medical schools but are supervised by the 24 specialty boards which certify post-graduate physicians in the various medical specialties. Several specialty boards made serious efforts to incorporate ethics teaching into residency training.

In 1978, I was invited to serve as consultant to the American Board of Internal Medicine, which oversees the largest residency training in the country. The Board decided to stimulate interest in ethics by adding ethics questions to the certifying examination that concludes residency and qualifies the resident as a specialist in internal medicine. The questions were intended to inspire residency directors to introduce ethics instruction into their training programs. During the five years that I worked with the Board, I drafted questions and sat in the intense meetings of the exam-writing committees, attempting to shape the slippery stuff called ethics into the tight molds of multiple-choice questions. In 1981, the board initiated a wider project—an evaluation of the humanistic qualities of the internist. A subcommittee was appointed with the charge of defining those humanistic qualities desirable in an internist and of suggesting methods that would support and assess these qualities. Presence of such qualities were to be considered part of the "clinical competence" that residents were expected to demonstrate at the conclusion of their training. Subsequently, a *Guide to Awareness and Evaluation of Humanistic Qualities in the Internist* was published in 1985, which defined the desirable qualities of integrity, respect and compassion, and proposed ways of heightening sensitivity to them. Other specialty boards have encouraged the introduction of ethics into their training programs.[34]

Twenty years after the Hastings Conference on Teaching, medical ethics is an established part of medical education. The style of teaching is still as varied as it was in the early days. Nonetheless, a strong preference for the practical over the theoretical, for case discussion over lecture, and for real-world problems over possible ones, mark the educational philosophy at the end of the eighties.

As bioethics assumed the characteristics of a discipline, and as medical schools set up courses, graduate education preparing teachers and scholars became desirable. The first graduate program was inaugurated in 1974 at the University of Tennessee under the direction of Glen Graber, a philosopher, and David Thomasma, a theologian. A program leading to the doctorate in philosophy with a concentration on bioethics began at Georgetown University in 1976. These programs attracted students from the humanities and the sciences, immersed them in the topics and theories of bioethics, and encouraged them to devise analytic methods of analysis and expression. Several fellowship programs, such as those sponsored by the National Endowment for the Humanities at The Hastings Center and at The Institute for Human Values in Medicine, provided similar opportunities for more advanced scholars and professionals. The Intensive Bioethics Course at Georgetown and other similar short educational programs for professionals reached out to physicians, nurses, and educators.

The discourse in the classroom, whether with graduate students, medical students, or undergraduates, contributed to the disciplinary nature of bioethics. As teachers stand before (or sit among) their students, they are forced to bring into focus theories, principles, methods, and cases. They must prepare a syllabus that provides an orderly presentation of the issues. Abstract words are pushed into definitions; discussions are forced into logical form; questions are pressed toward answers. As we saw in Chapter 10, myriads of textbooks and articles flowed from these teaching activities, putting the discourse into print. So, as bioethics moved from the airing of the issues in the era of conferences to the more focused debates of task forces and commissions and finally into the didactic regimen of the curriculum, it took on the shape of a discipline. But classroom bioethics did more than contribute to the disciplinary character of bioethics; it gave many persons who were not bioethicists an appreciation of the issues and a language to speak articulately about them. Many of those persons carried their newly acquired talents into their practice as health professionals.

Hospital Ethics Committees

Another form of discourse was carried on outside the classroom—the deliberations of committees that evaluated research and the hospital ethics committees. Although committee discourse lacked the structure of pedagogy, it had a purpose and direction that distinguished it from simple conversation. As we have seen in Chapter 5, institutions receiving federal funds for biomedical research were required to establish institutional review boards (IRBs) for the oversight of experimentation with human subjects. Participants on those IRBs learned the vocabulary and grammar necessary to evaluate the ethics of a research protocol. In the mid-1970s, another innovation appeared in some hospitals, the ethics committee. For a number of years, Catholic hospitals had already maintained "medico-moral" committees, pursuant to the Catholic Hospital Association's *Ethical and Religious Directives* issued in 1949.[35] These committees, usually comprised of several physicians, several nursing sisters, and, perhaps, the hospital chaplain, were charged with assuring that Catholic teaching on such matters as contraception, sterilization, abortion, and euthanasia were faithfully observed.

In 1975, pediatrician Karen Teel recommended the establishment of hospital ethics committees. She was particularly concerned about the difficult decisions facing those who cared for impaired newborns; her essay made obvious reference to the Johns Hopkins baby. Dr. Teel suggested that rather than leaving these decisions to the parents alone, who may be unable to make an unbiased decision, or to the physicians alone, who are not authorized to make them, an ethics committee be established that would "provide a regular forum for more input and dialogue in individual situations and to allow the responsibility for these judgments to be shared." Dr. Teel mistakenly believed that "many hospitals had established an ethics committee composed of physicians, social workers, attorneys and theologians (known irreverently in some circles as the 'God Squad')." She was apparently thinking of the Seattle dialysis-selection committee; very few hospitals, outside of the Catholic institutions, had such committees. Despite this factual error, the New Jersey justices sitting on the *Quinlan* case were impressed by Dr. Teel's proposal. They cited her article and then described something quite different from what she had recommended; namely, a committee of physicians competent to make an accurate neurological prognosis for a patient in the state in which Karen Ann lay.[36] Following the New Jersey court's endorsement of ethics committees, several other legal cases mentioned the committee concept—sometimes to repudiate it;[37] sometimes to recommend it.[38]

Despite the judicial interest in ethics committees, the concept did not rapidly move beyond the law. In 1983, Dr. Stuart Youngner reported to the President's Commission that "[committees] have not been widely adopted as a means of handling medical ethics problems. Only 1% of hospitals in this country—none with fewer than 200 beds—have such committees. Furthermore, the committees that do exist are not involved in large numbers of cases. Existing committees reviewed an average of one case per year."[39] The Commission gave a push to the concept and published as an appendix to *Deciding To Forego Life-Sustaining Treatment* a model statute on the role and composition of hospital ethics committees prepared by the American Society of Law and Medicine.[40] Following the Commission's endorsement, the number of ethics committees doubled between 1983 and 1985, from 26% of reporting hospitals to 60%.[41]

These proliferating committees were set an odd task. Unlike the standard hospital committees, such as the pathology committee or the credentials committee, the ethics committee had no well-defined task to perform; they were ordered to think about ethics, probably the vaguest and most controversial of topics. The medico-morals committees of Catholic hospitals had clear Catholic teaching and the *Ethical and Religious Directives* to guide them; the institutional review boards had been given a set of federal regulations and the principles of *The Belmont Report* to orient their thinking. The ethics committees had no similar touchstones beyond, perhaps, the skimpy code of the AMA. If the bewildered members were given any orientation, it was likely that the hospital attorney taught them a bit about the well-publicized legal cases, such as *Quinlan*, and a philosophy professor from a local college explained, in short form, ethical theory. Some fortunate committees may have had a member who subscribed to the *Hastings Center Report* or who had taken the Georgetown intensive course. Thus, members could be informed that a growing literature about the problems of medical ethics was available and that some of it might be found in the hospital's library. In general, however, the duties and agenda for the novel ethics committees were amorphous; their members were sent off to do ethics on their own.

The early committees gave some meaning to their existence by formulating hospital policy about cardiac resuscitation which, as we saw in Chapter 8, created considerable perplexity. After framing DNR policies, some committees went on to the more difficult yet pressing question of hospital policy about foregoing life-sustaining treatment. Certain bold committees invited their hospital's physicians to submit cases to them for consultation, an invitation that was met with some skepticism by medical staff, but often enough welcomed in particularly difficult cases. As they worked at these tasks, committees became adept at research into the issues. They requested improved library resources and sought consultation from bioethicists where those rare creatures were available. Above all, they sought education: across the country, local networks of ethics committees arose, pooling resources to invite ethicists for occasional conferences on issues such as living wills, refusal of care, life support, and so forth. Some committees undertook programs of ethics education for their institutions. An organization to assist in the formation of committees and in their education was created and a journal was founded to serve their needs.[42] In hundreds of hospital ethics committees, discourse about ethics went on; thousands of persons became familiar with the issues and arguments. When asked to consider a question, many committees had already developed the competence to respond in an informed and orderly manner.[43]

In 1982, Moffitt Hospital of the University of California, San Francisco, established an ethics committee, which was instigated by the Medicaid official who was assigned to review patient records after the installation of the diagnostic related group (DRG) method of hospital payment. The official, a retired dermatologist, realized that some patients in intensive care units surpassed the allowed days of hospitalization and suggested to the administrator of the hospital that a committee be established to review these cases and advise him on the suitability of continued care. Although not a physician, I was asked to chair the committee, which was made up of five physicians and one nursing supervisor. Since I had shared in the President's Commission deliberations, I was able to provide my colleagues with some general ideas about the function of committees. It was quickly obvious that some method for reviewing the cases was needed. I had been searching for just such a method, with the help of several young physicians who were doing fellowships with me, Drs. Christine Cassel, Bernard Lo, and Henry

Perkins. At the same time, Drs. Mark Siegler and William Winslade and I had just finished writing *Clinical Ethics*. Out of these discussions emerged a method of reviewing cases by examining, in order, medical indications, patient preferences, quality of life, and contextual features. Our UCSF medical ethics committee adopted this method, giving to the random conversation so often characteristic of ethics discussion a shape and a direction. I subsequently taught this method to many newly formed ethics committees. Other bioethicists also helped committees develop a more informed and formal discourse.

Ethics committees proliferated during the 1980s. Their quality was, it appears, very diverse.[44] In 1987, Bernard Lo wrote a critical article about the function of these new committees, suggesting that they suffered from bias, were tainted by "group think," and had little in the way of standard procedures to deal with the problems that were proposed to them.[45] Lo's criticisms were probably deserved; still, the committees became part of hospital life. In some places, they are moribund; in others, they are vibrant. When they are vibrant, the ethics committees advance bioethical discourse.

Clinical Ethics

Ethics committees, while often composed of clinicians, sat outside the intensive care units, clinics, and hospital rooms where the problems that they discussed actually occurred. The real world of "who lives? who dies?" beckoned to bioethics. A few early bioethicists judged that they needed to learn the actual pace and pulse of medical life and felt that, once they learned what went on in hospitals, they could teach ethics within the clinical setting, and even offer some advice about how decisions should be formulated. Some physicians welcomed this participation in their clinical work; others found it intolerable. Every bioethicist has stories of being welcomed or being ignored as he or she entered the clinics and wards. I was one of the fortunate ones who found a welcome. I entered the clinical world within several years of my arrival at UCSF, first in the intensive care nursery, then in the cancer center and in the adult intensive care unit. I learned much in those settings and discovered that medicine was not difficult to learn if one does not have to diagnose and treat patients. I became familiar with the vocabulary and understood the rudiments of the complex clinical problems. I was occasionally asked to comment on a problem and, from clumsy beginnings, I grew more confident that what I said could be heard in those settings.[46] In the mid-1970s, several other bioethicists immersed themselves in clinical settings: John Fletcher was at the NIH Clinical Center, George Kanoti at the Cleveland Clinic, Ruth Macklin at several New York hospitals, and Terrance Ackerman was at St. Jude's Children's Research Hospital in Memphis. The NIH-funded project, Philosophers in Medical Centers, began in 1976.[47]

Philosophers and theologians were gingerly stepping into the clinical setting, but few were clear about exactly what their place was among the physicians, nurses, residents, and medical students, as they visited the bedsides of patients on morning rounds or met in conferences to discuss their care. Certainly, the ethicists had no clinical expertise and, in the beginning, they had no skill at turning their theoretical knowledge about utilitarianism and deontology into practical advice that the team caring for the patient could use. Yet, they accommodated themselves to the clinical setting and began to participate in its discourse. Most of the hospitals where bioethicists were situated were teaching hospitals, and in such places, the clinical discourse about patient care is, inevitably, teaching. So bioethicists began to teach there, together with the medical and nursing faculty who presided over the clinics.

Dr. Mark Siegler of the Pritzker School of Medicine, University of Chicago, used the phrase "clinical ethics" in a 1978 article, "The legacy of Osler: teaching clinical ethics at the bedside" (Joseph Fletcher may have invented the phrase).[48] The term "clinical ethics" masks an ambiguity. It can refer either to the incorporation of explicit ethical considerations in physicians' decisions about patient care or to the ethical interpretation and analysis of clinical decisions. In the first sense, only physicians or other clinicians "do" clinical ethics; in the second, other persons, such as philosophers or theologians, participate in shaping and criticizing clinical decisions. This latter activity constitutes ethics consultation, an activity that became increasingly common in the late 1970s.

In *Clinical Ethics* (1982) Mark Siegler, William Winslade, and I defined clinical ethics as "the identification, analysis and resolution of moral problems that arise in the care of a particular patient. . . . Clinical ethics is inextricably linked to the physician's primary task, deciding on and carrying out the best clinical care for a particular individual in a particular set of circumstances."[49] We attempted to bring the general ethical considerations that were being shaped in the growing literature of bioethics into the regular decision-making of physicians caring for patients. Printed in a format that could be slipped into the pocket of the clinician's white coat, *Clinical Ethics* proposed a method of analysis that was closer, we felt, to the reasoning of clinicians than to the speculations of philosophers. Dr. Robert Petersdorf, a leading medical educator, contributed the preface. Remarking that most books on ethics are too theoretical for the practical needs of physicians, he commented: "This little book handles ethical problems in medicine quite differently. Jointly authored by an ethicist, a clinician and a lawyer, it attacks ethical problems in real life terms. . . . The advice the authors give is consonant with good common sense, generally accepted ethical teachings, and legal statutes."[50] We were pleased by Dr. Petersdorf's accolade, but we knew how difficult it was to forge advice that was practical and consonant with common sense, ethics, and law. This was the task all clinical ethics consultants took upon themselves.

In 1985, John Fletcher and I sponsored a meeting in Washington, D.C., at which some fifty active consultants convened and agreed to form an association, The Society for Bioethics Consultation. At that meeting, Lawrence McCullough made a remark that summed up the challenge of the clinical ethicist: "I was educated as a philosopher, whose goal is to show how complex simple questions are: that is just what clinicians do not want to hear!" The daily work of ethics consultation was vividly described by a journalist who followed bioethicist Ruth Macklin on her rounds and conferences in the affiliated hospitals of New York's Albert Einstein College of Medicine. The cover article in *The New York Times Magazine* described in detail Dr. Macklin's skillful participation in the discussions of physicians and nurses and families over agonizing cases. While some physicians failed to appreciate the value of this work, most were eager to avail themselves of the lucidity and logic of Macklin's discourse. One of those physicians is quoted: "The more you hang out with people like Ruth, the more you see the value of turning something over and over. You'll still make errors, but maybe less serious ones."[51]

Community Discourse

The phrase "society must decide" was often heard in the conferences and commissions where bioethical questions were raised, yet no mechanism existed to elicit the decisions of society about major ethical issues. In the early 1980s, a concerted effort to engage ordinary people in life and death decisions was made in Oregon. The state had suffered a severe economic depression and many of its residents had lost health insurance coverage. A Governor's Conference on Health Care for the Medically Poor was convened by a state agency, the Oregon Health Council. The discussions at the conference stimulated the creation of a nonprofit educational foundation called Oregon Health Decisions. Led by a Portland, Oregon, physician, Dr. Ralph Crawshaw, and a bioethicist, Dr. Michael Garland, the foundation raised funds, recruited and trained volunteers, made contacts with various health agencies, and reached into communities through existing organizations such as Rotary Clubs, Chambers of Commerce, and churches. A two-day workshop trained volunteers in the major bioethical issues, and during the next six months, these volunteers, together with staff, conducted some three hundred meetings involving some five thousand Oregonians.

The participants, drawn from a wide spectrum of Oregon's citizens, discussed issues such as the autonomy of patients, care at the end of life, access to health care, and allocation of resources. The discussions were aimed toward conclusions that would reflect the values of the participants. A Citizens' Health Care Parliament of citizen representatives was held in October 1984, to review the community reports and to prepare a comprehensive final report. Oregon Health Decisions inspired considerable enthusiasm among the public, which felt that its process had focused "disparate medical, technical, social, ethical, economic and psychological issues into an understandable community consensus from which public policy can develop."[52] The experiment was replicated in other states with funding from the Prudential Foundation and other sources.

Oregon Health Decisions' deliberations did not remain inert. Several years after the conclusion of the project, the state legislature, faced with a decision about funding expensive organ transplantation, sought community consultation and in the succeeding years, initiated the most ambitious program for public contribution to health policy that the nation had seen.[53] That story lies beyond the bounds of this history but the concerted effort to create a "peoples' bioethics" reveals a feature of bioethics that the academic and professional viewpoint often misses. Theories and principles often fail to capture the values held by the public. When provided the opportunity, and with some prompting, people express those values and thus provide the moral basis for policy and decision. Philosopher Jonathan Moreno, commenting on the Oregon process, says, "This project . . . falls into a tradition in recent liberal political philosophy that can be associated with John Dewey. Dewey was strongly influenced by town meeting democracy. . . . Community consultation is arguably a requirement of liberal democracy, so that members of the polity have the opportunity to express themselves on substantive moral questions, the answers to which are certain to affect them."[54]

Movements as Discourse

American life is filled with movements. The abolition movement, the temperance movement, the women's suffrage movement, the labor movement, and many others, were causes powerful enough to enlist the enthusiasm and energy of many persons to change social institutions. Movements are not political parties or legal entities or organizations; they transcend these structures, using them as they see fit to attain their ends. Movements are great cascades of public discourse that rush toward public policy. People caught in those cascades—and even those who stand beside them—learn much about the cause, its rationale, and its aims. Although one occasionally hears the phrase "bioethics movement," the phrase is hyperbole: bioethics has shown nothing like the power and persuasiveness of the great American movements. Still, two genuine movements have contributed to bioethics: the patients' rights movement and the women's rights movement.

It is difficult to generate a movement on behalf of patients' rights. Patients are too transitory to become deeply engaged in being patients, and most people who have been patients would prefer to forget rather than perpetuate the experience. Nonetheless, some persons, particularly those with chronic conditions, and their families, have formed organizations that advocate for their better treatment and place in health care and in society. During the debates over the Baby Doe rules, the National Association for Handicapped Persons raised its voice and had a place at the legislative conference that fashioned the rules. Persons with HIV/AIDS have also formed remarkably effective organizations.

No movement on behalf of patients' rights emerged until the National Welfare Rights Organization (NWRO), which was formed during the 1960s as a grass-roots advocacy group for persons on welfare, took up the issue. NWRO influenced the policies of President Johnson's War on Poverty. When, in 1969, the Joint Commission on Accreditation of Hospitals (JCHO) invited the public to suggest changes in the standards for hospital accreditation, NWRO responded (perhaps to the dismay of JCHO). In the confrontational manner popular in the 1960s, NWRO forwarded twenty-six demands for changes that would protect the rights of patients. They insisted on grievance procedures for patients with complaints against hospitals, representation of patients on hospital boards, nondiscrimination, and prompt response to a call for nursing assistance. Some of these demands found their way into the JCHO accreditation manual.

In 1972, the American Hospital Association adopted a Patients' Bill of Rights. This document guaranteed, among other things, respectful care, information, privacy, and a problem irritatingly familiar to most patients, the right to an explanation of their bills. During the next few years, many states incorporated these rights into health legislation or regulation. Hospitals printed the Bill of Rights in brochures provided to patients on admission and proudly exhibited these brochures to the JCHO accreditation teams. Otherwise, the Patients' Bill of Rights was hardly a revolutionary document. It was, in fact, something of a moral fraud, for the rights contained therein were not wrest from a tyrant by an aroused and offended people but were defined and granted by *noblesse oblige,* with a content, extent, and duration at the will of the grantor. Dr. Willard Gaylin of The Hastings Center harshly criticized the Patients' Bill of Rights, describing it as "the thief lecturing his victim on self-protection." The Bill of Rights, he said, was nothing more than hospitals returning to patients the legal rights that hospitals had previously stolen from them.[55]

Uninspiring as the Patients' Bill of Rights was, it contained the germ of a bioethical dispute. One of its provisions guaranteed the "right to refuse treatment to the extent permitted by law." The extent permitted by law was not entirely clear in 1974; the leading court cases were yet to come and the recommendations of the President's Commission regarding the autonomy of patients were almost a decade in the future. The Patients' Bill of Rights, perhaps unwittingly, granted a right about which there would be much bioethical discourse and legal argument. A second seed of dispute lay in the very title, "Bill of Rights." In the United States, the Bill of Rights protects individual states and individual citizens from intrusions by the federal government. Other bills of rights, which proliferate in every part of American life, not only declare the rights of the parties that issue them but also set those parties apart from others, drawing lines over which each party must not step. While hospitals, as increasingly powerful organizations, needed limits set to their power over those who were their often unwilling and vulnerable inhabitants, doctors had always thought of themselves as being the friends and guardians of their patients. Although the Patients' Bill of Rights spoke to the hospital directly, many doctors heard its provisions as an accusation against them. Paul Starr writes: "[Patients' rights] raised radical questions about the prerogatives of the doctor's role. Implicit was a belief that the interests of doctors and patients frequently diverged and hence that patients needed protection. . . . Some doctors did not appreciate this signal of distrust."[56] This reading of patients' rights as moral entitlements against their doctors' authoritarianism and paternalism became a common notion in the discourse of bioethics.

The feminist movement had a dynamism and consistency that the patients' rights movement lacked. Through the 1950s, many women expressed discontent with the role of contented wife and mother as defined by post-World War II America. Women who had been employed in the war effort found themselves the first to be fired in favor of returning men. The worlds of higher education and careers which opened to male veterans still discriminated against women. Women who participated in great numbers in the movement for racial equality wondered whether they themselves were unequal. Betty Friedan's *Feminine Mystique*, published in 1963, gave voice to these stirrings. She chose her title to give a "name for whatever it was that kept us from using our rights, that made us feel guilty about anything we did not as our husband's wives . . . but as people. . . . All the things that kept [women] from being full people in our society would have to be changed."[57]

Among the things that needed to be changed was the culture of health care. Over half the patients who visited doctors were women; doctors were overwhelmingly male. The predominant providers of hospital care were women nurses who were subordinate in authority and economics to male doctors. Many women, reflecting on the quality of their care, came to believe that they were being denied information and participation and, worse, that their needs were being defined from an exclusively male viewpoint. Reproduction, sexuality, and the physical and physiological gender differences were particularly sensitive areas. Childbirth had become medicalized; bearing a baby was not a disease, as it had been made to appear by modern obstetrics. Most women who sought abortions, which was generally illegal until 1973, were put at great medical risk.

Some women took matters into their own hands. In 1969, the Chicago Women's Liberation Union organized a referral service for abortion and trained laywomen and nurses to do the procedure. In the same year, a group of Boston women formed a discussion group to educate themselves about women's health problems. They decided that women had to be able "to do something about doctors who were condescending, paternalistic, judgmental and non-informative." The group evolved into the Boston Women's Health Book Collective and published *Our Bodies, Our Selves*, a compendium of information and advice about gynecology, sexuality, reproduction, and other health issues.[58] The book became a bestseller and inspired many women and women's groups to take a more assertive role in their own health care. The value of autonomy, which theoretical bioethics extolled, was made real. At the same time, the concern and cooperation of women working together for their collective good foreshadowed another value that bioethics had yet to discover—"the ethics of caring."

In 1983, Harvard professor of educational psychology Carol Gilligan published a book that would greatly influence academic thought about moral reasoning and gently push moral philosophy in fresh directions. *In a Different Voice* proposed that the moral understanding and attitudes of women developed differently from those of men.[59] Women value caring and the fostering of relationships; men value justice and freely entered agreements. These fundamental differences in moral perception inspire quite different moral perspectives for the genders. The application of Gilligan's thesis to bioethics was first noted by those working in nursing ethics, but soon the ethics of caring began to be mentioned as a balance to the ethics of autonomy, which had dominated bioethics. In the years beyond the borders of this history, many women working in bioethics brought these feminist perspectives into the mainstream.⁶⁰

Media Bioethics

This history has been filled with references to news stories (and would be filled with references to television were that media not so ephemeral). The life of bioethics in the United States is recorded in such stories. Many of the news stories in the 1970s, such as the events at Tuskegee, Willowbrook, and the Jewish Chronic Disease Hospital, were exposés of scandals. The next generations of stories, such as the tragedies of Karen Ann Quinlan, Baby Doe, Baby Fae, and Barney Clark, were exposés of the dilemmas of technology. Arthur Caplan, the current face and voice of bioethics in the media, contends that the agenda of bioethics has been set by the media: after the scandals and exposés, the bioethicists appeared with their comments and criticisms. There may be some truth to this view, but it is equally plausible to assert that the media events merely punctuated a flow of discourse that was already moving; the concern over life-support, expressed by Dr. Haid to Pope Pius XII predated the Karen Ann Quinlan case, the Artificial Heart Panel deliberated before Barney Clark's operation. Yet, the events that elicit heart-wrenching sympathy, startling astonishment, or morbid fascination may provide more momentum to public discourse than does philosophical speculation about the moral questions raised by technological advances in contemporary society—Congress would not have created the National Commission apart from the outrage over the Tuskegee Study and the fetal research in Helsinki.

The media have not only publicized bioethics by showcasing its events. The media have also shaped the perception of bioethics' practitioners, both for themselves and for the public, as experts in an area where expertise is difficult to justify. According to Caplan, "Bioethicists are torn in two directions. The public face of bioethics makes Americans nervous because they dislike ethical experts. The bioethicists being put in the role of experts are nervous because they know that there cannot be expertise without theory or without consensus about the foundations of the field."⁶¹ And inevitably, given the instantaneous nature of media, the serious and sustained discourse necessary for deliberation about moral issues is chopped into fragments; the sound-bites that bedevil politicians have also demeaned bioethics.

Nevertheless, media, particularly television, have contributed to the education of the public and to public discourse about bioethical dilemmas. Several Public Broadcasting System productions have presented these dilemmas in dramatic ways. One of the first of these was an excellent series, "Hard Choices," produced by Seattle's KCTS/TV, the University of Washington's PBS station and shown nationally in 1981. "Hard Choices" was written and directed by a young woman, Sandy Walker, who was so captivated by the issues that she left a promising media career to enter the University of Washington

School of Medicine. Another influential series was "Managing Our Miracles," produced by Fred Friendly, in which he and Harvard law professor Arthur Miller quizzed and cross-examined panels of experts from various fields on the tough questions of bioethics. Programs such as these contributed to the public discourse of bioethics.

Conclusion

Bioethics has grown both as a discipline and as a public discourse, and both are intricately related to each other. The public discourse provides the subject matter for the discipline of bioethics: while we often point to the new science and technology as the cause of bioethics, it is actually the discourse about the uses of science and technology—the differing views and values about human life that informs individual and social judgment about those innovations—that gives rise to bioethics. When the public discourse, initiated in the conferences of the 1960s, was transported into government forums and classrooms, it was subjected to more stringent intellectual analysis with a view toward the formation of public policy and a teachable curriculum. The discipline and the discourse exist in synergy, and both draw their vigor from the surrounding ethos of American culture. The concluding chapter of this history will forage in the vast fields of the American ethos for hints about why bioethics grew and flourished in the United States.

Notes for Chapter 11

1. Jay Katz, "Disclosure and consent in psychiatric practice: mission impossible?" in Charles K. Hofling (ed.), *Law and Ethics in the Practice of Psychiatry* (New York: Brunner/Mazel, 1980), pp. 91–117, quote on p. 98; Martin S. Pernick, "The patient's role in medical decision-making: a social history of informed consent in medical therapy," in President's Commission for the Study of Ethical Problems in Medicine and Biomedical and Behavioral Research, *Making Health Care Decisions*, vol. 3 (Washington, D.C.: U.S. Government Printing Office, 1983), pp. 1–35, quote on p. 3. See also Jay Katz, *The Silent World of Doctor and Patient* (New York: Free Press, 1984); Ruth R. Faden and Tom L. Beauchamp, *A History and Theory of Informed Consent* (New York: Oxford University Press, 1986).
2. Plato, *Laws* IV, 720.
3. Hippocrates, *Precepts*, IX.
4. Hippocrates, *Decorum*, XVI.
5. Lateran IV, ch. 23, in Henry Denzinger and Adolf Schoenmetzer, *Enchiridion Symbolorum Definitionum et Declarationum de Rebus Fidei et Morum* (Rome and New York: Herder, 1965), 815.
6. Thomas Percival, "Notes and illustrations," in Chauncey Leake (ed.), *Percival's Medical Ethics* (Baltimore: Williams and Wilkins, 1927), p. 194; Percival is arguing against his friend, Reverend Thomas Gisborne. The prominent medical moralist of the early 17th century, Rodrigo a Castro, presents an elaborate defense of the therapeutic privilege in *Medicus Politicus* (Hamburg, 1614), III, 9. Dr. Worthington Hooker refutes Percival in "Truth in our intercourse with the

sick," *Physician and Patient* (New York: Baker and Scribner, 1849), ch xvii. See also Richard Cabot, "Truth and falsity in medicine," *American Medicine* 5 (1903): 344–349.

7. James Boswell, *Boswell's Life of Johnson* (London and New York: Henry Frowde, 1904), vol. II, p. 560. Johnson said this exactly six months before the day he died; Percival quotes the good doctor only to dismiss his complaint. See *Percival's Medical Ethics*, p. 183.

8. *Schloendorff v Society of New York Hospitals* 211 NY 125 105 N.E. 92 (1914). Despite Justice Cardozo's eloquent language, Mrs. Schloendorff, who had had a fibroid tumor removed after having given consent only for an exploratory operation, lost her case.

9. *Salgo v Leland Stanford Jr. University* 317 P 2nd 170 Cal 1st Dist Ct. App. (1957).

10. *Natanson v Kline*, 186 Kan 392, 350 P.2d 1093 (1960).

11. *Canterbury v Spence*, 464 F 2d 772 (DC Cir 1972). A California case, *Cobbs v Grant*, and a Rhode Island case, *Wilkenson v Vesey*, were decided in the same year and affirmed the same principle. See *Cobbs v Grant* 8 Cal. 3d 229, 502 P.2d 1, 104 Cal.reptr. 505 (1972). On the evolution of the legal concept, see Marjorie M. Shultz, "From informed consent to patient choice: a new protected right," *The Yale Law Review* 95 (1985): 219–295 and Faden and Beauchamp, *A History and Theory of Informed Consent*, chapter 4.

12. Principle 1 of *The Nuremberg Code, Trials of War Criminals before the Nuremberg Military Tribunals Under Council Control Law No. 10,* Vol. 2 (Washington, D.C.: U.S. Government Printing Office, 1949), pp. 181–182.

13. Hans Jonas, "Philosophical reflections on experimentation with human subjects," *Daedalus* 98 (1969): 236.

14. John C. Fletcher, "Realities of patient consent to medical research," *Hastings Center Report* 1 (1973): 39–49, quote on p. 41. The article originally appeared as "Human experimentation: ethics in the consent situation," *Law and Contemporary Problems* 34 (1967): 620–649, and was based on his Union Theological Seminary doctoral dissertation.

15. Jay Katz, "Reservations about Panel Report on Charge I," *Final Report of the Tuskegee Syphilis Study Ad Hoc Advisory Panel* (Washington, D.C.: U.S. Public Health Service, 1973), reprinted in Stanley Joel Reiser, Arthur J. Dyck, and William J. Curran (eds.), *Ethics in Medicine* (Cambridge, Mass.: The MIT Press, 1977), p. 320.

16. Paul Ramsey, *The Patient as Person: Explorations in Medical Ethics* (New Haven: Yale University Press, 1970), pp. 2, 5, 6, 11.

17. Robert M. Veatch, "Three theories of informed consent: philosophical foundations and policy implications," in National Commission for the Protection of Human Subjects of Biomedical and Behavioral Research, *The Belmont Report: Ethical Principles and Guidelines for the Protection of Human Subjects of Research*, Appendix II, pp. 1–56, quote on p. 26.

18. President's Commission, *Making Health Care Decisions*, p. 36.

19. Jay Katz, "Limping is no sin: reflections on making health care decisions," *Cardozo Law Review* 6 (1984): 243–266, pp. 243, 266.

20. Katz, *The Silent World of Doctor and Patient*; see also Jay Katz, "Informed consent: a fairy tale? Law's vision." *University of Pittsburgh Law Review* 39 (1977): 144.

21. *American Medical Times* (February 2, 1861), pp. 82–83, cited in Annette Dula, "Teaching Medical Ethics: A Study in Applied Philosophy," Ed.D. dissertation, Harvard University, 1987, p. 29.

22. In the 1920s, Dr. Park White, Professor of Pediatrics at Washington University, St. Louis, instituted what may have been one of the first modern ethics courses, giving seven lectures on the AMA Code, advertising, honesty, medical finances, physician etiquette, quacks, eugenics, euthanasia, and birth control. See Park J. White, "A course in professional conduct," *Journal of the American Medical Association* 88 (1927): 1751, cited in Dula, "Teaching Medical Ethics," p. 30. See also Arthur Dean Bevan, "The need of teaching medical ethics," *Journal of the American*

Medical Association 88 (1927): 617–619; Chester R. Burns, "Medical ethics and jurisprudence," in Ronald L. Numbers (ed.), *The Education of American Physicians: Historical Essays* (Berkeley: University of California Press, 1980), pp. 273–289; Carleton B. Chapman, "On the definition and teaching of the medical ethnic," *New England Journal of Medicine* 301 (1979): 630–636.

23. Robert M. Veatch, "National survey of the teaching of medical ethics," in Veatch, Willard Gaylin, and Councilman Morgan (eds.), *The Teaching of Medical Ethics* (Hastings-on-Hudson: Institute of Society, Ethics, and the Life Sciences, 1973), pp. 97–102.

24. Robert Veatch, personal interview, Oct. 25, 1995.

25. Susan M. Kegeles, Albert R. Jonsen, and Andrew Jameton, "A course for senior medical students in the responsibilities of medical practice," *Journal of Medical Education* 60 (1985): 876–878; Albert R. Jonsen, "Medical ethics teaching programs at the University of California, San Francisco, and the University of Washington," *Academic Medicine* 64 (1989): 718–722.

26. Robert M. Veatch and Sharmon Sollitto, "Medical ethics teaching: report of a national survey," *Journal of the American Medical Association* 235 (1976): 1030–1033.

27. Janet Bickel (ed.), *Integrating Human Values Teaching Programs into Medical Students' Clinical Education: Project Report to AAMC* (Washington, D.C.: AAMC, 1986); T. K. McElhinney and E. D. Pellegrino (eds.), *The Humanities and Human Values in Medical Schools: A Ten Year Overview* (Washington, D.C.: Society for Health and Human Values, 1982); Steven H. Miles, Laura Weiss Lane, Janet Bickel, Robert M. Walker, and Christine Cassel, "Medical ethics education: coming of age," *Academic Medicine* 64 (1989): 705–714.

28. Edmund D. Pellegrino, "Medical ethics, education and the physician's image," *Journal of the American Medical Association* 235 (1976): 1043–1044.

29. Albert R. Jonsen and Charles Culver, "Teaching of bioethics in medical school," in *The Teaching of Bioethics: Report of the Commission on the Teaching of Bioethics* (Hastings-on-Hudson: Institute of Society, Ethics and the Life Sciences, 1976), pp. 25–31.

30. C. M. Culver, D. K. Clouser, B. Gert, H. Brody, J. Fletcher, A. Jonsen, L. Kopelman, J. Lynn, M. Siegler, and D. Wikler, "Basic curricular goals in medical ethics," *New England Journal of Medicine* 312 (1985): 253–256.

31. Mark Siegler, A. G. Rezler, and K. J. Connel, "Using simulated case studies to evaluate a clinical ethics course for junior students," *Journal of Medical Education* 57 (1982): 380–385; Donnie J. Self, F. D. Walinsky, and D. C. Baldwin, "The effect of teaching medical ethics on medical students' moral reasoning," *Academic Medicine* 64 (1989): 755–759; Albert R. Jonsen and Andrew Jameton, "Evaluation of curriculum in medical ethics in schools of medicine: report to the National Endowment for the Humanities and the Josiah Macy Jr. Foundation," (NEH-C-80-12, 1983, unpublished).

32. Donnie J. Self and Evi Davenport, "Measurement of moral development in medicine," in Albert R. Jonsen (ed.), *Honesty in Learning, Fairness in Teaching: The Problem of Academic Dishonesty in Medical Education* (New York: Josiah Macy, Jr., Foundation, 1995), pp. 42–51. See also D. Baldwin, S. Daugherty, and D. J. Self, "Changes in moral reasoning during medical school," *Academic Medicine* 66, Suppl. (1991): 51–53.

33. Edmund D. Pellegrino, Richard J. Hart, Sharon R. Henderson, Stephen E. Loeb, and Gary Edwards, "Relevance and utility of courses in medical ethics," *Journal of the American Medical Association* 253 (1985): 49–53, quotes on pp. 49, 50, 51.

34. Subcommittee on Evaluation of Humanistic Qualities in the Internist, "Evaluation of humanistic qualities in the internist," *Annals of Internal Medicine* 99 (1983): 720–724; American Board of Internal Medicine, *A Guide to Awareness and Evaluation of Humanistic Qualities in the Internist* (Philadelphia: American Board of Internal Medicine, 1985); Jay A. Jacobson, Susan W. Tolle, Carol Stocking, and Mark Siegler, "Internal medicine residents' preferences regarding medical ethics education," *Academic Medicine* 64 (1989): 760–764; Steven A. Wartman and Dan

W. Brock, "The development of a medical ethics curriculum in a general internal medicine residency program," *Academic Medicine* 64 (1989): 751–754. For examples of other specialties, see Joanna M. Cain, Thomas Elkins, and Paul F. Bernard, "The Status of Ethics Education in Obstetrics and Gynecology," *Obstetrics and Gynecology* 83, no. 2 (1994), pp. 315–320; American Board of Pediatrics, Medical Ethics Subcommittee, "Teaching and evaluation of interpersonal skills and ethical decisionmaking in pediatrics," *Pediatrics* 79 (1987): 829–833.

35. "Ethical and religious directives," *Linacre Quarterly* 15 (July–October 1949): 1–9; revised in 1955 and 1971.

36. Karen Teel, "The physician's dilemma: a doctor's view: what the law should be," *Baylor Law Review* 27 (1975): 6–10; discussed in *In The Matter of Quinlan*, 70 N.J. 10, 355 A.2d 647 (1976), pp. 668–669.

37. *Superintendent of Belchertown State School v Saikewicz*, 373 Mass. 728, 370 NE.2d 417 (1977).

38. *In re Colyer*, 99 Wn.2d 114, 660 P.2d 738 (1983).

39. Stuart J. Youngner, David L. Jackson, Claudia Coulton, et al., "A national survey of hospital ethics committees," in President's Commission for the Study of Ethical Problems in Medicine and Biomedical and Behavioral Research, *Deciding to Forego Life-Sustaining Treatment: A Report on the Ethical, Medical, and Legal Issues in Treatment Decisions*, Appendix F (Washington, D.C.: U.S. Government Printing Office, 1983), pp. 443–449, quote on p. 448. The survey was also published in *Critical Care Medicine* 11 (1983): 902–905.

40. Mary Beth Prosnitz, "A model bill to establish hospital ethics committees," in President's Commission, *Deciding to Forego Life-Sustaining Treatment*, Appendix F, pp. 439–442.

41. "Ethics committees double since '83," *Hospitals* 59 (1985): 60, 64.

42. M. B. West and Joan Gibson, "Facilitating medical ethics case review: what an ethics committee can learn from mediation and facilitation techniques," *Cambridge Quarterly of Health Care Ethics* 1 (1992): 63–74.

43. Stuart J. Youngner, Claudia Coulton, Barbara W. Juknialis, and David L. Jackson, "Patients' attitudes toward hospital ethics committees," *Law, Medicine, Health Care* 12 (1984): 21–25; Richard A. McCormick, "Ethics committees: promise or peril?" *Law, Medicine, and Health Care* 12 (1984): 150–155; Jonathan D. Moreno, *Deciding Together: Bioethics and Moral Consensus* (New York: Oxford University Press, 1995).

44. In 1993, Judith Ross and her colleagues estimated that 4,000 ethics committees functioned in all sorts of institutions, but they found little information about their activities and their efficacy. Judith Wilson Ross, et al., *Health Care Ethics Committees: The Next Generation* (Chicago: American Hospital Publishing Co., 1993).

45. Bernard Lo, "Behind closed doors," *New England Journal of Medicine* 317 (1987): 46–49.

46. Albert R. Jonsen, "Can an ethicist be a consultant?" in Virginia Abernathy (ed.), *Frontiers in Medical Ethics: Applications in a Medical Setting*, (Cambridge, Mass.: Ballinger, 1980), pp. 157–171; "Watching the doctor," *New England Journal of Medicine* 308 (1983): 1531–1535.

47. William Ruddick (ed.), *Philosophers in Medical Centers* (New York: The Society for Philosophy and Public Affairs, 1980).

48. Mark Siegler, "The legacy of Osler: teaching clinical ethics at the bedside," *Journal of the American Medical Association* 293 (1978): 951; Mark Siegler, "Clinical ethics and clinical medicine," *Archives of Internal Medicine* 139 (1979): 914. In a 1976 commencement address at the University of Minnesota School of Medicine, Fletcher said that physicians preferred his method of "clinical ethics," or deciding the ethics on a case by case basis, to the more abstract "rule ethics." See John C. Fletcher and Howard Brody, "Clinical ethics," in Warren T. Reich (ed.), *Encyclopedia of Bioethics*, revised ed. (New York: Simon and Schuster, 1995), vol. I, p. 399.

49. Albert R. Jonsen, Mark Siegler, and William J. Winslade, *Clinical Ethics*, 1st ed. (New York: Macmillan Publishing Company, 1982), pp. 2–3.

50. Robert G. Petersdorf, "Foreword," in Jonsen et al., *Clinical Ethics*, p. vii.

51. Katherine Bouton, "Painful decisions: the role of the medical ethicist," *New York Times*, August 5, 1990, 65; Ruth Macklin, *Mortal Choices: Ethical Dilemmas in Modern Medicine* (Boston: Houghton-Mifflin, 1987).

52. Ralph Crawshaw, Michael Garland, Brian Hines, and Caroline Lobitz, "Oregon Health Decisions: an experiment with community informed consent," *Journal of the American Medical Association* 254 (1985): 3213–3216, p. 3215; Ralph Crawshaw and Michael Garland, *Society Must Decide: Ethics and Health Care Choices in Oregon* (Salem: Oregon Health Decisions, 1985).

53. Charles J. Dougherty, "Setting health care priorities: Oregon's next steps. A conference report," *Hastings Center Report* 21, no. 3 (1991): S1–S10; David C. Hadorn, "The Oregon priority-setting exercise: quality of life and public policy," *Hastings Center Report* 21, no. 3 (1991): S11–S16.

54. Moreno, *Deciding Together*, p. 70.

55. Willard Gaylin, cited in William J. Curran, "The patients' bill of rights becomes law," *New England Journal of Medicine* 290 (1974): 32–33. See George J. Annas, *The Rights of Hospital Patients: The Basic ACLU Guide to Hospital Patient's Rights* (New York: Discus Books, 1975), revised in 1989; Annas and Joseph M. Healey, Jr., "The patient rights advocate: redefining the doctor–patient relationship in the hospital context," *Vanderbilt Law Review* 27 (1974): 243–269.

56. Paul Starr, *The Social Transformation of American Medicine* (New York: Basic Books, 1982), p. 390.

57. Betty Friedan, *The Feminine Mystique,* cited in John Blum, *Years of Discord* (New York: W.W. Norton, 1991), p. 275.

58. Boston Women's Health Book Collective, *Our Bodies, Our Selves* (New York: Simon and Schuster, 1973), revised in 1976 and 1992.

59. Carol Gilligan, *In a Different Voice: Psychological Theory and Women's Development* (Cambridge: Harvard University Press, 1982). See also Nel Noddings, *Caring: A Feminine Approach to Ethics and Moral Education* (Berkeley: University of California Press, 1984).

60. Susan Sherwin, *No Longer Patient: Feminist Ethics and Health Care* (Philadelphia: Temple University, 1992); Helen Bequaert Holmes and Laura M. Purdy (eds.), *Feminist Perspectives in Medical Ethics* (Bloomington: Indiana University Press, 1992); Susan M. Wolf (ed.), *Feminism and Bioethics: Beyond Reproduction* (New York: Oxford University Press, 1996).

61. Caplan, "What bioethics brought to the public," (paper read at the Birth of Bioethics Conference, Seattle, Wa., Sept. 23–24, 1992), transcript, p. 519.

12

Bioethics—American and Elsewhere

The story of bioethics that we have told is largely an American one. Apart from several brief visits to Great Britain for the Ciba conferences and the birth of Baby Louise Brown, and a trip to Australia to investigate the way they treat embryos "down under," we have dwelt largely within U.S. borders. But of course, bioethics does not exist only in the United States. In 1997, as this book is being written, there is an International Association of Bioethics, whose founders were Australian bioethicists. The Council for International Organizations of Medical Sciences (CIOMS), associated with the World Health Organization and UNESCO, has demonstrated interest in bioethics for many years and has issued international guidelines on many topics, including transplantation, the definition of death, and human research. Since 1985, the Council of Europe has had a Committee of Experts on Bioethical Issues which, with wide international consultation, composed a *Convention for Bioethics* containing guidelines on major bioethical issues. UNESCO formed an International Bioethics Committee in 1993. The European Community and its legislative arm, the European Parliament, have formulated bioethics policy and sponsored bioethical studies. Centers and institutes of bioethics exist worldwide, from Bonn to Beijing and from Bangkok to Buenos Aires. The 1994 UNESCO Directory lists 498 such centers outside the United States.[1] The second edition of the *Encyclopedia of Bioethics*, published in 1995, contains many articles on historical, theoretical, and practical bioethics around the world in different nations and cultures.[2] Clearly, bioethics is a worldwide phenomenon. And yet, in Dan Callahan's words, "Bioethics is a native grown American product, which did emerge elsewhere but finds uniquely fertile ground in the U.S."[3] This chapter briefly reviews bioethics elsewhere and then asks why it grows the way it has in the United States.

Bioethics Outside the U.S.

International bioethics began more than a decade after the birth of bioethics in the United States.[4] American bioethicists once naively thought that the bioethical seeds that sprouted in the United States had wafted across borders and taken root in other nations. It soon became clear that bioethics in other societies is, if not a different species, certainly a varietal. The review which follows concentrates on bioethics in continental Europe.

The word "bioethics" is found in the titles of organizations, committees, conferences, and publications throughout the world. It is not, however, universally loved. To Europeans speaking the romance languages, the American neologism suggests an ethics based on biology, implying an unacceptable moral materialism. French, Italian, and Spanish scholars prefer terms such as *éthique biomédicale,* or *etica biomedica* or, at best, *bioética médica.*[5] The word has an even more sinister meaning in Germany, where some understand it as "an uncritical and ideological defense of any biotechnology . . . or on a par with a dangerous pro-euthanasia movement."[6] Despite these dissents, which reflect linguistic and cultural differences, bioethics is now a generally accepted term for reflection, private and public, on the social implications of medicine and science.

The topics of that reflection are essentially the same across national boundaries, although emphases differ. Experimentation with human subjects is a universal concern. The Nazi research in concentration camps burned more deeply into the European conscience than it did into the American, although it may have been NIH Director Shannon's 1966 Policy and Procedure Order that stimulated the international establishment of committees to review research protocols.[7] Genetics and reproductive science is an issue everywhere: many policy statements from international bodies and a considerable body of national law, which is often quite restrictive, addresses these questions. A major project of the UNESCO International Bioethics Committee has been the preparation of an Universal Declaration of the Human Genome and Human Rights which proclaims the human genome to be "the common heritage of humanity," and proposes principles to guard against eugenic practices and discriminatory and bellicose uses.[8] The attention to genetics is even greater in Europe than it is in the United States, most probably because Nazi eugenic ideology brought disaster more terrible than did the rather mild eugenics movement in America. So much attention is paid to genetics and reproduction in European bioethics that one scholar commented that many people there think bioethics is synonymous with reproductive morality.[9] Care of the dying is also a universal issue, although the discussion of euthanasia takes a strikingly different form in different countries. The Netherlands' open debate and civil tolerance regarding assisted suicide contrasts with German reticence and even violent repudiation of debate.[10] The problem of allocation of scarce health resources is a common topic that looks very different in the developed countries, where the scarce resource is tax money to finance highly expensive health care, from that in Africa, South America, and Southeast Asia, where the most basic medical care and public health protection are absent. It is notable, for example, that Thailand's bioethics center is situated within the Center of Human Resource Development at Mahidol University, Bangkok.[11]

Although similar in name and concerns, bioethics outside the U.S. has origins, methods, and traditions that distinguish it from bioethics in the United States.[12] The origins of European bioethics are more closely associated with denominational religion and academic theology than are those of American bioethics. While theologians were attracted to bioethics in America, in Europe, Catholic and Protestant theological circles initiated the questions about the new medicine and science. Questions were formulated in the terms familiar to these religious traditions,[13] and until the late 1980s, all European bioethics centers were religiously affiliated. These origins, however, do not guarantee peaceful co-existence between religious and secular bioethics. Unlike the smooth integration seen in America (an integration that some criticize as an absorption), in Europe strongly felt differences divide bioethics based on theological premises from secular bioethics.[14] Similarly, European bioethics knows patterns of socialized health care that have never touched the United States. Many decades of universal availability of health care to the citizens of most European nations color views about the value of both persons and medicine. The ideal of solidarity, the communal responsibility to help those in need, has religious and socialist roots that pervade bioethical thinking across Europe. Solidarity is a European bioethical principle that has only a weak reflection in the American principle of justice.

Principles obviously have a place in the bioethical method wherever it is found. The standard principles of American bioethics, respect for autonomy, beneficence, nonmaleficence, and justice, are cited everywhere, perhaps because of the welcome given to foreign scholars at the Kennedy Institute where these principles were framed.[15] However, these principles are often criticized as inadequate and even inappropriate. European scholars have suggested alternatives: for example, liberty, therapeutic wholeness, and social subsidiarity.[16] Justice is often reinterpreted as solidarity. The principle of respect for the autonomy of persons particularly perplexes bioethicists outside the United States. They find the American interpretation of this Kantian notion peculiar. While bioethics everywhere aims at securing the rights of individuals in health care and rejects the medical paternalism that has often been even more oppressive in non-American cultures, the strong emphasis given to personal autonomy seems an exaggeration. It is, says Patrick Verspieren, "an excessive reaction against paternalism to give an absolute primacy to autonomy and to affirm that the sick person has the right to decide by himself his choices and the rules that should be applied to him." He believes that the American notion of autonomy, particularly as expressed by H. Tristram Engelhardt, is a way of absolving physicians of their responsibility for the sick.[17]

The problem with the American principles can be traced, according to many scholars, to the relative poverty of ethical theory in American bioethics. They praise Engelhardt, Veatch, and Pellegrino and Thomasma for their theoretical tentatives but judge them either misguided or inadequate. They hardly count as ethical theory the conventional Anglo-American duo of formalism and utilitarianism. They assert that an ethical theory must grow from an ontological or phenomenological theory of human nature. Modern European philosophy has a rich store of such reflection in the work of Paul Ricoeur, Jürgen Habermas, Karl Apel, and others. Spanish bioethicist Diego Gracia, for example, builds his clinical bioethics partly on the doctrine of his teacher Xavier Zubiri, who weaves an original personalism and phenomenology out of the strands of Husserl's and Scheler's thought, and partly on the historical interpretation of the medical relationship elaborated by his other teacher, Pedro Laín Entralgo.[18] In his view, only a deep and solid theory of human nature and human community, reflecting the human condition and its cultural history, can support ethical reflection about medicine, science, and health care. Gracia calls the American method "soft" because it relies only on strategic or tactical reasoning about the interests of individuals. The European method is "hard," seeking to "take account of the totality of the person implicated in the problem, who is himself obliged to include the totality of humanity."[19] These are theoretical realms unfamiliar to most American bioethicists.

Theory invades even the world of practical bioethics. The Comité Consultatif National d'Éthique Pour les Sciences de la Vie et de la Santé, established by President Mitterrand in 1983, has been prolific, issuing opinions on almost every topic in bioethics. Its members were persuaded from the beginning to undertake a method of deliberation based on the theories of Habermas and Apel, as interpreted by one of their members, philosopher Lucien Séve.[20] This method requires wide and deep reflection and dialogue with all concerned parties. As a result of this wide consultation and deep reflection the CCNE "is becoming an active center of public morality in the life of people."[21] As we have seen, the several American commissions worked without any explicit theoretical commitments.

The cultural, philosophical, and medical traditions that nurture American bioethics are notably different from their European counterparts; for example, European bioethics has distinctly theological origins. The religious morality behind the American ethos is the same Judeo-Christian morality that pervades European history but the horrifying religious wars of the seventeenth century left scars still unhealed in the European mentality. The Reformation created stark divisions not only between faiths but also between nations and regions occupied by the diverse faithful. The European Enlightenment inspired a disdain for religion and religious institutions quite unlike the Enlightenment ideas welcomed in America that sponsored a deism many Americans found compatible with organized religion. Europe's 19th century was an intellectual and political reprise of the religious military campaigns of the 17th century: the liberal and conservative movements were marked by deeply antagonistic religious and secular partisanship that their nominal American counterparts never felt. "The . . . issue that bioethics must face in Europe is its relationship with religious ethics," say several scholars.[22] This has not been a major issue in American bioethics where religious ethics and philosophical ethics have not only collaborated but have even melded in the formation of bioethics.

Other cultural traditions and historical experiences which serve as the background for ethical thought—what we will describe as "ethos" later in this chapter—are profoundly different. Those who came to the American colonies left behind a Europe disrupted by several centuries of almost continual warfare, as nation states and regimes established themselves. The devastating conflicts have left marks on the lands and cultures where they were waged. The French Revolution, fought not for religious or dynastic hegemony but for a moral cause, degenerated into a debacle from which the nation long struggled to salvage its worthy aims. Nazi, Fascist, and Communist ideologies have demolished freedoms and slaughtered millions. These experiences, which have no American analogue, with the exception, perhaps, of the Civil War, temper the European enthusiasm for new ventures, whereas the American ethos embraces innovation. Caution and protection from excess color the European ethical attitude. Even the philosophical literature that nourishes ethics reflects pessimism about the moral power of humanity. American moral philosophy has no counterparts to Schopenhauer, Kierkegaard, and Unamuno.

There are, then, many differences between the bioethics that was born in the United States and the bioethics that came into being elsewhere a decade or so later. We have looked almost exclusively at Europe. Asian and African bioethics is still more distinct, since cultural and religious traditions, as well social and economic conditions, are so different from those of the western world.[23] Yet, when the time comes to formulate transnational policy, remarkably broad consensus has been found among these diverse views. Grounds for agreement can often be found despite local emphases on certain values or local perceptions of the seriousness of certain problems. Statements of international groups on human experimentation, on genetics and reproductive science, and on the rights of patients and duties of governments to protect the health of their people, reflect quite similar values. Conferences that summon bioethicists from many nations give voice to many differences of opinion and perspective but frequently converge in their conclusions. Despite the common topics and the converging conclusions, however, we might still ask why bioethics began first in the United States and whether its American roots give it a particular vigor.

Bioethics and the Historians

At the Birth of Bioethics Conference, three medical historians, David Rothman, Daniel Fox, and Stanley Reiser, offered their interpretations of why bioethics was born in the United States.[24] All three historians suggested that the medical enterprise that grew so greatly in size, capability, and wealth had become the private domain of the professionals who had the knowledge and skill to use its technology. These professionals not only worked within that enterprise; they also dictated its directions, policies, and values. The many others who had interests in the enterprise—patients, the public, and the government—were excluded from decisions about directions, policies, and values. The title of

Rothman's book, *Strangers at the Bedside: How Law and Bioethics Transformed Medical Decision Making*, appropriately describes this situation, although it is often assumed that the bioethicists and lawyers are the strangers who appear in the patient's room with their unwanted advice. Rothman does designate these newcomers as strangers, but not until he has demonstrated how physicians themselves had become strangers to their patients: "the doctor had become a stranger . . . levels of trust had diminished . . . technology placed the doctor's hands more often on dials than on patients." The estrangement of physician from patient made room for others who had never before been parties to the medical relationship. These "outsiders to medicine" now "defined the social and ethical questions facing the profession and set forth the norms that should govern it."[25]

In Reiser's view, the technology that is the engine of the complex enterprise of health care increasingly absorbed the physician's attention. The power and potentiality of the machine defined the purposes of medicine. Subsequently, the values which the institution of medicine and health care should serve, and which patients expect, are diminished; the technology and its science dominate. These values must be regained with the help of persons who are not so thoroughly invested in the technologies. Only then will we direct the technology rather than the technology directing us.

Fox offered an intriguing analogy between the rise of bioethics and the movement for control of nuclear weapons, both of which occurred at the same time in American history. He saw the health care enterprise as an almost irresistible defense establishment in a cold war on disease: its "hawks" press for greater power and authority and incessantly build their arsenals, and the "doves" challenge those plans, not by militant opposition but by asserting values that are compelling within the wider society. Each of these historians sees bioethics as a response to the effects that technologized medicine has on the relation between patients and physicians and between medicine and society; patients become less than persons, partners in research become "subjects," the technological imperative drives the practice of medicine and shapes its institutions, and the masters of technology dictate decisions and policies.

This is a plausible view. Its plausibility is corroborated by the histories of particular bioethical issues related in previous chapters. Yet the interpretation must go further. Technologized medicine swept across the developed world and touched the shores of the underdeveloped world. Was its reception in the United States—with a warm embrace and a cautious bioethics—different from its reception in Europe, Latin America, Asia, and Africa? Why did the response take the form of an ethics? Why did the ethics assume the theoretical and methodological shape that it did? Why do the public and professional discourses follow the course that they do? Why did bioethics begin in the U.S. a decade or more before it appeared in other nations? Is the ethics, as discipline and as discourse, different in American bioethics from that in the bioethics existing elsewhere? At the Birth of Bioethics Conference, Dan Callahan added two reasons that move us closer to answering these questions. He suggested that "the emergence of bioethics dovetailed very nicely with the reigning political liberalism of the educated classes in America." He also proposed that "medicine, previously very much a closed world, was cracked open to public scrutiny by virtue of the large amounts of public money, of public interest and sometimes of scandals within medicine."[26] These two suggestions deserve reflection.

American Liberalism and Bioethics

Callahan knows, of course, how difficult it is to define liberalism but, in shorthand, he did so in terms of market system economy and an emphasis on individual freedom politically and culturally. The liberal tradition in America runs wide and deep, deeper than the rift between liberal and conservative that is common in contemporary parlance and wider than the meaning of liberalism in European political life. Louis Hartz's classic study, *The Liberal Tradition in America*, propounds the thesis that liberalism is marked indelibly by the founding fathers' dedication to Locke's interpretation of the social contract, which creates civil society by the consent of freely contracting individuals in a state of nature. Their contract was framed, not by what John Adams once described as "the canon and feudal law," but by self-evident principles of equality and individual rights.[27]

This original liberal vision, while it took democratic and Whiggish/republican, conservative and radical, populist, and capitalist forms, has been the fundamental assumption of the American culture. This belief constituted a liberalism unquestionably flawed—its concept of equality only slowly recognized others who were not landholding men, and its concept of rights long excluded Blacks, first in their inhumane condition as slaves, then in their discriminated condition as second-class citizens. Yet it was a liberalism thoroughly different from the liberalism of Britain and Western Europe, which was shaped by opposition to canon and feudal law. These ancient laws built strong citadels of privilege and enchained populations with unchallengeable beliefs and unchangeable status. The liberal movement that grew in Europe through the 18th and 19th centuries aimed at liberation from those constraints. American liberalism never fought against these powerful opponents. "There has never been a 'liberal movement' or a real 'liberal party' in America," wrote Hartz, "we have only had the American Way of Life, a nationalist articulation of Locke, which usually does not know that Locke himself is involved."[28]

American liberalism emphasizes equality and autonomy. It has often been noted that equality must necessarily remain imperfect and unrealized when it must cohabit with autonomy. But they have lived together, sometimes in strife and often in dialectic tension. As equality has remained imperfect, autonomy has never been seen as absolute. The autonomous American of history (like the autonomous Greek cities of antiquity) has espoused a code of law. Decalogue and Constitution, covenants and ordinances have stood in the background of American autonomy. Indeed, in a paradoxical way, laws have been authoritative because they were agreed to. American autonomy has never been antinomian.

There is also a liberalism more narrow than this broad American spirit and more confined to recent American history, which, in its political manifestation, marks the New Deal of Roosevelt, the New Frontier of Kennedy, and the Great Society of Johnson. The narrower liberal mentality began to take unique shape at the end of the nineteenth century in the Progressive movement which undertook reforms to restore faith in American opportunity and applied governmental power as never before to enforce those reforms. The Progressive movement appeared as the nation was becoming urbanized and industrialized. Capitalism, originally rooted in the liberated enterprise of individuals working to save, saving to invest, and investing to grow, became the massive power of combines and monopolies, ruthlessly attempting to control business and finance. Capitalism had become an ideology that, as it grasped the American mind, began to create contradictions in the culture.[29] Individuals, who, in principle, were free masters of their fate, had to be controlled for efficiency; communities, which were voluntary associations of citizens, had to be organized for production. Opportunity, meant to be open to all, was captured by a powerful few. Moral values suited to the small community and fostered by religion, such as charity, generosity, and simplicity, were pushed aside by acquisitive virtues and single-minded entrepreneurial zeal. Masses of immigrants, crowded into teeming slums, were exploited by industrialists and politicians alike. Government at every level was tainted by corruption. Consequently, strong impulses toward economic, political, and social reform began to spring from the grass roots, forming a movement with the general name of Progressivism. Many prominent persons, among them politicians ranging from Republican Theodore Roosevelt to Democrat Woodrow Wilson, and philosophers such as William James and John Dewey, associated themselves with the movement, and a Progressive political party was formed. Progressivism, which had many ideas but no definitive ideology, was intensely moral in tone. One historian writes, "The 'pragmatic' leanings [of the progressivists] were combined with a high moral fervor against business and political corruption, a Christian socialist abhorrence of gross materialism and inequality, a moralistic disdain for intemperance of any sort."[30]

The liberalism of the New Deal carried this mentality beyond reform. Government and the power of its laws and money had to pull the nation out of economic depression and reshape institutions in the private sector, such as banking and farming, so that economic catastrophes would never return. The landmark of New Deal liberalism was the passage of the Social Security Act in 1935. Although these programs were in the service of the liberal ethos, many critics judged that they favored equality above autonomy and government authority above liberty, thus fostering a new, narrower conservatism than the nation had known. Kennedy's liberalism, which was more pragmatic than philosophical, was announced in his inaugural address, which summoned the nation to a "battle . . . against the common enemies of man: tyranny, poverty, disease and war itself."[31] Yet, there lurked a fatal ambiguity in these words. The battle against tyranny, in the form of Soviet communism, was fought in ways that the liberal mentality would regret, and the battle against war itself, ironically, led the nation into war. The battles against poverty and disease were nonetheless in the true liberal spirit.

Kennedy began these battles; Johnson pursued them with notable victories: the "war on poverty" was fought with broad increases in Social Security coverage, expansion of Aid to Families with Dependent Children, the establishment of the Office of Economic Opportunity, and above all, the enactment of Medicare and Medicaid in 1965. All these programs contributed to a significant decrease in the number of Americans living below the poverty line, from 17% in 1965 to 11% in 1973. The Great Society also attacked racial discrimination with the Civil Rights Act of 1964 and the Voting Rights Act of 1965, and by executive orders on affirmative action and federal support of desegregation of schools and facilities. The long battle against racial discrimination, led bravely by Dr. Martin Luther King and dramatized in the events of Selma, Alabama, in the early months of 1965, was now "legitimized" by the authority of the federal government. By this time, the American liberal spirit, which underlies all political views, had become associated primarily with a single political strategy and with the Democratic party.

The liberal social policies of the Kennedy and Johnson administrations were anticipated by the liberal judicial stance of the Supreme Court with President Eisenhower's appointment of Earl Warren as Chief Justice in 1954 ("biggest damn fool mistake I ever made," said the conservative President). Warren was a moderate Republican, a man of independent mind and commitment to "ethical imperatives . . . he held a set of values that he believed represented moral truths about decent, civilized life. It was inconceivable to Warren that these values should not be embodied in constitutional principles. . . . Indeed, Warren felt bound, as a judge, to consider ethical imperatives in his adjudication."[32] Warren's commitment to ethical imperatives and his Court's propensity to depart from its traditional judicial restraint led to a series of momentous liberal decisions on racial segregation, voting rights, rights of criminal defendants, school prayer, and personal privacy.[33] These decisions, which moved American law in a decidedly liberal direction, formed a constellation of cases that significantly affirmed the liberal mentality. Thus, from the New Deal onward, a contemporary liberalism took shape in contrast to a contemporary conservatism—the former being dedicated to the alleviation of social and economic structures that inhibited personal liberty; the latter devoted to the preservation of those very structures as the necessary conditions for personal liberty. Both views were rooted in the fundamental liberal spirit of the nation, but each had a profoundly different vision of its cultural and political incarnation.

The liberal mentality of the 1960s was deeply affronted by the escalation of the war in Southeast Asia. The escalation that had begun covertly during the Kennedy administration slowly infiltrated the public consciousness, generating confusion, dismay, and dissent. In November 1965, dissent brought thirty thousand people to Washington, D.C., and during the next five years, dissent turned to confrontation, often violent. On April 30, 1970, President Nixon announced to the nation that he had authorized the bombing of Cambodia, and four days later a peaceful protest at Kent State University in Ohio was met by military force, leaving four students dead. The civil discord over the war was matched by racial discord that also escalated into violence. On August 11, 1965, one week after President Johnson had signed the Voting Rights Act, the ghetto of Watts in Los Angeles erupted in riot and flames. During the next summer, Black ghettos in Chicago and Cleveland burned, and in the following summer Tampa, Cincinnati, Atlanta, Newark, and Detroit were in ruins. These "long, hot summers" proved that access to the vote was not enough to cure the deep problems endemic to the African American community. When, on April 4, 1968, Dr. Martin Luther King, Jr. was assassinated, riots again broke out across the country; this time Washington, D.C., suffered the worst of them. These violent events, together with the Black radicalism that accompanied them, conflicted the liberal spirit. While favoring social change, the liberal spirit cannot abide violence.

These political and legal events reflected the liberal mentality, which both inspired them and was troubled by them. In addition, a number of eloquent spokespersons for liberal analysis of American society made their contributions during the decades after World War II. David Reisman's *The Lonely Crowd: A Study of the Changing American Character* (1950) described American life as moving from the inner-directedness of purpose and principle to an other-directedness generated by fictive values of a consumer society. C. Wright Mills's *The Power Elite* (1956) proposed that the mediocre domestic and foreign policy of the country derived from the mediocre minds of three reinforcing elites—corporate, government, and military. John Kenneth Galbraith's *The Affluent Society* (1958) taught that America's consumer society wasted resources while the public sector and its needs were left to starve. Michael Harrington's *The Other America: Poverty in the United States* (1962) revealed the "culture of poverty" in which millions of Americans—children, the aged, minorities, migrants—continued to dwell amidst the nation's abundance. Betty Friedan's *Feminine Mystique* (1963) exposed the frustration of women whose abilities and aspirations were distorted by a male-dominated culture.

Other authors, like Paul Goodman, Herbert Marcuse, and Norman O. Brown, savagely criticized the oppressive structures of the social and psychic worlds. Popular novelists like Kurt Vonnegut, Joseph Heller, and Ralph Ellison exposed the hypocrisy, cynicism, and insanity of American life. These authors pictured American life, which appeared complacent and prosperous, as trapped by social strictures and conventions from which it had to be "liberated." All this became a part of the liberal mentality of the time. These authors were often on the bookshelves of graduate students in those days; I read these books while I was studying ethics at Yale. They were hardly treatises on theological or philosophical ethics (with the exception of Marcuse's works), but they strongly affected my views of the culture in which I was to teach ethics.

Many of the pioneer bioethicists were products of this liberalism; they were enthusiasts for the domestic social policies of the New Deal, the New Frontier, and the Great

Society, and opponents of the foreign policies of the New Frontier and the Great Society. The first bioethicist, Joseph Fletcher, was an activist for the rights of labor and the poor. Other early bioethicists were at the universities as graduate students or as junior faculty during the intense years of student unrest between 1964 and 1970. It was impossible to ignore the turmoil and difficult not to associate with the liberal protest. John Fletcher, a minister in the conservative Episcopal church of the South, threw himself into the civil rights movement. Bob Veatch joined the Peace Corps soon after its establishment and served in Africa; as a graduate student at Harvard, he devoted energy to the anti-war and civil rights movements. Norman Daniels was a vigorous anti-war activist. Jim Childress's doctoral dissertation was an ethical justification of conscientious objection to war. As a Yale graduate student in March 1965, I was active in the Civil Rights movement. Four years later, as a Jesuit faculty member in a conservative Jesuit university, I counseled Catholic students, who were not eligible for conscientious objector status in the early years of the war, in forming their conscience against conscription. Many other early bioethicists, I am sure, were pro civil rights and against the war.[34]

The fact that a number of the bioethical pioneers came of age in an intensely liberal culture does not yet explain their attraction to bioethics. Nor does the "reigning political liberalism of the educated classes in America," in Callahan's phrase, explain the emergence of bioethics—it may be a necessary condition but it is not a sufficient one. After all, the moral opprobrium of racial segregation and discrimination and the moral repugnance against an unjust war are far more serious moral questions than the issues of bioethics. The deaths of soldiers without a cause and of civilians caught in a crossfire are more difficult to justify than withdrawal of life support from a person in an intensive care unit. The inequalities visited on persons of color are far more offensive than those suffered by patients who are sorted into second-class medicine. The problems bioethics confronted were, by contrast with the war and racism, relatively benign. Still, the liberal mentality of many early bioethicists, with its reinforced concern for rights of individuals and its acquired distrust of authority, was ready to find compromised rights and misused authority in the world of medicine. As Bob Veatch says, "I moved easily from civil rights to patients' rights."[35]

Dan Fox's analogy between bioethics and the nuclear arms control movement suggested that professional and scientific medicine had arrogated to itself power over health care. Americans are suspicious of any enterprise too tightly controlled by a closed group. That suspicion fell on government during the Jacksonian era, on industry in the Progressive era, and on the military during the war in Southeast Asia. In the American ethos, the direction into the future should be guided not only by the experts (in Fox's analogy, the defense establishment) but by all who have an interest in that future. The decisions about policies that affect individuals should be made by those individuals, not just by the policy-makers, and those decisions should be made in ways that allow for expressions of individual values within a general movement toward a common good. The world of medicine had affronted those fundamental liberal values.

Public Scrutiny of Medicine

The medical establishment, like the defense establishment, had grown large, very visible, and even showy. This visibility, as Dan Callahan noted, invited public scrutiny.[36] He associates this scrutiny with the large infusion of government funding into medicine and research in the post-war years. Medicine, which had been a cottage industry before World War II, was building into a major enterprise, much of it supported by public money. The Congress invested large amounts of money, first in research, then in underwriting the building of community hospitals through the Hill-Burton Act, then by directing a significant stream of tax money into two unprecedented programs of health insurance, Medicare and Medicaid. The public funding of human research, in particular, demanded that medical research assume an unaccustomed visibility and adopt practices that its scientists might never have adopted if left to themselves. Many states opened state-supported medical schools. Americans have always demanded accountability from those who receive public money. The American liberal spirit, in all its political forms, places a moral value on the probity of governments established by the common will and for the common good. Medicine had never before been so intimate with government and government money, and now it had to assume accountability.

Private money, as well, was flowing into medicine and health care. Pharmaceutical companies, entranced by advancing science and enticed by the power of advertising to open markets, grew apace. Philanthropy endowed splendid new hospitals. Health insurance became a profitable new line of business for life and casualty insurance companies. The large sums of money attached to medicine and health care made them bigger and more noticeable. In addition, medicine began to show off. In the years after World War II, the walls that had shut medicine from the public view were deliberately knocked down. Technological innovations were announced in the media with great fanfare, and magnificent research centers were built for medical science. The modest medical schools of prewar days were built into shining laboratory complexes, and hospitals, once simple buildings of several floors, sprouted into skyscrapers. Physicians' incomes increased, moving them into the upper-middle economic strata. Now manifestly more prosperous than their predecessors, doctors became persons of prominence and appeared on the new television as compassionate heroes. Medicine was no longer practiced only in the privacy of the consulting room or the surgical suite; it was produced in the media. Medicine sought public attention; public scrutiny, particularly when things went wrong, was inevitable. Americans like things big, but bigness, particularly when it is showy, elicits suspicion of abuse of power. Medicine had become a public enterprise yet, because of the American liberal spirit and mentality, it was susceptible to scrutiny. Bioethics was just around the corner.

The American Ethos

The theses of the three historians and Callahan's suggestions move us toward an answer to the question why bioethics began in the United States and took the form that it did in the United States during the 1960s and 1970s. American medicine had become large, complex, technical, and rich and the control of its policies and practices was closely held by its practitioners. The traditional liberal spirit of Americans, sharpened by the fight for civil rights and against the war, looked with suspicion on this medical-technical complex. Still, this thesis does not explain why that suspicion took the form of ethics. The civil rights and the anti-war movements were certainly inspired by moral sentiments and commitments but they did not create an ethical discipline. In both movements, the moral lines were in general clearly drawn, once the war could no longer be defended as a just war against communist domination and before reaction to affirmative action raised questions of reverse discrimination. Genuine moral problems arose in foreign and domestic policy and the students of ethics who were energized by these problems explored them, but no disciplinary equivalent of bioethics appeared. In these concluding pages, I want to reflect on why the reaction to American medicine took the form of American bioethics.

My reflections converge in a hypothesis: there is an American ethos that shapes the way in which Americans think about morality, and that ethos transformed the response to American medicine into a discipline and discourse called bioethics. Ignoring the reams of scholarly debate about the word "ethos" and about such analogues as national character, I mean by ethos the characteristic way in which a people interpret their history, their social world, and their physical environment in order to formulate convictions and opinions about what is good and right. Ethos is not the actual behavior of a people, as an anthropologist might describe it. It is the panorama of ideas and ideals by which a people judge themselves when they attempt to justify or explain or repudiate behavior. Nor is ethos the collection of rules and principles that are invoked. It is the matrix in which those rules, principles, and values are formed. I give the name ethos to what philosopher Charles Taylor has described as the "background picture of our spiritual nature and predicament that lies behind some of the moral and spiritual intuitions of our contemporaries."[37]

By "Americans," I mean the people who have inhabited the land now called the United States from its colonial times until today, and who have created its complex culture and shared in it, to a greater or lesser degree. This vast population encompasses the Puritans, with their intensely religious mission to create God's kingdom in New England, the Cavaliers, with their worldly dreams of wealth in the southern colonies, and the wretched Africans cruelly imported to create the landowners' wealth. It includes the Scottish and German immigrants moving into the middle colonies and the Catholic French drifting down from Quebec and dwelling in the Louisiana territory, as well as the Catholic Hispanics in the Southwest. The Irish arriving in the early nineteenth century and the Italians and eastern Europeans, including many Jews, coming in the latter half, swelled the crowd. People from Asia were enticed to labor but given cool welcome. During all this movement, the peoples native to the land were pushed to the margins. Each of these groups brought religious beliefs and moral convictions; some promoted their cultures into the foreground and others cherished theirs among themselves.

Across these distinct peoples broad social, intellectual, and political currents flowed, sometimes sweeping away particular beliefs but more often catching them into the current, making a common, although not uniform, culture. Among the social movements were the dynamic religious revivals called "Awakenings" that swept across the colonies and states periodically in the eighteenth and nineteenth centuries and the abolition effort that galvanized and divided the nation not long after its beginning. Intellectual trends, such as Enlightenment thought that strongly influenced early American politics and religion, and scientific and social Darwinism, captured the imagination of the educated public. Political causes, such as Progressivism, which challenged corrupt government and avaricious industry, and civil rights activism, which challenged the structures built by racism, altered the culture. Movements of people into the West and South of the continent not only filled the land but also created a mythology of its destiny. The cataclysm of the Civil War paradoxically cemented the nation that it had rent apart.

My thesis, then, is that the American ethos is a way of thinking about ethics that differs somewhat from ways followed by those who have not lived, as a people, through the American experience.[38] This is a thesis that is, at one end, a truism, and at the other, a complex, highly contentious, and ultimately unprovable assertion. Somewhere in the middle I hope to stake out enough common ground to build a case for my explanation of why bioethics was born in the United States and why American bioethics took the form that it did. There are, I believe, three facets of the American ethos that exert a powerful influence on all American thought about morality. I call these three facets moralism, meliorism, and individualism.

Morality consists of rules for behavior, standards for motives, and ideals of achievement. What these are and how they are imparted and sanctioned may differ from culture to culture but they are usually relatively clear constituents of a culture's life. Moralism implies something more than morality. The *Oxford English Dictionary* defines "moralism" as "addiction to moralizing" and then tells us that "moralizing" is "the act of making moral." Moral addicts are familiar enough: persons who must make everything—eating ice-cream, playing cards, table manners—into a matter of morality. Such folks often appear stern, censorious, even fanatic. However, it is not quite so clear what "making moral" means, because behind the phrase lurks the difficult philosophical question about the range and scope and definition of morality itself. Are there aspects of life that are not susceptible to moral assessment? However one might answer this question, it appears that, in the course of human affairs, the constituents of morality have often been applied to some institutions and withheld from others. Art, politics, commerce, entertainment, warfare, labor, and some forms of sexuality have been morally ignored in some cultures and embraced by moral constraints in others. In some cultures, a pan-moralism prevails in which every movement, thought, and endeavor is surrounded by moral standards and sanctioned by moral judgments; in other cultures, moral notions of right and wrong highlight certain endeavors but hardly touch others.

My hypothesis is that the American ethos is strongly tempted to endow various aspects of life with moral meaning in a capricious way. The colonial Puritans revered the morality of the Old Testament, in which God's command touched not only stealing, lying and killing, swearing and sacrificing, but eating and drinking, planting and gathering, working and resting. Puritan morality was close to a pan-moralism, which is difficult to sustain, particularly when strangers arrive in its closed world and soon even the "Chosen" fall away. Thirty years after the founding of Massachusetts colony, its Puritan divines met in synod to deplore "a decline in the spiritual intensity and social inclusiveness of religious observance . . . [and] the spiritual state of the 'rising generation.' "[39] At the time of the Revolution, it is estimated that only between four and seven percent of the people of the new nation were officially church members. As Martin Marty writes, "While religion was deeply stamped in colonial institutions and minds, few bothered to be observant."[40] The cool rational morality of the Enlightenment stressed honest intention in interpersonal conduct and dispensed with a rule-bound construction of the most secret corners of life. The paragon of the American Enlightenment, Thomas Jefferson, was intensely interested in morality but skeptical of the "Moral Sciences." Moral sense, or conscience, was as much a natural part of every human as were arms and legs, and like those limbs, it could be strengthened by exercise, but only of a certain kind: "State a moral case to a ploughman and a professor. The former will decide it as well, and often better than the latter, because he has not been led astray by artificial rules."[41] Moral sentiment would find its way easily to the proper places where it needed to be exercised. Thus the shadow of morality was lifted from large segments of life that could now be lived as business, politics, and entertainment. The moral preaching of the Awakenings and the evangelical missionaries could not abide this reduced moral agenda and railed not only against the traditional sins but against activities not condemned in the Decalogue, such as gambling, dancing, and drinking. Progressivism, Catholic social doctrine, and the Social Gospel encompassed American economic and commercial life with moral imperatives. Contemporary American life is to this day filled with moralizing: diet and exercise, smoking, media entertainment, welfare policy, and environmental concerns have been incorporated into the sphere of morality. This "moralizing" of aspects of life entails the application of familiar moral rules to new circumstances which they sometimes fit awkwardly, or it entails the invention of new moral rules cut for the problems at hand.

Moralizing not only imports the concepts of morality into various aspects of life, it also imparts to those aspects an energy and passion that is characteristic of moral sentiment. It has never been difficult to engage Americans in a cause by making it a moral crusade. Abolition of slavery, prohibition of alcohol, universal suffrage, and safety of food and water supplies are issues that contain moral value but, in American history they have been thoroughly moralized, raised out of the political or economic or health realm to the higher plane of moral imperative which, presumably, overrides all other considerations. This is praiseworthy when the causes touch deep human values, and attention to those values can be galvanized only by defining them as moral issues.[42] The American ethos, in my view, has a tendency to seize on aspects of life and endow them with moral meaning, precepts, and passion. It is not always clear why certain aspects are chosen and it is not always certain that the moral attribution will be maintained. But while it is, the chosen aspect of life will occupy central attention in the nation's moral life.

Moral Meliorism

It is often noted that the American spirit envisions and aspires to a future always better than the present. The term "meliorism" is sometimes applied to that spirit and evidence of it can be found everywhere in American history. Texts of the Old Testament are filled with divine exhortations such as, "Depart and go up hence . . . unto the land which I swear unto Abraham, to Isaac, and to Jacob, saying, Unto thy seed I will give it. And I will send an angel before thee and I will drive out the Canaanite, the Amorite and the Hittite . . . into a land flowing with milk and honey"(Ex. 33:1–3). The Puritan colonists saw in these texts about Israel's destiny, uttered to ancient Hebrews, the intimation of a divine destiny for their entry into the new world. American preachers and politicians converted these words into an American message, incessantly announcing to Americans that they had a mission, a destiny, a challenge.[43] When journalist John L. O'Sullivan proclaimed in 1845 that "our manifest destiny is to overspread the continent allotted by Providence," he captioned a message already familiar to Americans.[44] They would inhabit the land, civilize it, and make it prosper. The obstacles of dense forests, towering mountains, broad rivers (and indwelling peoples) would be overcome. Metaphors of conquest and progress fill the American vocabulary of the eighteenth and nineteenth centuries. The people are charged with moral missions, some noble, some (in our eyes) base. The subjugation along with the conversion of indigenous people was preached as a moral mission; failing those goals, not a few Christians felt that these people, like the Canaanites, should be driven out. The abolition of black slavery was preached with equal passion by evangelical voices in the northern states. Later in American life, suffrage for women and prohibition of alcohol, social justice for laboring persons, and the persecution of communists were moral causes that inspired devotion and sacrifice. The mission to make a future often led to brutality, greed, and destruction, but it attained the status of a moral ideal that had the power to create an ethos in light of which intentions and conduct could be judged.

The melioristic ethos—current situations can and should be made better—lingered long after the Puritans proclaimed that they were legates of a providential mission. It was augmented by the Enlightenment's rational belief in progress, given scientific credibility by the evolutionary hypothesis and political energy by Progressivism and, in the twentieth century, was seemingly confirmed by America's political, military, and economic ascendancy among nations. The recurrent failures, disappointments, depressions, and crises that racked American life never radically shook that faith, until the ambiguous ending of the Korean war and the double disgrace of Vietnam and Watergate. American ethics, in its academic and homiletic forms, has reflected the meliorism of this ethos. From Edwards to Emerson, through James and Dewey, the ultimate goal was always something beyond the present and was achievable by human striving, with or without God's grace.

Moral Individualism

American meliorism is not a metaphysical or cosmic ride into a better future. Progress is not inevitably written into the history of humans; it must be made by the hard work of individuals. This belief is another mark of the American ethos: it is individualistic. From the beginning, each person counts as one and no more than one, a free agent, expected to become responsible and to make one's own way in the world. The Calvinist doctrine of personal salvation, the broader Christian affirmation that each soul was infinitely precious in the eyes of God, the evangelical call for personal commitment to Jesus, the Enlightenment espousal of natural law rights, capitalism which, despite its intrinsic need to control its workers and crush competitors, idolized free enterprise—all of these created a vital sense that moral worth and moral responsibility resided not in the collectivity but in the individual. Collectivities, such as communities and churches, were cherished less as the source of worth than as places where individual worth could be fostered and rewarded. Class was not honored among these collectivities or, when it was by a few, it was condemned as snobbery by the many. "We are all of one estate," said a democrat of the early nineteenth century, "we are all commoners."[45] The omission of native Americans and African Americans from this formula called for tortured rationalizations or rigorous banishment from mind. The omission of women was justified by endowing them with mystic maternal and wifely virtues.

This individualism is not an atomistic, antinomic moral chaos. While it is true that individuals are equal and their free choices about how they shall live should be honored, individuals are expected to cooperate in effecting the better future that American meliorism envisions. Meliorism and individualism are linked by agreements between free persons. The better future toward which good persons strive may not be a clear vision but it is out there, and it will be attained by the actions of individuals which must, in some fashion, be brought into concert: free persons must work together. It is expected that free and equal persons, given the opportunity to debate a problem, will find a mutually acceptable resolution. This image, sanctified in the New England town meeting, was applicable to morality as well as to politics. As we are frequently reminded, Alexis de Tocqueville was astonished by the penchant of Americans to join associations for all sorts of purposes, some frivolous but many melioristic. Even the churches of Protestant America became what churches had never been—free associations of believers who could join and leave at will but who, while together, would collaborate not only in activities but even in creating worship and doctrine. All these associations are little compacts, small covenants, minor contracts whereby persons agree to work together; consent creates and continues communities. Even though consent is at their roots, certain moral conditions limit the structure they can take: associations must be democratic not tyrannical, free not forced, peaceable not violent. The American ethos is marked by a contractual individualism.

The moralism of the American ethos might seem incompatible with this melioristic, individualistic ethos. If the ethos always looks toward a new and better future, and if that future is accomplished by the free choices of individuals agreeing to cooperate in its pursuit, then logically it would seem that moral standards move at the will of those who are moving ahead in their quest for a better situation. If the primary moral qualifiers of their activities are the procedural ones of democracy, freedom, and peace, the contents of any moral standards would seem to be determined only by the choices of those willing to abide by those procedures. Yet, throughout American history, preachers and teachers, parents and philosophers, and even politicians have alluded to "morality" in a way more substantive than procedural. Even figures as open to progress and freedom as Emerson, James, and Dewey were far from antinomian. Emerson, ever a proponent of moral innovation, still feared the disruptions that might follow innovation, and wrote in his private journal, "Beware of antinomianism."[46] Although expressions vary with the times, the same virtues are consistently extolled: loyalty to one's country and companions, obedience to one's parents and legitimate authorities, respect for law and lawful institutions, fidelity and restraint in sexual life, temperance and modesty in social behavior, and honesty in business activities.

The description of the American ethos that I have given may seem to some readers hopelessly naïve and incorrect. Had Americans ever been that way, they are not now, these critics might say; we are now cynical, anarchistic, morally adrift. There is evidence aplenty for this criticism. Still, I stand by my description for three reasons. First, my meaning of ethos does not depict people as they are but as they seek to be. Cynicism, cruelty, and exploitation, so often found in American life, have never been ethical ideals. Second, I contend that even the current moral disarray that can be seen in American life reflects that ethos, either as an exaggeration or as a partial repudiation of it, and neither can be understood without recourse to the original, embedded American ethos. Third, and more to the purpose of this book, the early bioethicists grew up in the ethos that I have described, and much of the content and style of bioethics is marked by it.

Bioethics and the American Ethos

It is time to return to the question, why an American bioethics and how does it differ from all other bioethics? The answer lies, I believe, in the American ethos: a destiny to make life better than it is and a conviction that it is possible to do so, a faith in the value of individuals and their capacity to reach consensual agreements, and a vague but genuine commitment to a conventional morality.

When concerns about the new medicine were first expressed and bioethics began to form around them, American medicine had long identified itself as a moral enterprise. Moralism had captured American medicine long before bioethics. In the mid-nineteenth century American physicians were seen as "humbugs," quarrelsome competitors, and worse, as poisoners and butchers. The newly founded American Medical Association endeavored to restore public respect and confidence by improving the ethics of the profession. The profession armed its members with a code of ethics even before it was able to give them an effective pharmacopoeia and, even as medicine was becoming more useful, the moral reputation of physicians guaranteed that its new capability would be rightly used. Recall the country doctor who appeared in the opening pages of this book: Dr. Ceriani was the beneficiary of that effort. By his day, the moral probity of the American physician was beyond doubt and the profession enjoyed a moral reputation unprecedented in the history of medicine. The public viewed their physicians as "insightful and caring men who could minister and bring relief to the barren lives of others."[47] Even though moral reality may not have equaled moral reputation, American medicine had been touched by the moralism of the American ethos and had greatly benefited from it.

Medicine was also caught by the melioristic ethos. The world of science and medicine, as it appeared after World War II, showed the American people a future of better health and better health care. The technologies that came in large part from the victorious war effort were being converted to peace and health. The general optimism of the post-war era, with its economic growth and its social mobility, embraced the future. Scientists had always been creators of the American future; now physicians, wearing the white laboratory coat, joined them. Making a better world in which infectious disease was eradicated and illnesses such as fatal cardiac and kidney conditions were alleviated, was easily incorporated into the American ethos as an ethical imperative. Physician scientists had to make it so; the people could then enjoy another right, the right to health.

Medicine was becoming technological and Americans, always entranced by technology, took to artificial kidneys, heart–lung bypass machines, and powerful imaging equipment just as they had to the telegraph, telephone, and automobile. Savants who warned of the dangers of technology, such as French theologian Jacques Ellul and American writer Louis Mumford, were little heeded. Even after Hiroshima, the terrifying power of atomic energy did not terrify Americans: the bomb, they thought, was used rightly, would probably never have to be used again, and the science behind it could and would be turned to peaceful uses. Although Rachel Carson's 1962 *Silent Spring* did awaken concern about industrial pesticides, and other environmental problems, such as polluted water and smog, began to tarnish the reputation of technology, there was little anti-technology sentiment in the United States. During the early years of bioethics the technological optimism that had prevailed throughout American history persisted. Ivan Illich's shocking claim that modern medicine had become "a major threat to health . . . expropriating the power of the individual to heal himself and to shape his or her environment" caused a stir but hardly dimmed the melioristic glow that suffused the medicine of that time.[48]

"Miracle" described the new medical interventions that appeared from time to time—the "wonder drugs" and "artificial organs" and transplantation—and soon became, as a true miracle never does, a common designation of everyday medicine. When President Johnson signed the Medicare bill, he exclaimed, "no longer will older Americans be denied the healing miracles of modern medicine."[49] Even if the transformed medicine of the era was not made up of literal miracles, it offered genuine progress in diagnosis and therapy, and much of that therapy was unquestionably life saving and extending. In the fashion of a traditional miracle, it attracted admiration. Medicine, for so long stuck in its past, was now magnified under the glass of the melioristic ethos. From an art that could, as the old motto went, "sometimes heal, often relieve, comfort always," medicine became a science that was expected usually to save, consistently to heal, and always to relieve. When it failed to do so for this or that sick patient, disappointment rather than resignation was the reaction; when it failed on a wider scale, as in the thalidomide tragedy, shock and anger was the response. Medicine was now assigned the task of creating a better future. It is only after reading reams of praise for the new scientific medicine, which brought health and happiness, that the querulous complaints of the few prominent scientists and physicians, which we heard at the beginning of the story of bioethics, make sense. The problems were faults in the miracle.

The early conferences about medical ethics basked in the glow of medical progress. Participants congratulated each other on the panoply of new scientific understanding and technological medicine that they had brought to the world. At the same time, a second characteristic of American moralism could never be expunged. The participants at conferences, after the eulogies, asked the question of conscience, "but in all this, is there anything that is not permitted? Are there things we should not pursue? Are there limits we should impose upon ourselves? For, after all, even our progress seems to be doing some harm." Once the doubts about progress's total benignity were raised, a host of questions followed. Meliorism and moralism converged and the task began of writing a new list of commandments that could confine progress within moral limitations and, at the same time, not inhibit its rush toward better health and life.

The two earliest bioethicists took different paths at the crossroads in the American ethos posted Meliorism and Moralism. Joseph Fletcher blessed the forces of progress while Paul Ramsey warned about progress's illusions. Fletcher, planted firmly in the meliorism of the American ethos, affirmed that new things would advance human good and saw ethics as the willingness to accept the new medical technology with a reasonable awareness of possible misuse. Ramsey glimpsed, as any Calvinist should, the power of evil hidden even in the good. He played the prophet, pointing to the moral problems that plague all progress and urging rules that would contain those problems. Joseph Fletcher endorsed the vision of advance toward human betterment with cautions about possible tyrannies; Paul Ramsey preached the supremacy of the moral imperatives that must guide and sometimes curtail those advances. Yet both men honored the autonomy and rights of individuals; both conceived of contracts and covenants as moral instruments to protect freedom and rights. Both were essentially American moralists: Fletcher followed in the tradition of James and Dewey (and even of his Anglican ancestor, the theological utilitarian Archdeacon Paley, once so popular in America). Ramsey walked in the tradition of Jonathan Edwards and Reinhold Niebuhr. Contemporary bioethicists sometimes criticize Fletcher's benign blessing and praise Ramsey's prophetic stance, but they have marched, somewhat waveringly, behind both leaders.

Medicine was particularly easy to interpret within the ethos of meliorism and moralism. Scientific medicine was clearly melioristic, pushing toward a better, healthier future for individuals and society. At the same time, medicine had inherited from its long tradition multiple maxims about right and wrong. Physicians were commanded not to harm, not to molest their patients sexually nor to take advantage of their weakness. Even more, the American medical profession had defined itself by its moral attributes. As medicine's new capabilities endowed physicians with new powers over disease, bringing at the same time new harms, the old rules needed to be renovated. As medicine enlarged its technical control over life and death, its traditional views about what made for a good life and a good death needed to be enhanced by the views of those persons whose lives and deaths medicine affected.

This renovation was relatively benign. While the work of sharpening the commandments that should govern medicine and science aroused considerable interest, it did not, at first, stimulate great passions. Bioethics moved with a certain tranquillity through the tempestuous moral turmoil of racism and warfare that was contemporaneous with its origins. There were issues that deservedly did stir great moral passion. When bioethics encountered the immorality of racial discrimination, as it did in the Tuskegee affair, those passions were aroused. Similarly, when the ethics of caring for the dying came anywhere near the moral disgust for killing, it had to move with extreme caution to avoid conflagration. Abortion, always a matter of conscience for doctors and patients, was caught up in almost irrational crusades. Still, the work of revising the commandments of medical morality in such a way as to permit, even encourage, medical progress was done in a relatively quiet way.

The bioethical protest against the domination of medicine by technologized professionals aimed at preserving the progress that these professionals had effected and, at the same time, at giving direction of that progress to all individuals who have an interest in it. The protest was a peaceable one for several reasons. First, the world of health care is, in general, a peaceful place, occupied by sick patients, concerned families, and serious doctors and nurses. It is a world filled with anxiety, fear, tension, and intensity but it is free of violence. Second, the world of health care encountered the protest with a long tradition of ethics, which it willingly and proudly affirmed. The call by outsiders to freshen that tradition so that it could accommodate the new biology and the new medicine might be irritating but it could not easily be ignored—even less when insiders also raised the call. The peaceable protest was accomplished through another intrinsically quiet means: the testing of principles and values within medical tradition against other values that, while they might be alien to the tradition, were congenial to the broader ethos within which it now lived. For example, the principle of autonomy had never been prominently displayed within the long tradition of medicine, but American practitioners could hardly fail to recognize its essentially American character. Bioethics, in its disciplinary form, was a conceptual protest against the "medical establishment," one that the establishment could understand and, at least in its broad proposals, accept.

Early bioethicists did encounter some opposition from physicians and scientists. American physicians had enjoyed at least a half century of prestige and almost unquestioned authority. The arrival of "strangers" to dictate the terms of their relationship to patients was, for many, an unwelcome, irritating advent. Indeed, the traditional ethics of medicine, as they saw it, was more venerable and respectable than the unrealistic pieties and abstract principles of theologians and philosophers. Many, perhaps most, medical practitioners and medical scientists were honestly dedicated to the welfare of their patients and were sincerely motivated by the desire to cure disease and to improve the health of patients and populations. Those who strayed from the old moral paths took familiar enough detours: practitioners were enticed by the wealth that new techniques and financial forms could bring; scientists were lured by fame and the prestige of the Prize.

Nevertheless, physicians did know that they worked within a profession marked by a long tradition of ethics; discussion of the updating and refining of that tradition, if the need was manifest (and many physicians readily admitted that it was), was not unpalatable. Indeed, to some physicians, it was enticing. Franz Ingelfinger, a leading voice of American medicine, wrote a stinging criticism of "the unethical in medical ethics," which he concluded with the conciliatory words, "If medical ethics is to achieve its goal of imbuing medical research and practice with a loftier morality. . . . The physician must become more aware of the ethicist and *visa versa.* . . . Unless integrations of this type are aggressively sought, ethics will not exercise the influence it should have in medical research and practice, and medical ethics will continue to be tainted by unethical exploitation."[50] The integrations of which Ingelfinger wrote—constant intercourse in clinical and research settings, seminars and continuing education, and local discussion groups—did occur, and mutual awareness grew throughout the profession. The "strangers," philosophers and theologians, were actually hired by the premier institutions of American medicine, its medical schools, and asked to make that constant intercourse a constituent of curriculum. While this might be viewed cynically, as medicine's attempt to co-opt its critics, it can equally be seen as the move of a moralized profession to deal with its melioristic future. Bioethics has not been incorporated into medicine's educational world elsewhere to the extent that it has in the United States. By incorporation into American medical faculties, the discourse about the new medicine was shaped into an academic discipline as nowhere else.

The problems that bioethics found were not the radical corruptions that critics like Illich condemned. They were flaws in genuinely beneficial developments. The technological ability to save and sustain life, to correct inherited defects, to discover new possibilities for cure, to remedy infertility and to control fertility are all human goods for which humans have long yearned. These scientific advances also have undesirable consequences and can be misused for undesirable ends. These developments create, as the early theological commentators saw, moral ambiguity. The ethical problem is how to enjoy the benefit without the detriment or how to unravel the ambiguity so that the least detrimental effects flow from the benefits. Bioethics was a needed adjunct to the publicity of the new medicine and science: it was a commitment to take seriously the adverse effects of medical and scientific progress, an acknowledgment that medical "miracles" are indeed marvelous but marred.

The technological advances and their ambiguities captured the attention of early bioethicists, just as they entranced the public and endowed physicians with unprecedented power. Bioethicists also recognized that the vastly expanded, technologized, and costly health care system was depriving many persons of access and making care very expensive. Their liberal mentality, attuned to the moral obligation of institutions to serve the public, worried about justice and fairness. Still, bioethics hardly touched the deeper issues of the ends and purposes of medicine. Callahan, who has been among the few to call for such an examination, has said, "Bioethics has never been a critic of the ends of medicine. . . . It accepted those ends and has worked on the moral means of gaining those ends."[51] This reluctance to criticize the ends of medicine can be cynically explained as the opportunism of bioethicists who discovered that they could live better in the wealthy environs of medical schools than in the poverty of philosophy departments and vicarages. Less cynically, the adoption of bioethics as a part of the medical curriculum and the employment of many bioethicists as medical school professors did dampen the critical spirit—bioethicists were colleagues rather than critics of medicine's practitioners. At the same time, that collegiality did introduce an internal critical spirit into the minds of many practitioners, into the performance of institutions, and into the formulation of policy that otherwise would not have appeared.

Commentators on the American ethos have often noted that liberalism, while reformist, is not revolutionary. The liberal mentality, although perceiving the distortion of institutions, remains convinced that they can be reformed piece by piece rather than wholesale. A revolution requires a clear, often dazzling vision of its ultimate goals. The American ethos, as I have described it, does not try too hard to define its ultimate goals and values; it postulates a better situation that can be realized by cooperating free persons acting democratically, freely, and peaceably. The steps toward that better situation are taken incrementally and are designed as they go. Laws, guidelines, policies, and regulations, issuing from different sources with differing authority, provide provisional direction. Behind this incrementalism stands the idea that interested persons can contract their way into the future. This is a concept of ethics compatible with the American ethos and reflected in the pragmatic ethics of James and Dewey. The bioethics that developed within American moralism and meliorism is also marked by the incremental obligations that arise from individuals contracting to resolve difficult problems. This results in a form of ethics quite foreign to those unfamiliar with the American ethos and for whom moral obligations rest not on the choices of individuals but on deep structures of human nature.

The renovation of the old ethics of medicine was accomplished by the equivalent of contracts, concords, and covenants. Most of these instruments, like the social contracts of Locke and Rousseau and Rawls, were metaphorical. They represented the tacit acceptance by professionals of a redefined relationship with their patients, who now entered their care not as abject petitioners for their skills but as persons with the right to determine how those skills were to be applied. Some of the covenants were more explicit. Policies issued by professional organizations guided physicians in their dealings with the dying patient or the patient with dangerous infection. Law imposed the duty of informed consent on the practitioner and even more rigorously on researchers. Organ transplantation proceeded within a set of implicit and explicit covenants with society to assure that access was fair and that harvest of organs was not coerced. The sciences of genetics and reproduction, still too young to be tightly confined by rule, wondered how far it should leap beyond conventional moral understandings.

Even though utilitarianism has intermittently attracted American thinkers, and American pragmatism is often interpreted as disguised utilitarianism, the bioethical examination of various problems has never led to policies designed exclusively by the utilitarian principle. The definition of death, the allocation of organs and other scarce resources, research with human subjects, and the application of genetic and reproductive science—all susceptible to utilitarian manipulation—have been surrounded by restrictions and limitations more deontological than utilitarian. The harsh judgment of an Italian theologian, Elio Sgreccia, who distinguishes between a European bioethics based on personalist theory and the *philosophia perennis* and an American bioethics "whose inadequate ethical theory risks being lured into utilitarianism, if not into a nazi biologism," seems unwarranted.[52] As we have seen, even in the absence of grand theory, American bioethics has not succumbed to utilitarianism. This is due, I think, to the constant correction of meliorism by moralism. It reflects the moralistic constraints on the melioristic impulse.

These many tacit and explicit covenants give the world of medicine and biological science an appearance quite different from that of forty years ago. The technologies of today's world are different but, more importantly, the use of these technologies is surrounded by a new moral appreciation. David Rothman concludes his *Strangers at the Bedside* with the judgment, "The record since 1966, I believe, makes a convincing case for a fundamental transformation in the substance as well as the style of medical decision making."[53] There will be many arguments about how fundamental that transformation has been, but I believe Rothman is right.

This is the vision that emerges from the history of bioethics in the United States. The vision is, of course, idealized and it is never realized exactly as described. Still, these general features emerge in each issue that has generated bioethical discourse and benefited from bioethical analysis. The utilitarian principle—that the promotion of the general good can morally override individual good—is restrained. The individual is placed at the center of value; claims for an overriding social good must be justified in particular cases. The advances in technology and the complex organizational structures that must be built to accommodate them are accepted, but with provisos that require respect for conventional moral imperatives (even though what those imperatives are might be disputed). Medicine's progress has been encouraged yet moral limits have been set. The authority to determine the course of one's care has been allocated to the individual patient and authority within health care has been dispersed to those who have an interest in it, rather than to those who utilize its technologies. Resolutions of problems are tentative but given transitional sanction by policy and regulation. This is American bioethics.

Notes to Chapter 12

1. Comité international de bioéthique, *Répertoire de l'UNESCO sur les Comités et/ou les Instituts de bioéthique* (Paris 1994).

2. The best survey of international bioethics is found in the articles under the heading, "Medical ethics, history of," in Warren T. Reich (ed.), *Encyclopedia of Bioethics*, 2nd ed. (New York: Simon & Schuster Macmillan, 1995), vol. III, pp. 1439–1646, together with articles on the ethical systems of particular religions and cultures. Useful summaries can be found in B. Andrew Lustig, Baruch A. Brody, and H. Tristram Engelhardt, Jr. (eds.), *Bioethics Yearbook Vol. 4: Regional Developments*, 1992–1993 (Dordrecht: Kluwer Academic Press, 1994). Some representative books are: from Great Britain, Ranaan Gillon, *Philosophical Medical Ethics* (Chichester: Wiley, 1986) and Alastair Campbell, *Moral Dilemmas in Medicine* (Edinburgh: Churchill Livingston, 1972); from Spain, Diego Gracia, *Fundamentos de Bioética* (Madrid: Eudema Universidad, 1989); from Italy, C. Romano and G. Grassiani (eds.), *Bioetica* (Torino: UTEP, 1995) and Maurizio Mori (ed.), *La Bioetica: Questioni Morali e Politiche per il Futuro dell' Uomo* (Milano: Politeia, 1991); from Germany, Ludger Honnefelder and Günter Rager, *Ärtzliches Urteilen und Handeln: Zur Grundlegung einer medizinischen Ethik* (Frankfurt am Main and Leipzig: Insel Verlag, 1994).

3. Daniel Callahan, "Why America accepted bioethics," Birth of Bioethics Conference, (Seattle, Wa., Sept. 24–25, 1992), transcript pp. 354–373.

4. An exception to this generalization is the founding of the London Medical Group by Canon Edward Shotter in 1963, which later developed into the Institute of Medical Ethics in Great Britain.

5. Interview with Pére Patrick Verspieren, Director, Department of Bioethics, Centre Sevrés, Paris, April 17, 1996. See Anne Marie Moulin, "Medical ethics in France: the latest great politi-

cal debate," *Theoretical Medicine* 9 (1988): 271–285; Sandro Spinsanti, *Etica bio-medica* (Milan: Paoline, 1987). The Dutch word, "Gezondheidsethiek" strikes a nice balance.

6. Bettina Schöne-Seifert, Hans-Martin Sass, Laura Jane Bishop, and Alberto Bondolfi, "Medical ethics, history of, German-speaking countries," in Reich, *Encyclopedia of Bioethics*, vol. 3, pp. 1579–1589, p. 1580.

7. See Chapter 5 of this volume. Shannon's policy was communicated to the World Health Organization which stimulated review committees in various countries. Dr. Zbigniew Bankowski, who was the organizer of this effort, says that the Shannon policy "had a major impact on world bioethics." Interview with Dr. Bankowski, Director, CIOMS, Geneva, April 30, 1996.

8. UNESCO International Bioethics Committee, *Universal Declaration on the Human Genome and Human Rights*, Paris, December 3, 1997.

9. Interview with Pére Verspieren, Paris, April 17, 1996.

10. Bettina Schöne-Seifert and Klaus-Peter Rippe, "Silencing the Singer: antibioethics in Germany." *Hastings Center Report* 21 (1991): 20–27.

11. See Pinit Ratanakul, "Bioethics in Thailand: the struggle for Buddhist solutions," *Journal of Medicine and Philosophy* 13 (1988): 301–312.

12. These thoughts on origins, methods, and traditions derive from an interview with Dr. Maurice de Wachter, long-term president of the Association Européenne des Centres d'Éthique Médicale, Paris, April 20, 1996.

13. The remarks cited from the leading European theologians, Helmut Thielicke (Chapter 1) and Karl Rahner (Chapter 2) exemplify these religious formulations of ethical questions.

14. Interviews with Sandro Spinsanti, Rome, May 13, 1996 and with Maurizio Mori, Rome, May 14, 1996. See Maurizio Mori, "La bioetica: che cos'è, quand'è nata, e perché. Osservazioni per un chiarimento della "natura" della bioetica e del dibattito italiano in materia. *Bioetica* 1 (1993): 115–143 and the riposte by Paolo Cattorini, Roberto Mordacci, Daniela Morelli, Massimo Reichlin, and Roberto Sala, "Sulla natura e le origini della bioetica: una risposta a Maurizio Mori, *Bioetica* 2 (1994): 325–345.

15. Among the many scholars from abroad who have studied and taught at The Kennedy Institute are Francisco Abel of Spain, Rihito Kimura of Japan, and Hans-Martin Sass of Germany. The Hastings Center has also welcomed many foreign scholars and has been particularly hospitable to those from eastern and central European countries.

16. Elio Sgreccia, *Bioetica: Manuale per medici e biologi* (Milano: Vita e Pensieri, 1988).

17. Patrick Verspieren, "Respecter et promouvoir l'autonomie du malade," in *À la Recherche des Contours de l'Autonomie et du Champ de la Liberté dan les Relation Médecin-Malade: Colloque "Dignité Humaine—Perte de Dignité," Revue d'Ethique et Theologie Morale* 192 (1995), pp. 43–56, suppl. See also Jean-Marie Thévoz, "L'autonomie, positivité et limites," in the same collection, pp. 25–42.

18. Diego Gracia, *Fundamentos de Bioética* (Madrid: Eudema, 1988), especially pp. 369–382.

19. Gracia, "Bioetica clinica," in Sandro Spinsanti (ed.) *Bioetica e Antropologia Medica* (Rome: La Nuova Italia Scientifica, 1991), pp. 43–68.

20. Comité Consultatif National d'Éthique pour les Sciences de la Vie et de la Santé, *Les Avis de 1983 à 1993* (Paris: INSERM, 1993); Lucien Séve, *Recherche biomédicale et respect de la person humaine* (Paris: Documentation Française, 1988).

21. François Malherbe, "Orientamenti e tendenze della bioetica nell'area linguistica francese" in Corrado Viafora and Alberto Bondolfi (eds.), *Vent'anni di bioetica: Idee, protagonisti, instituzioni* (Padova: Fondazione Lanza e Gregoriana Libreria Editrice, 1990), pp. 199–235. Cited in Diego Gracia and Teresa Gracia, "Medical ethics, history of, southern Europe," in Reich, *Encyclopedia of Bioethics*, vol. 3, p. 1561.

22. Dietrich von Engelhardt and Sandro Spinsanti, "Medical ethics, history of, Europe," in Reich, *Encyclopedia of Bioethics,* vol. III, p. 1556. This issue is particularly significant in the vigorous world of Italian bioethics where centers and professorships sponsored by the Catholic church take quite different views on many issues than do the secular bioethicists. See reference 14.

23. We have also not commented on bioethics in Canada and the United Kingdom. There are differences, but the common English language with its exchange of literature tends to effect broad similarities. We have neglected the active world of Scandanavian bioethics which also, in my view, shares many Anglo-American characteristics.

24. David Rothman, Daniel Fox, Stanley Reiser, "Three views of the history of bioethics," Birth of Bioethics Conference, pp. 438–452, 453–464, 465–480.

25. David J. Rothman, *Strangers at the Bedside: A History of How Law and Bioethics Trans-formed Medical Decision Making* (New York: Basic Books, 1991), pp. 257, 247.

26. Daniel Callahan, "Why America accepted bioethics," (paper read at the Birth of Bioethics Conference, Seattle, Wa., Sept. 23–24, 1992), transcript pp. 354–373.

27. Louis Hartz, *The Liberal Tradition in America: An Interpretation of American Political Thought since the Revolution* (New York: Harcourt, Brace and World, 1955), pp. 6, 37. The John Adams quotation is from "Dissertation on the Canon and Feudal Law," *Works of John Adams*, ed. C. F. Adams (Boston, 1856), vol. iii, pp. 447–465.

28. Hartz, *The Liberal Tradition in America*, pp. 10–11.

29. See Daniel Bell, *The Cultural Contradictions of Capitalism* (New York: Basic Books, 1976).

30. James McGregor Burns, *The American Experience* (New York: Knopf, 1982, 1985, 1989), vol. 3, p. 246.

31. Cited in John Morton Blum, *Years of Discord: American Politics and Society, 1961–1974* (New York: W. W. Norton, 1991), p. 26.

32. G. Edward White, *Earl Warren: A Public Life* (New York: Oxford University Press, 1982), quoted in Blum, *Years of Discord*, p. 188.

33. Principal among those decisions were *Brown v Board of Education* (1954), which de-clared school segregation unconstitutional and was followed by a series of cases that dismantled on constitutional grounds the legal rationale for all racial segregation; *Engle v Vitale* (1963) de-clared officially mandated prayer in public schools to be a violation of the establishment of reli-gion clause of the Constitution; *Griswold v Connecticut* (1965) struck down a state law that pro-hibited sale, prescription, or use of contraceptives, and *Roe v Wade* (1974) invalidated state laws prohibiting abortion; *Gomillion v Lightfoot* (1960) and *Baker v Carr* (1962) declared unconstitu-tional electoral practices that denied "one vote" to "one man." A series of decisions from *Mallory v United States* (1954) through *Miranda v Arizona* (1966) invalidated police practices that con-travened the rights of the accused and jeopardized due process.

34. The political allegiances of early bioethicists are more complex than this simple general-ization intimates; for example, Paul Ramsey defended the Vietnam war long after others had turned against it; Stanley Hauerwas passionately espouses pacifism and racial justice, but cher-ishes many conservative values.

35. Robert Veatch, interview, October 25, 1995.

36. Daniel Callahan, Birth of Bioethics Conference, p. 365.

37. Charles Taylor, *Sources of the Self. The Making of the Modern Identity* (Cambridge, Mass.: Harvard University Press, 1989), p. 3. I suppose my sense of the American ethos has an affinity with the notion of common morality that has come to play as an important, though not entirely clear, role in the later versions of Beauchamp and Childress, *Principles of Biomedical Ethics*; see particularly pp. 100–111 of the 4th edition. Strangely enough, ethicists do not dwell

much on what I have called "ethos." The work of Taylor, Stuart Hampshire, Bernard Williams, Stephen Toulmin, and the late Alan Donagan have instructed my thinking in this regard.

38. It is, of course, presumptuous to address so complex a subject as the American ethos. My ideas are drawn from reading over the years and this note acknowledges some sources from which I have formed my view of the American ethos. James MacGregor Burns, *The American Experiment* (New York: Knopf, 1982, 1985 and 1989) and Daniel J. Boorstein *The Americans* (New York: Random House, 1958, 1965, and 1973) are my principal sources for American history. Perry Miller, *The New England Mind: The Seventeenth Century* (Cambridge, Mass.: Harvard University Press, 1954) and Henry Steele Commager, *The American Mind: An Interpretation of American Thought and Character Since the 1880s* (New Haven: Yale University Press, 1950) influenced my understanding of the beginning and latter part of the American ethos. Martin E. Marty, *Righteous Empire: The Protestant Experience in America* (New York: Dial Press, 1970) and James Turner, *Without God, Without Creed: The Origins of Unbelief in America* (Baltimore: The Johns Hopkins Press, 1985) were particularly helpful in tracing religious history. Henry F. May, *The Enlightenment in America* (New York: Oxford University Press, 1976) shows how the European Enlightenment was translated into an American idiom. Louis Hartz's *The Liberal Tradition in America: An Interpretation of American Political Thought since the Revolution* (New York: Harcourt, Brace and World, 1955) is a classic on the topic. Charles E. Rosenberg, *No Other Gods: On Science and American Social Thought* (Baltimore: The Johns Hopkins Press, 1961) puts the emergence of science in its American content. Richard Hofstadter, *Social Darwinism in American Thought* (New York: G. Braziller, 1955) and Paul Lawrence Farber, *The Temptations of Evolutionary Ethics* (Berkeley and Los Angeles: University of California Press, 1994) are useful guides to the place of science in American culture. John Morton Blum, in *Years of Discord: American Politics and Society, 1961–1974* (New York: W. W. Norton, 1991) recalls the social, cultural, and political scene in which bioethics was born.

39. James A. Henretta and Gregory H. Nobles, *Evolution and Revolution: American Society, 1600–1820* (Lexington, Mass.: D. C. Heath, 1987), p. 39.

40. Marty, *Righteous Empire*, p. 38.

41. Thomas Jefferson, *Writings of Thomas Jefferson*, ed. Albert Ellery Bergh (Washington, D.C.: Thomas Jefferson Memorial Association, 1907, vol. VI, p. 257, cited in Daniel J. Boorstin, *The Lost World of Thomas Jefferson* (Chicago: University of Chicago Press, 1948), p. 141.

42. It may seem strange to include the abolition of slavery as an issue that has been moralized. Modern people can hardly see slavery as anything but a moral abomination. Yet, in many cultures and climes, it has been morally sanctioned even by the most morally stringent: Stoicism tolerated slavery even in the light of a theory of universal equality, courageous defenders of the liberty of Amerindians, such as Fra Bartolomeo de las Casas and the Portuguese Jesuits saw no moral problem with African slavery. See, for example, Dauril Alden, *The Making of an Enterprise. The Society of Jesus in Portugal, Its Empire and Beyond, 1540–1750* (Stanford: Stanford University Press, 1996), chapters 19, 20. It took enormous effort for British and American antislavery advocates to "moralize" the issue in the first half of the 19th century.

43. See Marty, *Righteous Empire*.

44. John Louis O'Sullivan, *United States Magazine and Democratic Review*, July–August, 1845. See Frederick Merk, *Manifest Destiny and Mission in American History* (New York: Alfred A. Knopf, 1963).

45. Hartz, *The Liberal Tradition in America*, p. 108. The speaker was a certain General Root.

46. Sacvan Bercovitch, *The Puritan Origins of the American Self* (New Haven: Yale University Press, 1975), p. 175.

47. Richard Malmsheimer, *"Doctors Only" The Evolving Image of the American Physician. Contributions in Medical Studies*, No. 25 (New York: Greenwood Press), p. 99. See also Ronald

Numbers, "The fall and rise of the American medical profession," in Ronald Numbers and Judith Leavitt (eds.), *Sickness and Health in America* (Madison: University of Wisconsin Press, 1985).

48. Ivan Illich, *Medical Nemesis: The Expropriation of Health* (New York: Pantheon Books, 1976), pp. 1, 9.

49. Quoted in Blum, *Years of Discord*, p. 175.

50. J. Franz Ingelfinger, "The unethical in medical ethics," *Annals of Internal Medicine* 83 (1975): 264–269, p. 269.

51. Daniel Callahan, Birth of Bioethics Conference, p. 369; "Shattuck lecture: contemporary biomedical ethics," *New England Journal of Medicine* 302 (1980): 1228–1255; "Aging and the ends of medicine," *Annals of the New York Academy of Sciences* 530 (1988): 125–132; *Setting Limits: Medical Goals in an Aging Society* (New York: Simon and Schuster, 1988).

52. Elio Sgreccia, "Il ruolo della bioetica nella formazione del medico europeo," *Medicina e morale* 6 (1990), p. 1123. Cited in Mori, "La bioetica," p. 141.

53. Rothman, *Strangers at the Bedside*, p. 251.

Epilogue

I chose 1987 as the terminus of this history, although I have occasionally slipped over the line. During the decade since 1987, however, the discipline and discourse have not only moved ahead; they have changed direction in significant ways. Any field that comments on actuality, as bioethics does, is necessarily moved by events and inventions, and the decade has been filled with advances in medicine and science, as well as new forms of health care delivery and policy, that called for commentary. At the same time, the leading ideas that form the discipline have come under scrutiny; the theory, principles, and practices that evolved during the first decades do not seem to measure up to the new questions.[1]

Several personal events prompted me to choose 1987 as the conclusion of my account of the origins of bioethics. In those events, I saw signs of the challenges that would force bioethicists to examine the shape they had given their discipline during its formative years. These events also serve as a short prelude to the years after 1987 that will, in due course, merit their own history. Whoever writes that history will find bioethics a much more complex and diverse field than I have described in this book. It may, in fact, be inadvisable for that future historian to attempt a comprehensive history, since the topics and the theories may have fractured so far that many particular histories, rather than a single one, will be needed to comprehend them. During most of my career, I was what might be called a general practitioner of bioethics, capable of commenting on a wide range of issues, from medical experimentation to termination of life support. Now, it seems, bioethicists must be specialists—expert in the ethics of genetics or the ethics of health policy or the ethics of the health care industry. They may be identified with distinct theories: foundationalist, deconstructionist, feminist, or cultural. These directions began to become clear at the end of the 1980s and the personal events that I recall below are their intimations.

In 1987, the UCSF Division of Medical Ethics sponsored a conference called "The Meaning of AIDS."[2] The AIDS epidemic had begun some five years earlier and San Francisco was an epicenter. We were intimately involved in the agonizing ethical problems that the epidemic thrust upon health care providers and patients. Although April 11, 1983, was not the start of the AIDS epidemic in the United States, it was the day on which two events that defined the epidemic took place. On that day, *Newsweek* splashed across its cover: "EPIDEMIC: The Mysterious and Deadly Disease Called AIDS May Be the Public-Health Threat of the Century. How Did It Start? How Can It Be Stopped?"[3] Randy Shilts, an historian of the epidemic, says of that issue of *Newsweek*, "with AIDS finally ensconced as a legitimate news story, an avalanche of coverage began." On the same day, Dr. Robert Gallo, a National Institutes of Health scientist, announced to the first National Cancer Institute conference on AIDS that he suspected that a retrovirus was the causal agent of the syndrome. That announcement, states Shilts, "was later cited by the officials of the National Cancer Institute as the turning point, the time that the Institute became firmly committed to finding the cause of acquired immune deficiency syndrome." By April 1983, 1,295 Americans had contracted AIDS; 492 had died and unknown thousands more harbored the lethal virus.[4]

Two years before, physicians around the country had begun to see unusual symptoms in young male patients: fatigue, fever, wasting, swollen lymph nodes, incessant respiratory and other infections, and uncommon skin cancers. Some impairment in the immune system and a possible infectious agent were suspected. Often, the patients with these perplexing symptoms were gay men. In May 1981, the newsletter of the Centers for Disease Control, *Morbidity and Mortality Weekly Report*, reported under the headline "Pneumocystis pneumonia—Los Angeles" that "5 young men, all active homosexuals, were treated for biopsy-confirmed Pneumocystis carinii pneumonia . . . two of the patients died."[5] During 1982, interested physicians constructed a clinical diagnosis to which the ugly acronym GRID, Gay-Related Immunodeficiency, was applied. As reports filtered into the Centers for Disease Control (CDC) in Atlanta, it became apparent that persons other than gay men were also affected. Persons who had received blood transfusions or regularly used blood products for treatment of hemophilia were among the affected. By mid-1982, more than 500 cases of the disease had been reported; shockingly, over half of those were already dead. At a July 27, 1992, meeting of CDC, NIH, and FDA officials and others, the acronym GRID, clearly no longer appropriate, was discarded in favor of AIDS, acquired immune deficiency syndrome.

My own institution, The University of California, San Francisco, and one of its teaching hospitals, San Francisco General Hospital, felt the first tremors of the AIDS epidemic. I recall a Faculty Club lunch sometime in the late spring of 1982 at which a group of professors listened with fascination as Dr. Marcus Conant, Professor of Dermatology, told us that he had seen half a dozen young men with a rare skin cancer, Kaposi's sarcoma, characteristically seen only in elderly Eastern European men. He had consulted with oncologist Dr. Paul A. Volberding at San Francisco General Hospital, who was equally puzzled. Soon thereafter I left San Francisco to spend a sabbatical year at Oxford University. When I returned, I found myself in the midst of an epidemic with extraordinary ethical implications. During 1982, a much clearer clinical picture of AIDS had emerged; the gay community started to realize that it was being decimated by a lethal epidemic; public health officials became concerned and slowly began to organize a response; and the public learned, in fragmented and often distorted ways, that a plague was abroad in the land.

San Francisco General Hospital established the first AIDS ward in the nation. After my return from sabbatical leave, Dr. Volberding invited me to a clinical conference to discuss whether a patient who had recovered from a bout of pneumocystis pneumonia should be intubated a second time, given the almost hopeless prospect of a second rescue. Dr. Volberding's wife, Dr. Molly Cooke, invited me to talk with her medical residents about the duty to care for patients even when it put caregivers at risk of contracting disease. Dr. Cooke, Dr. Barbara A. Koenig, and I collaborated to write an article about ethical problems in the care of AIDS patients. We discussed four problems that we had encountered: the duty of health personnel to treat AIDS patients even at risk to themselves, the appropriate level of care during critical episodes, the protection of confidentiality of persons with HIV infection, and the allocation of resources to research and care. Although our article, which was published in an obscure journal, was not much noticed, its topics anticipated the central agenda for ethics and AIDS.[6]

Other serious questions were on that agenda. San Francisco's Irwin Memorial Blood Bank tried to formulate a policy about screening blood donors in a city where many donors were gay men who were deeply concerned about their privacy. San Francisco's Department of Public Health battled to close the city's gay baths, against the opposition of some leaders of the gay community who saw the move less as a measure of public health than as a brand of stigmatization. San Francisco General Hospital struggled to develop a policy for resuscitation of persons suspected of being infected. I was involved in each of these discussions, learning first hand the legitimacy of the gay community's fear of stigmatization and discrimination, and the conflicting need to devise effective protection from the spreading infection. I also saw the anger and frustration at the studied indifference of the Reagan administration to the need for aggressive scientific research and expanded clinical care.

In May 1985, The Hastings Center initiated the Research Group on AIDS: Public Health and Civil Liberties. A Hastings' staffer, Dr. Ron Bayer, became the most prominent commentator on the ethical issues raised by the epidemic.[7] Sometime in 1986, Bayer and some of his associates on the Hastings Task Force visited San Francisco. I assembled a group of our local experts to talk with them. At that meeting, I became aware, as never before, of the "dual" epidemic. Our San Francisco patients were almost exclusively gay men; the Hastings visitors, many of whom were from the New York area, had seen not only patients who were gay men but also many who were IV drug users, a population hardly visible in our AIDS ward. We left that meeting with the realization that these diverse populations posed quite different ethical questions and, as the epidemic devastated lives and communities over the next years, those questions became obvious.[8]

The spring 1986 meeting of the Society for Health and Human Values was held in San Francisco, and my colleagues, Eric Juengst and Barbara Koenig, organized it around the theme The Meaning of AIDS: Implications for Medical Science, Clinical Practice, and Public Policy.[9] The title could have included "and for Bioethics," since the AIDS epidemic opened a new era for the discipline. Appearing toward the end of the forty years I have chosen as the formative period for bioethics, the epidemic is a mirror for the changing questions and style of bioethics that marked the decade that lies beyond our history. It would be an exaggeration to claim that AIDS alone drove those changes; many other influences—intellectual, medical, cultural, and economic—pushed the emerging discipline. Still, the ominous force of an epidemic gave momentum to its directions.

An epidemic is not just the increased incidence of a disease affecting individuals; it is a disruption of society. The sickness and death of individuals, occurring in unusual numbers, ripple out, fragmenting communities, weakening institutions, confounding customs and law, and challenging the courage and charity of the people among whom the epidemic rages. Medical ethics had encountered epidemics before but bioethics was born in an era when epidemic disease was thought to have been banished in the developed world. During the first two decades of its existence, bioethics dealt with a medicine focused on the treatment of individuals. The questions raised by experimentation, transplantation, care of the dying, genetics, and reproduction were framed in terms of the rights and autonomy of individuals. A major epidemic called for a wider view, comprising the welfare of populations as well as the care of individuals. It invited bioethics to become a social philosophy.

Medicine was prepared to diagnose and characterize HIV/AIDS because of progress in virology, immunology, and epidemiology during the prior decades. Medicine was unprepared to treat or cure this devastating disease. Quickly, scientists went to work to find drugs and vaccines that would attack the virus or palliate its effects. Essentially all therapy was experimental and all patients were, by definition, experimental subjects, "protected" from the risks of experimentation by the concepts and rules that bioethics had helped shape during its formative period. Those affected by HIV/AIDS felt cold comfort in that protection; they demanded to be experimental subjects, with access to emerging treatments, willing to take the risks in the face of certain death. The right to be an experimental subject was an innovative claim.

Persons with AIDS faced inevitable death. Consistent efforts to delay death, while sometimes successful, were doomed to futility. A medicine that had become confident of its ability to conquer all threats found itself frustrated, and the ethical implications of futility troubled physicians, patients, and researchers. Futility entered the vocabulary of bioethics. Those who faced that futility most starkly, the patients, often decided that they preferred a quick and easy end to the lingering, wasting death. The ethics surrounding assisted suicide was pushed to the front of the ethics of caring for the dying.

During the campaigns for legalization of assisted suicide in Washington State (1991), California (1992), and Oregon (1994), advocates from the gay community were in the forefront.

AIDS devastated a population characterized by sexual preference. Although that population, so diverse in age, social class, and economic status, and so dispersed across the nation, could barely be called a "community" at the inception of the epidemic, it began to coalesce around the common tragedy. Voices strengthened by this cohesion spoke out to demand better care, more intense research, and protection against discrimination. By quiet pressure and raucous demonstration, the gay community took control of its fate, forcing policy decisions to be made with the community's interests in mind. At the same time, personal narratives of illness, courage, loss, and determination gave vivid reality to the lives of those who lived in the midst of the epidemic.

As AIDS came into the ken of bioethics, it evoked the need for better ways to think about the individual's relation to the community. Not only did the carefully crafted ethics of research and the ethics of care for the dying have to be revisited, but community—as carrier of distinct cultures, source of power, and repositories of strength for individuals—had to be introduced into bioethical reflections as a balance to individualism. Narratives from those communities and from individuals supplemented the spare logic of bioethical analysis. The diverse cultural beliefs that inspire these communities enriched the monotone of Western ethnocentricity that prevailed in bioethics. Realization that communities live within natural and made environments, and that the health of persons cannot be extracted from the health of environments, summoned bioethicists to examine the world beyond human life. A bioethics barely born was already challenged to mature in ways different than its origins promised.

During 1986, I collaborated with my colleague, Dr. Eric Juengst, in writing an ethics chapter that appeared in the National Academy of Sciences report, *Mapping and Sequencing the Human Genome*.[10] Our chapter said that the ambitious scientific project posed no ethical problems that had not already surfaced in the field of genetics. Now, a decade later, Juengst and I would probably reword that conclusion. In 1988, Congress launched the Human Genome Project by appropriating funds to the Department of Energy and to the National Institutes of Health. The beginning of that story is recounted in Chapter 6. The Genome Project has opened a new path for bioethics, as medicine moves inexorably into the molecular medicine of the next millennium.

That path, like the one opened by the AIDS epidemic, leads toward an expanded view of community. Genetics is about kinship; genetic information is not about the individual alone but about all others who share his or her genetic makeup. Problems about confidentiality are confounded when other parties not only have an interest in the information but also hold its source as an intrinsic part of themselves. Confidentiality also takes on a new dimension when the power of predictability of disease becomes greater: who has the right to know that an employee or an insuree or a relative is likely to have a future of sickness? How is information, gathered from and interpretable only through communities, to be used for screening and testing of individuals? These questions are, on their face, matters of policy but, in their depths, they are ethical problems that require a richer and deeper appreciation of communal responsibility than initial bioethics had fostered. Those ethicists who make genetics their specialty are invited to think about ethics in a way that does not fit comfortably into the individualism of the American ethos.

Genetic and reproductive science have revived the earlier debates about cloning. The debate between Lederberg and Ramsey was exciting and amusing but, since cloning was so speculative, the loud arguments soon faded and the ethics of cloning humans became only a footnote in the new field of bioethics. In 1993, scientists at George Washington University announced that they had cloned several human embryos which had briefly survived. While their cloning was actually embryo splitting rather than transplant of adult genetic material into an egg, it had a similar result, the making of genetically identical copies. Again, the ethicists cloned the arguments of twenty years before. The National Advisory Board on Ethics and Reproduction (NABER), of which I was then chair, produced a balanced report on embryo splitting and genetic transplanting. The report found some modest values in the form of cloning called embryo splitting: at least it could benefit women who sought assisted reproduction. Instead of extracting multiple oocytes with many somewhat risky procedures, a single oocyte could be split several ways. But the National Advisory Board saw no value that would justify human cloning by genetic transplantation.

On February 27, 1997, the journal *Nature* carried an article obscurely titled, "Viable offspring derived from fetal and adult mammalian cells," by a Scottish scientist, Dr. Ian Wilmut. That obscure title got a quick translation into journalese: *The New York Times* headlined, "After Many Years and Missteps, a Dazzling Cloning Breakthrough."[11] Dr. Wilmut had taken a skin cell from the mammary glands of a 6-year-old Finn Dorset ewe, extracted the nucleus, and transferred it to the enucleated ovum of a Scottish Blackface ewe. The ovum was implanted in the fallopian tube of another ewe and carried to term. A pretty, fatherless lamb was born 148 days later. She was named Dolly, after Dolly Parton.

Ethicists were interviewed and they repeated the arguments of the old debate. President Clinton imposed a temporary ban on human cloning and ordered the National Bioethics Advisory Commission to produce recommendations in short order. The Commission duly complied with advice that permitted scientific research on cloning but prohibited implantation of cloned human embryos into a womb for gestation. But with Dolly in her pen, and more Dollys and the cloned calves and piglets that are sure to come, people will be fascinated by human cloning. Somewhere, somehow, despite government rules, a scientist will copy a human—probably himself or herself. (NABER called such a prospect "bizarre, narcissistic and ethically impoverished.")

Cloning aims at more than making copies. Science is now seeking techniques to modify genetic structures themselves, cutting out the pieces that are defective and grafting in good parts. While these techniques are far from perfected, they are in the making. The real value of cloning would come from the ability to make the genome (the genetic blueprint) do better things and then to copy those genomes. This, and the less dramatic forms of gene therapy, have the potential of designing human beings to suit models and purposes. The bioethicists who contemplate the powers of genetic and reproductive science are challenged not only to understand the science itself but also to generate a stronger picture of human nature and normalcy than they now have in mind. They are even challenged to more deeply appreciate animal nature, since animals can now be congeners with humans through cloned production of human enzymes and organs.

1987 was the year in which Stephen Toulmin and I published *The Abuse of Casuistry*.[12] We advocated a revival of the antique mode of moral analysis called casuistry as a way of dealing with the clinical cases that are the substance of clinical bioethics. Our book stimulated a conversation that had already begun as murmurings among bioethicists, just starting to wonder about the methods then used by scholars in the field. The introduction of an old method in new garb gave focus to the conversation, and soon articles and books were appearing that embraced or repudiated or cautiously accepted casuistry. This discussion became part of a broader conversation over the theoretical basis for bioethics. What was pejoratively named "principalism" became the foil not just for casuistry but for a variety of other contenders for a place in bioethical theory. Always in ferment, as we have seen in Chapter 10, the intramural discussion about theory intensified in the 1990s. Many writers expressed concern that bioethics was working with an impoverished theoretical mentality. Three perspectives, in particular, seemed neglected: feminist ethical theory, appreciation of cultural diversity and the value of narrative in grasping moral reality.

It seems inevitable that bioethicists will reach for more elaborate and powerful concepts of ethics, moral life, and moral discourse than they originally employed. Philosophical ethics and religious ethics have advanced significantly since the days in which they provided the elements of bioethics. Although deconstructionist and anti-fundamentalist critiques of ethics have done damage, they have also inspired creative responses. Bioethics, which "saved the life of ethics" by turning ethics toward the practical problems of life, may again contribute to general philosophical and theological ethics by entering into a more intensive dialogue with its parent disciplines.

Finally, in 1987, I encountered for the first time a for-profit health care system when Humana Hospital Corporation asked me to participate in an evaluation of their Artificial Heart Implant Program. I was amazed to discover that Humana planned to market this experimental procedure as a "loss-leader" for its programs in cardiac care. For-profit hospitals had only recently appeared in the health care world and their business philosophy and *modus operandi* were vigorously debated.[13] The debates raised questions about whether the profit motive would impair quality of care and how a profit oriented hospital would fulfill community obligations, especially care for the poor. These questions anticipated the much wider arguments that raged during the early 1990s, as the for-profit hospital was dwarfed by massive integrated systems of care. The concept of managed care, first exemplified in the few health maintenance organizations, such as

Kaiser-Permanente in California and Group Health Cooperative of Puget Sound, expanded into an omnipurpose solution to the delivery of care and the containment of costs and, as "managed competition," became the centerpiece of President Clinton's ill-fated health reform legislation. Novel forms of payment for health care and payment to providers challenged the settled ethical concept of the physician as fiduciary and the melee of the marketplace obscured responsibility for the care of the poor.

Justice was the neglected sibling among the principles of bioethics, always acknowledged but seldom given significant tasks or much praise. Bioethics had so concentrated on the relationship between patient and physician that the wider world of fair and just institutions were neglected. Organ transplantation, with its problem of distribution, was the sole bioethical problem that insistently invoked the principle of justice. Now the entire health care system had become a classic problem of justice: how are persons given their due, in accord with need, merit, and contribution when investors, employers, providers, subscribers, and patients all claimed their just share. Bioethicists who studied the problem met new partners in the discourse: health care administrators, economists, health planners, and policy analysts. Bioethicists were forced to understand the inner workings of insurance, finance, business, and government regulations. The other discussants were invited to understand the principles and power of ethical discourse. Bioethics and business ethics entered into uneasy dialogue.

Bioethics has been a busy place since 1987. Issues keep arriving for the consideration of bioethicists; the work is never boring. The issues have stressed the theoretical shape that bioethics took during its formative years. In particular, the individualism and the importance of autonomy that so effectively dealt with the major problems of the first decades, such as medical paternalism, human experimentation, and organ procurement, have been pushed toward conceptions of community and justice that are demanded by questions in genetics and health policy. I have no doubt that my younger colleagues will sculpt new shapes for bioethics. I hope that, as they do so, they do not forget that bioethics is a discipline and discourse meant to be used by persons who make decisions about life and death. Their creative and critical reshaping of the discipline must not make it so malleable that those seeking guidance can no longer discern outlines of problems or directions toward solutions. This would return bioethics to the amorphous debates of its beginnings.

One lesson should be clear from this history. Whatever the issues posed to the future bioethics and whatever the theories, principles and styles future bioethicists bring to those issues, the insistent move of science and medicine toward new discoveries and techniques raises questions that are at first uncertainties and then worries about how those innovations will fit into our familiar world. If those questions are to be answered in ways that help us to benefit from the innovations and at the same time preserve what we value about our familiar world, the questions must be articulated with clarity and the various responses honestly expressed. Any future bioethics should remain faithful to that task.

Some thirty years ago, as I was about to begin my career in bioethics, I visited the

Accademia in Florence to view Michelangelo's David. I was stunned by the scene in the great hall. Leading up to the splendid perfection of the David is a row of hulking stones called "the slaves." Half-human figures struggle out of the blocks, their amorphous shapes in startling contrast to the chiseled proportions of the statue standing at the head of the hall. In reflection, I find in this scene an image for what bioethics has been and, I hope, will be. The work of bioethics is to shape amorphous questions into clear ones. We hardly attain the symmetry of the David but we are challenged to draw out of diffuse concerns the dimensions of a problem that people can see sharply and debate reasonably.

Notes to Epilogue

1. One index of the growth of bioethics is the appearance and survival of seven new journals since 1987: *Bioethics* (1987), *Medical Humanities Review* (1987), *Journal of Medical Humanities* (1989), *Journal of Clinical Ethics* (1990), *Kennedy Institute of Ethics Journal* (1991), *Cambridge Quarterly of Healthcare Ethics* (1992), and *Christian Bioethics* (1996). The *Bibliography of Bioethics* expands each year, from a slim 225 pages in 1975 to a hefty 782 pages in 1995. LeRoy Walters and Tamar Kahn (eds.), *The Bibliography of Bioethics* (Washington, D.C.: Kennedy Institute of Ethics, annual).

2. Eric T. Juengst and Barbara A. Koenig (eds.), *The Meaning of AIDS: Implications for Medical Science, Clinical Practice, and Public Health Policy* (New York: Praeger, 1989).

3. Quoted in Randy Shilts, *And the Band Played On* (New York: St. Martin's Press, 1987), p. 267.

4. Shilts, *And the Band Played On*, p. 271.

5. "Pneumocystic Pneumonia—Los Angeles," *Morbidity and Mortality Weekly Report* 30 (June 5, 1981): 250.

6. Albert R. Jonsen, Molly Cooke, and Barbara A. Koenig, "AIDS and ethics," *Issues in Science and Technology* 2 (1986): 56–65. Only about six articles appeared from 1982 to 1985. The earliest article on AIDS and ethics is, I believe, from my UCSF colleagues, R. Steinbrock, B. Lo, J. W. Dilley, and P. A. Volberding, "Ethical dilemmas in caring for patients with acquired immunodeficiency syndrome," *Annals of Internal Medicine* 103 (November 1985): 787–790; see special supplement to *Hastings Center Report*, Carol Levine and Joyce Bermel (eds.), "AIDS: the emerging ethical dilemmas," 15, no. 4 (1985): S1–S36. In late 1986, a flood of articles appeared.

7. Levine and Bermel, "AIDS: Emerging ethical dilemmas," and AIDS: public health and civil liberties," *Hastings Center Report* 16, no. 6 (1986): S1–S36. See also Ronald Bayer, *Private Acts and Social Consequences: AIDS and the Politics of Public Health* (New York: Free Press, 1989).

8. Albert R. Jonsen and Jeff Stryker (eds.), *The Social Impact of AIDS in the United States* (Washington, D.C.: National Academy Press, 1993).

9. Juengst and Koenig, *The Meaning of AIDS*.

10. National Research Council (U.S.) Committee on Mapping and Sequencing the Human Genome, *Mapping and Sequencing the Human Genome* (Washington, D.C.: National Academy Press, 1988), pp. 99–104.

11. I. Wilmut, A. E. Schnieke, J. McWhir, A. J. Kind and K. H. S. Campbell, "Viable offspring

derived from fetal and adult mammalian cells," *Nature* 385 (1997): 810–813; Michael Specter and Gina Kolata, "After many years and missteps, a dazzling cloning breakthrough," *The New York Times*, March 3, 1997: A1, 10–13.

12. Albert R. Jonsen and Stephen Toulmin, *The Abuse of Casuistry: A History of Moral Reasoning* (Berkeley: University of California Press, 1988).

13. Bradford H. Gray (ed.), *For-Profit Enterprise in Health Care* (Washington, D.C.: National Academy Press, 1986).

Index